# Principles of Animal Nutrition and Feeds

(Revised Edition of Animal Nutrition)

# Principles of Animal Nutrition and Feeds

(Revised Edition of Animal Nutrition)

**GC Banerjee**
MSc (Ag) AH & Dairy Sc, PhD (Ani. Sc.), Cornell, USA
Professor of Animal Nutrition
Bidhan Chandra Krishi Viswavidyalaya
West Bengal

**Oxford & IBH Publishing Co. Pvt. Ltd.**
New Delhi
( *A Unit of* **CBS Publishers & Distributors** Pvt Ltd )

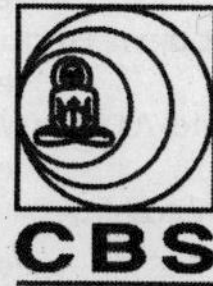


**CBS Publishers & Distributors** Pvt Ltd
**New Delhi • Bengaluru • Chennai • Kochi • Kolkata • Mumbai**
**Hyderabad • Jharkhand • Nagpur • Patna • Pune • Uttarakhand**

**This is a** revised edition of
Principles of Animal Nutrition and Feeds


Reprint: 2018 2019 2021

ISBN 978-81-204-0191-4


**OXFORD & IBH**
New Delhi
*(A Unit of CBS Publishers & Distributors Pvt Ltd)*

**CBS Publishers & Distributors** Pvt Ltd
204 FIE, Patparganj Industrial Area, Delhi 110 092
E-mail: delhi@cbspd.com, cbspubs@airtelmail.in
Ph: 4934 4934 Fax: 4934 4935 Website: www.cbspd.com
e-mail: publishing@cbspd.com; publicity@cbspd.com

*Branches*

- **Bengaluru:** Seema House 2975, 17th Cross, K.R. Road, Banasankari 2nd Stage, Bengaluru 560 070, Karnataka
  Ph: +91-80-26771678/79 Fax: +91-80-26771680 e-mail: bangalore@cbspd.com
- **Chennai:** No. 7, Subbaraya Street, Shenoy Nagar, Chennai 600 030, Tamil Nadu
  Ph: +91-44-26680620, 26681266 Fax: +91-44-42032115 e-mail: chennai@cbspd.com
- **Kochi:** Ashana House, 39/1904, AM Thomas Road, Valanjambalam, Ernakulam 682 016, Kochi, Kerala
  Ph: +91-484-4059061-65,67 Fax: +91-484-4059065 e-mail: kochi@cbspd.com
- **Kolkata:** No. 6/B, Ground Floor, Rameswar Shaw Road, Kolkata-700014 (West Bengal), India
  Ph: +91-33-2289-1126, 2289-1127, 2289-1128 e-mail: kolkata@cbspd.com
- **Mumbai:** 83-C, Dr E Moses Road, Worli, Mumbai-400018, Maharashtra
  Ph: +91-22-24902340/41 Fax: +91-22-24902342 e-mail: mumbai@cbspd.com

*Representatives*

| | | | | | |
|---|---|---|---|---|---|
| • **Hyderabad** | 0-9885175004 | • **Jharkhand** | 0-9811541605 | • **Nagpur** | 0-9021734563 |
| • **Patna** | 0-9334159340 | • **Pune** | 0-9623451994 | • **Uttarakhand** | 0-9716462459 |

*Printed at* Chaman Interprises, Daryaganj, India

*The book is dedicated to my devoted wife,*
ARATI

*whose patience and assistance aided its completion and to our two sons*
JOY and DEBJIT

*who also had to share the pain on many occasions for bringing the book out.*

# CONTENTS

**PART II. PRINCIPLES OF ANIMAL NUTRITION**

# PREFACE

The rapid changes in the scientific know-how of the science of Animal Nutrition which have taken place in the past decade, and since the publication of my book *Animal Nutrition* in 1978, have motivated the publication of this completely revised and enlarged edition, now entitled *Feeds and Principles of Animal Nutrition.*

The book is divided into two main sections. The first part exclusively covers Feeds. Although the feedstuff varies in all parts of the world, the basic information and principles remain the same and are applicable to most countries.

The second part deals with the Principles of Nutrition. We are at the point now where almost all essential nutrients have been defined. It is possible that some other mineral elements may eventually be determined to be essential and it is also possible that one or more vitamins may be added to the present list. However, all of the currently known nutrients appear to be adequate to sustain animals on purified diets, and therefore, any unidentified nutrients surely are not too important, or if required, are done so in extremely small amounts. This is not to say that all of the nutritionally-related problems have been solved because much remains to be learnt about nutrition and infectious disease, nutrition and many different stresses, and about various nutritional interrelationships.

In any event, with a book of this type there is always a question of how much and what type of detail to present to the reader. The author's preconception of the audience for the book may or may not be correct. Consequently, it is a matter of picking and choosing what to include or exclude. More space could have been allotted on any of the subjects. For some readers there may be more information on nutrient metabolism than they might desire. Others will probably wish for more complete coverage in either Part I or Part II.

Regardless of the approach, some areas of topics must be slighted in order to keep the size of the book within the bounds and at a reasonable cost. Whatever the deficiencies of this book may be, it is hoped that it will serve a useful purpose by covering in broad scope a complicated and voluminous subject, and that it will serve to guide the student through the important areas of basic and applied animal nutrition and feeds.

I wish to express my grateful appreciation to some of my colleagues in the Department of Animal Nutrition of Bidhan Chandra Krishi Viswavidyalaya, Dr. Lalmohan Mandal, Dr. Samirendra Biswas, Dr. Narayan Chakraborty, Dr. Tapan Kr. Ghosh and Dr. Gautam Samanta for their constructive criticisms.

I would also like to expreses a special thanks to my wife Mrs. Arati Banerjee who shared all my problems and worked with me as I wrote this book.

Department of Animal Nutrition,
Bidhan Chandra Krishi Viswavidyalaya,
MOHANPUR (Nadia) West Bengal, India.

G. C. BANERJEE

## DEFINITION OF NUTRITION AND ALLIED TERMS

**Nutrition**

In dictionary terms, it is defined as "series of processes by which an organism takes in and assimilates feed for promoting growth and replacing worn or injured tissues".

Thus the science of nutrition not only involves the physiological and biochemical phenomenons of ingestion, digestion, absorption of various nutrients to all over the body cells but also encompasses the processes of excretion of waste products of metabolism from the body. By the processes of various chemical reactions individual nutrients are deposited in body tissues for further or immediate utilisation in various body activities including participation as components of animal products.

It is evident that to understand the nature of the nutrients themselves, to grasp the way in which they perform their roles, to perceive the consequences of their deficiency or of their imbalance in the diet, and to be able to prepare nutritionally adequate diets, it is necessary to call upon subject matter ordinarily considered a part of chemistry, biochemistry, physiology, endocrinology, microbiology, or biophysics. Because of genetic variability among animals, statistics are frequently needed to interpret observations in which both genetic and nutritional factors are involved.

**Nutrient**

The chemical substances found in feed materials are necessary for the maintenance, production and health of animals. The chief classes of nutrients include (i) 25 carbodydrates, (ii) 15 fatty acids, (iii) 20 amino acids, (iv) 15 essential and 10 *probably essential* minerals, (v) 20 vitamins, and (vi) water.

**Nutriment**

Anything that promotes growth or development.

**Nutriture**

Nutritional status.

**Nutritious**

Substances which promote growth and participate in repairing tissues of the body.

**Nutritionist**

A specialist in the problems of nutrition.

**Nourish**

To feed an animal with substances necessary to life and growth.

**Feed (or feedstuff)**

Food of animals comprising any naturally occurring ingredient or material fed to animals for the purpose of sustaining growth and development. The term is exclusively used for animals. In case of humans it is food while for animal it is termed as feed.

**Diet**

A regulated selection of a feed ingredient or mixture of ingredients including water, which is consumed by animals on a prescribed schedule. A balanced diet supplies all nutrients needed for normal health and productive functions.

**Ingredients**

Any of the feed items that a mixture is made of.

**Ration**

A fixed amount of feed for one animal, fed for a definite period, usually for a 24-hour period.

**Balanced ration**

The ration which provides an animal with the proper amount, proportion and variety of all the required nutrients to keep the animal in its form to perform best in respect of production and health.

# PRINCIPLES OF ANIMAL NUTRITION AND FEEDS

# Part I : FEEDS

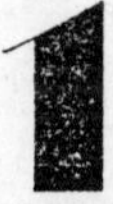

# CLASSIFICATION OF FEEDSTUFFS AND ROUGHAGES

Livestock feeds are generally classified according to the amount of a specific nutrient they furnish in the ration. They are divided into two general classes—*roughages* and ***concentrates.*** Roughages are bulky feeds containing relatively large amount of less digestible material i.e., crude fiber more than 18 per cent and low (about 60 per cent) in T.D.N. on air dry basis. Concentrates are feeds which contain relatively smaller amount (less than 18 per cent) of fiber and have a comparatively high digestibility and as a result higher nutritive value having more than 60 per cent T.D.N.

The number of substances used as feeding stuff to different species of livestock may exceed over 2,000 items. All that is being attempted in this section is to indicate the outlines of classification of the conventional feeds into broad categories and to give typical examples of different groups under this classification.

**Nature of Roughages**

To most livestock feeders, a roughage is a bulky feed that has a low weight/unit of volume. This is probably the best means of classifying a feedstuff as a roughage, but any means of classifying roughages has its limitations since, due to the nature of products we are dealing with, there is a great variability in physical and chemical composition. Most feedstuffs classed as roughages have a high crude fiber (CF) content and a low digestibility of nutrients such as crude protein and enegry. If we attempt to classify all feedstuffs as roughages that have >18% CF and/or with low digestibility, immediately we find exceptions. Corn silage is a good example; nearly always it has >18% CF, but the TDN content of well-eared corn silage is about 70% on a dry basis. Lush young grass is another example. Although its weight/unit volume may be relatively low and fiber content relatively high, its digestibility is quite high. Soybean hulls are another exception for ruminants.

Most roughages have a high content of cell-wall material. The cell-wall fraction may have a highly variable composition, but contains appreciable amounts of lignin, cellulose, hemicellulose, pectin, polyuronides, silica and other components. In contrast, roughages generally are low in readily available carbohydrates as compared to cereal grains.

The amount of lignin is a critical factor with respect to digestibility. Lignin is an amorphous material which is associated closely with the fibrous carbohydrates of the cell wall of plant tissue. It limits fiber digestibility, probably because of the physical barrier between digestive enzymes and the carbohydrate in question. Removal of lignin with chemical methods increases digestibility greatly by rumen microorganisms and, probably, by caecal organisms. Lignin content of plant tissue increases gradually with maturity of the plant and a high negative correlation exists between lignin content and digestibility, particularly for grasses, although somewhat less for legumes. There is evidence that the silica content of plant tissue is related negatively to fiber digestibility.

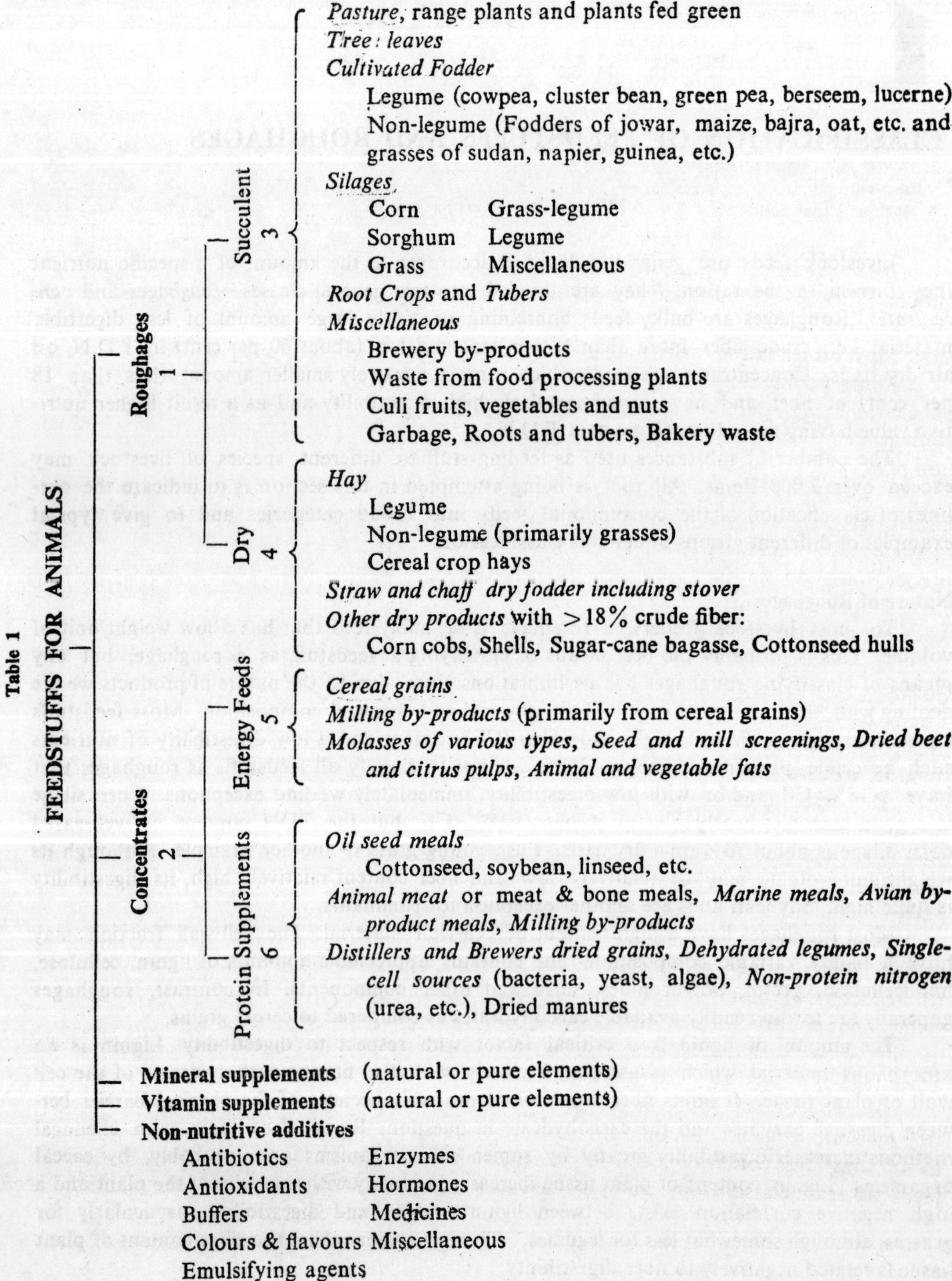

Table 1

**FEEDSTUFFS FOR ANIMALS**

- **Roughages** 1
  - Succulent 3
    - *Pasture*, range plants and plants fed green
    - *Tree leaves*
    - *Cultivated Fodder*
      - Legume (cowpea, cluster bean, green pea, berseem, lucerne)
      - Non-legume (Fodders of jowar, maize, bajra, oat, etc. and grasses of sudan, napier, guinea, etc.)
    - *Silages*
      - Corn, Sorghum, Grass, Grass-legume, Legume, Miscellaneous
    - *Root Crops* and *Tubers*
    - *Miscellaneous*
      - Brewery by-products
      - Waste from food processing plants
      - Cull fruits, vegetables and nuts
      - Garbage, Roots and tubers, Bakery waste
  - Dry 4
    - *Hay*
      - Legume
      - Non-legume (primarily grasses)
      - Cereal crop hays
    - *Straw and chaff dry fodder including stover*
    - *Other dry products* with >18% crude fiber:
      - Corn cobs, Shells, Sugar-cane bagasse, Cottonseed hulls
- **Concentrates** 2
  - Energy Feeds 5
    - *Cereal grains*
    - *Milling by-products* (primarily from cereal grains)
    - *Molasses of various types, Seed and mill screenings, Dried beet and citrus pulps, Animal and vegetable fats*
  - Protein Supplements 6
    - *Oil seed meals*
      - Cottonseed, soybean, linseed, etc.
    - *Animal meat* or meat & bone meals, *Marine meals, Avian by-product meals, Milling by-products*
    - *Distillers and Brewers dried grains, Dehydrated legumes, Single-cell sources* (bacteria, yeast, algae), *Non-protein nitrogen* (urea, etc.), Dried manures
- **Mineral supplements** (natural or pure elements)
- **Vitamin supplements** (natural or pure elements)
- **Non-nutritive additives**
  - Antibiotics, Antioxidants, Buffers, Colours & flavours, Emulsifying agents, Enzymes, Hormones, Medicines, Miscellaneous

1. Feed consisting of bulky and course plants or plant parts, containing a hign-fiber content and low total digestible nutrients, arbitrarily defined as feed with over 18% C.F. and under 60% TDN.
2. A broad classification of feedstuffs which are high in NFE and TDN but low in crude fiber (under 18%).
3. A condition of plants characterised by juiciness, freshness and tenderness, making them appetising to animals.
4. Feeds in the dry state that are bulky and low in weight per unit volume; usually they contain more than 18% CF and relatively low in energy.
5. Feeds that are high in energy and low in fiber (under 18%), and that generally contain less than 20% protein.
6. Products that contain more than 20% protein or protein equivalent.

The protein, mineral and vitamin contents of roughages are highly variable. Legumes may have 20% or more crude protein content, although a third or more may be in the form of non-protein N. Other roughages, such as straw, may have only 3-4% crude protein. Most others fall between these two extremes.

Mineral content may be exceedingly variable; most roughages are relatively good sources of Ca and Mg, particularly legumes. P content is apt to be moderate to low. and K content high; the trace minerals vary greatly depending on plant species, soil and fertilization practices.

The kind of roughage, the method of harvesting, and the degree of maturity at the time of harvesting are very important criteria influencing the nutritive value. Legumes and grasses cut at a late stage of maturity may not have more than half the value per tonne of those cut at the proper time. As an example, lucerne cut when only a few flowers are showing will supply 15 to 20 per cent more digestible nutrients and from 25 to 30 per cent more proteins than when cut after it reaches full bloom.

In overall nutritional terms, roughages may range from very good nutrient sources (lush young grass, legumes, high-quality silage) to very poor feeds (straws, hulls, some browse). The nutritional value of the very poor often can be improved considerably by proper supplementation or by some feed preparatory methods. However, the feeder must use some judgement in selecting the appropriate roughage for a given class and species of animal.

The amount of roughage incorporated in a ration depends largely upon intensity of production of the particular animal being fed. Non-ruminants without functional caecum utilise very little roughage. On the other hand, ruminants and non-ruminants with functional caecums are generally given at least a small amount of roughage to maintain healthy, functional gastrointestinal activity.

Non-ruminants with functional caecums, such as swine, can utilise limited amounts of forage. When swine are on maintenance levels, forages, can be included in the formulation to reduce feed costs. Some forage, such as high quality lucerne, is frequently fed to swine and poultry for its high vitamin content. For dairy cattle for every 10 kg of good quality greens, 1 kg concentrate can be cut from the concentrate quota with the additional advantage of dry matter, TDN, minerals and vitamins in favour of greens.

Roughages are subdivided into two major groups—succulent and dry, based upon the moisture content. Succulent feeds usually contain moisture from 60-90 per cent, whereas dry roughages contain only 10-15 per cent moisture. For the sake of convenience, succulent feeds are again classified into various types such as pasture, cultivated fodder crops, tree leaves, silage and root crops. Dry roughages have been further classified as hay and straw based on the nutritive vaiues and methods of preparation.

## SUCCULENT ROUGHAGES

### A. Pasture

In the management and feeding of almost all types of farm animals, the great importance of feeding through grazing has been recognised at all times and in all the countries of the world. In fact this is the only natural way of feeding livestock at a minimum cost. Of the total area of 328.8 million hectares of the Indian Union, only 8.6 million hectares are under permanent pastures and grazing lands. In India most of the grazing land are situated on undulating and hilly areas and in semiarid and arid tracts. The Indian grass cover have been classified into five groups as below:

1. *Sehima-Dichanthium type*

This type spreads over the whole of peninsular India, including the Central India Plateau, the Chhota Nagpur plateau and the Aravali ranges, comprising the states of Gujarat, Maharashtra, Madhya Pradesh, Orissa, Andhra Pradesh, Karnataka, Tamil Nadu, Kerala and also south West Bengal, southern Bihar and the southern hill portions of Uttar Pradesh and Rajasthan. The most important grass species are:

*Sehima nervosum, Dichanthium annulatum, D. carricosum, D. nodosum, Eremopogon foveolatus, Heteropogon contortus, Iseilama laxum, Chrysopogon fulvus, Cymbopogon coloratus, Cynodon dactylon etc.*

2. *Dichanthium-Cenchrus-Lasiurus type*

This types spreads over arid and semi-arid sub-tropical regions comprising of northern Gujarat, the whole of Rajasthan, excluding the Aravalli ranges in the south, western Uttar Pradesh., Delhi, Punjab and Haryana. The principal grass species are *Cenchrus ciliaris; C. setigerus; Cynodon dactylon, Eremopogon foveolatus, Lasiurs sindicus, Sporobotus marginatus, Dicanthium annulatum and Eleusine compressa etc.*

3. *Phragmites-Saccharum-Imperata type*

This cover type occurs throughout the Gangetic Plain, the Brahamaputra valley and extends westwards into plains of the Punjab comprising of states of Manipur, Assam, Tripura, West Bengal, Bihar, Uttar Pradesh, Delhi and Haryana. This cover is found mostly on water logged soils having poor drainage. The most important grass species are : *Imperata cylindrica, Phragmites karka, Saccharum arundinaceum, S. bengalense, S. spontaneum, Cynodon dactylon, Paspalum conjugatum etc.*

4. *Themeda-Arudinella type*

This cover type occurs in the entire northern and north-western mountain tract in the states of Manipur, Assam, West Bengal, Uttar Pradesh, Punjab, Himachal Pradesh and Jammu and Kashmir. The upper limit for this cover appears to be around 2100 m above mean sea level. The principal grass species are: *Arunainella begalensis, A. nepalensis, Chrysopogon fulvus, Themeda anathera etc.*

5. *Temperate Alpine type*

This type occurs at elevations above 2100 m in west and 1500 m in the east of the whole Himalayan region. The grass vegetation of this cover type are: *Agropyron canaliculatum, Agrostis canina, A. filipes, Andropogon trists, Dactylis glomerata, Phleum alpinum, Poa pratensis, Stipa concinna, Festuca lucide* etc.

Pasture lands may be divided into two main groups, *natural grassland,* which includes rough and hill grazing, and *cultivated grassland,* which may be further subdivided into permanent and temporary pastures. The permanent pasture is intended to remain as grass indefinitely whereas temporary pasture forms part of a rotation of crops.

*Natural grasslands*: It is estimated that half of the world's cattle population graze on natural pastures. There is great scope for improving these pastures by easing the grazing pressure during the dry season. The botanical composition of these grasslands can be changed by controlled grazing, fertilizing, mowing, seasonal burning, etc. The provision of drinking water at close intervals and of feed supplements during the dry season will help to increase the productivity of natural pastures. This type of grassland is usually continually grazed and is found mainly in the drier tropics where rainfall is inadequate and soils are deficient for arable crops. These grasslands usually contain trees and shrubs which provide useful shade and valuable browse, especially during the dry season.

*Cultivated grasslands*: The grasses in these pastures have been planted or sown, very often in conjunction with legumes. The pasture is mostly used intensively by rotational grazing or strip grazing. When grazed rotationally, the grassland is typically subdivided into paddocks, and the animals move systematically from one paddock to another at intervals of perhaps 4 to 6 days. The aim of this system is to use the pasture when it is at its most productive stage. Strip grazing is more intensive and makes use of an electric fence which is moved progressively along the paddock. The area on which the animals can graze is changed once or twice a day. This method minimizes trampling losses. Zero-grazing or soiling is a method in which high-producing grasses sensitive to trampling can be used and the land utilized to its maximum capacity. With this method, herbage is cut each day and brought to the animals which are in confinement.

**Nutrients in Pasture**

The composition of pasture dry matter is extremely variable; for example, the crude protein content may range from 3 per cent in very mature herbage to over 30 per cent in young heavily fertilised grass. The crude fiber content is inversely related to crude protein content and may range from 20 to as much as 40 per cent in very mature samples. Moisture content is high in early stages of growth (75 to 85%) and falls as the plant mature to about 60 per cent. The soluble carbohydrates of grasses include fructans—inulin and levan and the sugars glucose, fructose, sucrose, raffinose and stachyose. Their total concentration in the dry matter varies 5 to 30 per cent. The cellulose is between 20 to 30 per cent while hemicelluloses vary from 10 to 30 per cent. Both these polysaccharides increase with maturity; so also does the lignin. The lipid content of pasture rarely exceeds 4 per cent of the dry matter. The mineral content varies with species, stage of growth, soil type, amount of fertiliser applied etc. Green herbage is exceptionally rich in carotene, the precursor of vitamin A and quantities as high as 55 mg per 100 grams of dry matter of young green crops.

Nutritionally the legumes are frequently superior to grasses in protein and mineral content (particularly calcium, phosphorus, magnesium, copper and cobalt), and their nutritive value falls less with age.

**B. Cultivated Fodder Crops**

In the absence of sufficient grazing ground of good quality for maintaining cattle, sheep, goat on pasture all the year round, the importance of growing fodder crops to provide feed economically for production of milk and for draught animals, need no special emphasis. For the sake of convenience, these are classified into two groups—leguminous and non-leguminous. Among leguminous fodders, cowpea (*Vigna catjang*), cluster bean (*Guar*; *Cyamopsis psoraloides*), are the most common *kharif* leguminous crops. They contain from 2-3 per cent D.C.P. and about 10 per cent T.D.N. on fresh basis and yield about 100 quintal of forage per acre. Berseem (*Trifolinm alexandrinum*) and lucerne (*Medicago sativa*) are two other common leguminous fodder in India. The former is an annual crop, grown during the rabi season; the latter is a perennial one having maximum growth in winter and spring but is retarded during the monsoon. Both these crops can yield over 30 quintals per acre in 5-6 cuttings. The disadvantage is that, both the fodders are liable to produce "bloat" if given in large quantities and thus it is advisable that they should always be given along with some dry fodder. Lucerne and berseem contain on an average 2.5 to 3 per cent D.C.P. and 12 per cent T.D.N. on fresh basis. The phosphorus content of these two forages are poor and thus have wide calcium to phosphorus ratio. It is advisable to supplement a ration containing a large amount of leguminous fodder with a limited quantity of wheat or rice bran.

Among non-leguminous fodder jowar (*Sorghum vulgare*), maize (*Zea mays*) and sudan grass (*Sorghum sudanense*) are most common *kharif fodder*. Yield ranges from 100-200 quintals per acre. Most of the fodders belonging to this group (non-legume *kharif*) are having 0.5-1 per cent D.C.P. and 11-15 per cent T.D.N. except maize, which is the nutritious of all, having 1 per cent D.C.P. and 17 per cent T.D.N. on fresh basis. An improved variety of Bajra *Pennisetum typhoides*) named as I.C. 2291, has been evolved by I.C.A.R., which has a protein content of 2.5 per cent on fresh basis and the yield is about 65 tonnes per acre in 4 cuts. Among the *Rabi* non-leguminous fodder crops, oats (*Avena sativa*) and barley (*Hordeum vulgare*) are the most important. Of these two, oat is by far excellent for milch cattle. It has 2 per cent D.C.P. and 17 per cent T.D.N. on fresh basis. Non-leguminous perennial fodder crops consists of Napier grass (*Pennisetum purpureum*), Hybrid Napier grass (cross between Napier and Bajra), Guinea grass (*Panicum maximum*), Para grass (*Brachiaria mutica*).

All these grasses flourish vigorously during summer and rainy seasons. About 4-6 cuttings can be taken under north Indian conditions so that an annual yield of 30-40 tonnes per acre is the yield. Two to three animals can be maintained per acre on these grasses.

Details of cultivation of fodder crops have been discussed in Chapter 2.

**C. Tree Leaves**

The utilization of tree leaves for feeding to livestock is not common. They are, however, used for feeding sheep and goats, and are sometimes fed to cattle during periods of fodder crisis. In the early stages of their growth, leaves contain fairly high amounts of crude protein and a comparatively low percentage of crude fiber. As maturity progresses, there is a gradual decrease in protein content with a concomitant increase in crude fiber. The tree leaves and shrubs are generally rich in calcium but poor in phosphorus.

1. *Jack fruit* (*Artocarpus heterophyllus*)

A tree up to 15 m high with stiff, 3-lobed leaves on young shoots. The fruits are green and clump-formed with a papillate surface. They grow all along the trunk of the tree. The fruits are an important food in the Eastern Tropics. The leaves are relished by the goat, sheep and cattle and fed particularly in Kerala, Maharashtra, Orissa and West Bengal.

Fresh leaf : As % of dry matter

| D. M. | C. P. | C. F. | Ash | EE | NFE | Ca | P |
|---|---|---|---|---|---|---|---|
| 53.0 | 18.5 | 26.2 | 10.2 | 5.0 | 40.0 | 2.00 | 0.11 |

2. *Neem* (*Azadirachta indica*)

Neem trees grow throughout South and South East Asia. The tree remains green all the year round and is draught resistant. Although the leaves are not relished by normal livestock, but buffaloes are found to consume about 5 kg per day.

Fresh leaf : As % of dry matter

| C. P. | C. F. | Ash | EE | NFE | Ca | P |
|---|---|---|---|---|---|---|
| 15.4 | 12.7 | 11.2 | 4.2 | 56.5 | 2.65 | 0.24 |

3. *Mowra* (*Bassia latifolia* also as *Madhuca indica*)

A large deciduous tree with a short trunk, spreading branches and a large rounded crown. Flowers are used as vegetable and as source of alcohol. The cake from the oilseed is used as fertilizer. Cattle eat the leaves, flowers and fruit.

Fresh leaf : As % of dry matter

| C. P. | C. F. | Ash | EE | NFE | Ca | P |
|---|---|---|---|---|---|---|
| 9.1 | 18.7 | 7.8 | 4.1 | 60.3 | 1.53 | 0.22 |

4. *Indian Kapok or Red silk cotton tree* (*Bombax malabaricum*)

A tree native to India cultivated for the fine, lustrous material (kapok) obtained from the seed hairs. The flowers are collected for human consumption. The leaves which are 5 to 8 cm long are felted with star shaped hairs. These, together with the twigs, are lopped for fodder.

Fresh leaf : As % of dry matter

| CP | CF | Ash | EE | NFE | Ca | P |
|---|---|---|---|---|---|---|
| 12.6 | 22.3 | 9.3 | 6.4 | 49.4 | 2.70 | 0.19 |

5. *Coffee* (*Coffea arabica*)

The dark, glossy green leaves of the coffee bush are, in some areas, dried and included in concentrates for cattle. The leaves are reported as palatable and can be fed without any unfavourable side effects. It has been claimed that feeding of coffee leaves extends the lactation period.

Dried leaf : As % of dry matter

| DM | CP | CF | Ash | EE | NFE | Ca | P |
|---|---|---|---|---|---|---|---|
| 93.6 | 9.9 | 18.7 | 13.0 | 5.9 | 52.5 | — | — |

6. *Banyan* (*Ficus benghalensis*)

A large tree, which can have a huge crown of horizontal branches covering as much as 200 square metres. The crown is supported by aerial roots. It is often planted as shade tree. The leaves are relished by sheep, goat, cattle and buffaloes.

Fresh leaf : As % of dry matter

| CP | CF | Ash | EE | NFE | Ca | P |
|---|---|---|---|---|---|---|
| 9.7 | 22.6 | 14.4 | 2.9 | 50.4 | 2.56 | 0.19 |

7. *Fig* (*Ficus carica*)

A small spreading shrubby tree with large leaves, native to Asia, but now cultivated in sub-tropical countries also. The leaves can be used as fodder for cattle and should be collected as soon as the fruit has been harvested and before yellowing begins.

Fresh leaf : As % of dry matter

| DM | CP | CF | Ash | EE | NFE | Ca | P |
|---|---|---|---|---|---|---|---|
| 34.2 | 14.2 | 17.1 | 16.7 | 5.9 | 46.1 | 3.16 | 0.16 |

8. *Peepal* (*Ficus religiosa*)

A large glabrous tree with leathery, shining, broad based, pointed leaves. Commonly grown as an avenue tree. Although the palatability and nutritive value of peepal leaves is not very good but still the leaves and branches are extensively lopped for fodder.

Fresh leaf : As % on dry matter basis

| CP | CF | Ash | EE | NFE | Ca | P |
|---|---|---|---|---|---|---|
| 9.0 | 15.9 | 20.0 | 2.7 | 52.4 | 2.97 | 0.21 |

Stage of maturity terms used in the NRC feed names.[a]

| Preferred maturity term | Definition | Comparable term |
|---|---|---|
| Germinated | Resumption of growth by the embryo in a seed after a period of dormancy | Sprouted |
| Early leaf | Stage at which the plant reaches 1/3 of its growth before blooming | Fresh new growth, very immature |
| Immature | Period between 1/3 and 2/3 of its growth before blooming (this may include fall aftermath) | Prebud stage, young before boot, before heading out |
| Prebloom | Stage including the last third of growth before blooming | Bud, bud stage, budding plants, in bud, pre-flowering, before bloom, heading to in bloom, boot heads just showing |
| Early bloom | Period between initiation of bloom up to stage at which 1/10 of the plants are in bloom | Up to 1/10 bloom, initial bloom, heading out, in head |
| Mid-bloom | Period during which 1/10 to 2/3 of the plants are in bloom | Bloom, flowering plants, flowering, half bloom, in bloom |
| Full bloom | When 2/3 or more of the plants are in bloom | 3/4 to full bloom |
| Late bloom | When blossoms begin to dry and fall and seeds begin to form | Seed developing, 15 days after silking, before milk, early pod |
| Milk stage | Seeds well formed, but soft and immature | Post bloom to early seed, pod stage, early seed, in tassel, fruiting |
| Dough stage | Stage at which the seeds are soft and immature | Seeds dough, seed well developed, nearly mature |
| Mature | Stage at which the plant would normally be harvested for seed | Fruiting plants, fruiting, in seed, well matured, dough to glazing, kernels ripe |
| Over ripe | Stage after the plant is mature, seeds are ripe and initial weathering has taken place (applies mostly to range plants) | Late seed, ripe, very mature, well matured |
| Dormant | Plants cured on the stem, seeds have been cast and weathering has taken place (applies mostly to range plants) | Seeds cast, mature and weathered |

[a]Harris et al (1967)

9. *Babool or gum arabic tree (Acacia arabica)*

Grows in dry regions but can also endure floods. The pods and leaves are excellent fodder. Besides being a browse tree, the pods are also collected for supplement to dairy cattle. Babool is also used in rotation with grass in order to improve the soil. The pods are reported to contain tannic acid.

As % of dry matter

| | CP | CF | Ash | EE | NFE | Ca | P |
|---|---|---|---|---|---|---|---|
| Fresh leaf | 12.9 | 11.3 | 6.4 | 12.6 | 56.8 | 1.14 | 0.18 |
| Pods | 13.1 | 12.3 | 5.3 | 2.3 | 67.0 | 1.09 | 0.28 |

**D. Root Crops and Tubers**

The main characteristics of root crops are their high moisture content (70-90%) and low crude fibre content (5-12%). The organic matter of roots consists mainly of sugars and is of high digestibility. Roots are generally low in crude protein content. The composition is influenced by season, fertilizer dose, variety of the species etc. Root crops like turnips, swedes, mangolds, fodder beet, carrots are used extensively in U.K. and in other European countries for feeding during winter, when other succulent fodders are not available.

Tubers differ from the root crops in containing either starch or fructan instead of sucrose as the main storage carbohydrate. They have higher dry matter and lower crude fibre contents and consequently are most suitable than roots for feeding to pigs and poultry. Potatoes, cassava, sweet potatoes and jerusalem artichoke are some of the examples of tubers. In India feeding root crops and tubers are not in practice.

**E. Silage**

The most economical method of raising livestock is to feed them on grasses and legumes directly from the fields. Seasonal influences, however, limit the supply of these feeds at a uniform rate throughout the year. They are, therefore, conserved as hay or silage for use at the time of crisis. Details of silage making and its nutritive values have been given in Chapter 3.

## DRY ROUGHAGES

**A. Hay**

A method of conserving green crops is that of hay making. The aim in hay making is to reduce the moisture content of the green crop up to 15-20 per cent to inhibit the action of plant and microbial enzymes. Thus a green crop in a mature state is preserved for a long time. According to the type of forages which are dried, hays are categorised as leguminous, or non-leguminous. Among the leguminous plants, the most suitable is lucerne (known as alfalfa in U.S.A.). Properly prepared lucerne hay contains 14-15 per cent of DCP and 50 per cent TDN Berseem and cowpea are more difficult to be converted into hay. The former has got a hollow stem, while the latter has very thick stem both of which make drying a difficult process. Non-legume hays made from grasses are not as good feeds as legume hays. These are less palatable and contain less protein, mineral matters and vitamins than legume hays.

The details of preparation and nutritive value are given in Chapter 3.

**B. Straw, Bhusa and Karbi**

Inadequate production of green fodder in the country compelled the farmers to utilize dry roughages as livestock feed particularly for the ruminants. In one estimate it has been found that in the country there are about 310 million tons of these dry roughages produced annually. Among those straw, bhusa, karbi and hay are noteworthy. In all developed countries feeding of high quality hay is in practice. Straws are never fed to their livestock but are usually used as bedding. The position in South East Asian countries is quite different. Due to unavailability of high quality dry roughages, straw, bhusa and karbi form the major bulk of livestock feed. Obviously feeding of inferior quality dry roughage is reflected in low production.

Farmers utilize these poor quality dry roughages as energy feed which unfortunately varies between 40 to 50 per cent in digestible energy. Voluntary intake of animals is so low that it is barely sufficient to yield adequate energy (100 kcal per $kg^{0.75}$ per day) to meet their maintenance needs. For some roughages more energy is spent by the animal in chewing and digesting the roughages than what the animal derives from the dry roughages. The DCP and TDN content of some common dry roughages are given below on dry matter basis:

| Dry roughages | % on dry matter | |
|---|---|---|
| | DCP | TDN |
| Paddy straw | 0.2 | 45.9 |
| Wheat straw | 0.0 | 48.3 |
| Ragi straw | 0.2 | 50.0 |
| Grām bhusa | 2.2 | 21.0 |
| Bajra karbi | 0.8 | 48.0 |
| Jowar karbi | 1.0 | 51.0 |

The poor nutritive value of these roughages may be attributed to the following facts:

1. The digestibility of straw is limited due to the formation of strong physical and/or chemical bonds between lignin and the structural polysaccharides (hemicellulose and cellulose). Although cellulose by itself has a highly ordered crystalline structure, it has a very strong association with lignin with the result that even the most potent cellulosic enzymes can not have easy access to the cellulose unless the bondage between lignin and cellulose is broken. The lignin thus acts as a barrier in the efficient utilisation of cellulosic plant materials even as a source of energy. Whether the inhibitory mechanism involves the presence of lignin-cellulosic or lignin-hemicellulosic chemical bonds or the three dimensional macromolecular lignin network by itself acts as a protective barrier in the efficient utilisation of cellulose as a source of energy is yet to be fully understood and established.
2. Crystalline structure of cellulose is also responsible for low digestibility of cellulose.
3. Highly deficient in other nutrients like minerals, vitamins, fatty acids and in proteins. The minimum crude protein requirement for efficient lignocellulose breakdown of

roughages fed as the sole diet is claimed to be from 3.8 to 5.0 per cent.

4. High silica content of straw is known to depress organic matter digestibility.
5. Due to dustiness of straw the total intake is markedly affected.

In some cases it is economical to increase the nutritive value of all types of poor quality roughages by physical, chemical, or biological treatments.

**Physical Treatments**

These are (i) soaking of straw and karbis in fresh water for 2 hours before feeding. The process, makes it succulent and palatable, (ii) grinding, (iii) ball-milling, (iv) steaming under pressure, and (v) pelleting.

**Chemical Treatments**

These are (i) treating straw with acid, (ii) sodium hydroxide, (iii) ammonia, (iv) calcium hydroxide, (v) chlorine, and (vi) ozone.

Details of some of the physical and chemical methods have been described in Chapter 8.

Apart from the above treatments, further improvement in the nutritive value of all poor quality roughages have also confirmed when these are fed (A) mixed with good quality nutritious green leguminous fodders such as berseem, lucerne and cowpea in the ratio of 1 : 4 and with non-legumes such as oat, maize and hybrid napier in the ratio of 1 : 5. The method increases the voluntary intake by about 25 per cent along with increased digestibility: (B) ensiling with green forages. Some of the combinations are given below.

**Table 2**
**Ratio of the Fodders in the Silage**

| Sr. No. | Fodder | Ratio | Molasses kg/qt. | Common salt kg/qt. | Urea kg/qt. |
|---|---|---|---|---|---|
| 1. | Berseem+wheat straw/karbis | 5 : 2 | 4 | — | — |
| 2. | Oats+wheat straw/karbis | 5 : 1 | — | 1 | 0.5 |
| 3. | Maize+wheat straw/karbis | 6 : 1 | — | 1 | 0.5 |
| 4. | Jowar+cowpea+wheat straw | 2 : 1 : 1 | — | — | 0.5 |
| 5, | Lucerne+wheat straw/karbis | 3 : 1 | 4 | — | — |
| 6. | Maize+cowpea+wheat straw | 2 : 1 : 1 | — | 1 | 0.5 |

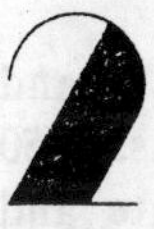

# GREEN FORAGES

Forages and roughages are coarse bulky feeds with more than 18 per cent crude fibre and low indigestible nutrients (NFE is approximately 40 per cent) such as crude protein and energy. It has a high content of cell wall materials.

Forages are grown for feeding domestic animals reared on a farm. Domestic animals are either allowed to graze for themselves or simultaneously are also fed to supplement grazing with cut grass in stalls. The green forages that are cut and fed in fresh condition to the animals are termed as *soiling* of crops. Although forage and fodder crops are synonymous terms, yet the latter is referred to cultivated forage crops which may be either cereals or legumes.

### Importance and Present Position of Forage Crops in Animal Nutrition

Among so many secrets of success in a dairy farm, daily feeding of green forage is probably the first item. The practise maintains the normal health and reproduction of all herbivores. The longevity and production are adversely affected when cattle are reared either without green or with poor quality forage, even though it may be provided with the best quality of concentrates. Such animals usually give birth to weak, deformed or blind calves. Green forages are also praised for their overall cooling effect on the body due to the nature of being easily digestible, more palatable, being slightly laxative in action and above all provide fresh nutrients in a most natural form resulting in efficient utilisation of the feed without any strain on the body organs.

Unfortunately, at present about 90 per cent of the herbivores in India subsist on naturally growing grasses, which are of low nutritive value, and moreover the amount available to the herbivores are far less than the requirement. For better health and high production, the animals, especially the ruminants must be fed either with additional cultivated forage crops (fodder) or with concentrate feeds. Unfortunately, India cannot afford to feed the bulk of the ration as concentrates because of tremendous scarcity due to low production and high demand, firstly to meet the requirement of 700 million human population, and secondly, feeding concentrates at a higher level without sufficient green forages, adversely affects the digestive system of the animals in the long run. On the other hand *animals yielding as high as 10 litres of milk can easily be maintained solely on green fodders without any complaint.* By this the feed costs (taking market prices of all feeds) are reduced by 20 per cent over a normal dry roughage (straw) and concentrate ration. It is a well known fact that for any livestock farm, feeding alone involves about 60-75 per cent of the total expenditure. The amount will be proportionately on the higher side as the amount of concentrate ingredients are increased in their ration for the supply of energy, minerals and vitamin requirements of the animals. Considering an average cost per quintal of concentrate and green fodder @ Rs. 180.00 and Rs. 10.00 respectively, the cost of DCP per kg will then be about Rs. 12.50 and Rs. 4.50 while that of TDN per kg will be Rs. 5.50 and Re. 1.00 respectively from concentrate and fodder.

It may be noted that high yielding animals have a greater feed conversion efficiency than low yielders, although the feed inputs required by the former are much higher than the latter.

**Table 3**

**Requirement of dry matter, protein and energy to produce 1 litre of milk**

| | Feed Dry-matter (kg) | Crude Protein (g) | TDN (kg) | Gross Energetic Efficiency (output/input ratio) % |
|---|---|---|---|---|
| Deshi cow | 6.31 | 734 | 3.51 | 5.91 |
| Buffaloes | 2.03 | 250 | 1.35 | 19.56 |
| Sahiwall | 1.10 | 136 | 0.66 | 28.23 |
| Karan-Swiss cow | 1.07 | 133 | 0.65 | 29.14 |

To have maximum economy in milk production up to 10 litres, all nutrient requirements may be met by feeding forages alone while for high yielders to meet the extra demand for energy, supplementation of grains will be required.

The composition of green forages varies due to various factors such as soil type, rainfall, varieties of plants, and altitude, but from average values the following comments may be made:

1) These are highly digestible mostly when harvested at a proper time (55-65 per cent).

2) The crude protein may range from as little as 3 per cent in very mature forages to over 30 per cent in young heavily fertilised grass (on dry matter basis).

3) The soluble carbohydrates of grasses include fructans and the sugar glucose, fructose, sucrose, raffinose etc. ranging in the dry matter from 4 per cent to 30 per cent. The cellulose is generally within the range of 20-30 per cent while hemicellulose may vary from 10-30 per cent of the dry matter.

4) Grass proteins are particularly rich in ariginine, and also contain glutamic acid and lysine.

5) Lipid content hardly exceeds 4 per cent.

6) The mineral content of pasture is very much dependent on soil type, stage of growth, species and cultivation of conditions.

7) Green forages are excellent sources of carotene, the precursor of vitamin A, and quantities as high as 250 mg/kg may be present in the dry matter.

Thus a dairy farmer will be economically in a safe position if he maintains his cattle mostly on forages. If one has irrigation facilities, he may adopt intensive crop rotations for the production of quality fodders. Under suitable crop rotation as much as 1,500-2,000 quintals of green fodder per hectare is the average annual harvest. The amount is sufficient to maintain about 8-10 adult animals when fed @ 55-60 kg fodder daily. Further, green fodder is best utilised when it is fed chaffed.

At present, the dairy cattle in villages is maintained mostly on naturally growing grasses supplemented at best with straw, *bhusa* or *karbi*—which are all nutritionally very poor. The chronic situation has resulted in an average per capita consumption of milk in India as 142 grams against the minimum requirement of 210 grams/head/day as recommended by the Indian Council of Medical Research. Lack of adequate supply of quality fodders alone is the main constraint in achieving any increased milk production in India.

According to the National Commission on Agriculture (1976), there is a shortage of about 44 per cent of concentrates, 44 per cent green fodder and 38 per cent of dry fodder. Projecting the population for 1982 and working out the energy and proteinre quirement, it was seen that the deficiency of these two components amount to 37 and 34 per cent respectively and in terms of roughages and concentrates it comes to 36 and 44 per cent respectively.

In spite of the research and development efforts for improving cultivated fodder production and improvement of range and common grazing lands, there has not been any serious increase in feed resource from these sources. Rather, there has been a reduction in the effective area available for grazing and the quality of grazing resources, because of the diversion of lands earlier available under natural vegetation for cultivation of dryland crops. This has forced the livestock to the poorer grazing areas, and in consequence has not only resulted in serious problems of soil erosion but also in poor nutrition of the livestock and thus their reduced production.

Realising this fact the country has established seven regional stations in different agro-climatic regions with the objective of achieving quick transfer of technology on all aspects of fodder production, conservation and utilisation and to assist the state agencies in the conduct of their extension programme on scientific lines. Introduction of high yielding varieties of fodder crops has resulted in increased fodder production by the small farmers. Cultivation of berseem in winter is now practised in the Kashmir Valley. A new agro-technology now enables the farmer to utilise his paddy fallows without in any way disturbing paddy cultivation.

A significant breakthrough has been achieved in the production of pasture legume seeds for use in grassland development. New varieties such as *Stylosanthes hamata* and *S. scabra. S. viscesa*, have been introduced and large scale seed multiplication undertaken for distribution to the forest departments, areas of drought prone programme and other interested agencies.

Improved varieties of fodder seeds are being multiplied at the Central Fodder Seed Production Farm, Hesserghata. Through rigorous selection a high yielding variety of fodder maize has been evolved which is capable of high seed yield as well. The production of foundation/certified seeds of the recommended high yielding varieties was further stepped up by the regional stations and the seed farm. The fodder minikit demonstration programme has been intensified to cover all States and the Union territories and over 24,100 kits were supplied during the *Kharif* and *rabi* reasons.

Considering the importance of forage crops so far discussed, a farmer should not think of having a dairy farm without sufficient provision of growing fodder throughout the years. We, therefore, need better forage crop varieties, both annual and perennial with higher nutrient yield potential per unit area and unit times for maximising animal products including milk, wool, meat, eggs etc.

India has the largest cattle population in the world. It was 182 million of cattle, and 63 million of buffaloes in 1984. The figure shows a gradual increase of cattle and buffalo population in the country. Simultaneously, the human population is also increasing day by day, and at present land has to provide food for over 700 million of human population in addition to the load of feeding an enormous number of low productive bovine population. Because growing food and cash crops are more profitable, major lands have been diverted towards cultivation of such crops resulting in inadequate production of green fodder. For obvious reasons the condition of the cattle population is becoming very poor.

The cultivated fodders occupy only 6.91 million hectares, which is less than 5 per cent of the area under cultivation in the country. It is only in a few States like the Punjab where the percentage of area under irrigated cultivated fodder is around 10 per cent. If proper steps are not taken the future of India's livestock cannot be satisfactory. More areas are required to be brought under fodder crops for more production of green fodder to maintain the health of the cattle as well as to increase the milk production. It may be noted that the economics of livestock production based on cultivated fodder production is much better than feeding of low quality roughages/crop residues supplemented with concentrates.

With the extension of irrigation facilities and of high yielding varieties of food crops, intensive cropping can be practiced in all types of holding in which forage crops can be accommodated in the cropping programme without risking the production of food and other crops. To augment milk production, it is therefore, imperative to regenerate the existing grazing areas by adopting better management practises and also to increase the area under cultivated fodder crops and establishment of pastures wherever possible.

In this connection, the estimated requirements of feeds *vis-a-vis* availability by 2,000 A.D. as estimated by the National Commission on Agriculture, 1976 is given below:

**Table 4**

**Estimated requirements of feeds *vis-a-vis* availability in 2000 A.D.**

(million tonnes)

| | Requirement | Availability | Excess/deficit |
|---|---|---|---|
| Concentrates of plant origin | 82.8 | 77.05 | (—) 5.75 |
| Green fodder | 594.8 | 575.0 | (—)19.8 |
| Dry fodder | 373.0 | 356.8 | (—)16.2 |

The position shown here is again on the deficit line but somewhat better than previous years. The improvement was postulated by the committee only on assumptions that from now onwards all emphasis will be given on (A) the reduction of feed requirements and simultaneously (B) by increasing the feed supply which is discussed in brief as below:

### A. Reduction of feed requirements of animals

1) By progressive elimination of unproductive animals.
2) By sharing bullocks by two or more farmers.
3) By feeding balanced ration to all stock.
4) By maintaining animals having low unproductive period of life, namely the age till attainment of maturity and calving intervals.
5) By reducing parasitic infection.

## B. Increasing feed supply

1) Considering the present cattle and buffalo population, forage requirement @ 20.00 kg/head/day will be around 50 million tonnes, for this an additional area of one million hectares should be brought under irrigated fodder production.

2) By increasing the growth of fodder crops by utilising (a) fallow land, (b) land on river side, (c) land on road and railway sides, (d) uncultivable waste and forest areas.

3) By planting more of shrubs. Camels, sheep and goats in particular obtain a major portion of their nutrient requirements from leaves of trees and shrubs such as *Jharbari*, *Babul*, *Kanthal*, fig etc.

4) By adopting a judicious crop rotation pattern, so that farmers periodically can grow fodder crops without affecting their main commercial crops.

## Cultivation of Forage and Pasture Crops

Most of the forage and pasture crops belong to two families, namely, Gramineae and Leguminosae. There are a few other forage crops which fall under families, such as Cruciferae (rape and turnip), Umbelliferae (carrot) and Compositae (sunflower). Like food and other crops, due care has to be exercised for the cultivation of forage crops in respect of seed bed preparation, selection of cultivars, seed rate, sowing, manuring, irrigation, drainage, weeding and harvesting.

Plant protection chemicals should be used cautiously to guard against ill effects on livestock. For the cultivation of leguminous forage crops, seeds should be inoculated with appropriate bacterial culture to encourage nodulation in roots by *rhizobium* for the fixation of atmospheric nitrogen and higher production of forage.

## Graminaceous Crops

### OAT (*AVENA SATIVA* LINN.)

*Genus* : *Avena L.*
$2n = 42$

It is a crop of western countries and widely grown in all parts of India. A stout erect annual cereal grows up to 1 m high, is extensively used for fodder production, and is very good for hay or silage preparation.

This is a rabi crop grown for soiling and hay, and occupies a large area in military fodder farms, particularly for consumption by horses. The land for its cultivation should be well drained and fertile. It is sown in October or November with seed rate 60-70 kg per hectare. Nitrogen fertilisation at 60-75 kg per hectare is recommended. The crop cannot withstand drought and it should be irrigated when necessary. Mixed cropping with berseem or lucerne may be practised. For soiling purposes, the crop should be harvested at milk stage and for hay, at the soft dough stage. Oat may give more than one cut if sown early. The average yield of green fodder is 200 quintals per hectare and it can rise up to 400 quintals per hectare under better management.

*Improved varieties*:—Kent, Weston-11, Fulghum, Fos 1/29, Algerian, IGFRI-S-54.

## PARA GRASS (*BRACHIARIA MUTICA* STAPF.)

*Genus* : *Brachiaria Griseb* (*Gramineae*)

2n = 36 Synonyms : Mauritius grass, California grass, Giant Couch.

The grass is a native of Brazil, but has now been cultivated in many other warm countries. It is now growing widely in the Haringhata Farm in West Bengal, Aarey Milk Colony in Bombay, Bangalore, Kerala State and many other places in India.

It is a water loving perennial, tropical, exotic grass and widely cultivated in India. It has very long trailing stems rising to 2.5 m with broad hairy leaves. It can be grown on all types of soil but thrives better in moist and water logged soils. It is propagated exclusively from cuttings, having two or three nodes in each and planted with the break of the monsoon. The forage can be harvested three months after planting and subsequently, at one month intervals, depending on climate and management. The green yield varies from 1,500 to 2,000 quintals per hectare per annum.

## ANJAN GRASS (*CENCHRUS CILIARIS.*)

*Genus* : *Cenchrus Linn* (*Gramineae*)

2n = 32 Synonym : Indian sandbur

It is an indigenous perennial grass and now it is cultivated in Rajasthan, the Punjab, Madras and in other drier parts of India. It is an erect annual growing from 15 to 60 cm in height.

A tufted perennial grass it is used for pasture, soiling and hay. It is adapted to arid and semi-arid regions of India and grows on all types of soil. As a forage crop, it is sown or broadcast, using a seed rate of 5 kg per hectare. A cross between Rajasthan and American types, known as "*Pusa Giant Anjan*" remains green throughout the year under extremes of drought and temperature.

*Improved varieties* :—IGFRI-S-3108 and Palsana.

## RHODES GRASS (*CHLORIS GAYANA*)

*Genus* : *Chloris gayana Kungh* (*Rhodes grass*)

2n = 20

This perennial grass is a native of South-Africa. Fine stemmed, leafy, turf-forming perennial grows up to 150 cm high. It is a, drought resistant, exotic grass, cultivated in India since 1915 for soiling, hay and pasturage. It grows everywhere except in clayey and water-logged soils. The grass is propagated through seeds, using 8 to 9 kg per hectare. It responds to irrigation and fertilisation. The first cutting is usually taken after three months of sowing and subsequent cuts can be taken at one month intervals, depending on the growth of the crop. This crop is generally grown in pasture.

## TEOSINTE (*EUCHLAENA MEXICANA.*)

*Genus* : *Euchlaena Schrad.* (*Gramineae*)

2n = 20 Synonym : Buffalo grass.

Native of Central America and Mexico and is considered to be the wild ancestor of maize.

It is a coarse, tall growing (2.5-4 m), annual, exotic grass, cultivated since 1893 for soiling, hay and silage. Unlike maize, it tillers freely. It grows well in warm regions with high humidity and rainfall. It is generally sown late in the *kharif* season to meet the scarcity of green fodder in October and November. The seed is sown or broadcast, using a seed rate of 50 to 60 kg per hectare. It responds to manuring like maize. The forage can be harvested at soft dough stage for quality and yield. The average yield of green fodder is 400 quintals per hectare.

## BLUE PANIC (*PANICUM ANTIDOTALE* RETZ.)

*Genus* : *Panicum antidotale Retz.*
$2n = 18$ Synonym : Giant panic grass.

This grass grows wild in Rajasthan and the north-western regions of India, but its fodder value was first recognised in Australia. A vigorous, much branched perennial with wiry stems grows up to 2.5 m or more with blue green leaves.

It is a good pasture crop, also grown for soiling and hay, is coarse, quick growing leafy, perennial grass propagated by stem cuttings or seeds. Blue panic is adapted to varied soil and climatic conditions and is resistant to drought but prefers sandy loams. Due to its quick regeneration the forage can be harvested after establishment at intervals of 20 to 25 days.

## GUINEA GRASS (*PANICUM MAXIMUM* JACQ.)

*Genus* : *Panicum Linn.*
$2n=18$. Synonyms : Colonial grass, Tanganyika grass.

The grass is a native of tropical Africa but has now spread to many other countries, like Australia, the Philippines and the Southern States of the U.S.A.

A tufted, tall (2 to 3 m), perennial grass, introduced from tropical Africa in 1793, it is cultivated for soiling, pasturage, hay and silage. The forage is palatable to all classes of livestock. Guinea grass is drought resistant and suited to varied soil and climatic conditions, but not to waterlogged or cold climates. It is generally propagated vegetatively through rootstock, planted 90×45 cm in February. It may also be grown from seeds. Replanting should be done after three to five years to ensure good production. It responds to high manuring and irrigation. The first cut of green fodder is taken two and half months after planting and subsequently at six to eight weeks intervals, depending on growth and management. The yield of green fodder is 600 to 1250 quintals per hectare per annum.

## DINANATH GRASS (*PENNISETUM PEDICELLATUM* TRIN.)

*Genus* : *Pennisetum L., Rich.* (*Gramineae*)

The grass had been growing wild in the Chhota Nagpur and Gaya district of Bihar as well as in some parts of peninsular India but its fodder value was first recognised in Africa and in Australia.

Highly branched, leafy, annual, it grows up to 1.5 to 2.5 m in height. The introduced varieties from Africa and the perennial varieties (CSIRO No. 7968) are much superior to the indigenous types in performance. This grass is mainly cultivated for soiling and pasturage. It grows in all types of soils during *kharif* season. The seed is sown or broadcast at 10 kg per hectare. The perennial variety responds to heavy manuring and irrigation. The green fodder is harvested about 80 days after sowing and at 60 days' interval afterwards. The yield of green fodder varies from 500 to 750 quintals per hectare.

## THIN NAPIR (*PENNISETUM POLYSTACHYON* SCH.)

*Genus* : *Pennisetum polystachyon Sch.*
$2n=54$ Synonyms : China grass, Kyasuwa

Thin Napier first came into prominence at the Hebbal Farm in Bangalore in the forties as a very drought resistant grass.

It is a perennial, profuse tillering, tall (2 m) grass, adapted to warm and humid climatic regions of India. The grass is chiefly cultivated for soiling purposes and is propagated through seed sown in rows 30 cm apart, using clean seed at the rate of 5 kg per hectare and also vegetatively. It combines very well with perennial legumes in grass legume mixtures. About 750 to 1000 quintals of green fodder per hectare may be obtained in five to six cuts per annum.

## NAPIER GRASS (*PENNISETUM PURPUREUM SCHUM.*)

*Genus* : *Pennisetum L. Rich* (*Gramineae*)
$2n=28$ . Synonyms : Elephant grass, Uganda grass

Col. Napier first drew attention to the fodder. The crop is a native of South Africa, and the name of this grass has become Napier grass after Col. Napier.

Napier is a robust, perennial, tall (2-3 m) profuse tillering, exotic grass, cultivated in India since 1912 for soiling and silage. It thrives well in warm and humid climate in fertile loamy soil. It is propagated vegetatively like sugar cane though sets planted in furrows one metre apart or through rooted stock planted 1 m × 50 cm. For good production replanting after five to six years is recommended. The grass responds to heavy manuring and irrigation. The first cut of green fodder is taken three months after planting and subsequent cuts at six or eight weeks interval, according to growth and palatability of the forage. The yield ranges from 1000 to 1500 quintals per hectare per annum. "Giant Napier" or "Hybrid Napier" or Napier × barja (*Pennisetum typhoides*) cross is gradually replacing Napier grass as a forage crop. Its yielding capacity and water requirements are higher than Napier grass. Though the oxalic acid content of the forage has been found to be about 4 per cent, no ill effects on livestock have been reported. It is a very high yielding grass; liberal manuring pays in the long run. To compensate the low yield in winter and to make the fodder more balanced, berseem or lucerne may be grown in between the rows with irrigation. Once the grass is established, five to six cuts may be taken in a year. The first cut should be made at ground level to encourage tillering and subsequent cuts may be done 15 to 20 cm above the ground level. It gives 1500 to 2000 quintals of green fodder per hectare per annum.

*Improved varieties* : NB-21, BN-1 and BN-2

## BAZRA (*PENNISETUM TYPHOIDEUM*)

*Genus*: *Pennisetum Typhoideum.*
$2n=14$ Synonyms: Pearl millet, Indian millet, Bulrush millet, Horse millet.

Usually it was grown only for grain. Subsequently it was introduced as green forage.

It is a drought resistant tall erect with stems up to 3 m high annual crop primarily cultivated as a millet crop in arid and semi-arid regions of India, but also grown for soiling purpose in drier tracts. It generally succeeds where other forage crops fail. It is sown or broadcast with seed rate of 12 to 15 kg per hectare during the *kharif* season. It is harvested for forage at full bloom stage, yielding 250 to 300 quintals per hectare of green fodder. Improved varieties: Anand KMF 7264, MB-2, HB-3.

## SUDAN GRASS (*SORGHUM SUDANESE*)

*Genus*: *Sorghum vulgare, var. Sudanese.*
$2n=20$

Though it is claimed that this grass has been grown in Egypt from very early times, the value of this grass was first noted in Sudan in 1909. It was also introduced in the U.S.A. at about the same time.

A profuse tillering leafy, tall (3 m) annual, exotic grass, cultivated in India since 1920 for soiling, hay and pasturage due to its high growth rate, this grass serves as an emergency forage crop. It is a drought and heat resistant summer crop, not exacting in soil requirements. The seed is shown in rows 45 cm apart on broadcast with seed rate 20 and 40 kg per hectare respectively. It responds to high manuring and irrigation. The crop can also be cultivated mixed with *kharif* legumes. The forage can be harvested any time between heading to full bloom stage. The yield of green fodder ranges between 450 to 550 quintals per hectare according to management. Prussic acid poisoning in livestock has been reported when the forage is harvested and fed at the young stage due to the presence of a glucosiderrin. For this reason, cattle should not be allowed to graze on Sudan grass in the young stage.

## SORGHUM (*SORGHUM VULGARE* PERS.)

*Genus*: *Sorghum Moench* (*Gramineae.*)
$2n=20$ Synonyms: Milo, Hegari, Kafir, Guinea corn, Dari, Jowar.

It has been in cultivation since very ancient times in all regions of the tropics where rainfall is low and uncertain. Sorghum is believed to be indigenous to Africa, although both India and China have claimed to be the home of at least certain varieties of sorghum.

Sorghum or jowar is one of the best drought and heat resistant *kharif* forage crops grown for soilage, silage and hay. Deep fertile sandy loam soil is suitable for this crop, but it can also be grown in well drained heavy soil. The seed is sown or broadcast at 30 to 40 kg per hectare. It can either be grown as a pure crop or mixed with legumes. For good yield and palatability, the forage should be harvested at the flowering stage. The yield of green fodder varies from 250 to 500 quintals per hectare according to management. Prussic acid poisoning has been reported in livestock by feeding the forage harvested at the young stage or after drought. Mature green fodder, hay and silage are safe for feeding purposes.

## MAIZE (*ZEA MAYS* L.)

*Genus* : *Zea Limu* (*Gramineae.*)
2*n*=20

Its origin is in Mexico and it has been cultivated from pre-historic times by the aboriginal people of America. In India its cultivation is popular for grain as well as for fodder.

Maize is a *kharif* crop cultivated both for grain and as a forage crop. It is one of the earliest introductions from America, grown in warm and moist regions of India for green fodder and silage. Well drained fertile soil is suitable for its cultivation. The seed is sown or broadcast at 40 to 60 kg per hectare. Mixed cropping with *kharif* legumes is also practised. The crop responds to manuring and irrigation. For soiling purposes, the crop can be harvested at any stage and for silage, at dough stage. The yield varies between 300 to 400 quintals per hectare.

Improved varieties :—Ganga-2, 5, 7, Ganga 101, Adecuba and Composite.

### Leguminous Crops

## CLUSTERBEAN (*CYAMOPSIS TETRAGONOLOBUS* L. TAUB.)

*Genus* : *Cyamopsis DC.*
2*n*=14 Synonym : Guar

It is an indigenous crop to India and cultivated in all parts of India. An annual, erect herb, 1-2 m high with trifoliate leaves and rose coloured flowers.

Clusterbean or *guar* is a drought resistant *kharif* soiling crop, also grown as a vegetable crop and suitable for cultivation in arid and semi-arid regions. The seed is sown in rows 30 cm apart or broadcast, using a seed rate of 28 and 45 kg per hectare respectively. Mixed cropping with sorghum is usually followed for forage purposes. It responds to phosphate fertilisation and irrigation. For soiling purposes, the crop is harvested from bloom to pod formation stage. The yield of green fodder ranges from 100 to 200 quintals per hectare according to management.

Improved varieties. No. 2, FS 277, Durgapen Safed, AG 111.

## SOYBEAN (*GLYCINE* MAX *SIEB.* AND ZUCC.)

*Genus* : *Glycine Linn.*
2*n*=40, 80 Synonyms : Soja bean, Manchurian bean.

The crop is native of Central Asia and is one of the important crops of China, Japan and Mongolia. It has been cultivated in the hilly areas of India.

A summer annual herb up to 100 cm high usually erect but some varieties twine. The wnole plant is covered by fine brown or grey hair. The trifoliate leaves usually drop before the seeds are mature.

Soybean is a *kharif* grain crop, also cultivated for soiling purposes and hay making. It thrives well in warm and moist climate, in well drained loamy soil. The seed is broadcast at the rate of 25 to 30 kg per hectare. Mixed cropping with sudan grass. maize or sorghum is also practised. Soybean responds to phosphate fertilisation and seed innoculation with bacterial culture. The green fodder is harvested after pod formation and the yield varies from 200 to 300 quintals per hectare.

## LUCERNE (*MEDICAGO SATIVA* L.)

*Genus* : *Medicago Linn.*

2*n*=16, 32, 64   Synonyms : Alfalfa, Purple medick, Snail clover, Chilean clover.

Lucerne is a native of South-Western Asia. It is now grown all over the world. Lucerne is grown under irrigated conditions in India.

Lucerne or alfalfa is a deep rooted perennial herb and is the oldest among the cultivated forage crops of the world. It is grown in the eastern region of India as a winter annual. Lucerne is a crop of semi-arid tract and fairly resistant to extremes of heat and cold, but does not thrive well under high temperature in a moist climate. It grows well on all types of soil, provided it is not waterlogged. Lucerne can be sown any time during the winter season, preferably in October or November to ensure high production. In regions with unfavourable climatic conditions during *kharif* season, through which the crop fails to persist, as in West Bengal, broadcast sowing is recommended using a seed rate of 20 to 25 kg per hectare. For longer stand of the crop under favourable climatic conditions and to facilitate intercultivation, line sowing at 40 to 50 cm apart with seed rate of 12 kg per hectare should be done. The crop responds to phosphate fertilisation and seed inoculation with bacterial culture. It should be given light and frequent irrigation in dry season. Eight to ten cuttings of green fodder can be taken per annum, which according to management yields varies from 750 to 1000 quintals per hectare when grown as perennial.

Improved varieties : Sirsa 9 (T-9), LGL 1, Anand 1 and 2, Sri Ganganagar, IGFRI-S-244 and IGFRI-S-54.

## RICE BEAN (*PHASEOLUS CALCARATUS.*)

*Genus* : *Phaseolus calcaratus Roxb.*

2*n*=22   Synonym : Red bean

It is a native of India and has now been cultivated in eastern parts of India particularly, West Bengal.

Rice bean is a drought resistant fodder and fluorishes on comparatively poor soils where other legumes fail. It is short-lived, very hairy, twining fodder with yellow flowers and cylindrical pods. The legume is very profitably cultivated on *aman* paddy lands in summer months and also as a catch crop in between *kharif* and *rabi* crops. In highland the legume is also cultivated in August and September and a good quantity of green fodder is taken during the scarcity months of December and January without any irrigation. When the soil condition permits, the legume is also sown during November and December in the paddy fields; the crop remains dormant during the cold months but with the spring rains it makes a luxuriant growth for harvesting in early May. In fact, it may be sown in any time of the year. The fine, penetrating roots and the leafy growth has made the plant also useful for soil cover as well as for green manure.

It is usually sown from March to September. The seed rate is 25 to 30 kg per hectare.

A higher seeding rate of 30 to 35 kg per hectare is recommended when it is grown as catch crop for getting fodder within 50 to 60 days. The seeds are sown or broadcast after two or three ploughings. No special culture is ordinarily required for its cultivation.

The crop needs fertilisation with superphosphate at 50 to 60 kg of $P_2O_5$ per hectare. Normally, for its cultivation during *kharif* no irrigation is necessary but for early sowing in March one irrigation before sowing may be given.

The crop is ready for harvest 70 to 80 days after sowing when a yield of 200 to 220 quintals of green fodder per hectare is obtained. The advantage of this crop is that for its prolonged vegetative growth. A higher yield up to 350 quintals per hectare may be available if harvested after 120 to 130 days of sowing. The crop is usually cut once but a second cut is possible if the first one is taken as lopping.

For raising the seed crop the best time of sowing is late August or early September. It flowers in late December or early January and the pods mature by the end of February. The crop is harvested in the morning hours when wet with dew to avoid shattering of the pods. The seed yield varies from 15 to 20 quintal per hectare. As the legume is highly susceptible to frost, the seed crop should be raised in frost-free areas. After the harvest of the seed crop a thick mat of litter is left on the field, which when ploughed down adds a good amount of organic matter to the soil.

## KUDZU VINE (*PUERARIA THUNBERGIANA*)

*Genus* : *Pueraria DC.*
$2n = 22$

It is a native of the East Indies and has become very popular for forage and soil conservation. Kudzu has become very common in the eastern part of India also. A woody perennial vine with leaves resembling those of grapes. In one summer its shoots will grow to a length of 10 m.

Kudzu is a perennial drought resistant legume suitable for pasturage and also for soiling and conservation of soil. It grows on all soils under varied climatic conditions. Its growth is prolific throughout, except in winter when it remains dormant. Kudzu vine is propagated vegetatively through crowns removed from mature vines in December-January.

## BERSEEM (*TRIFOLIUM ALEXANDRINUM*.)

*Genus* : *Trifolium*
$2n=16$ Synonym : Egyptian clover.

It is a native of Egypt and is also cultivated in Syria and Persia. It was introduced in India during the years 1904 to 1961. Now, Berseem is a prominent legume in irrigated areas of different parts of the country.

Berseem as a soiling and hay crop is rated as a very nutritious forage and it also has a remarkable capacity of building up soil fertility, resistant to alkaline soils. It is a *rabi* crop, tolerant to alkali and grows on all types of soil in regions with mild cold weather. It needs copious irrigation. The sowing starts in October-November when the night temperature falls to 18.5°C. The seed is soaked over-night in water and broadcast at 20-22 kg per hectare in standing water held in small compartments. Rhizobial inoculation of seed is essential for fields which did not carry berseem previously. Light and frequent irrigations should be given according to the soil and climatic conditions. Berseem responds remarkably to phosphate fertilisation. The first cutting of green fodder is ready about 45 days after sowing; subsequent cuts may be taken at 30 days' interval. The number of cuts depends on the duration of winter season, as the plant perishes with the approach of hot weather. The yield ranges from 50 to 100 tonnes per hectare, depending on the number of cuttings and management. Good production of forage in the first cutting can be ensured by mixing seeds of tetraploid berseem at sowing with the commonly cultivated varieties.

Improved varieties : Mescavi, Tetraploid berseem and IGFRI-S-99-1

## WHITE CLOVER (*TRIFOLIUM REPENS.*)

*Genus* : *Trifolium L.*
$2n=32$

This species is native to Europe and is grown as pasture crop.

This fodder is of recent introduction which has shown great potentiality as a winter annual for soiling, hay and pasturage. It prefers clay and silt loam soils and has the capacity to withstand high temperatures of early summer. Scarified inoculated seed is sown or broadcast at 5 kg per hectare. A good stand of white clover having white flower can be obtained in succeeding seasons from the volunteer crop through self sown seeds. Reseeding, except in poor patches, is not necessary. Irrigation is given immediately after sowing and subsequently at 15 to 20 days' interval according to soil and climatic conditions. White clover responds to phosphate and potassic fertilisation and to liming in acidic soils. The first cutting is taken 60 to 65 days after sowing (ten days earlier in case of volunteer crop) and subsequently at 25 to 30 days' interval. In West Bengal, four cuts with an average yield of 300 quintals per hectare have been recorded.

Improved varieties : E.L. 82 (Tasmania), Strain-A (Haringhata), E.L. 34 (Louisiana), E.L. 19 (A 2309-I.A.R.I.).

## CENTRO (*CENTROSEMA PUBESCENS.*)

*Genus* : *Centrosema* Synonym : Butterly pea

Centrosema is one of the most promising perennial legumes for pasture lands. Its potentiality of producing profuse viable seeds and quick regeneration capacity with vigorous growth made this legume popular as a component in grass-legume mixtures (pasture). Centro flourishes best in areas receiving over 125 cm of annual rainfall. It has a deep and extensive root system and can stand long drought, but has never become adapted in the areas receiving less than 100 cm of rainfall. It is essentially a crop for warm and humid climate. Centro does not grow in cooler climate even when moisture and light factors are adequate. The crop is quite tolerant to shade when well established. Centro will climb anything it encounters and often is seen climbing on trees. The crop is useful for smothering weeds and is a good cover crop to control soil erosion. Centro grows well when sown alone but as a component in the pasture mixtures its compatability with perennial grasses provides high tonnage of mixed fodder. It can also withstand heavy grazing and frequent cutting. The crop once established will continue to grow for several years. Centro is adaptable to all types of soils and grows well on fertile loams. It is moderately tolerant to acid soils.

Under irrigated conditions, seeds are sown in March and April with light irrigation, but under rainfed conditions, sowing is done with the early showers in May. Late sowing is not recommended as the weeds interfere with the establishment of seedlings. For sowing centro alone or in mixture with grasses, the land should be prepared thoroughly in the month of February and March by incorporating into the soil five to eight tonnes of farmyard manure per hectare. Before sowing the seeds should be treated with concentrated $H_2SO_4$ for 15 to 20 minutes at 80°C to remove the hardness of the seed coat to accelerate germination. The seeds treated with acid should be washed and dried before sowing. The seed may be drilled or broadcast at a depth of about 3-4 cm. The seeding rate is about 8-12 kg per hectare when grown in mixture and 15-20 kg for the pure crop. Once established it will continue to grow for a long period even up to 10 to 15 years. Besides farmyard manure, an annual application of 100-150 kg of $P_2O_5$ per hectare is essential for getting high tonnage of fodder.

The crop takes about six months for establishment and naturally one or two cuts may be available and the yield will, therefore, not be normal in the first year of its establishment. Regeneration ability is very quick and when once established the subsequent cuts are generally taken at seven to eight weeks's intervals. The fodder is harvested 15-20 cm above the ground level. In the winter months (December-February) the growth of this crop is poor and no cut is available at that time. On an average this legume gives 300-350 quintals of green fodder per hectare in four to five cuts.

## STYLO (*STYLOSANTHES GUIANENSIS.*)

*Genus* : *Stylosanthes Swartz*. Synonym : Brazilian lucerne.

The grass is a native of South America and this perennial grass has a wide range of adaptability which has been grown successfully on many soil types, but it flourishes well in lataritic soil. The crop is a good pasture legume. The average yield of the crop is 40 to 50 quintals per hectare in the first cut and in subsequent cuts the yield is comparatively more.

## COWPEA (*VIGNA SINENSIS.*)

*Genus* : *Vigna Savi*
$2n=22$ Synonyms: Black-eye pea, Cultivated cowpea, Lobia.

It is a crop of Central Africa but it is claimed to be indigenous to India as well. The crop is widely cultivated in all parts of India.

A trailing or bushy, vigorous-growing annual with large seeds, blue-purple to white flowers, oval to heart-shaped leaves and flattened, 10-20 cm long pods, it has a medium to late maturity (70-140 days).

Cowpea or *lobia* is a quick growing *kharif* crop, the green pods of which are used as vegetable, but green vines with pods serve as an excellent forage for livestock, especially the milch cattle. It is adapted to varied soils with good drainage. It is sensitive to cold, but withstands drought. It can be sown with the onset of spring; the seed is broadcast at 45 to 55 kg per hectare mixed with annual *kharif* gramineous forage crops. The green fodder is harvested after the formation of pods and the yield ranges from 200 to 300 quintals per hectare depending on management.

Improved varieties : HFC 42-1, IGFRI-S-450, IGFRI-S- 457, Russian Giant, EC 4216, FOS 1, CO 1 and No. 10.

## GROW FORAGES ALL ROUND THE YEAR

The availability of green succulent and nutritious fodder all round the year constitutes the major key to the success of all dairy enterprises. For this forage production should be increased in a systematic manner either as intensive production where the land is utilised exclusively for fodder all throughout the year or in a mixed farming system where land is utilised in a balanced way for the production of fodder and grain/cash crops simultaneously following a scientific rotational practice. In different parts of the country, the cropping pattern varied depending upon the agro-climatic conditions, the land topography, adaptability and the socio-economic conditions, etc. Accordingly the potential cropping pattern for the year round under intensive production of forages as well as rotation along with food and cash crops are discussed as per different zones of India.

### North-Eastern Zone

**(Sikkim, Manipur, Tripura, Assam, West Bengal, Orissa, Bihar and Eastern U.P.).**

### SUITABLE CROP VARIETIES AND ROTATION FOR THE REGION

*A. Kharif Forage*

Sorghum—Pusa chari/M.P. chari.
Rice bean, Moth, Horse gram (Tetraploid).
Cowpea—Russian Giant, Meerut, EC 4216 Co-I.
Maize for forage—Ganga-2, 5, 7, Ganga-101, Adecuba and composite.
Dinanath grass—$T_3$, $T_{15}$, $T_{10}$, $T_{14}$.
Bajra—K 674, K 677, L 72.
Hybrid Napier—NB-21, BN-1 and BN-2.

*B. Rabi Forage*

Berseem : Pusa Giant, Mascave.
Lucerne : T 8 and T 9.
Sarson : Japan rape.

*C. Pasture Grasses and Legumes*

(*a*) Plains/valleys : Anjan grass, Para grass, Spear grass, Thin napier, Marvel grass, Styles, Centre.
(*b*) Hills : Orchard grass, Fescues, Rye grass, Red clover, White clover.

## WEST BENGAL

1. *For intensive forage production* :

Unirrigated highland : (*a*) Jowar/Bajra/Maize-Rice bean.
Irrigated highland : (*b*) Maize-M.P. Chari-Berseem +Mustard/Lucerne+Oats.
(*c*) Maize/Jowar-Berseem +Mustard/Lucerne+Oats.

2. *Mixed farming system* :

Unirrigated : (*a*) Summer Paddy/Jute-Rice bean.
Irrigated : (*b*) Jute/Summer Paddy-Winter Paddy-Berseem+Oats.

## ORISSA

1. *For intensive forage production* :

Unirrigated : (*a*) M.P. Chari/Dinanath grass/Maize-Cowpea/Horse green.
Irrigated : (*b*) Hybrid Napier (NB-21) Berseem.

2. *Mixed farming system* :

Unirrigated : (*a*) Maize (Fodder)-Paddy.
Irrigated : (*b*) Maize+Cowpea/Jowar-Potato-Sesamum
(*c*) Paddy-Maize-Cowpea.

## TRIPURA

1. *For intensive forage production* :

Unirrigated : (*a*) Maize/Maize+Cowpea-Cowpea.
(*b*) Hybrid Napier (NB-21)-Rice bean.
(*c*) Dinanath grass+Cowpea-Fallow.

2. *Mixed farming system* :

Unirrigated : Maize+Cowpea-Cowpea Seeds-Sunflower (oil).

## BIHAR

1. *For intensive forage production* :

Unirrigated : (*a*) Dinanath grass-Cowpea.
(*b*) Maize/Jowar-Cowpea.
Irrigated : (*a*) Hybrid Napier (NB-21)-Berseem.
(*b*) Maize+Cowpea-Dinanath grass-Oats.
(*c*) Maize+Cowpea-Jowar-Berseem+Japan Rape.

*2. Mixed farming system :*

Unirrigated : Jowar/Maize-Gram-Bajra+Cowpea.

Irrigated : (*a*) Paddy-Berseem-Maize+Cowpea.
(*b*) Paddy-Sarson-Wheat.

EASTERN U.P.

*1. For intensive forage production :*

Unirrigated : (*a*) Maize+Cowpea/M.P. Chari-Cowpea.
(*b*) M.P. Chari-Phaseolus Spp.

Irrigated : (*a*) Hybrid Napier (NB-21)-Berseem.
(*b*) Maize+Cowpea-Jowar-Berseem.

*2. Mixed farming system :*

Unirrigated : (*a*) M.P. Chari-Gram.
(*b*) Jowar+Cowpea-Barley.

Irrigated : (*a*) Paddy-Berseem-Maize+ Cowpea.
(*b*) Maize (grain)-Berseem-Bajra+Cowpea.

**North and North-Western Zone**

(Jammu-Kashmir, Himachal Pradesh, Punjab, Haryana, Rajasthan, Western U.P. and Delhi).

SUITABLE CROP VARIETIES AND ROTATION FOR THE REGION

| | |
|---|---|
| Berseem | — Mascave. |
| Oats | — Kent, HFO 114. |
| Lucerne | — Type 9. |
| Rape LG | — Chinese cabbage. |
| Hybrid Napier | NB-21. |
| Sorghum | — J.S. 220, SS 59-3 and M.P. Chari, SL 44 (in Central Punjab) and Rio (in U.P.). |
| Bajra | — L 72, K 677, D 1941, D 2291 are the new strains. |
| Cowpeas | — FOS 1, K 397, 42-1, EC 4216, Cowpea 74, Russian Giant. |
| Guar | — FOS 277. |
| Maize | — Vijay and Ganga safed for plains & Maize local for Hills. |

*1. For intensive forage production :*

Irrigated : (*a*) Maize+Cowpea-Jowar+Cowpea-Berseem+Sarson.
(*b*) Hybrid Napier (NB-21)+Cowpea-Berseem+Sarson.
(*c*) Hybrid Napier-Lucerne.
(*d*) M.P. Chari-Berseem.
(*e*) Bajra+Cowpea-Maize+Cowpea-Oats+Chinese Cabbage. (For desert area of Rajasthan).

2. *Mixed farming system* :

Irrigated : (*a*) Hybrid Napier (NB-21)-Berseem.
(*b*) NB-21+M.P. Chari+Bajra+Maize+Cowpea-Berseem+Mustard.
(*c*) Maize+Cowpea-Maize+Cowpea. Maize+Cowpea+Tesinte-Oats +Mustard.
(*d*) Maize+Cowpea-Bajra+Cowpea-Berseem-Rape/Berseem+Oats

HILL REGION

(*a*) Maize+Cowpea-Turnip-Oats+Pea
(*b*) Maize+Cowpea-Oats+Lucerne+Japan Rape.
(*c*) Maize+Cowpea-Berseem+Japan Rape+Oats.

HIGHER ALTITUDE

Red clover+White clover+Lobium.

## Central Zone

(South Western parts of Uttar Pradesh, South Eastern Rajasthan, whole of M.P., Maharashtra and Gujarat).

SUITABLE CROP ROTATION FOR THE REGION

*For Intensive Forage Production*:

Irrigated : (*a*) Hyb. Napier+Cowpea-Berseem+Sarson.
(*b*) Maize+Cowpea/M.P. Chari-Berseem+Sarson.
(*c*) Hybrid Napier alone.
(*d*) Hyb. Napier+Guar/Cowpea-Lucerne.
(*e*) Hyb. Napier+Cowpea-Berseem-Cowpea.
(*f*) Hyb. Napier+Cowpea-Berseem.
(*g*) Maize+Cowpea-Berseem.
(*h*) Jowar+Cowpea-Oats.
(*i*) Hyb. Napier-Sesloania/Subabul.

SUITABLE VARIETIES FOR THE REGION

| FORAGE | GUJARAT | M.P. | MAHARASHTRA | U.P. |
|---|---|---|---|---|
| *Hy. Napier* | N.B. 21, 5, B.N. 6 | N.B. 17 | E.B. 4 | N.B. 21, 35. |
| *Maize* | Ganga 5 Ganga Safed-2, Teosinte | Ganga-5 | Ganga Safed-2, Deccan double Teosinte | Ganga-5 |

| FORAGE | GUJARAT | M.P. | MAHARASHTRA | U.P. |
|---|---|---|---|---|
| *Oats* | Kent, 37/14 Western-11 | Kent, Brunkar-10 | Kent | IGFRI-2688, 3021, 3018. |
| *Lucerne* | Anand-2 IGFRI-54 | MPL-2 | Sirsa-9 Poona 1 B | IGFRI-244 IGFRI-54 |
| *Berseem* | Mascave, Chhindwara | Jawahar-1 | — | IGFRI-99-1 |
| *Cowpea* | NP 3, Col. IGFRI-457, IGFRI-998 C-14-20, C-24 | 53 RG, IGFRI-457 Russian Giant J.C.-21 | MPK-1 | Summer-IGFRI-450, 457, Kharif-985, 978, C-24. |
| *Sarson* | Japan variety T-16 IGFRI-I.M. 100 | IGFRI-I.M. 100 IGFRI-S-2276-5 | — | IGFRI-I.M.-100 |
| | | *Low input areas/dryland farming* | | |
| *Sorghum* | MP. Chari S. 1049 | J-69, G-287, Vidasha-68-1 | Nilwa, MB 5-1 S-10-49 M.P. Chari. | M.P. Chari IGFRI-5-427, IGFRI-S-452 |
| *Bajra* | Anand KMF 7264 | M.B.-2 HB-3 | HB-3 | HB-3 |
| *Guar* | Anand No-2, 277 | 277 | — | — |
| *Marvel* | IGFRI-495, 10, IGFRI-495-5 Anand-65 | | MARVEL-8 MARVEL-40 | IGFRI-495-1, IGFRI-495-5 |
| *Dinanth grass* | P P 38, 42 | | | IGFRI-3808 966-1 |
| *Anjan* | | IGFRI-3108 | | IGFRI-3108 |

## South Zone

(Andhra Pradesh, Karnataka, Tamilnadu and Kerala)

## SUITABLE CROP VARIETIES AND ROTATION FOR THE REGION

1. Sondhi Jowar (all states)
2. Al-14-8 (Karnataka)
3. J-Sed-3 (Karnataka)
4. K-3 Cholam (Tamil Nadu)
5. N.l. (Nandyal) A.P.
6. Co-11 (Tamil Nadu)
7. Teosinte (all states).

*1. For intensive forage production* :

Irrigated : (*a*) Maize+Cowpea-Maize-Berseem+Oats.

(b) M.P. Chari-Cowpea-Berseem+Oats.

(c) Maize+Jowar/Bajra-Berseem/Lucerne.

(d) Synthetic Maize/Teosinte/M.P. Chari/Bajra-Berseem+Oats/Lucerne+Oats.

*2. Mixed farming System* :

(a) Sunnhemp/Fodder Metha (Tetraploid) for fodder purpose.

(b) M.P. Chari-Maize+Cowpea.

(c) Hybrid Napier/Guinea grass-Berseem/Lucerne-NB-21.

Costal region of Kerela and Goa. Fodder crops in between plantation crop.

(a) Guinea grass/NB-21/Sataria/Centrosema/Desmodium/Stylos/Dolichos axillaris/Kudzu/Velvet bean.

(b) In Sugar cane field short duration legume like Cowpea/Trilobus/field bean may be grown.

(c) In low area Dinanath grass (P. pedicellatum)+Horse grass/Siratro may be grown.

Land of undulating topography, gravelly with lesser short deposit.

(a) Dinanath grass (b) Horse grass.

COSTAL ANDHRA AREA

Waterlogged area : Para grass.

Sandy stips : (a) Blue Panic+Siratro/Centro.

(b) Coastal bermuda+Seratro/Styles.

(c) Dinanath-I-15+Horse grass.

(d) Hybrid Napier+Siratro.

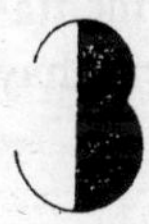

# CONSERVATION OF FORAGE CROPS

India has the largest livestock population in the world. F.A.O.'s projected estimate in 1984 indicated that there are 182 m cattle, 63 m buffaloes, 8.6 m pigs, 41.7 m sheep, 78 m goats and 150 m chickens, giving almost one L.S.U. (livestock units) per hectare of total land area and 1.7 L.S.U. per hectare of arable land. The grasses and other fodders, and feed available in the country are in deficit for all these animals. There is a shortage of 36 and 44 per cent of roughages and concentrates respectively. The shortage of green fodder is also to the extent of 44 per cent of the requirement.

The country has a total land area of 328.8 million hectares, of which 143 million hectares is under cultivation and of this about 60 million hectares (gross) is irrigated. Less than 5 per cent of the irrigated area is under fodder crops. The area is again extremely disproportionate to the minimum requirement in several States. Assam having a bovine population of about 16,000 heads per hectare of cultivated fodders, followed by Kerala and West Bengal with about 8,000. The figures for Bihar, Himachal Pradesh have about 1,750 and 800 respectively. The position in the States of the Punjab, Haryana, Rajasthan, western Uttar Pradesh is encouraging as they have about 12 bovine per hectare. The so called permanent pasture (13.1 million hectare) is mostly confined to Madhya Pradesh, Maharastra, Karnataka, Andhra Pradesh, Rajasthan, Orissa, Himachal Pradesh and Tamilnadu and is overstocked and overgrazed (20-25 bovines per hectare); and even the grazing land such as the forests occupies an area of nearly 75 m hectares which is about 22.8 per cent of the total geographical area of our country.

To meet the requirement of the growing human population, it is necessary that the production of milk, meat and other animal products is increased at a rapid rate. One of the important factors through which this can be achieved is by increasing animal feeds for further conversion into products.

The rainfall in India is seasonal. As a result abundant grass is available in the rainy season, all of which is not properly utilised. We can also produce a good amount of fodder during this season with proper selection of the plant material and proper cultural practises. To satisfy the needs of the stock during the lean months, namely, November-December and April to June, an adequate amount of the surplus grass available during the rainy season must be conserved. The ideal and simple method of conversion is to drive off the moisture in the fresh grass with artificial heat and store the product as dried fodder for use when required. Unfortunately, considerable capital expenditure is involved. In practise the moisture in grass is reduced through exposure to sun and wind, and hay is obtained. This process is simple in theory but is fraught with difficulties in practise.

To combine cheapness and simplicity, and yet ensure at the same time a product of high feeding value and virtually independent of weather conditions at the time, natural fermentation must be used and the process of ensilage adopted. There lies the choice of the farmer—hay or silage.

## HAY MAKING

Hay refers to grasses or legumes that are harvested, dried and stored as 85-90 per cent dry matter. High quality hay is green in colour, leafy and pliable and free from mustiness. When harvested in the proper physiological stage of growth and well cured to 20 per cent or less moisture at the time of storing, hay can be utilised as an excellent feed for dairy cattle, particularly when fodder is scarce or pasturage is insufficient.

Indian hay is seldom taken in the sense in which this term is understood in the western countries. It consists of dry grass on which the seed has ripened and leaves have usually been shed. In feeding value, it mostly corresponds to the straw of cereals rather than to hay made before the seed has ripened. During the later part of the monsoon season, when grass is ready to be cut for hay (the only time when grass is available for hay making,) the weather is often so wet that hay making cannot be attempted. At the end of the monsoon season when there is still some chance of making hay from some good quality grasses that may be left, cultivators are too busy in making preparation for *rabi* sowing.

As will appear from the above, hay making is scarcely practiced in our country. Successful hay making is done to some extent on military farms where economic considerations are not important, but even this hay is of very inferior quality because of the strong action of the sun. Other places where hay making is being practiced are some of the Government farms. Hay making by private farms whether big or small is almost unknown for reasons given above.

### Principles of hay making

The principle involved in hay making is to reduce the water content of the herbage so that it can safely be stored in mass without undergoing fermentation or becoming mouldy. This must be accomplished in such a manner that the hay is not leached by rain and that the loss of leaves is kept at a minimum. Good, well-cured hay makes an excellent forage for all types of livestock on a dairy farm, particularly at times when good quality green fodder is not available or that the green fodder available is too succulent and feeding of dry fodder in addition is essential to keep the stomach of the animal replete.

### Requisites of good quality hay

1) Good hay should be leafy. It has been found that leaves are richer in food value compared to other parts of the plant. The leaves are generally rich in proteins, vitamins and minerals. Loss of leaves in hay making would mean deterioration in feeding value of the ultimate product.

2) It should be prepared out of herbage, cut at a stage nearing maturity, preferably at the flowering stage when it has the maximum of nutrients. Delay in cutting would mean losses of a part of nutrients which would be used up by the plant in seed formation.

3) It should be green in colour. The green colour of leaves indicates the amount of carotene which is a precursor of vitamin A.

4) It should be soft and pliable.

5) It should be free from dust and moulds.

6) It should be free from weeds and stubbles.

7) It should have the smell and aroma characteristic of the crop from which it is made.

8) The moisture percentage in hay should not exceed 15 per cent.

9) Hay of average quality will usually run from 25-30 per cent crude fibre and 45-60 per cent TDN.

10) Hay is primarily a cattle, buffalo, horse, sheep and goat feed. Very little of hay of any kind is ever fed to swine.

## KINDS OF HAY

**1. Legume hay**

Good legume hay has many characteristics that make it of special value to the dairy cattle. It has a higher percentage of digestible nutrients. It has more of digestible proteins because of the high protein content. Furthermore, the proteins of legumes are of superior quality as compared to proteins from other plants. Well-cured legume hays are higher in vitamin contents. They are particularly rich in carotene and may even contain vitamin D. They are also a rich source of vitamin E. The legume hays are particularly rich in calcium and are generally palatable. Among various leguminous fodder crops lucerne, berseem, cowpea and soybean hays are considered first.

**2. Non-legume hay**

Non-legume hays made from grasses are inferior to legume hays. They are, as a rule, less palatable and contain less proteins minerals and vitamins than the legume hays. Non-legume hays have the advantage over legume hays because their outturn per hectare is more than that of legume hays and the former can be grown easily.

Hays made from green crops like oats and barley, compare very favourably with the other grass hays. For good quality hay making these crops should be harvested in the milk stage. They are low in proteins and minerals, but rich in carbohydrates.

**3. Mixed hay**

Hay prepared from mixed crops of legumes and non-legume is known as mixed hay. The composition of such a kind of hay will depend on the proportion of the different species grown as a mixed crop. Such a crop is generally cut earlier because of the variation in the seeding time of the mixed crops. If harvested early, cereals are generally richer in proteins.

## Harvesting of the crop for hay making

There has been much discussion concerning the best time for harvesting a crop for hay making. The crop should be harvested during the day time after the dew has dried off so that plants when spread over the ground may dry evenly. Another factor which needs attention is that the field should not be wet, othewise uniform drying will not be effected.

One of the common mistakes made in making hay is to let the crop ripen too much before cutting. The crop cut early is higher in protein, lower in crude fibre, contains more of vitamins, is more palatable and will shatter less. The best time for cutting a crop for hay making is when it is one-third to a half in blossom.

Recently, new types of hay collection machinery have been introduced in developed countries. These roll the hay into large bundles or gather it into small stacks that can be mechanically handled. Such machinery would be uneconomical in countries like India where there are a limited number of large farms.

**Curing for hay**

In curing, it is necessary that the herbage should be saved from bleaching by the sun and as far as possible, leaves preserved from shattering. The maximum quantity of moisture should be evaporated, so that it can be stored without generation of heat and consequent loss of nutrients.

For reasonably rapid curing and production of high quality hay, it is best to let the herbage lie in the field for a few hours until it is well wilted or about one-fourth to one-third cured. It should be raked into small loose heaps known as windrows. If good weather continues, the hay is cured in windrows alone. When the weather is such that the hay cures slowly, it may be advisable to turn over the windrows partly after a few hours in order to hasten curing. Turning may also be necessary if the hay is wet by rain when in windrows. Besides field curing, hay can be cured by hanging the herbage on tripods, and on farm fences. In artificial curing, the material is placed in a suitable chamber where it comes in contact with heated air and exposure is regulated depending on the material and the temperature.

To avoid serious losses of leaves in very dry seasons, it may be necessary to handle the hay early in the morning before it has become too dry. Hay when ready for storing, should not contain more than 20 per cent moisture and preferably not more than 15 per cent, if it is to be stored in large quantities. If there is more moisture, it will generate heat and fermentation will take place causing loss of nutrients.

A very simple technique for making berseem or lucerne hay without loss of leaves has been developed by the Animal Nutrition department of Haryana Agricultural University involves : (a) cutting berseem or lucerne in pre-bloom or bud stage, (b) chopping fresh forage and spreading it in thin layer of four to five inches on a smooth clean surface, (c) stirring the drying forage frequently, (d) gathering of leaves and chopped stem together. Any storage normally used for wheat *bhoosa* can be used for this chopped hay.

**Losses of nutrients in hay making**

Some nutrients are always lost in field curing of hay, but under favourable conditions this loss is not too much. Drying of green forage at ordinary temperature reduces its digestibility. If the plants are dried without fermentation or bleaching, they contain a high percentage of nutrients.

The losses in nutrient value in hay making are :

1) Losses due to late cutting.
2) Losses of leaves by shattering.

3) Losses of vitamins due to leaching and fermentation.

4) Losses of soluble nutrients by leaching in heavy rain.

### 1. Losses Due to Late Cutting

Late cutting means greater lignification and lower carbohydrate and protein digestibility while cutting early suffers from low yield and high moisture content of the forages meant for hay making.

### 2. Losses by Shattering

The loss due to shattering of leaves and finer parts in hay making is of importance, especially in the case of legumes. The leaves are much richer in digestible nutrients than the stem and hence losses by shattering materially decrease the nutritive value of hay. To avoid these losses, hay should never be overdried or handled during warm periods of the day.

### 3. Losses of Vitamins

In the process of drying, much of the green colouring matter containing carotene, a precursor of vitamin A is lost with bleaching. In general, the carotene content of freshly cured hay is proportional to the greenness. With severe bleaching, more than 90 per cent of carotene may be destroyed.

### 4. Losses in Fermentation

In fermentation of hay, some of the organic nutrients like starch and sugars are oxidised into $CO_2$ and water. If drying is prolonged because of unfavourable weather conditions, changes brought about by the activity of bacteria and fungi may occur. Mouldy hay is not only unpalatable but also may be harmful for animals as well as for persons handling the hays due to the presence of mycotoxins. Very often such hays contain actinomycetes, responsible for the allergic condition in man known as "Farmer's Lung". One of the ways to prevent the development of mould growth is to spray propionic acid uniformly on entire hay. In general, it is not uncommon to find patches of mouldy hay in a stack resulting from uneven drying.

### 5. Losses by Leaching

If hay is almost cured and is exposed to heavy and prolonged rains, especially when it is in the field, severe losses may occur through leaching. Unless the rain is so heavy as to soak the material, losses by leaching will not occur. For this reason losses will be much less even in heavy rains if the hay is in good sized windrows.

**Storage of hay**

Hay is usually stored in stacks in this country. Care should be taken that the hay is in a good and dry condition before it is stored. It should be stacked in a shady place where there is no danger of fire. The stacks should be made at an elevated place. Machines are also available for baling the hay. Baled (a large package or bundle) materials occupy less space.

**Brown hay**

Sometimes because of very unfavourable weather conditions, good hay cannot be obtained by the ordinary method of curing. Under such circumstances, hay is allowed to dry until about 50 per cent moisture has been removed and then it is packed in stacks or piles. Fermentation takes place and the hay may become very hot; the temperature however, should not be allowed to exceed 80°C. There are great losses in the nutritive value on account of fermentation. These losses range from 30 to 40 per cent. Such hay is often quite palatable.

**Biochemical changes during preparation and storage of hay**

During the time of harvesting there is a sudden interruption of the transpiration stream. The shutting off of the water supply from the roots and a continued evaporation from the leaf surface leads to wilting, drying and death of the plant. However, while the forage is being dried, plant respiratory enzyme activity will continue resulting in the oxidation of some valuable plant nutrients. The process also continues during the storage period. The biochemical changes during preparation and storage of hay at ambient temperature are discussed below :

1. CARBOHYDRATES

The water soluble carbohydrates in the crop which are highly digestible will be oxidised to $CO_2$ and $H_2O$, with the production of heat leading to loss of dry matter. The greatest loss comprises glucose and fructose with some decrease in sucrose.

Among organic acids, malic, citric and succinic acids have been found to decrease during wilting.

2. NITROGENOUS CONSTITUENTS

During the drying process, losses observed with nitrogenous substances are insignificant. Total soluble nitrogen mostly of amino acids as opposed to protein nitrogen increases as a result of proteases.

Cyanogenic glycosides of *jowar*, white clover and few other forages have been shown to lose their toxicity property during drying which may be due to denaturation of the enzymes responsible for liberation of hydrocyanic acid.

3. VITAMINS

Slow drying in sun under normal temperature has been found to cause a loss of 80 per cent carotene mostly due to action of lipoxidase. The obvious change is a loss of plant pigments. However, rapid drying tends to protect the carotene content due to quick inactivation of the concerned enzyme.

The exposure of ultraviolet rays of sun converts ergosterol into ergocalciferol (vitamin $D_2$) in plants. Thus the process of hay making by sun drying increases the value of vitamin D.

Vitamin E is quite high in green leaves particularly during the flowering period. However, matured forages are lower and dried hays are still lower in vitamin E activity. The difference may be partly due to the lower leaf-stem ratio of the matured plants.

Hay stored at higher moisture content (more than 20 per cent) may undergo enough fermentation to result marked temperature increases (largely because of growth of thermophilic moulds), which may cause browning and, sometimes spontaneous combustion. Excess heating or moulding results in a marked reduction in digestibility of protein and energy. Ample evidence shows that rapid drying, provided it is not accompanied by excessively hot temperatures, results in the least changes in chemical components of forage.

Thus. we see that drying may not have any great effect on forage utilisation. However, in practice we must expect some loss of leaves in plants and reduced soluble carbohydrates. Hay, if made from moderately mature plants, will have lower protein and digestible energy than young herbage, but is apt to be better than very mature herbage. Nutritive properties of hays are, then, similar to those of forages, but with slightly to greatly reduced values depending on freedom from weather damage and method of harvesting.

Little interest is taken in India in conserving surplus grasses as hay, possibly because during the monsoons, when surplus grasses are available, hay making becomes difficult due to adverse weather conditions. By the time the monsoon is over, the grasses are in a late stage of maturity, and their nutritive value deteriorates.

## SILAGE MAKING

*What is silage*? Silage is a fermented feed resulting from the storage of high moisture crops, usually green forages, under anaerobic conditions in a structure known as a silo.

*What is ensiling*? It is also referred to as ensilage. The name actually stands for all physical and chemical changes that take place when forage or feed with sufficient moisture are stored in a silo in the absence of air. The entire ensiling process requires two to three weeks for converting forage into silage.

*What is silo*? A silo is an airtight to semi-airtight structure designed for the storage and preservation of high moisture feeds as silage. Silos are of different types.

**Characteristics of silo pits**

1) That its size should be decided on the basis of the number and kind of animals to be fed daily, the length of the feeding period, and the amount of forage available for ensiling.

2) That it excludes air from the stored material including entrance of air around the doors of tower silos.

3) That side walls be straight and smooth in order to prevent the formation of air pockets which may retard the normal microbial fermentation.

4) That it be of adequate depth, thereby making for better packing and less surface area to total mass exposed.

5) That the walls should be strong and rigid in order to withstand the pressure which develops inside the pit as fermentation takes place. Note that silage made from cut grass will exert from a half to two and a half times as much pressure on the walls as does maize silage. Reinforcement of walls will be desired.

6) That adequate provision be made for the escape of surplus juices, either by a drain or by a gravel bottom.

7) That it be conveniently located and accessible in all kinds of weather, from the standpoint of both filling and feeding.

8) That silo pits (not tower type) are always located preferably at the highest spot on the farm to avoid water seepage.

The kind of silo and the choice of construction material should be determined primarily by economics. Silos may be classified as follows :

I. *Conventional upright (tower) silos*

1) Concrete stave (thin, shaped strips of concrete set edge to edge to form the wall).

2) Wood stave.
3) Tile block.
4) Brick.

II. *Gastight (oxygen-limiting) silos*
1) Concrete stave.
2) Brick.

III. *Pit silos*

IV. *Horizontal silos*
1) Trench silos (below ground level).
2) Bunker silos (above ground level).

V. *Temporary silos*
1) Plastic or polyethylene bag silos
2) Modified trench-stack silos

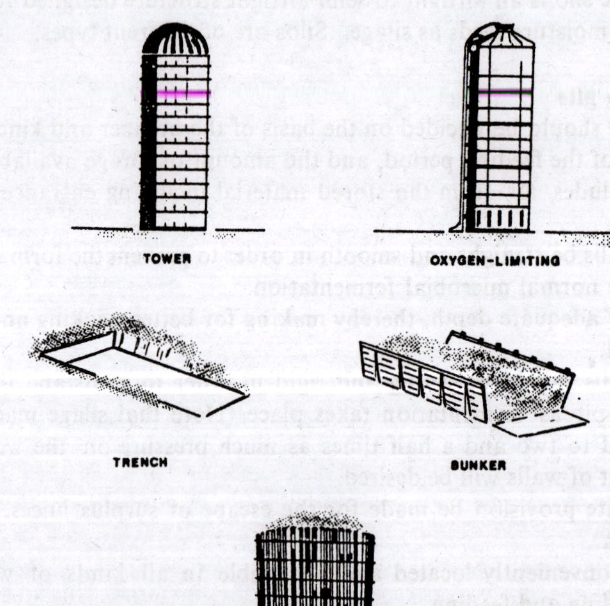


**Fig. 1** Kinds of silos: (1) tower silo, (2) oxygen-limiting, (3) trench silo, (4) bunker (aboveground level), and (5) enclosed stack silo. The latter two are both aboveground temporary silos.

### Conventional Upright (Tower) Silos

Being a permanent farm structure, a silo should be constructed to withstand long usage. Among advantages of such silos are: (1) durability, (2) minimum top and side spoilage, (3) well adapted to automation (loading and unloading machinery).

The only disadvantage is the cost of making it. Under only large commercial dairy farms this type of silo may be thought of. Most present day conventional upright silos are made of reinforced poured concrete or of concrete staves.

All upright silos are circular in shape and equipped with a series of doors about 2 ft. square approximately every 6 ft. up one side of the silo. These are closed as the silo is filled and opened and as the silo is emptied. Recent developments in construction of tower silos have been made in bottom unloaders and large diameter features (24-30 ft.)

For effective preservation of silage, the forage should contain between 25 and 35 per cent dry matter. The size varies from about 12-20 ft. in diameter and 40-80 ft. in length.

### Gastight or Airtight or Sealed Silos

These silos resemble conventional tower silos, but they are more expensive because of their construction to make the tower completely free from oxygen.

Gastight silos are designed for forages having as high as 50-75 per cent dry matter or for the storage of high moisture grain containing 60-75 per cent dry matter

### Pit Silos

A pit silo is shaped like the tower silo, but inverted into the ground. It resembles a well. This type of silo can be made only in places where the water table is low enough that the silo will not fill with water that is in semi-arid or in arid regions.

In comparison with tower silos, pit silos have the following advantages: (1) they are never damaged by storm, (2) require less reinforcing. Among disadvantages: (1) they are dangerous, due to the frequent presence of suffocating $CO_2$, (2) considerable work is involved in removing the silage.

### Horizontal Silos

Only two types of horizontal silos will be discussed herein, trench silos and bunker silos.

#### *Trench silo*

At a comparatively low cost this type of silo can be constructed quickly. It is most popular in areas where the weather is not too severe and where there is good drainage. A trench silo should be wider at the top than at the bottom, and the bottom should slope away from one end so that excess juices will drain off if material with high moisture content is ensiled.

*Advantages* : Low initial cost and ease of construction.

*Disadvantages* : In comparison with the tower type it will require larger space to seal.

When filling is completed, the top should be carefully sealed by polyethylene, plastic or by wet straw mixed with mud or by saw dust to make it air tight.

*Bunker silos*

As a labour saving measure, bunker type of silos above the ground (or slightly recessed) usually with concrete floors are generally catching the attention of many farmers.

**Size of silo to build**

| Number of adult cow | Diameter of silo in metre | Height of silo in metre | Tonnes of silage |
|---|---|---|---|
| 12 | 3.05 | 7.93 | 39.4 |
| 20 | 3.66 | 8.23 | 56.4 |
| 30 | 4.27 | 9.14 | 84.6 |
| 50 | 5.49 | 10.68 | 141.0 |
| 100 | 6.10 | 11.89 | 282.0 |

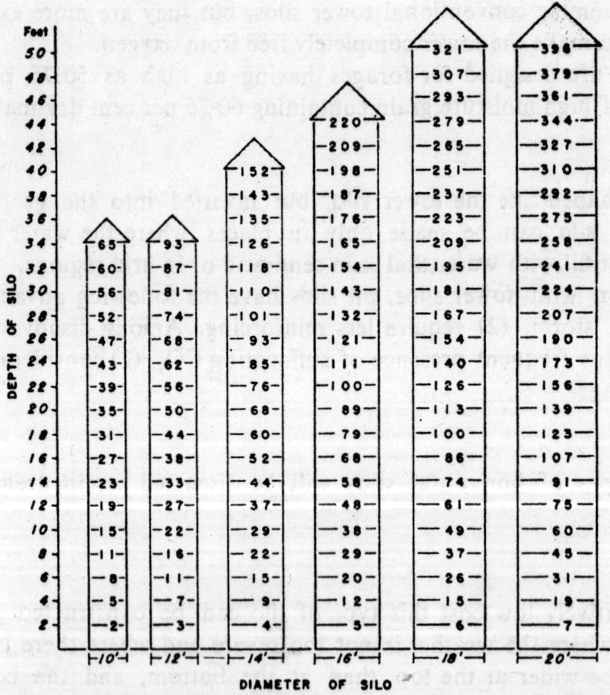


**Fig. 2** Capacity in tons of settled corn silage in tower silos of varying sizes. See Table 5 for tabular material.

## Kinds of crops used for silage

Practically any crop having sufficient soluble carbohydrates and moisture to produce the desired quantities of acids may be made into silage. The most commonly used silage crops

Tahle 5

## GUIDE FOR ESTIMATING AMOUNT OF SILAGE IN A TOWER TYPE SILO[1]

| Depth of Settled Silage | Total Quantity of Settled Silage, from the Top to the Depth Indicated, in Silos Having a Diameter of: | | | | | |
|---|---|---|---|---|---|---|
| | 10 Feet | 12 Feet | 14 Feet | 16 Feet | 18 Feet | 20 Feet |
| (ft) | (tons) | | | | | |
| 1 | 1 | 1 | 1 | 2 | 2 | 3 |
| 2 | 2 | 3 | 4 | 5 | 6 | 7 |
| 3 | 3 | 5 | 6 | 8 | 10 | 13 |
| 4 | 5 | 7 | 9 | 12 | 15 | 19 |
| 5 | 6 | 9 | 12 | 16 | 20 | 25 |
| 6 | 8 | 11 | 15 | 20 | 26 | 31 |
| 7 | 10 | 14 | 19 | 25 | 31 | 38 |
| 8 | 11 | 16 | 22 | 29 | 37 | 45 |
| 9 | 13 | 19 | 26 | 34 | 43 | 53 |
| 10 | 15 | 22 | 29 | 38 | 49 | 60 |
| 11 | 17 | 24 | 33 | 43 | 55 | 67 |
| 12 | 19 | 27 | 37 | 48 | 61 | 75 |
| 13 | 21 | 30 | 41 | 53 | 67 | 83 |
| 14 | 23 | 33 | 44 | 58 | 74 | 91 |
| 15 | 25 | 36 | 48 | 63 | 80 | 99 |
| 16 | 27 | 38 | 52 | 68 | 86 | 107 |
| 17 | 29 | 41 | 56 | 73 | 93 | 115 |
| 18 | 31 | 44 | 60 | 79 | 100 | 123 |
| 19 | 33 | 47 | 64 | 84 | 106 | 131 |
| 20 | 35 | 50 | 68 | 89 | 113 | 139 |
| 21 | 37 | 53 | 72 | 94 | 120 | 148 |
| 22 | 39 | 56 | 76 | 100 | 126 | 156 |
| 23 | 41 | 59 | 81 | 105 | 133 | 164 |
| 24 | 43 | 62 | 85 | 111 | 140 | 173 |
| 25 | 45 | 65 | 89 | 116 | 147 | 181 |
| 26 | 47 | 68 | 93 | 121 | 154 | 190 |
| 27 | 50 | 71 | 97 | 127 | 161 | 198 |
| 28 | 52 | 74 | 101 | 132 | 167 | 207 |
| 29 | 54 | 77 | 105 | 138 | 174 | 215 |
| 30 | 56 | 81 | 110 | 143 | 181 | 224 |
| 31 | 58 | 84 | 114 | 149 | 188 | 232 |
| 32 | 60 | 87 | 118 | 154 | 195 | 241 |
| 33 | 62 | 90 | 122 | 160 | 202 | 249 |
| 34 | 65 | 93 | 126 | 165 | 209 | 258 |
| 35 | 67 | 96 | 131 | 171 | 216 | 267 |
| 36 | — | — | 135 | 176 | 223 | 275 |
| 37 | — | — | 139 | 182 | 230 | 284 |
| 38 | — | — | 143 | 187 | 237 | 292 |
| 39 | — | — | 148 | 193 | 244 | 301 |
| 40 | — | — | 152 | 198 | 251 | 310 |
| 41 | — | — | — | 204 | 258 | 318 |
| 42 | — | — | — | 209 | 265 | 327 |
| 43 | — | — | — | 215 | 272 | 335 |
| 44 | — | — | — | 220 | 279 | 344 |
| 45 | — | — | — | 226 | 286 | 353 |
| 46 | — | — | — | — | 293 | 361 |
| 47 | — | — | — | — | 300 | 370 |
| 48 | — | — | — | — | 307 | 379 |
| 49 | — | — | — | — | 314 | 387 |
| 50 | — | — | — | — | 321 | 396 |

[1]This tabular material was used as a basis for Fig. 2

are : among graminaceous crops, maize, sorghum, sudan grass, bajra, hybrid, napier etc. Out of all, maize and sorghum are supposed to be the best crops for silage making. So far leguminous crops are concerned, lucerne, berseem and cowpea, they are not suitable for silage making but after giving some treatments they may also be converted into good quality silage. For preserving leguminous crops which have less percentages of sugar, the fodder is sprinkled with a solution of molasses in water at every one-third metre of filling to provide the necessary amount of sugar for silage making. Gramiaceous forage crops can be mixed with legumes for making silage of good quality.

**Preparation of forage for making silage**

In addition to using a sound silo of proper size, those who make good silage generally harvest at the proper stage of maturity, cut to proper length, control the moisture content, add an additive or preservative when needed, fill rapidly, distribute forage uniformly in the silo, and seal the silo. Each of these factors are briefly described as below.

HARVEST AT PROPER STAGE OF MATURITY

The crop for silage making is generally harvested at the flowering stage when it has the maximum amount of nutrients. For maize this is about the early dent stage (well matured stage, normally harvested for seed) of maturity and for sorghum the late dough stage (stage at which the seeds are soft and immature) at the earliest. Silage materials containing less than 25 per cent dry matter (more than 75 per cent moisture) will form a very sour silage and will usually lose significant amounts of silage juices during storage, involving a considerable loss of nutrients. Thus plants for silage making may be allowed to mature till the dry matter content attains 35-40 per cent.

CUT TO PROPER LENGTH

The length of the cut sections affects the packing and, hence, the quality of the silage. Silage crops usually vary from a fraction of an inch to over an inch in length. Grass silages require to be more finely chopped than maize or sorghum. Wilted and dry forages and forage with hollow stems should be chopped more finely than forage of high moisture content, thus permitting more thorough packing and eliminating most air pockets.

CONTROL THE MOISTURE CONTENT

Practical experience has indicated that 35-40 per cent dry matter that is 60-65 per cent is the best moisture content for most crops to be ensiled.

Forage containing more than 60-65 per cent moisture (1) is heavier and more costly to handle than is necessary; (2) is apt to produce slimy, putrid silage, due to the presence of butyric and other undesirable acids; (3) will have excessive seepage of the juices and some loss of nutrients, except carotene, from the silo; (4) will result in excessive deterioration in the silo walls due to the high acidity; and, (5) will exert high pressure on the silo walls.

The high moisture content of the silage may be lowered by any one or a combination of the following methods:

1) *Conditioning—wilting*: The method is suitable for making of grass silage. Conditioning and/or wilting for three to four hours on a good drying day may reduce 10-15 per cent reduction of moisture content.

2) *Adding dry hay or straw*: During poor wilting weather, the moisture content of grass forage can be reduced within the desired range by adding 5-20 per cent straw.

3) *Combining high and low moisture crops*: By mixing at a calculated ratio between high and low moisture crops, the forage may be made into desired moisture content.

4) *Adding dry preservative*: Dry preservatives as ground grains, maize and cob meal, dried molasses etc. will reduce moisture content.

If the crop is over-ripe and too dry when cut, or if it becomes over-wilted, it will be necessary to add water to the silo after fine chopping and during packing.

## Add an Additive or Preservative When Needed

Addition of additives or preservatives serve one or more of the following purposes:

(1) Add nutrients; (2) provide fermentable carbohydrates; (3) furnish additional acids; (4) inhibit undesirable types of bacteria and moulds; (5) reduce the amount of oxygen present, directly or indirectly; (6) reduce the moisture content of the silage; and (7) absorb some acids which might otherwise be lost in seepage: (8) increase nitrogen content.

Some common additives and preservatives are discussed below:

1) *Molasses*: Some green forages such as legumes and certain grasses are rather low in sugar content. Adding molasses definitely improves the quality of silage by increasing lactic and acetic acid production. It also increases the palatability and nutritive value of the silage. Molasses may be added (3.5 to 4 per cent of the green weight of the forage) in either liquid or dehydrated form. Molasses and starches when added in the form of grains supply the silage bacteria with ample food so that fermentation proceeds normally.

2) *Urea*: Adding urea at a level of 0.5 per cent of fresh forages has several advantages including a way to feed urea more uniformly throughout the day than when it is fed with concentrates at particular times. The very idea of adding urea is to enrich the silage with nitrogen as cereal forages are mostly deficient in this element.

3) *Limestone*: This is calcium carbonate and may be added at a level of 0.5 to 1.0 per cent to maize silage to increase acid production. It neutralises some of the initial acids as they are formed allowing the lactic acid bacteria to perform longer and to produce more desirable acids.

4) *Sodium metabisulphite*: Sulphur dioxide ($SO_2$ a gas) is a very antibacterial preservative. It also improves carotene content.

5) *Organic acids*: Propionic and formic acids are used for enhancing preservation of forages without the loss of palatability. These are costly and when added, the following guidelines may be observed:

i) Add 1 per cent propionic acid to the forage in the field at the time of harvest or at the chopper.

ii) Limit the presence of oxygen by using a sound, well built silo.

iii) Prevent dilution of organic acid treated silage by rain and cover it with plastic when it is stored outside.

6) *Bacterial cultures*: Silage preservatives containing cultures of acid-forming bacteria like *Lactobacillus acidophilus*, *Torulopsis* sp., and *Bacillus subtilis*, are added to silage crops. The basis for including these as a preservative is to provide an inoculum or to increase the number of bacteria for helping rapid fermentation.

### FILL RAPIDLY

Once silo filling is started, it should be rapid, say within two days or less. For creating the desired type of anaerobic condition inside the silo, the forages during filling should be compressed. Never fill a silo when it is raining.

### DISTRIBUTE FORAGE UNIFORMLY IN THE SILO

Again in order to avoid the presence of air pockets and spoilage, chopped forage should uniformly be distributed in the silo and packed well.

### SEALING OF SILO

For maintaining the silo anaerobic it is a must to stop the entrance of atmospheric air in the silo. This may be done as follows: (1) Level the top and tramp the last few feet, especially near the walls. (2) Cover the top by using any type of insulator like mud, plastic or loose earth. (3) For bunker or trench silo apply sufficient load on top to facilitate compactness.

Within a period of two to three weeks the forages will be converted into silage. The silage may be taken out of the silo from the top in case of tower and trench silos and from the front side in case of a bunker silo. After opening it becomes necessary to feed a pit completely. A two to four inch layer of silage must be removed daily. In case the silage is not used for livestock feed immediately after its preparation, the accumulation of by-products of bacterial metabolism will tend to preserve the forage material as silage for an indefinite period unless air is permitted to enter.

## How silage is formed ?

When the green, chopped forge is first stored in a compact mass in a silo, the living plant cells continue to respire, thus rapidly using up the oxygen in the trapped air and giving off $CO_2$. In about four or five hours the free oxygen is all used up, but the $CO_2$ increases rapidly for about 48 hours, when it comprises from 60-70 per cent of the silo gases. Subsequent to this time due to production of other metabolites including various gases like $CO_2$, $CH_4$, CO, NO, $NO_2$ etc., the amount of $CO_2$ begins to decrease.

This condition will promote optimum production of organic acids primarily lactic, acetic and formic by bacteria to prevent decomposition. Eventually the acids will kill the bacteria and preserve the silage as long as (may be 10-15 years) anaerobic conditions are maintained.

### Silage microbiology

The plant forage carries with it a large number of aerobic fungi and bacteria. The activity of aerobic microorganisms gradually ceased with the development of anaerobic conditions. The situation is further favoured by rise of temperature of about 80 to 85°F near the bottom and about 100°F for about 15 days and then gradually decreases. If air gets into the silage, the temperature may rise to 130°F. The heat is caused by bacterial fermentation, and by the presence of sufficient readily available carbohydrate, by moisture content of 60 to 65 per cent for the growth of anaerobic bacteria such as *Lactobacillus*, *Leuconostoc*, *Streptococcus*, *Escherichia*, *Klebsiella*, *Bacillus*, *Clostridium* and *Padiococcus*. Being facultative anaerobes, yeasts present in the silo contents also proliferate. Of course the lactic acid bacteria dominates all except in formic acid treated silage. However, the anerobes increase very rapidly, frequently to hundreds or thousand of millions per milliliter of the juice. These bacteria, or enzymes produced by them, and enzymes from the cut plant material, attack the sugars and other food material, breaking them down into organic acids, principally lactic, acetic and formic, some ethyl alcohol, some gases like $CO_2$, $CH_4$, CO, NO, $NO_2$.

It has been found that besides the sugars, 25 per cent of the pentosans and 25 per cent of the starch contained in the forage are changed as a result of four months ensiling. Much of it is changed to organic acids, and some of it is used for food for the bacteria and is built up into compounds in their bodies. In this process, some of the proteins of the green forage are also broken down into amino acids and will not affect the nutritive value of feed proteins, but in badly preserved material the amino acids are broken down further to various amines such as tryptamine, putrescine, histamine, phenylethylamine etc., which at higher concentration may be harmful to the consuming animals.

When the acid in the silage is about pH 4.0, bacteria cease to multiphy and will bring in reduction of their number hence the action of the enzymes stops, with the result that no more acid is developed, putrefaction ceases, and, if air does not gain entrance, the silage will keep for long periods with but very little change.

**Characteristics of a good silage**

1. VERY GOOD SILAGE

It is clean, the taste is acidic, and has no butyric acid, no moulds, no sliminess nor proteolysis. The pH is between 3.5 and 4.2. The amount of ammoniacal nitrogen should be less than 10 per cent of the total nitrogen. Uniform in moisture and green or brownish in colour. Taste is pleasing, not bitter or sharp.

2. GOOD SILAGE

The taste is acidic. There may be traces of butyric acid. The pH is between 4.2 and 4.5. The amount of ammoniacal nitrogen is 10-15 per cent of the total nitrogen. Other points same as of very good silage.

3. FAIR SILAGE

The silage is mixed with a little amount of butyric acid. There may be slight proteolysis along with some mould. The pH is between 4.5 and 4.8. Ammoniacal nitrogen is 15-20 per cent of the total nitrogen. Colour of silage varies between tobacco brown to dark brown.

4. POOR SILAGE

It has a bad smell due to high butyric acid and high proteolysis. The silage may be infested with moulds. Less acidity, pH is above 4.8. The amount of ammoniacal nitrogen is more than 20 per cent. Colour tends to be blackish and should not be fed.

In Germany, a widely used method of grading silage requires determination of lactic, butyric and acetic acid contents along with pH values. It gives the final classification on the basis of scores (Fleig's value). Briefly a particular silage is assigned scores according to its pH and fatty acid content as given in Table and is graded according to its total score. If the silage is of very good quality its total score will range between 44 and 50, if poor it will have no more than 19 points. Similarly, satisfactory and moderately made silage will have scores in between 30-36 and 20-29, respectively.

**Table 6**

**German method of grading silage**

| pH | Points | Lactic acid* | Points | Acetic acid* | Points | Butyric acid* | Points |
|---|---|---|---|---|---|---|---|
| 3.50—3.79 | 9 | Over 60 | 20 | Under 30 | 10 | 0.0—0.1 | 10 |
| 3 80—4.2 | 10 | 60—55.1 | 18 | 30.1—34 | 9 | 0.1—2.5 | 9 |
| 4.21—4.4 | 9 | 55—50.1 | 16 | 34.1—38 | 8 | 2.51—5.0 | 8 |
| 4 41—4.6 | 8 | 50—45.1 | 14 | 38.1—42 | 7 | 5.01—7.5 | 7 |
| 4.61—4.8 | 7 | 45—40.1 | 12 | 42.1—46 | 6 | 7.51—10.0 | 6 |
| 4.81—5.0 | 6 | 40—35.1 | 10 | 46.1—50 | 5 | 10.01—15.0 | 5 |
| 5.01—5.2 | 5 | 35—30.1 | 8 | 50.1—54 | 4 | 15.01—20.0 | 4 |
| 5.21—5.4 | 4 | 30—25.1 | 6 | 54.1—58 | 3 | 20.01—25 | 3 |
| 5.41—5.6 | 3 | 25—20.1 | 4 | 58.1—62 | 2 | 25.01—35 | 2 |
| | | | | | | 35.01—45 | 1 |
| 5.61—5.8 | 2 | 20—15.1 | 2 | 62.1—66 | 1 | 45.01—55 | 0 |
| | | | | | | 55.01—60 | −5 |
| 5.81—6.0 | 1 | 15.0 & under | 0 | over 66 | 0 | 60.1 —65 | −10 |
| | | | | | | 65.01—over | −20 |

***Percentage of total acids**

## Advantages and disadvantages of silage

1) Green fodder can be kept in a succulent condition for a considerably long period. Silage furnishes high quality forage in any desired season of the year at a low expense. As there is an acute shortage of green fodder during the summer months, silage can meet this deficiency during that part of the year.

2) Grass silage preserves 85 per cent or more of the feed value of the crop, whereas hay making will preserve significantly less percentage of nutrients.

3) It is the most economical form in which the whole stalk of maize or sorghum can be processed and stored. On the other hand, a considerable part of this crop is wasted during the course of feeding in dry condition even if it is of good quality.

4) During the monsoon months, it becomes exceedingly difficult with dry grasses for making hay. Preserving the fodder as silage avoids this difficulty.

5) Weeding crops which tend to make poor hay may produce silage of good quality. The ensiling process kills practically all weeds that are present in the field because of their harvest before seed formation and thereby stopping dissemination of their seeds.

6) It is a very palatable feed and slightly laxative in nature.

7) It is a better source of protein and of certain vitamins, especially carotene, and perhaps some of the unknown factors, than dried forage.

8) With early removal of *khariff* crops from fields for silage making, enough time is available for preparing the land for the sowing of *rabi* crops which follow.

9) It makes for less waste, the entire plant being consumed, which is an important consideration with coarse, stemmy forages.

10) The produce from a given area can be stored in less space than dry fodder of the

same quantity. A cubic foot of silage contains about three times more dry weight of feed than a cubic foot of long hay stored in the mow.

11) It offers many advantages over pasture, including (a) no fencing required, (b) approximately one-third more forage from the same acreage, (c) harvesting at optimum maturity, (d) more uniform quality, and (e) closer observation of animals that are confined to a lot.

12) It helps to control weeds, which are often spread through hay or fodder.

Some of the disadvantages of silage are :

1) It requires a silo in comparison with the simpler methods of field curing and storing hay, this is likely to mean higher costs for small farmers.

2) It possess considerably less vitamin D than sun-cured hay.

3) It incurs an added expenditure when preservatives are necessary.

4) Extra labour is needed at silo filling time.

## Haylage

Haylage is a low moisture silage (40 to 45 per cent moisture) and is made from grass/or legume that is wilted to 40-45 per cent moisture content before ensiling. It is similar to silage except it is lower in moisture. For details, the chapter dealing with "Identifying feeds from their composition" written elsewhere in this book may be consulted.

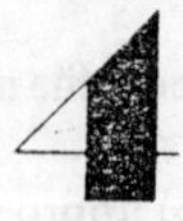

# POISONOUS PLANTS

A poisonous plant is one, which as a whole or a part thereof, under all or certain circumstances, when taken or brought in contact with an organism will exert a harmful effect or cause immediate death due to the presence of known or unknown chemical substances in it.

To list and describe all the plants known to have poisoned livestock in the tropics would require a volume of monumental proportions. In the Indo-Pakistan subcontinent alone, there are approximately 700 species listed. Some are known in every tropical area; some occur only in restricted areas in perhaps only one country.

**Predisposing factors**

Among the more important of the factors which affect the prevalence of poisoning by plants are:

1. *Season of year*: Some plants grow well in one season and are dormant in others. They may be highly toxic at the early stage of the new growth, when the flowers and seeds are forming at all seasons and at all stages of growth.

2. *Climate*: Generally, high humidity and temperature favours growth of poisonous plants and development of the poisonous principle in them, but this does not necessarily lead to a higher incidence of poisoning. Similar conditions favour the growth of palatable forage and so reduce the chances of animals ingesting the poisonous plant.

3. *Accessibility*: Many highly toxic plants seldom if ever cause poisoning because they are not readily accessible to livestock. They may grow in the depths of forests where livestock never go. Others grow throughout grazing areas and cause very high mortality. Others simulate the growing habits of forage plants and are intimately associated with them and consequently are accidentally consumed by the grazing animal.

4. *Palatability*: It is a relative term. Animals on a satisfactory plane of nutrition will not eat poisonous plants. Animals starving during drought will often graze on poisonous plants to appease their hunger. Some highly toxic plants are never consumed because of their unpalatability, which may be either due to bitterness, or the presence of spines, or the woodiness of the plant, or the presence of a repulsive aromatic smell, or the ability to cause blistering, or a rash around the mouth of the animal which has accidentally ingested the plant.

5. *Species and age of animal*: Some animal species are highly tolerant of some poisonous plants while others are susceptible. Pigs and horses are usually susceptible, but sheep and goats are more tolerant to most toxic plant species. Young animals are usually more susceptible.

6. *Familiarity*: Animals may become familiar with a poisonous plant through past association. Perhaps they have at one time ingested some of the plant, have been affected and

have connected cause and effect. Nevertheless, there are instances where animals have consumed poisonous plants, have been badly affected, have recovered, and have gone back and consumed more of the same plants, for some reason as yet unexplained.

7. *Part of the plant which is toxic*: Many plants are toxic in all their parts. Some only in one or two parts, for example the seeds or the flowers or the roots. Obviously if the seeds are toxic, animals will be affected only when seeds are present and this is again related to season. If only roots are toxic then cattle, sheep and horses are unlikely to be poisoned whereas pigs may be, because of their rooting habit.

8. *Parasitic fungi*: Poisonous fungi can invade and render toxic a plant which is itself harmless. Two of the better known ones are *Aspergillus flavus*, described under aflatoxicosis, and *Claviceps* spp. which attach themselves to grasses, mainly Paspalum spp. and render them highly toxic.

9. *Variability of toxic principle*: Many plants which are perfectly good forage under certain conditions of climate, soil type, or other as yet uncertain ecological factors, become highly toxic. This even applies to some well known grasses. These, under conditions of good growth followed by rapid wilt, produce large quantities of hydrocyanic acid. Some highly toxic plants when dried and treated in some way, are rendered harmless. Sometimes plants will change from the toxic to the non-toxic state or *vice versa* for no apparent reason.

10. *Soil type*: The type of soil has a marked influence on the toxicity or otherwise of plants which grow on it, and sharp divisions between environments where a poison plant does or does not grow can be due to an abrupt change of soil type, for example high selenium soils may be very clearly marked by the selenium 'accumulators' growing on them.

**Characteristic symptoms of plant poisoning**

The active principles of poison plants vary so widely in their chemical composition and in the symptoms produced that no specific guidelines can be laid down. Generally the effect of the poison is on more than one body system, but occasionally only one may be clearly affected so that there is some possibility of linking cause with effect. Nervous poisons are probably most commonly seen. They are usually in the form of overstimulation, such as occurs with the narcotics—these being present in many plants including *Datura*, and *Strychnos*. Stimulation may be followed by paralysis and finally death.

Irritant poisons produce skin blistering or dermatitis, such as, occur with many species of *Euphorbia* because of the milky fluid which they exude, or, various trees which may secrete juices with which animals accidentally come into contact. Other irritants are the hairs and cystalline spikes found in many plants that cause acute haemorrhagic gastroenteritis, such as many species of *Araceae*.

Muscular poisons mostly cardiac glycosides, similar to digitalis, directly affect the muscles and cause convulsions and paralysis. Plants containing the cardiac glycosides for example *Urginea* (squill) and *Strophanthus* (West African arrow poison) belong to this group. Blood poisons affect the red cells or the haemoglobin or plasma, causing jaundice, anaemia, cyanosis, and petechiation of mucous membranes. Examples are *Ricinus* (castor oil), *Manihot* (cassava) and *Abrus* (jequirity).

Photosensitisation affects animals ingesting plants containing substances, which apparently after circulating in the blood stream and passing thus to the unpigmented cutaneous tissue are acted upon by sunlight in such a way as to cause damage to the skin. An example is *Lantana.*

Cyanogenetic glycosides which owe their toxicity to the production of hydrocyanic acid by enzymes. This action occurs with some well known forage plants under certain conditions of climate, for example during changeable weather after rain has produced rapid growth by wilting. Examples are Sudan grass (*Sorghum halepense*) couch grass (*Cynodon dactylon*) and giant star (*C. plectostachyus*).

**Some common poisonous plants and plant material**

1. *Lantana*; Various species are involved, the most common being *Lantana camara*, a shrub with coarse branched stems having small curved prickles, rough toothed leaves and flower heads of yellow, red and white tubular flowers. It grows in most tropical countries and is notorious for its ability to escape from gardens where it is frequently grown as an ornamental. It flourishes in grassland. It is not particularly palatable to livestock, but is apparently often ingested accidentally.

Animals affected show severe jaundice and photosensitisation generally in the form of severe dermatitis, especially on light coloured areas. If large quantities are consumed, death from haemorrhagic gastroenteritis may occur before indications of photosensitisation are seen.

2. *Ratti Seeds—Abrus precatorius*: This plant grows in Asia, Australia and South America. It is a leguminous climber with red and black seeds, which are highly toxic. The toxic principle, a toxalbumin called abrin, causes blood poisoning, the main indications being violent purging, high temperature, shivering, incoordination and paralysis. The red and black colour seeds of ratti are used in India by goldsmiths as a measure.

3. *Castor oil plant—Ricinus communis*: This is another blood poisoning plant, also called '*palma christi*'. It occurs in all tropical areas. It is a shrub up to 3 m high with large palmate three or five pointed leaves. The flowers are small and yellow. The seeds, which look very similar to engorged ticks with various mottled markings, are in fact eaten by some tribes in Africa, after soaking and boiling, but in the untreated state they are toxic. Castor oil is obtained by pressing the seeds, the remaining 'castor cake' being rich in the toxic principle, a toxalbumin called '*ricin*'. The cake sometimes gets mixed into animal feeds by accident.

Affected horses show dullness and incoordination of gait followed by profuse sweating, tetanic spasms and a 'tumultuous' heart, the beat being reported as 'strong enough to shake the body' by one observer. There is profuse watery diarrhoea with all animals. Cattle may die in convulsions. Pigs show vomiting and diarrhoea, incoordination, abdominal pain, and cyonosis of ears, flanks and hams. Poultry become dull and droopy, with ruffled feathers and greyish coloured wattles and combs.

4. *Lilies*—Family *Liliaceae*: Most of the lilies are poisonous; they are also very unpalatable but many grow in pasture land and may be eaten accidentally. Moreover the bulb or underground tuber is often more poisonous than the above ground portion, and rooting pigs are liable to poisoning by this means.

Symptoms vary according to the lily involved but usually the glycosides or alkaloids which are the poisonous principle act on the heart and nervous system. When small quantities are eaten convulsions may be seen; with larger quantities the cardiac syndrome occurs before the nervous symptoms have time to develop. Vomiting and diarrhoea are commonly seen; ani-

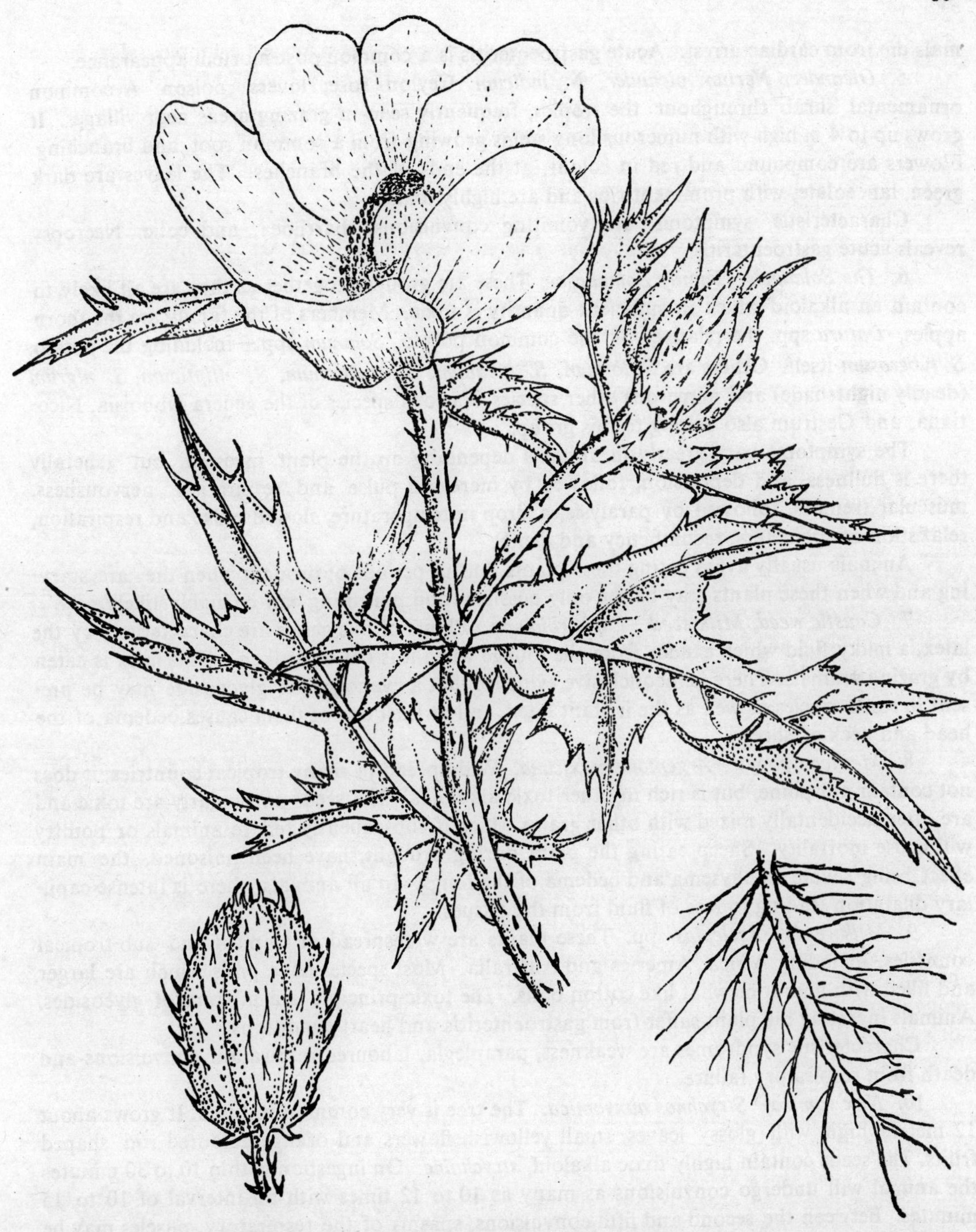

Fig. 3 *Argemone mexicana* Linn.

mals die from cardiac arrest. Acute gastroenteritis is a common post-mortem appearance.

5. *Oleander. Nerium oleander, N. indicum*: Ceylon rose; lovers' poison. A common ornamental shrub throughout the tropics, frequently seen in grazing areas near villages. It grows up to 4 m high with numerous long stems growing from a common root, and branching. Flowers are compound and red in colour, at the ends of the branches. The leaves are dark green, lanceolate, with prominent ribs and are highly toxic.

Characteristic symptoms are vomiting convulsions, diarrhoea, and colic. Necropsy reveals acute gastroenteritis.

6. *The Solanines—Family Solanaceae*: These are grouped together as they are all likely to contain an alkaloid which in sufficient quantity is toxic. Members of the family are the thorn apples, *Datura* spp. the relatives of the common potato, *Solanum* spp.—including the potato *S. tuberosum* itself. Others are *S. torvum, S. incanum, S. sturtianum, S. ellipticum, S. nigrum* (deadly nightshade) and numerous other species. Various species of the genera Duboisia, Nicotiana, and Cestrum also belong to this group.

The symptoms vary greatly in animals depending on the plant ingested, but generally there is dullness, and depression, followed by increased pulse and respiration, nervousness, muscular tremors, followed by paralysis, a drop in temperature, slowed pulse and respiration, relaxation of sphincters, recumbency and death.

Animals usually avoid eating these plants, but in periods of drought when they are starving and when these plants may be the only possible food poisoning can be highly likely.

7. *Caustic weed, Milk seed—Euphorbia* spp. Plants of this genus are characterised by the latex, a milky fluid which exudes from the foliage when it is cut or broken. This latex is eaten by grazing animals. There is inconclusive evidence that a cyanogenetic glyocoside may be present in some species as well as the irritant latex, and at least one of them causes oedema of the head and neck of sheep.

8. *Mexican poppy—Argemone mexicana.* Widespread in many tropical countries, it does not contain morphine, but is rich in other toxic alkaloids. The seeds particularly are toxic and are often accidentally mixed with other grains which if subsequently fed to animals or poultry will cause mortality. Sheep eating the plant during drought, have been poisoned, the main effect being severe emphysema and oedema of the lungs. In all animals, there is intense capillary dilatation leading to loss of fluid from the tissues.

9. *Milkweeds—Asclepias* spp. These plants are widespread in tropical and sub-tropical countries, including Africa, America and Australia. Most species have pods which are larger and filled with floss somewhat like cotton bolls. The toxic principle is a mixture of glycosides. Animals ingesting the plant suffer from gastroenteritis and heart conditions.

Characteristic syndromes are weakness, paraplegia, laboured respiration, convulsions and death from respiratory failure.

10. *Nux vomica—Strychnos nuxvomica.* The tree is very common in India. It grows about 12 meters high with glossy leaves, small yellowish flowers and orange coloured rod shaped fruits. The seeds contain highly toxic alkaloid, *strychnine*. On ingestion within 10 to 30 minutes the animal will undergo convulsions as many as 10 to 12 times with an interval of 10 to 15 minutes. Between the second and fifth convulsions, spasms of the respiratory muscles may be noted. During all such convulsions the animal dies.

The course of treatment includes the oral administration of activated charcoal followed by intravenous administration of a rapid action barbiturate.

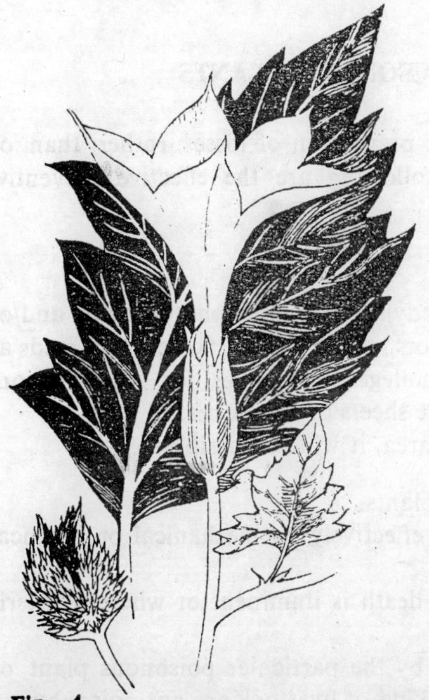

**Fig. 4**

Thorn apple (*Datura stramonium*), which is also known as Jamestown, or 'Jimson' weed. The flower may be white or purple. On the left is a fruit capsule. Well developed plants may be 5 ft high.

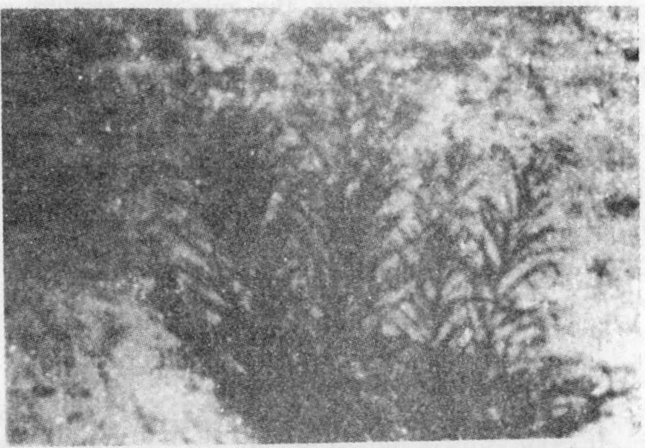

**Fig. 5** *Asclepias labriformis* (milkweed) Milkweeds grow in dry areas. A white gummy sap seeps from broken stems and leaves.

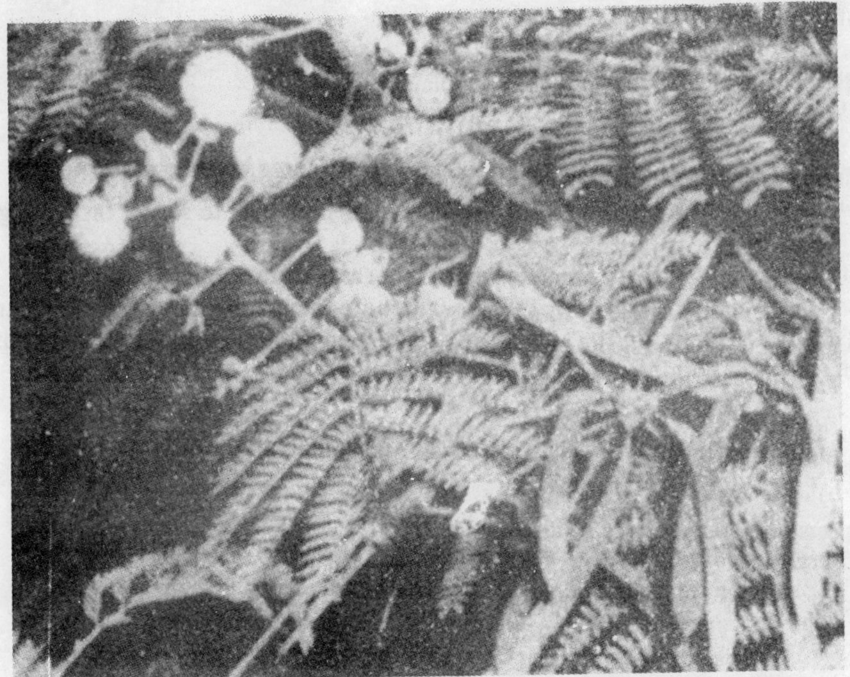

**Fig. 6** — *Leucaena leucocephala* (Lam.) de Wit.: foliage, flowers, pods.

## PREVENTING LOSSES FROM POISONOUS PLANTS

With poisonous plants, the emphasis should be on prevention of losses rather than on treatments, no matter how successful the latter. The following are the effective preventive measures:

1. **Know the poisonous plants common to the area**

This can ususally be accomplished through (a) studying drawings, photographs, and/or descriptions; (b) sending fresh whole plants including roots, stems, leaves, flowers and seeds as far as possible to the Botany department of nearby colleges/universities for identification. While carrying the plants, wrap the samples by polythene sheets or envelopes.

By identifying the poisonous plants common to the area, it will be possible—

(i) To avoid areas heavily infested with poisonous plants.
(ii) To control and eradicate the poisonous plants effectively by mechanical or chemical means.
(iii) To know what first aid to apply, specially when death is imminent or where a veterinarian is not readily available.
(iv) To graze with a class of livestock not harmed by the particular poisonous plant or plants. Many plants seriously poisonous to one kind of livestock are not poisonous to another.
(v) To shift the grazing season to a time when the plant is not dangerous. That is, some plants are poisonous at certain seasons of the year, but comparatively harmless at other seasons.

2. **Know the symptoms that generally indicate plant poisoning**

Such knowledge makes it possible to take early action.

3. **Provide supplemental feed during draughts, and after plants become mature**

Otherwise, hungry animals may eat poisonous plants in effort to satisfy their hunger.

4. **Avoid turning out very hungry animals where there are poisonous plants**

This caution especially applies to animals that have been recently shipped or transported from long distances. First feed the animals to satisfy their hunger or allow to graze sufficiently on an area free from poisonous plants.

5. **Remove animals from infested areas when plant poisoning strikes**

Hopefully, this will check further losses.

6. **Treat promptly, preferably by a veterinarian**

Rapid and proper treatment may save some animals.

## TREATMENT OF PLANT-POISONED ANIMALS

Unfortunately, plant-poisoned animals are not generally discovered in sufficient time to prevent loss. Thus, prevention is decidedly superior to treatment.

When trouble is encountered, the owner should immediately call a veterinarian. In the mean time, the animal should be (1) placed where adequate care and treatment can be given, (2) protected from excessive heat or cold, and (3) allowed to eat only feeds known to be safe.

The veterinarian may determine the kind of poisonous plant involved (1) by observing the symptoms, and/or (2) by finding out exactly what poisonous plant was eaten through looking over the grazing areas and/or hay and identifying leaves or other plant parts found in the animals digestive tract at the time of autopsy. Apart from searching for the poisonous plants, the veterinarian also suspect for other chemicals for poisoning reactions such as (1) *Arsenic*, which is used to control insects and weeds if consumed by any farm animal by mistake will cause restlessness, rapid breathing, muscular incoordination, blindness. Death in 3-4 hours to a week depending upon the amount of arsenic consumed. (2) *Ergot*, A parasitic fungus most commonly found in rye and in some hays. In ergot poisoning six different alkaloids are involved. Acute ergot poisoning caused by large quantities eaten at one time, may produce paralysis of the limbs and tongue, disturbance of the gastrointestinal tract and abortion. (3) *Lead poisoning*, It may get into the feed and water from contact with lead pipes, utensils or discharged storage batteries. Salivation, champing of the jaws, convulsions, coma and death. Sometimes faeces become very dark grey and be tinged with blood. Mature animals usually have diarrhoea and show incoordination specially in the hind limbs. (4) *Mercury*, It may get into the feed by consumption of seed grains treated with fungicides that contain mercury, for the control of fungus diseases of oats, wheat, barley and flax. It affects gastrointestine, kidney and nerve. Difficult to differentiate mercury from other poisons.

# 5

# CONCENTRATED FEEDS

## CONCENTRATES

**A concentrate is usually described as a feed or feed mixture which supplies primary nutrients (protein, carbohydrate and fat) at higher level but contains less than 18 percent crude fiber with low moisture. In general concentrates are feeds that are high in nitrogen-free-extract and TDN and low in crude fiber (CF).**

**On the basis of the crude protein (CP) content of air dry concentrates, these are classified as either *Energy rich Concentrates* when CP content is less than 18 percent or *Protein rich Concentrates* when the CP value exceeds 18 percent.**

### Energy rich Concentrates

**These are described under the following categories : (A) Grains and Seeds, (B) Mill by-products, (C) Molasses and (D) Roots.**

### A. Grains and Seeds

**Grains are seeds from cereal plants—members of the grass family, *Gramineae*. Cereal**

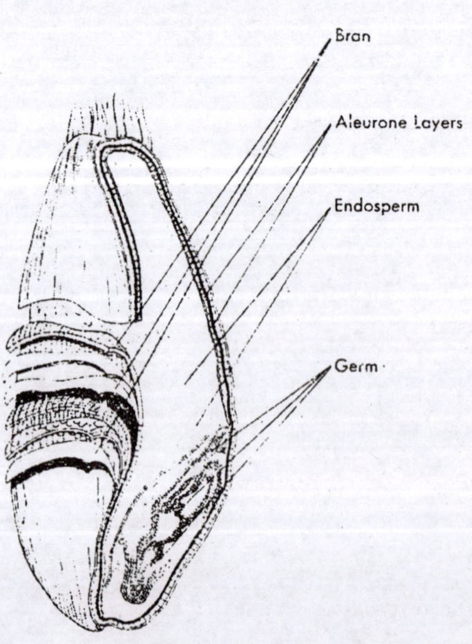


**Fig. 7** Whole wheat—cross section of grain.

*The Bran.* The brown outer layers. This part contains:

1. Bulk-forming carbohydrates.
2. B vitamins.
3. Minerals, especially iron.

*The Aleurone Layers.* The layers located right under the bran. They are rich in;

1. Proteins.
2. Phosphorus, a mineral.

*The Endosperm.* The white center. This consists mainly of:

1. Carbohydrates (starches and sugars).
2. Protein.

This is the part used in highly refined white flours. Less refined flours and refined cereals are made from this part and varying amounts of the aleurone layer.

*The Germ.* The heart of wheat (embryo). It is this part that sprouts and makes a new plant when put into the ground. It contains:

1. Thiamin (vitamin $B_1$). Wheat germ is one of the best food sources of thiamin.
2. Protein. This protein is of value comparable to the proteins of meat, milk, and cheese.
3. Other B vitamins.
4. Fat and the fat-soluble vitamin E.
5. Minerals, especially iron.
6. Carbohydrates.

grains are essentially carbohydrates, the main component of the dry matter being starch which is concentrated in the endosperm. All cereal crops are annuals (*Khariff*). By-products of harvested grains as chaff, stover, and straw are utilised as low quality forages for ruminant animals. Moreover, many of the grains are milled or processed in some manner, thereby creating additional by-products which can be fed to livestock with varying degrees of nutritive values. In our country except for poultry, swine and lactating dairy animals grains are not usually fed for livestock production because of high cost due to high demand by human beings.

The crude protein content of grains and seeds varies between 8-12% which again is deficient in lysine and methionine. The oil which is mostly present in the embryo is highest in oats

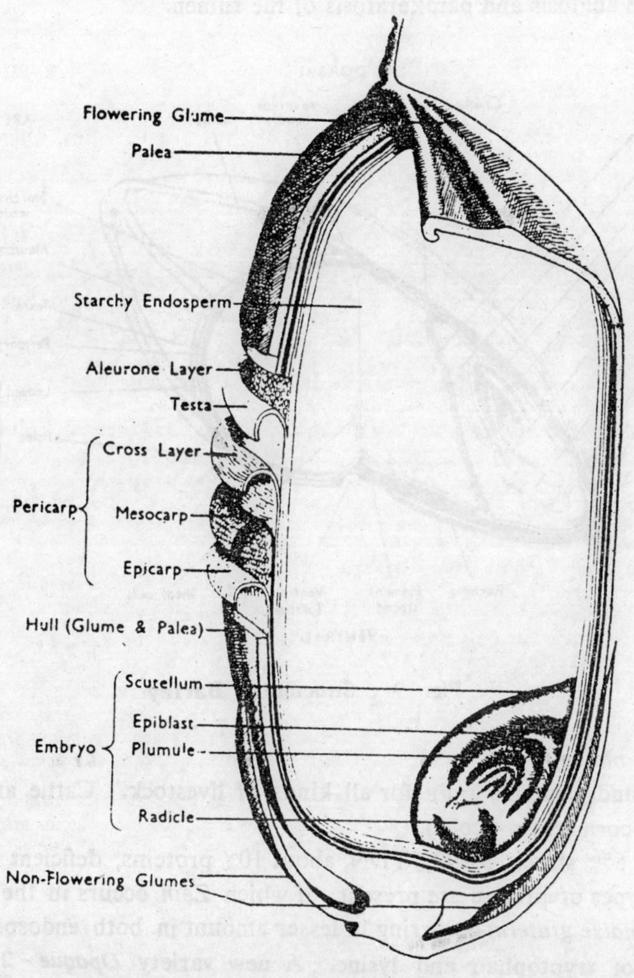


Fig. 8 Structure of Rice (*Oryza sativa*)

(4-6%) and lowest in wheat (1-2%). Cereal oils are unsaturated, the main fatty acids being linoleic and oleic, and because of this, cereals tend to become rancid quickly, and also produces soft body fat in non-ruminants. The crude fiber content of the hårvested grain is highest in oats and rice which contain a husk or hull formed from the inner and outer paleae (the inner and upper bract enclosing the grain) and is lowest in the nacked grains, wheat and maize. All cereals are deficient in vitamin D and in calcium (less than 0.15%) but are moderately rich in phosphorus (0.3 – 0.5%) and vitamin E.

Some problems are inharent in the use of grains ; among them (i) grains are most costly on a weight basis, (ii) must be processed before they can be fed (iii) extremely deficient in calcium and certain vitamins, (iv) in ruminants, high concentrate rations may cause digestive disturbances, such as acidosis and parakeratosis of the rumen.

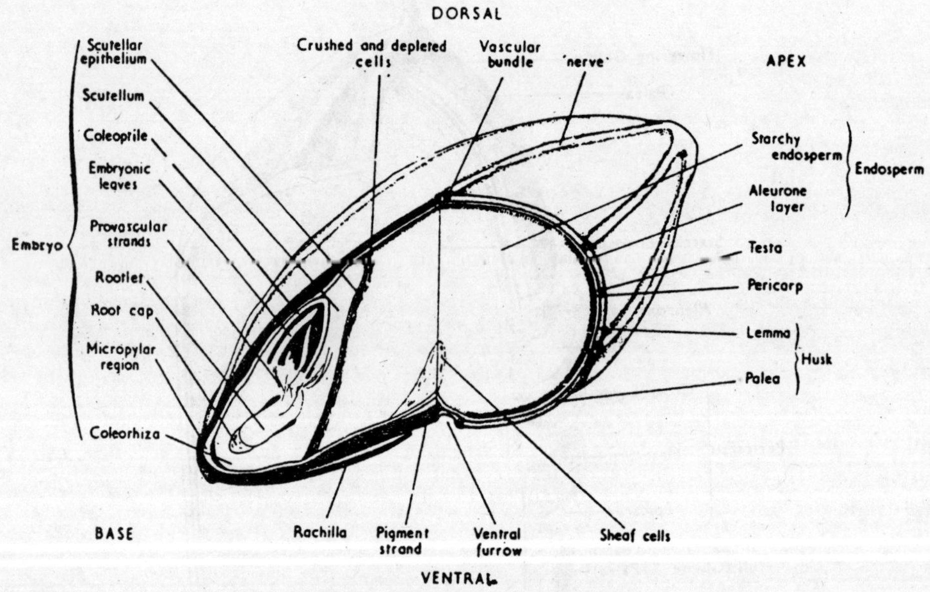


Fig. 9 Structure of Barley

**Maize or Corn (*Zea maize*)**

1. Most popular and palatable grain for all kinds of livestock. Cattle and sheep are often fed ground ear corn (grain + cobs).
2. Contains about 65% starch, 85-90% TDN, about 10% proteins, deficient in tryptophan and lysine. Two types of protein are present, of which *Zein* occurs in the endosperm. The other protein *maize glutelin* occurring in lesser amount in both endosperm and germ is a better source of tryptophan and lysine. A new variety *Opaque – 2* has been evolved having high lysine content. The other variety, *Floury – 2*, has both increased methionine and lysine.
3. Yellow maize is only grain with appreciable carotene.

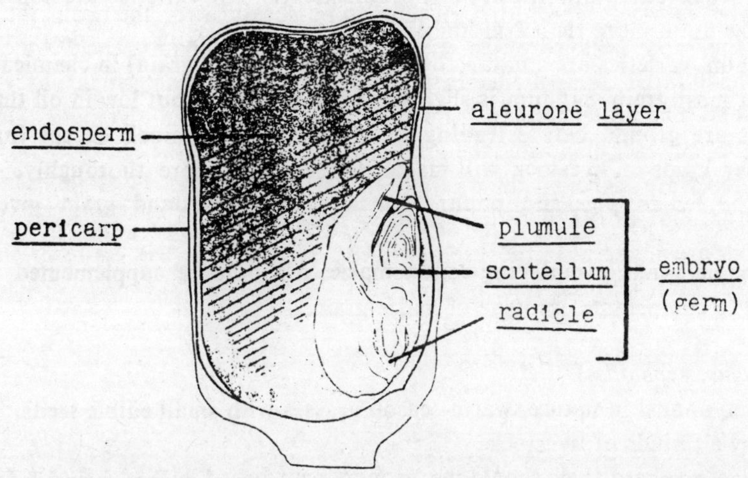


Fig. 10 Structure of Corn Kernal (Zea maize)

4. Extremely low in calcium and deficient in vitamin $B_{12}$ but fair in phosphorus content.

**Barley** (*Hordeum vulgare*)

1. A palatable but fibrous (7% CF) feed used along with or in place of oats in rations for horses, young growing stock and breeding animals including pigs.
2. Barley should always have the awns removed before they are offered to poultry or swine.
3. The grain may be used to replace up to one-half of the maize in rations for fattening animals without materially affecting their performance.
4. Barley is usually steam rolled (flaked), crimped or coarsely ground before feeding.
5. The crude protein varies from 8-12%.

**Oats** (*Avena sativa*)

1. Oats are higher than maize in CF (10-18% *vs* 2%) and accordingly lower in TDN (71% *vs* 87%).
2. Are usually rolled, crimped or ground for feeding.
3. Oats can be used for all farm animals. For pigs and poultry, ground oats have a considerably higher feeding value than whole oats. Hulled oats are more palatable but for cattle and older pigs it is usually not economical to hull the grain before feeding. The high fiber content limits the use of oats in pig and poultry and usually not more than 25% oats is included in rations for growing pigs, while ground oats of good quality are used upto 30% in rations for growing chickens and upto 50% in ration for layers.

**Sorghums** (*Sorghum vulgare*)

There are many varieties of sorghum but the composition of their grain does not differ enough to affect the feeding qualities to any great extent. All varieties are tall annual maize-like grasses grow up to more than 2 m high.

1. Most sorghum varieties are similar to shelled corn (maize grain) in chemical composition except that most grain sorghum is slightly higher in protein but low in oil than maize.
2. The grains are ground before feeding to all classes of livestock except for sheep which unlike other kinds of livestock will masticate the grains more thoroughly. Whole grains can also be fed to pigs and poultry but cracked or ground grain gives better feed efficiency.
3. When sorghum grain is replacing yellow maize, it should be supplemented with 3% dried green feed to compensate carotene of maize grain.

**Bajra** (*Pennesetum typhoides*)

This is a milet, annual in nature, warm-season grasses with small edible seeds.

1. Relished by all kinds of livestock.
2. As the seeds are hard they should be ground or crushed before being fed to cattle and hogs, while whole seeds or unthreshed bundles can be fed to poultry. Bajra grain which still has the hulls after threshing should be finely ground as otherwise the hard hulls will splinter into sharp fibers which can lead to internal irritation.
3. It resembles in feeding value to that of sorghum.
4. Crude protein ranges from 8-12%.
5. It is also rich in tannins.

**B. Mill by-products**

Quite often, the terms used to describe the various cereal by-products are confusing. Let us first discuss these terms along with some of the products commonly used as livestock feed.

1. *Bran*

Outer coarse coat (pericarp) of grain separated during processing e.g., rice bran, wheat bran, maize bran. Laxative in action. Rice bran must have 14% crude protein and less than 14% crude fiber. Protein content is about 8-18%.

2. *Flour*

Soft, finely ground meal of the grains. Consists primarily of gluten and starch from endosperm e.g., corn (maize) flour ; wheat flour ; sorghum flour etc. Sorghum grain flour must have less than 1% crude fiber while wheat flour may contain 1.5% CF. Flour contains about 16% protein.

3. *Germ*

It is the embryo of any seed. Wheat germ meal must contain at least 25% crude protein & 7% crude fat.

4. *Gluten*

When flour is washed to remove the starch, a tough, viscid, nitrogenous substance remains—this is known as gluten e.g., corn gluten, sorghum gluten. Gluten feed is generally not fed to non-ruminants due to bulkiness, poor quality protein and unpalatability. Protein content varies from 25-45% with CF from 4-8 percent.

5. *Grain screenings*

Small inperfect grains, weed seeds and other foreign material of value as a feed that is separated through the cleaning of grain with a screen. All cereal and legume grains are processed in this way and the by-products obtained therefrom. Protein percentage varies from 10-15% with 7-25% crude fiber. Quality varies according to percentage of weed seeds and other foreign material. Should be finely ground in order to kill noxious weed seeds.

6. *Groats*

Grain from which the hulls have been removed, e.g., oats ; rice etc. Improved feeding value over whole grain is achieved. Protein percentage varies from 8-16% while fiber is between 1-3 percent.

7. *Hulls*

Outer covering of grain. Generally not utilised as livestock feed.

8. *Malt sprouts*

The radicle of the embryo of the grain removed from sprouted and steamed whole grain e.g., barley, wheat, rye malt sprouts.

These are obtained as by-products of liquor processing. Barley sprouts used as livestock feed must contain 24% crude protein.

9. *Meal*

Feed ingredient of which the particle size is larger than flour, e.g., corn and oat meal contains protein between 9-18% and of C.F. between 3-10%. Oat meal must contain less than 4% fiber.

10. *Middlings*

A by-product of flour milling industry comprising several grades of granular particles consisting of varying proportions of bran, endosperm and germ, each of which contains different percentages of crude fiber.

The product is having protein percentage of 15-20% and that of CF is between 4-8 percent. Deficient in calcium, carotene and vitamin D.

11. *Polishings*

By-product of rice, consisting of a fine residue that accumulates during polishing of rice kernals after initial removal of hulls and bran. It contains about 10-15% protein, 12% fat, and CF between 3-4%. It is an excellent source of energy and vitamin B complex. Due to high fat content rancidity can pose problems.

It is an excellent feed ingredient for cattle, buffaloes, sheep, swine and poultry.

12. *Red dog*

By-product of milling spring wheat consists primarily of the aleurone with small amounts of flour and fine bran particles. Protein is about 17-20% with CF 2-4 percent.

13. *Shorts*

A by-product of flour milling consisting of a mixture of small particles of bran and germ, the aleurone layer and coarse fiber. It has protein percentage between 17-20% while that of CF is between 6-7 percent.

### C. Molasses

There are various types but all are concentrated water solutions of sugars, hemicelluloses, and minerals obtained usually as by-products of various manufacturing operations of the juices or extracts of selected plant materials.

**(a) Cane or blackstrap molasses**

This is the by-product of sugar industry from which a maximum of sugar has been extracted. About 25-50 kg of molasses results from production of 100 kg refined sugar. Cane molasses contains 3% protein, 10% ash comprising excellent source of minerals except phosphorous. It is also rich in niacin and pantothenic acid.

**(b) Beet molasses**

This product is obtained as a by-product of the manufacture of beet sugar. In making sugar from sugar beets, the beets are shredded into cossettes and the juice is extracted. In this process two valuable by-products are obtained, one is sugar beet and the other is beet pulp. Protein values are higher than cane molasses (6-10% *vs* 3%).

**(c) Citrus molasses**

When oranges or grape fruits are processed for juice or section, there remains 45-60 percent of their weight in the form of peel, rag and seeds as wastes. The liquid obtained from pressing these wastes contains between 10-15 percent soluble solids of which 50-70 percent is sugar. This material, which may amount for more than half of the total weight of the waste, can be concentrated into citrus molasses, which is normally a thick viscous liquid, dark brown to almost black in colour and has a bitter taste ! This bitter taste does not affect its usefulness in cattle feeding.

The molasses has got higher moisture content, 27-30%. On the other hand, protein content is about 14%.

**(d) Wood molasses**

By giving high pressure at high temperature in presence of dilute acid, wood is converted to molasses. After removal of the digester, the sugar solution is cooled to 138°C and neutralised with lime. The resulting sugar solution contains 5-6% simple sugars and is concentrated to syrup used for feeding. 1 ton of wood will yield about 0.5 tons of sugar.

In the manufacture of paper, fibre boards, pure cellulose from wood, there results an extract which contains soluble carbohydrates and minerals of the wood material which may also be processed into molasses for livestock feeding.

The molasses has a bitter taste but highly acceptable to cattle, particularly used for beef cattle.

**Use of Molasses in Livestock Feeding**

A. The different types of molasses are similar in feeding value and are available in both liquid and dehydrated forms.

B. Molasses is usually used in rations for cattle, buffaloes, sheep and horses

1. As a source of energy
2. As an appetisor
3. To reduce the dustiness of a ration
4. As a binder for pelleting
5. To stimulate rumen microbial activity
6. To supply unidentified factors
7. To provide a carrier for NPN and vitamins in liquid supplements
8. In the case of cane molasses, to provide trace minerals
9. In ruminant rations, molasses is restricted to the level of 10-15% of the ration. Excessive amounts of molasses (greater than 15%) will cause the feed to become messy as well as create digestive disturbance along with disrupted rumen microbial activity.
10. Poultry are rather sensitive to molasses as excess levels cause diarrhoea. Levels are restricted to from 2-5%.

**Molasses Brix**

The term is used in referring to the amount of sugar content of molasses.

Brix is determined by measuring the specific gravity of molasses, the value is then applied to a conversion table from which the level of sucrose (or degrees Brix) can be determined. As sugar content increases, degrees Brix likewise increases.

Since molasses also contains lipids, protein, inorganic salts, waxes, gums and other material, the Brix classification can often be misleading, because each of these components has an influence on the specific gravity of the solution. However, Brix value reflect the relative level of sugar present and so has over the years been used as a convenient basis for expressing molasses quality. Both cane and beet molasses have got generally 79.5 degree Brix.

**D. Roots and Tubers**

A root crop consists of the fleshy subterranean (underground) parts of a harvested plant, grown primarily for its sugar content and is normally not given to animals as such e.g., turnips, sugar beet, carrots, swedes, mangolds.

Tubers are short, thickend, fleshy stems usually formed underground such as e.g., potatoes, cassava, sweet potatoes etc. Tubers differ from the root crops in containing either starch or fructan instead of sucrose as the main storage carbohydrate. They have higher dry matter and lower crude fiber contents and consequently are more suitable than roots for feeding to pigs and poultry.

Root and tuber crops have traditionally been used more extensively as livestock feed in Europe. Due to large amounts of moisture (80 – 90%) in these feeds when fresh, only limited amounts are fed to high producing animals which requires considerable amount of dry matter.

The crude protein content is low and consists to a large extent of non-protein nitrogen. It is also poor in calcium and phosphorus content.

In India, the only tuber which is used in large scale as livestock feed is cassava tuber.

*Cassava* (*Manihot utilissma*) is a tropical shrubby perennial plant upto 4 m high with finger-like leaves. Cultivated for its edible roots. Cassava tubers are mainly used for the production of tapioca starch for human consumption although the tubers are often used as feed for cattle, pigs and poultry. Cassava root meal can be included upto 10% in rations for growing chicks and upto 20% in rations for layers with good results. For unknown reasons cassava meal seems to cause health problems when included in turkey rations. If the ration is supplemented with 0.15% methionine, the meal can constitute upto 50% of the poultry ration in substitution of maize. Cassava is usually limited to 20-30% of the pig ration.

The various other products obtained from cassava are discussed along with unconventional livestock feeds in India in this book.

*Toxicity*: Cassava roots must be processed very carefully by boiling or grating and squeezing, or grinding to a powder and then pressing as they contain two cyanogenetic glucosides (1) *Linamarin* and (2) *Lotaustralin*, which are acted upon enzymes readily liberate hydrocyanic acid (HCN). The peeled tubers contain much less HCN than unpeeled as most of the HCN is contained in the skin.

Varieties can be divided in two groups (1) Bitter varieties containing 0.02 – 0.03% HCN. Needs processing before used as feed ; (2) Sweet varieties, containing less than 0.01% HCN and can be used raw for feeding.

## Protein Rich Concentrates

Ingredients that contain more than 18 percent of their total weight in crude (total) protein are generally classified as protein feeds. Protein is one of the critical nutrients, particularly for young, rapidly growing animals and high producing adults, although it may be secondary to energy or other nutrients at times. In addition, protein supplements usually are more expensive than energy feeds, so optimal use is a must in any practical feeding system. The primary functions of protein feeds are to supply (1) those amino acids not provided in adequate amounts by the cereal portion of non-ruminant rations, or (2) nitrogen precursors of microbial protein in the case of ruminants.

Protein supplements may be further categorical according to source of origin as (1) plant proteins, (2) animal proteins (avian, mammalian and marine), (3) non-protein nitrogen, and (4) single-cell proteins.

### A. PLANT PROTEINS

#### Oilseed Meals

A number of oil bearing seeds are grown for vegetable oils for human food, and for paints and other industrial purposes. In processing these seeds, protein rich products of great value as livestock feeds are obtained. The by-products left after extraction of oil from oil seeds are used for feeding of all kinds of livestock. According to the method of processing use, cakes are classified into (i) *ghani*, (ii) expeller and (iii) solvent extracted. Of these, ghani-pressed cakes contain the maximum amount of ether extract while solvent extracted cakes contain trace of oil. Conversely the protein content is highest in solvent extracted cakes and lowest in the ghani cakes.

The seeds from which oil is to be removed is cracked and crushed to produce flakes (a small thin mass) of about 0.25 mm thick, which are cooked at temperature upto 104°C for 15-20 minutes. The temperature is then raised to about 110°115°C until the moisture content is reduced to about 3 percent. The material is then passed through a perforated horizontal cylinder in which revolves a screw of variable pitch. The residue is a by-product of oil extraction and usually has an oil content between 2.5 and 4.0 percent. The cylindrical presses used for extraction are called expellers and the method is referred to expeller process.

Oilseeds having oil content less than 35% is suitable for solvent extraction. If oilseeds having higher oil content is to be so treated, it first undergoes expeller syetem to lower the oil content to a suitable level. The first stage in solvent extraction is to crack the seeds and then crushed to produce flakes. After this the solvent like hexane is allowed to percolate through the flakes. The oil content of the cakes by this process is usually below 1% and it still contains some solvent, which is removed by heating.

Oilseed cakes (meals) are in general very good sources of protein, about 95% of the nitrogen is present as true protein. It usually has a digestibility of 75% to 95%. Certainly they are of poorer quality than the better animal proteins such as those of fish meal, meat meal, milk and eggs. Proteins of oilseed cakes have a low glutamic acid, cystine and methionine and a variable but usually low lysine content. The meals usually have a high phosphorus content, which tends to aggravate their generally low calcium content. They may provide good amount of B-vitamins but are poor sources of carotene and vitamin A.

The high temperatures and pressures of the expeller process may result in a lowering of digestibility and in denaturation of the protein, with a consequent lowering of its nutritive value. For ruminants such a denaturation may be beneficial owing to an associated reduction in degradability. The high temperatures and pressures also reduces most of the deleterious substances which might be present in oilcakes such as gossypol and goitrin Solvent extraction does not involve pressing or any high temperature and thus the protein value of the meal remains unaffected.

**Groundnut or Peanut Oil meal**

1. It is the most widely used high protein feed
2. The meal is usually made from the kernels (a grain or seed) ground to a meal with occasional use of whole pod when it is known as undecorticated groundnut meal
3. Its composition and feeding value vary considerably, depending on the quality of the nuts, the method of fat extraction used and the amount of hull included
4. It has about 45% protein and 10% oil in expeller variety
5. It is deficient in lysine, methionine and cystine
6. The cake is satisfactory as a source of protein for all kinds of livestock and poultry

7. Liable to contain a toxic factor—*Aflatoxin* a metabolite of the fungus *Aspergillus flavus* particularly in warm rainy season
8. The cake tends to become rancid specially in warm moist climate. It should not be stored longer than 6 weeks in the summer or 3-4 months in winter

**Linseed meal**

1. The meal is produced from flax seeds and the oil being a drying one used in paints, linoleum and soft soap
2. The cake is satisfactory for all classes of livestock except for poultry where if fed in more than 5%, it has a depressing effect on the growth. The toxicity can largely be eliminated by soaking the meal in water for 24 hours or by adding pyridoxin, one of the B vitamins
3. The meal has a very good reputation as a feed for ruminant animals due to high content (3-10%) of mucilage. The compound is capable of absorbing large amounts of water which results higher retention time in the rumen and give a better opportunity for microbial digestion. The lubricating character of the mucilage also protects the gut wall against mechanical damage and together with the bulkiness, regulates excretion, preventing constipation without causing looseness.
4. It is a satisfactory source of protein (about 35%) for almost all livestock. D.C.P. is about 30% with low T.D.N. (about 65%).
5. Immature linseed contains a small amount of a cyanogenetic glycoside, *linamarin*, and an associated enzyme, *linase*, which is capable of hydrolyzing it with the evaluation of hydrogen cyanide (HCN). Normal processing conditions however, destroy linase and most of the linamarin and the resultant meals are quite safe.

**Mustard Cake (*Sarson*)**

1. Widely used in many parts of India for cattle feeding.
2. Nutritive value is much less than that of groundnut cake. D.C.P. and T.D.N values are 27% and 74% respectively. It should preferably be mixed with other, more well-liked feeds. The deoiled type can be used for poultry upto 10 percent of the ration and for pigs the amount may go as high as 20 percent.
3. The calcium and phosphorus content are much higher, being about 0.6 percent and 1.0 percent.

**Cottonseed Cake**

1. It is an excellent high protein feed (about 40%) for ruminants but low in cystine, methionine and lysine.
2. The cake can also be used in pig and poultry rations if the free gossypol does not exceed 0.03 percent.
3. The free gossypol content of cottonseed meal decreased during processing. Expeller variety has about 200 to 500 mg free gossypol/kg, while deoiled type has about 1000 – 5,000 mg/kg.
4. In pig ration if the percentage of cottonseed meal exceeds 9%, it will kill the growing swine due to the presence of gossypol.

5. The cakes are available in two forms, (i) Whole pressed cottonseed cakes (i.e. undecorticated and (ii) Dehulled (decorticated, without hulls) cottonseed cakes containing less of fibers and more of proteins than the whole pressed type.
6. Today, glandless cottonseed, free of gossypol, is being grown in developed countries.
7. Gossypol is found bound to free amino groups in the seed protein or in a free form which can be extracted with solvents. The free gossypol is the toxic form. Gossypol toxicity can be prevented by addition of ferrous sulphate and other iron salts.

**Coconut meal (*Copra meal*)**

1. This is the by-product from the production of oil from the dried meats of coconuts and is available in many areas of the world
2. The crude protein content is low (20-26%), and poor in lysine and histidine
3. The oil content of coconut meal varies from 2.5 to 6.5%, the higher oilmeals tends to get rancidity and thus will cause diarrhoea. Hence low oil content type should be preferred
4. Due to poor quality of protein and high fiber, its use should be restricted in swine and poultry rations. If it is fed to monogastric, it should be supplemented with lysine and methionine
5. The lipid component of copra meal is very low in unsaturated fatty acids, hence the feeding of copra meal produces firm body fat in swine. Also dairymen use copra meal to produce a pleasant flavoured, rather hard (highly saturated) butterfat
6. The maximum safe amount for dairy cows seems to be 1.5 to 2 kg daily
7. The cake has the valuable property of absorbing upto half its own weight of molasses, and as a result is popular in compounding.

**Sesame meal (*Til cake*)**

1. Sesame oil meal is produced from what remains following the production of oil from sesame seed and the meal is extensively used for all classes of livestock including poultry
2. Protein content varies from 40-50% depending upon the variety used and the type of oil extraction. The protein is rich in arginine, leucine and methionine but is low in lysine
3. There are 3 varieties of til cakes, white, black and red grown at different seasons and in different parts of our country. Nutritive value is highest in white variety and lowest in the red variety cakes
4. Til cake is richest among all oil cakes in calcium content, being 2·3 percent but because of its high content of phytic acid, it appears to bind calcium so the amount of calcium in diets containing sesame meal should be increased
5. It has been used upto 15 percent, mixed with equal amount of groundnut cake in chicks ration.

**Soybean oil meal**

1. Soybean oil meal consists of fat extracted soybeans which have been ground to a meal and sometimes pelleted, has the highest nutritive value of any plant protein source, making up approximately, two thirds of the need of developed countries like U.S.A. and Canada

2. Most soybean oil meal is deoiled type
3. There are two grades : 44% and 49% protein
4. The protein contains all the indispensable amino acids, but the concentrations of cystine and methionine are sub-optimal
5. The cake is used for all kinds of livestock including poultry
6. As with most other oil seeds, soybeans have a number of toxic, stimulatory and inhibitory substances. For example, (i) a *goitrogenic material* is found in the meal and its long term use may result in goiter in some animal species, (ii) it also contains *antigens*, which are specially toxic to young pre-ruminants, (iii) a *trypsin inhibitor*, affects in digestibility of proteins specially in monogastric animals, (iv) a *haemogglutinin*, agglutinates red blood cells in rats, rabbits, and human beings but not in sheep and calves. Fortunately, these inhibitors and other factors like saponins are inactivated by proper heat treatment during processing
7. Soybeans also contain *genistein*, a plant estrogen, which may account, in some cases for part of its high growth inducing properties
8. Currently, there is interest in feeding whole soybeans after appropriate heat processing to inactivate the trypsin inhibitors (110°C for 3 minutes). This product is known in the feed trade as full fat soybean meal, it contains about 38% C.P., 18% fat and 5% C.F.

**Pulse Protein**

Pulses are the seeds of leguminous plants. They are used primarily for human consumption, but they may be fed to livestock at a time when it is available at a reasonable price. A listing of some important pulses used as livestock feed is given below :

Table 7

| *Name* | *Latin name* | *Crude Protein %* | *General comments* |
|---|---|---|---|
| **Beans—includes Kidney bean, Navy bean, Mung bean, Common bean, Dry bean,** | (*Phaseolus spp.*) | 20—28 | Many of these beans contain components which are harmful, if they are not processed properly. |
| **Cowpeas** | (*Vigna sinensis*) | 18—29 | Cooking or germinating seeds improves feeding value greatly. |
| **Field pea** | (*Pisum sativum*) | 22—29 | Highly palatable feed for all types of livestock. |
| **Soybeans** | (*Glycine max*) | 39—45 | Used primarily for production of vegetable oil and oilseed meal. Should be cooked before feeding to non-ruminants. |

All of the pulses contain components which possess antinutritional properties. Fortunately processing procedures, such as cooking, germination, and fermentation, can reduce risks of feeding pulses to livestock. Chemical factors present in various leguminous seeds are given in tabular form as below:

Table 8

| *Antinutritional factor* | *Mode of action* | *Comments* |
|---|---|---|
| Antivitamin factors | These factors render certain vitamins physiologically inactive | 1. Soybeans contain a rachitogenic factor & antivitamin $B_1$, factor.<br>2. Kidney beans contain an antagonist to Vit. E.<br>3. Cooking of the grains destroys these factors. |
| Cyanogens | Upon hydrolysis these compounds release HCN | 1. All legumes contain some cyanogens. |
| Lathyrogens | Nervous disorders and weakness in humans. | 1. Peas of the genus Lathyrus contain this.<br>2. Soaking & heat treatment will destroy the factor. |
| Phytohaemagglutins | Agglutinates RBC | 1. Found in all legumes.<br>2. Heat treatment is effective. |
| Protease inhibitors | Combine with trypsin forms inactive complex.<br>Causes hypertrophy of the pancreas. | 1. Found in all legumes seeds.<br>2. Heat treatment : autoclaving at 15 lb/sq in for 15-20 minutes.<br>3. Soaking followed by steaming.<br>4. Germination will cause detoxification. |
| Goitrogens | Enlargement of thyroid in rat and chicks. | 1. A number of feed ingredients including mustard oil cake, rapeseed cake, plant of the cabbage family e.g., cabbage, kale, turnips, cauliflower contain this factor.<br>2. Administration of iodides and heat treatment in some cases will help detoxification. |

**Brewer's Grains and Yeast.** In brewing, barely is first soaked and allowed to germinate. During this process, which is allowed for 6 days, there is development of a complete enzyme system for hydrolysing starch to dextrins and maltose. After this the grain or malt is dried, care being taken not to inactivate the enzymes. The sprouts are removed and are sold as *malt culms* or coombs. The dried malt is then passed through a process known as "mashing". The object of mashing is to promote enzymatic action on proteins and starch, the latter being converted to dextrins, maltose and small amount of other sugars. Water is sprayed onto this mixture and the temperature of the mash increased to about 65°C. After the mashing process is complete the sugary liquid or "wort" is drained off, leaving *brewer's grains* as residue and are sold wet or dried as food for farm animals. Dried grains contain 18 per cent crude protein and 15 per cent crude fiber.

The wort is then fermented in an open vassel with yeast for a number of days, during which time most of the sugars are converted to alcohol and $CO_2$. The yeast is filtered off, dried and sold as *brewer's yeast*. Dried yeast is rich protein concentrate containing about 42 percent crude protein. It is highly digestible and may be used for all classes of farm animals. It is a valuable source of B group of vitamins, is relatively rich in phosphorus but has a low calcium content.

## B. ANIMAL PROTEINS

Protein supplements derived from animal tissues are obtained primarily from inedible tissues, such as meat packing, from surplus milk by-products or from marine sources.

Many such compounds are difficult to process and store without some spoilage and nutrient loss. If not properly dried or heated to destroy disease producing bacteria they may be a source of infection. On the other hand, protein availability will be reduced and some nutrients are lost if the feed is heated excessively.

These materials are given to animals in much smaller amounts than the oilseed derivatives so far discussed, since they are not used primarily as sources of protein but to make good deficiencies of certain indispensable amino acids from which non-ruminant animals may suffer when they are fed on all vegetable protein diets. Due to high cost, large scale use of animal proteins become uneconomic.

### Meat meal or Meal scrap.

1. It is obtained from mammal tissue exclusive of hair, hoof, horn, stomach contents and hide trimmings by proper drying and grinding to which no otner matter nas been added, but which may have been preliminarily treated for the removal of fat and dried blood.
2. The product is normally used for swine and poultry.
3. Rich in crude protein (50-55%) and aṣh (21%) with high calcium about 8% and 4% phosphorus—but low in methionine and tryptophan.
4. Good sources of vitamins of B complex, specially riboflavin, choline, nicotinamide and $B_{12}$.

### Meat and Bone meal or scrap

1. The product is similar to meat scrap except it contains more bone, and consequently is higher in calcium and phosphorus and lower in protein, about 40%.
2. Used primarily in rations of swine and poultry.

### Blood meal

1. The meal is prepared by passing live steam through the blood until the temperature reaches 100°C. The treatment causes sterilization and the blood gets clotted. It is then

drained, pressed to express occluded serum, dried by steam heating and ground.

2. It has got high protein value, 80%, but the protein is lower in digestibility and quality than most other animal protein feeds. Poor in calcium and phosphorus content.
3. The meal is unpalatable and its use has resulted in reduced growth rates in poultry and it is not recommended for young stock. For older birds rates of inclusion are limited to about 1 to 2 percent.

**Feathermeal**

1. Poultry feathers are not digested by single stomach animals. However, when feathers are either processed under low pressure (130°C) for 2½ hours or under high pressure (145°C) for 30 minutes and dried at about 60°C and ground to pass a 20 mesh screen, the product is highly digestible.
2. The product is extremely high in protein, usually containing well over 80%.
3. Concentrates of dairy cattle may contain as high as 10%.
4. The product is used primarily in rations for swine and poultry.
5. Since feathermeal is deficient in several essential amino acids, it is customary to use the product upto 5% or less in the ration of poultry.

**Hatchery by-product meal**

1. Hatchery refuse consisting of infertile eggs, dead embryos, shells of hatched eggs and unsaleable chickens, can be made into a useful feed by cooking, drying and grinding.
2. Its high level of calcium (15-25%) limits its inclusion in ordinary diets but upto 5% level it can go with broiler type rations. It has got variable percentages of protein (45-55%) and fat (10-13%) depending upon the type of materials used.
3. It is used primarily in rations of swine and poultry.

**Fish meal**

1. Fish meal consists of fish or fish by-products which have been dried and ground into a meal.
2. There are several types depending on the type of fish and method of preparations.
3. Small scale production is made under rural condition in the following way : the fish or fish waste is ground or chopped, boiled for a short time and squeezed in cloth to get rid of water and excess oil. The residue is then dried in the sun.

   Another simple way is to dry fish materials directly under the sun on sea shore with an admixture of salt after removing alimentary tracts. The product is known as *'White fish meal'* and is made from fish which contains minimum fat.
4. The protein content of fish meal is usually around 60% with a digestibility of betwen 93 and 95 percent. Fish meal protein has a high content of lysine, methionine, and tryptophan. It has about 20 percent mineral content which is high in calcium (8%) and phosphorus (3.5%).
5. They are a good source of vitamins of the B complex, particularly choline, $B_{12}$ and riboflavin, and have an enhanced nutritional value because of their content of growth factors collectively known as *Animal Protein Factor* (APF).

6. For pigs and poultry fish meal has become a standard ingredient and is added to about 10% of the ration to make up for deficiencies of essential amino acids. Response from fish meal is greater than other protein sources in ruminants have been achieved but high cost makes it uneconomical.
7. Care must be taken to check the presence of urea, which is added as adulterant by uncrupulous businessmen with inferior type of fish meal to raise the nitrogen content.
8. Fish meals containing high levels of fat are considered to be of low quality. If they are incorporated into poultry feeds, they tend to impart a fishy flavour to poultry products. Also, problems of rancidity are greater in high-fat fish meals.

## C. NON-PROTEIN NITROGEN (NPN) FEEDSTUFFS

Feedstuffs which contain nitrogen in a form other than proteins or peptides are termed non-protein nitrogen (NPN). Organic NPN compounds would include ammonia, amides, amines, amino acids. Inorganic NPN compounds would include a variety of ammonium salts and ammoniated by-products. Of these urea dominates for feeding of animals with a functioning rumen as a substitute of protein feeds. Since microorganisms in the rumen of ruminant animals degrade dietary protein to synthesize microbial protein, similarly they degrade urea into ammonia which microbes utilise as the nitrogenous portion of the amino acids. For complete synthesis of amino acids, which will be utilized as polymer of proteins microbes needs carbon skeleton of amino acids. This will come from readily available carbohydrates. Thus for utilisation of urea or any other NPN compounds simultaneous ingestion of soluble carbohydrate is a must.

Crude protein is determined by multiplying the nitrogen content of a feed stuff by 6.25. Thus, urea having average of 45% nitrogen would have a crude protein equivalent of 281 percent.

Some of the non-protein nitrogenous sources being used successfully for ruminants are given below :

Table 9

**Some NPN sources for Ruminants**

| | Formula | $N_2$ (%) | Protein equivalent (%) |
|---|---|---|---|
| Ammonium acetate | $CH_3 CO_2 NH_4$ | 18 | 112 |
| Ammonium bicarbonate | $NH_4 H CO_3$ | 18 | 112 |
| Ammonium carbamate | $NH_2 CO_2 NH_4$ | 36 | 225 |
| Ammonium lactate | $CH_3 CHOH CO_2 NH_4$ | 13 | 81 |
| Biuret | $NH_2 CONHCO NH_2 H_2O$ | 35 | 219 |
| Urea | $(NH_2)_2 CO$ | 42-45 | 262-281 |
| Oilseed meals* | | 5.8-8.0 | 36-50 |

* Includes cottonseed, soybean, linseed, coconut and similar oil cakes.

## FACTORS AFFECTING UREA UTILISATION

The efficiency of urea utilisation is dependent on the composition of the ration and practical feed management.

**A. Composition of Ration**

1. Urea can effectively be used in high T. D. N. concentrates (greater than 75% T. D. N. on dry basis) when the crude protein level is below 12-13%. With low energy feeds (less than 60% feed on dry basis) urea may be fed when crude protein level is below 7%. Energy source must be provided by the feed so that carbon skeletons can be available for amination. Soluble carbohydrates are, by far, the most important precursors for these skeletons.
2. Minerals of the feed affect the utilisation of urea since many of them are constituents of key co-factors involved in the production of microbial protein. Additional sulphur in the form of sulphate must be provided as a precursor for the sulphur containing amino acids.
3. Feed additives have generally been shown to have little effect on urea utilisation.
4. Low levels of antibiotics generally added to feed are not sufficient to reduce urea utilisation significantly.

**B. Managerial Factors**

1. Animals started on a feed containing urea should be given an initial period of adaptation for the following purposes :
   - (*i*) The microbial population of the rumen is altered slowly, thus reducing the stress on the animal.
   - (*ii*) The rate of urea hydrolysis is reduced.
   - (*iii*) Microorganisms develop a greater ability to synthesise protein.
   - (*iv*) Animals have an opportunity to adjust to the taste of the feed.
2. Mixing of urea is an important factor in its ultimate conversion to protein. If it is improperly mixed, a serious threat of urea toxicity arises.
3. Frequency of feeding can affect the efficiency of urea utilisation. Urea should never be used in a feeding programme where feed containing urea is fed infrequently or fed two or three times weekly.

### METHODS OF FEEDING UREA

Urea can be provided by different methods and systems, with consideration given to the following factors : (*i*) protein needs of the animal as dictated by the type of production ; (*ii*) availability and cost of urea ; (*iii*) availability of energy sources and amount of plant protein being used (*iv*) cost of processing and mixing.

**1. Urea Mixed in Concentrates**

Most of the urea fed to growing and lactating dairy cattle and to finishing beef cattle is incorporated into the concentrate portion of the ration. Generally speaking, urea is not employed in amounts higher than 3% of the total concentrate feed or 1% of the total dry matter in the ration. The maximum safe limit is 136 grams of urea per animal over 260 kg body weight. Urea can be mixed in feed either as a powder or as an aqueous solution.

**2. Liquid Supplements**

This is a homogenous mixture of urea in the liquid molasses along with minerals and vitamins. Normally, it is prepared by completely dissolving 2.5 parts of urea in equal amount of water. The mixture is fortified with vitablend $AD_3$ at the rate of 25 grams per 100 kg of liquid feed. Common salt @ 1 part and mineral mixure @ 2 parts are sprinkled over 92 parts of sugarcane molasses. (2.5 parts urea + 2.5 parts water + 1 part salt + 2 parts mineral mixture + 92 parts molasses = 100). Special attention is required for the uniform mixing of urea solution in the liquid molasses. Undiluted urea-molasses liquid feed containing 65% or more dry matter can be safely stored for a long period. Animals started on a feed containing liquid molasses supplement should be given an initial period of 15 days as adaptation.

For initial 3 days feed your animals by substituting ¼th of the grain mixture with that of 500 ml of liquid feed after feeding concentrate part of the ration.

In the next 3 days substitute half of grain mixture with that of 1 kg. liquid feed.

From 7th day entire concentrate mixture may be substituted by offering liquid feed *ad libitum.* Animals should first be fed about 1 kg dry matter in the form of forage.

It is important to provide fresh drinking water at all times.

**3. Urea Mixed with Silage**

Another way of feeding urea to cattle—especially dairy cattle—is through the addition of urea to crops which are being ensiled. If chopped, whole maize plant is being ensiled at 35% to 40% dry matter, urea is then added at a level of 0.5% of wet material. This level should increase the crude protein level of the silage on a dry matter basis about 5 points.

**4. Urea Added to Dry Roughages**

Addition of urea molasses to straw has become popular for increasing nutritive value. A solution of 10 kg molasses and 2 kg urea in 10 kg of water is spread by a sprayer on straws in 100 kg lots and spread evenly under the sun over an area of 20 × 20 ft. The treated straws can form maintenance ration when supplied along with proper amount of 2% mineral and 1% salt and vitamin $AD_3$ mixture. About 8 kg of this enriched paddy straw per animal per day will supply sufficient nitrogen for the animals to synthesise the required amount of protein for maintenance.

**5. Urea in Salt Blocks**

Another simple way of supplying protein precursors to livestock on pasture is through the use of urea in salt licks or blocks. Numerous combinations of salt and urea are in use.

## GUIDELINES FOR USING UREA IN FEEDS

**A. Urea is best utilised in well-balanced, high energy rations.**

Urea is not well utilised in supplements to low quality roughages. The explanation is that the carbohydrates in grasses and hays appear to be so slowly available that the bacteria have difficulty in using the energy from roughages to make use of urea in preparing bacterial protein.

Other components of balanced feed include essential minerals and vitamins.

**B. Factors essential for optimum use of urea**

1. Mix the urea thoroughly.
2. Feed urea only to mature cattle, buffaloes, sheep and goat. Never feed it to monogastrics.
3. Provide a readily available energy source, such as molassess or grain.
4. Supply adequate and balanced levels of minerals.
5. Achieve a nitrogen-sulphur ratio not wider than 15 : 1.
6. Incorporate lucerne meal as a source of unidentified factors to stimulate the microbial synthesis of protein.
7. Include adequate salt for palatability ; 0.5% in complete rations and 3.5% in protein supplements.
8. Provide the proper level of vitamins particularly of vitamin A.
9. Accustom animals gradually to urea containing feeds (over a period of 5-7 days), feed at equal intervals.
10. Limit the intake of urea to recommended maximum level as below

*Sheep* : 1% of the dry matter in the ration (or one-third of the total nitrogen in the ration or 3% of the concentrate portion of the ration).

*Beef Cattle* : Urea may constitute upto one-third of the total protein of the ration. Total protein refers to the protein intake of the entire ration—including forage, grain and protein supplements.

*Dairy Cattle* : Lactating cows producing less than 20 litres of milk per day urea could constitute upto 2 percent of the concentrate mixture or upto 1 percent of the total hay. It was further recommended that no more than one-third of the protein requirements be met through the use of urea. For lactating cows yielding more than 20 litres of milk urea should not be fed. At this level of production, the microbes are unable to synthesise enough protein to meet the needs, thereby placing a premium on dietary protein which escapes ruminal fermentation (undegraded protein).

*Bulls, heifers and low-producing cows* :

1.5 to 2.0% of the concentrate mixture may be used as urea.

N.B.—Young calves and monogastric amimals should never be given urea.

**C. Toxicity**

When urea is fed at excessive levels, large amounts of ammonia are liberated in the rumen. Eventually, the pH of the ruminal fluid increases, thus facilitating the passage of ammonia across the rumen wall. If the levels of ammonia abosrbed are greater than the capacity of the liver to convert ammonia to urea, ammonia accumulates in the blood which when exceeds

1 mg/100 ml in cattle, the animal is under toxic condition. Such a condition may arise due to followings :

a. Poor mixing of urea in feed
b. Error in ration formulation
c. Inadequate period of adaptation
d. Low intake of water
e. Feeding of urea in conjunction with poor quality roughages
f. Rations that promote a high pH in ruminal fluid.

Symptoms of ammonia toxicity may include tetany, respiratory difficulty, bloat, excessive salivation, ataxia, convulsions and bellowing. If not promptly treated, death will follow in 30 minutes to 2.5 hours. The common treatment consists of drenching 20-40 litres of cold water which inihibits ureolytic activity of the rumen. Another way of curing is by drenching 4 litres of dilute acetic acids like vinegar along with cold water.

**Biuret**

The compound is produced by heating urea. The formula of the colourless crystalline compound is $NH_2CO.NH.CO.NH_2$. It contains 30 percent nitrogen, equivalent to 188 per cent of crude protein. A considerable period of adaptation is necessary for ruminants before the compound is effectively utilised. The compound is expensive and at present not produced in this country and moreover it is utilised by the ruminant less efficiently than urea. The advantage is that biuret is not toxic even at higher level.

**Poultry litters**

The composition varies, but on an average it contains about 5 percent nitrogen equivalent to about 31 per cent crude protein. The nitrogen is in the form of ureates. In concentrate diets, levels of inclusion may be as high as 35 per cent. The inclusion of poultry manure necessitates an allowance for extra energy and proper calcium and phosphorus inclusion.

**SINGLE-CELL PROTEIN (SCP)**

Single-cell protein (SCP) is obtained from single-cell organisms, such as yeast, bacteria and algae, that have been grown on specially prepared growth media. Production of this type of protein can be attained through the fermentation of petrolium derivatives or organic waste or through the culturing of photosynthetic organisms (algae) in special illuminated ponds. Microbes grow very fast. While 1,000 kg of livestock can produce a maximum of 1 kg protein in 24 hours, 1000 kg of yeast in the same period of time may increase to 5,000 kg of which half is edible protein

| | | *Time required to double the biomass* |
|---|---|---|
| Yeast and bacteria | ... | 20 min —2 hours |
| Algae | ... | 1 hour—2 days |
| Grass | ... | 1 to 2 weeks |
| Broilers | ... | 2 to 4 weeks |
| Growing pigs | ... | 4 to 6 weeks |
| Growing cattle | ... | 1 to 2 months |

1. *Bacteria*

Among various types of bacteria, *Methanomonas methanica* Sohngen has been more thoroughly investigated for single cell protein production. The bacteria are cultivated as a submerged culture in a water solution of mineral salts and as a source of nitrogen (ammonia or urea). Air and methane is bubbled through the liquid and stirred. A batch of culture is harvested after 3 days and yields about 12 grams wet bacteria per litre, the protein of which contains 70-80% balanced amino acids.

2. *Algae*

Three species of unicellular algae viz., *Chlorella vulgaris, Spirulina maxima* and *Scenedesmus obliquus* are of interest in the production of single cell protein. For growth algae requires $CO_2$, sunlight, nitrogen and minerals.

Algae meal, which is non-toxic is not fed to ruminants due to high cost but fed to pigs up to 10%. The protein value is comparable with that of meat and bone meal.

3. *Yeast and Mould*

While brewer's and distiller's yeast are usually *Saccharomyces cerevisiae*, yeast propagated specifically for animal feed is usually *Torulopsis utilis* (Torula yeast or fodder yeast) which grows very fast and can be grown on a variety of materials including press liquor obtained from paper industry and fruit wastes. Dried yeast is a valuable product and lacks the bitter taste of brewer's yeast.

Another type of yeast, *Candida lipolytica* are grown on paraffin fraction of petroleum oil. Yeasts grown on crude oil or paraffin extracted from oil are now commercially produced at several plants close to refineries. The fermentation takes place in an oil-water emulsion supplied with ammonia and mineral salts in presence of generous supply of oxygen.

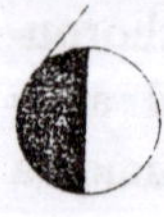

# USE OF UNCONVENTIONAL LIVESTOCK FEEDS IN INDIA

The importance of utilising the unconventional feeds to augment the existing resources of conventional livestock feed was recognised more than 30 years ago. India is facing a shortage of animal feeds and fodder which in terms of nutrients works out to 77 per cent D.C.P. and 62 per cent S.E. for feeding the livestock population. Moreover, this condition aggravates due to natural calamities like drought and flood. Recent studies indicated that quite a large number of agricultural by-products and industrial waste materials could be used for feeding livestock. Some of the unconventional livestock feeds used in India are described below:

*A. Vegetable protein sources*
*B. Animal protein sources*
*C. Energy sources*
*D. Other miscellaneous unconventional feeds*

## A. VEGETABLE PROTEIN SOURCES

### 1. Sunflower Meal

Indian work on Sunflower seed oil meal is limited but studies abroad indicate that decorticated sunflower seed oil meal in combination with other protein supplement is good for poultry. Recent move by the Government to locate areas for cultivation of sunflower seed is, therefore, welcomed by the animal nutritionists.

Good quality sunflower meal contains about 40–44 per cent high grade protein especially rich in methionine, but that made from unhulled seed has only 20 per cent protein. It has 2200-2610 Kcal of ME/kg. The expeller variety of sunflower meal or cake tends to produce soft pork and it also makes the butter soft if fed in large amounts in cows because of the character of the oil it contains. This can be used in cattle ration and safely included at 20 per cent level. Its effect is said to resemble linseed cake in dairy ration. Sunflower seed meal is a satisfactory substitute to groundnut cake in starter rations and it can replace 100 per cent GNC without any adverse effect on weight gain and feed efficiency. The meal can also be satisfactorily used in layers' ration. Studies indicated that it could be used in total replacement of groundnut cake without any adverse effect on egg production and egg weight.

### 2. Guar Meal

Guar is a drought resistant legume, and the meal, a by-product from the preparation of guar gum, is a potential source of protein. ME content is 2022-2274 Kcal of ME/kg. The two undesirable characteristics of guar meal are as below:

(i) Residual guar gum (Galactomannan)—may be as high as 18 per cent of the guar meal It is polysaccharide in nature which is neither digested nor absorbed.

(ii) Trypsin inhibitor.

It contains about 40-45 per cent protein and is a good source of amino acids. It is richer in lysine (2.55 per cent), cysteine (1.16 per cent) and glycine (4.61 per cent) than groundnut cake but comparable in respect of methionine content. It is also fairly rich in trace minerals.

Earlier experiments showed that it could be used in chick ration only up to 6.5 per cent; later it was found that up to 20 per cent guar meal could be used in chick ration if it is toasted and mixed with 0.1 per cent to 0.2 per cent cellulose enzyme. Substitution of 50 per cent guar meal (toasted) in replacement of groundnut cake was shown to give comparable performance in layers. High protein level in the mash is beneficial for its utilisation (i.e., depress the adverse effects of guar meal) in poultry.

Guar meal is not palatable to cattle since its inclusion at only 5 per cent level was refused at the initial phase by cows, although if accustomed, cows can accept rations containing as high as 15 per cent raw guar meal. Toasted guar meal, however, has not that acute palatability problem. Further, trypsin inhibitor factor is depressed. Higher levels of guar meal may cause diarrhoea, particularly in young calves. It is, therefore, always advisable to incorporate guar meal in the ration very gradually and once accustomed may be used as high as 10-15 per cent level in cows and 5-10 per cent level in calves.

### 3. Niger Cake

This is chiefly produced in Andhra Pradesh, Madhya Pradesh, Maharashtra and Orissa.

Niger cake compares well with other oil seed cakes in its chemical composition. It contains about 36 per cent crude protein and 5.98 per cent mineral matter, but contains about 14 to 18 per cent crude fibre. Its protein digestibility is about 80 per cent. It is richer in available lysine (400 mg/100 gms) and methionine content than groundnut cake. ME value varies between 2700-2800 Kcal/kg.

It is suggested that niger cake can completely replace groundnut cake on protein equivalent basis for the growing chicks and the two oil cakes have a complementary effect on chick growth with better efficiency in economics of feeding. The same is also true for layers, particularly if the fibre content of the ration is adjusted. Unfortunately not much studies have been made with the extracted variety of niger cake which is comparatively cheaper. Therefore, its suitability in feeding value will go a long way in economics of poultry rations.

The use of niger cake in cattle ration is also encouraging. Its inclusion in the cattle ration as high as 10 to 15 per cent is not uncommon. Unconfirmed reports suggest that higher levels may cause depression in total solids of milk. It is, therefore, advisable to include this along with other oil cakes like groundnut cake, copra cake, mustard cake, etc.

### 4. Karanja Cake

Pioneer work on the use of Karanja cake as livestock and poultry feed was first studied by L. Mandal and G.C. Banerjee at B.C. Krishi Viswavidyalaya in West Bengal, India.

Karanja seed grows widely in almost all the states of India especially in Mysore, Andhra Pradesh, Maharashtra, M.P., Bihar, West Bengal and Assam. So long the residual oil cakes are used as manure for paddy and rabi crops as a source of nitrogen.

Karanja cake is less palatable. It contains probably some polyphenolic compounds which have a deleterious effect on growth and production. The deoiled variety of karanja cake contains about 30 per cent crude protein and 60 per cent NFE, and only 6.66 per cent crude fibre. Its ME value as determined by Mandal and Banerjee as 2.20-2.34 Kcal/gm. Unfortunately, the expeller variety of karanja cake is not suitable for chickens since it results in high mortality, low feed consumption and poor growth whereas the deoiled variety is much better in growth response. It is moderately rich in all essential amino acids such as lysine (5.60 gm/100 gm of protein) methionine (0.99 gm/100 gm of protein).

Extracted karanja cake can be included in the ration replacing til cake to the extent of 30 per cent on protein equivalent basis in starters and growing chicks (18 week) with distinct economic advantage.

### 5. Neem Cake

The potential production of neem seed is estimated at 4.15 lakh tonnes. This can give 3.3 lakh tonnes of cake and 83,000 tonnes of oil every year provided this potentiality is fully utilized.

Neem cake contains 34 per cent protein while processed cake shows 48 per cent protein. Fibre content is only 4.4 per cent. The amino acid content in terms of lysine and methionine is also comparable to groundnut cake protein.

Neem cake as such is unpalatable and, therefore, it should be mixed with other well liked feed stuffs.

It is observed, however, that if this cake is introduced gradually then it can be included in the cattle ration about 15–20 per cent level. A few animals, however, may be reluctant to consume feeds at this level. 1 per cent inclusion, however, is a safe level.

Recent studies in poultry indicate that mixing of deoiled neem seed cake beyond 5 per cent level in replacement of groundnut cake causes high mortality in chicks. It is, however, of interest to note that Gupta et al. (1975) recommended use of processed neem seed meal at 20 per cent level in chicks and layers without any harmful effect.

### 6. Rubber Seed Cake

The total availability of rubber seed cake is about 1.5 lakh tonnes. The rubber pod contains three seeds which burst at maturity scattering its contents.

Rubber seed meal contains some cyanogenetic components. A good quality rubber seed cake contains about 30 per cent protein and 9-10 per cent ether extract. Fibre content of decorticated variety is, however, 5 per cent. D.C.P. content in cattle on fresh basis would be 18.6 per cent and T.D.N. 54 per cent, and for pigs 16.7 per cent D.C.P. and 78.8 per cent T.D.N. The material can successfully be used in the feed of cattle and pigs. It is suggested that rubber seed cake may be used at 10 per cent and 20 per cent level in concentrate mixture of pigs and calves without any deleterious effect on growth. It can be used in lactating cows at 20 per cent level in concentrate mixture. Rubber seed cake can also be used at a maximum level of 10 per cent in poultry ration without any adverse effect.

### 7. Sunnhemp Seed (*Crotolaria Juncea*)

The seed is grown throughout India but in most cases this is used as manure. In some parts, however, this is fed as fodder. After crushing this can be fed to cattle but feeding as such is not palatable. This can, however, be mixed with other palatable feed stuffs in a concentrate mixture and fed to cattle.

The nutritive value in terms of D.C.P. and T.D.N. is 30 per cent and 71 per cent respectively. Sunnhemp contains about 4.7 per cent lysine and 1.7 per cent methionine (on protein basis) and inclusion of this in chick ration at 80 per cent level resulted in improved growth rate.

### 8. Dhaincha Seed

This is a leguminous seed and is excellent in protein quality. It contains 30-33 per cent protein, and 8.32 per cent and 1.019 g/16 g N lysine and methionine respectively.

The seed cannot be used as such, as it contains deleterious factors like gum, trypsin inhibitor and tannin. Enzymic treatment as in the case of guar meal can improve the feeding value of this material. Recent studies indicated that deleterious factors can be removed by microbial fermentation. The growth rate of chicks fed on fermented dhaincha seed was almost similar to that of control. With the majority of seeds, the gum content and trypsin inhibitory activity increased while the tannin content decreased.

Fermentation by fungi decreases the gum content and trypsin inhibitory activity appreciably and increases the crude protein content of the seed.

Studies with dhaincha seed in cattle is limited. However, autoclaved dhaincha seed may be used in cattle in limited quantities.

### 9. Cassia Tora Seed

Available in plenty in Gujarat. Feeding this as part of the ration for milch cows has given encouraging results. Boiled cassia tora seeds up to the level of 15 per cent in the concentrate ration can safely be fed to milch cows. Cassia tora seeds (unboiled), however, can be incorporated up to the level of 10 per cent in concentrate mixture for cows without affecting milk yield and composition.

### 10. Kapok Seed Cake

It can be used as one of the components of cattle feed concentrate. D.C.P. and T.D.N. being 26 per cent and 69 per cent approximately.

### 11. Kidney Bean Chuni

Kidney bean chuni, a by-product from pulse, is a good source of cattle feed. It consists chiefly of broken kidney grains and kidney bean hulls. It contains 20.5 per cent crude protein, 7.8 per cent ether extract, 10.9 per cent crude fibre, 5.8 per cent NFE, 7 per cent ash, 0.52 per cent calcium and 0.34 per cent phosphorus. The D.C.P. and T.D.N. of the kidney bean chuni are 16.3 and 66.9 kg respectively per 100 kg dry matter. The much higher balance of nitrogen indicates that kidney bean chuni can be used as one of the protein supplements in the rations of young and milch animals.

### 12. Corn Gluten Meal

This feed consists chiefly of the dried residue from maize after the removal of the larger part of the starch and bran by the process employed in the wet milling manufacture of maize starch. Occasionally it may include maize oil meal. It contains protein from 50 to 60 per cent.

**13. Safflower Meal**

The meal is produced after removal of most of the hull and oil from safflower seed. In decorticated form it has about 40-45 per cent protein while the value goes down to about 18-20 if not decorticated. The 18-20 per cent protein safflower meals contains about 60 per cent hulls which limits its energy value and utilization in non-ruminants. Even the decorticated type contains about 14 per cent fibre. Safflower meal is low in lysine and methionine. It is always desirable that whenever safflower meal is fed to non-ruminants like pigs, it should be used in conjunction with other lysine rich protein concentrates.

## B. ANIMAL PROTEIN SOURCES

**1. Incubator Waste or Hatchery By-product Meal (HBPM)**

It is a mixture of egg shells, infertile and unhatched eggs which have been cooked, dried and powdered.

Broiler chicks when fed at levels of 3 or 6 per cent of the total ration with dried incubator waste proved a satisfactory substitute for meal or soyabean oil meal. Properly processed HBPM containing infertile eggs and eggs with dead embryos is found to replace 33 per cent fish neal and is a good supplement for increasing body weight of chicks.

**2. Liver Residue Meal**

This can profitably be used as animal protein supplement in place of fish meal. Liver residue can be favourably introduced in poultry rations at 10 per cent level or at 5 per cent level along with the same level of fish meal as an animal protein supplement. A good quality of liver residue meal should contain about 65 per cent protein, 5 per cent lysine, 1.2 per cent methionine and 1 per cent cystine apart from other amino acids.

**3. Frog Meal**

It is a leftover of the frog leg industry. It is suggested that it can replace fish meal twice by weight in poultry rations for growth as well as for egg production.

**4. Dried Poultry Manure**

So long poultry manure was considered as a fertiliser and was being exclusively used for that purpose. Droppings from poultry fed with high energy rations are likely to be rich in nitrogen and energy. Poultry droppings contain 60-90 per cent of urinary nitrogen as uric acid and 9-13 per cent as ammonium salts. The digestibility of nitrogen in pure droppings ranges from 70-85 per cent.

The composition varies, but on an average it contains about 5 per cent nitrogen, equivalent to about 31 per cent crude protein. Properly dried poultry manure can be used at 10-15 per cent level in chick and broiler rations with good results. If the fibre content is high, it is preferable to use the same at lower levels. The inclusion of poultry manure necessitates an allowance for extra energy and proper calcium and phosphorus inclusion.

Dried poultry manure can also be used in cattle ration with definite economic advantage. It is, however, not palatable and hence should be used with other palatable feed stuffs.

**5. Cow Dung Meal (Cow Manure)**

Attempt was made to replace cereals in poultry ration by dried cow-dung meal. It can be used at 10 per cent level satisfactorily in growing ration in replacement of maize. Sun dried sheep dung meal is recommended at 5 per cent level in starter mash. Sun dried manure is as effective as oven dried cow-dung manure. In layers 10 per cent inclusion of air on oven dried cow manure satisfactorily supported egg production, egg weight, body weight, hatchability and feed consumption.

**6. Shrimp Shell Powder (Prawn Waste)**

It is the waste product of shrimp processing industry. The crude protein content varies from 32 per cent to 43 per cent according to the source of supply. The soluble ash content is high. The calcium content is high (9.3 per cent) whereas the phosphorus is low (1.3 per cent). The salt content is only 3.7 per cent (chloride content expressed as sodium chloride). Depending on protein content, it is likely to replace fish meal at the maximum level of 5 per cent in broiler chickens.

**7. Crab Meal**

It is the well ground dried waste of the crab containing shell, viscera and part or all of the flesh. It usually contains 30 per cent protein (25 to 30 per cent) and 3 per cent salt, but must not contain less than 25 per cent crude protein and more than 7 per cent salt. It contains about 12 per cent fibre, 13 to 16 per cent calcium, 1.5 to 3.5 per cent phosphorus.

It can satisfactorily replace fish meal when the content and the ratio of calcium and phosphorus in the ration is adjusted.

**8. Poultry By-product Meal**

It is the ground product obtained after dry rendering or wet rendering process from parts of the carcass of slaughtered poultry, such as heads, feet, undeveloped eggs and intestines exclusive of feathers. It must not contain more than 16 per cent ash and not more than 4 per cent acid insoluble ash. It is an excellent source of protein (50–58 per cent) for chickens. It is also fairly rich in energy (2900 Kcal ME/kg), fat 10–13 per cent, calcium 3 per cent and phosphorus 2 per cent. It is fairly rich in minerals and provides unidentified growth factors. It can be used in broiler and layers rations. It is a good substitute of fish meal.

**9. Hydrolysed Poultry Feathers**

It is the product resulting from the treatment under pressure of clean, undecomposed feathers from slaughtered poultry. A minimum of 80 per cent of its crude protein must consist of "digestible protein". It is rich in protein (80-86 per cent), fairly rich in energy and is said to possess unidentified growth factor which is inorganic in nature. But the protein is severely deficient in methionine, lysine, histidine and tryptophan. This product, therefore, should be used judiciously with other protein supplements to balance the amino acid deficiencies. Feather meal can replace 2 per cent fish meal and 2 per cent dried whey in poultry ration satisfactorily.

### 10. Squilla Meal

It is obtained from the fisheries industries and appears to be one of the promising by-products. This product is very rich in protein (37.6 per cent). Calcium content is very high, about 10 per cent while comparatively it contains low phosphorus, being 2.0 per cent only.

### 11. Processed Fish Ensilage

Fish ensilage contains 31.18 per cent crude protein, 4.66 per cent ether extract, 10.63 per cent crude fibre, and 32.29 per cent total carbohydrates. The mineral contents namely Ca and P present are 3.20 and 1.97 per cent respectively. The nutritive value in terms of D.C.P., T.D.N. and S.E. work out to 19.41, 53.79 and 57.82 per cent respectively. The nitrogen balance is positive.

## C. ENERGY SOURCES

### 1. Sal Seed Meal

Sal seed meal or sal seed cake is a by-product obtained after the extraction of oil from sal seed for industrial use. The maximum potential yield of sal seed all over the country would be 56, 80, 000 tonnes. Sal seed is a good source of fat which can be used as substitute extender for cocoa, butter and soap industry. The meal left over is a good source of carbohydrate and contains fairly good amount of tannins. It is interesting to note that the extracted sal seed meal in addition to a small amount of oil, contains substantial amount of starch which can be a good source of energy and can be incorporated in animal feed.

Sal seed meal contains abount 8–9 per cent protein, 12–16 per cent oil and 2-3 per cent fibre. Sal seed is very rich in N.F.E. fraction (70–72 per cent) while meal contains about 85 per cent. It is rich in tannin content which varies from 8–12 per cent. Due to this large tannin content the energy present in the meal is not released for utilisation in the animals. Besides tannic acid, there might be certain other alkaloids or some other substances which might prove detrimental to growth and production.

Sal seed meal does not have D.C.P. Protein is not available to the animals. T.D.N. is about 55 per cent of maize. Its use as a source of T.D.N. should be limited to a maximum level of 20 per cent of concentrate mixture for maintenance and growth. However, ISI has recommended use of sal seed meal at 10 per cent level in cattle concentrate mixture after having taken all points into consideration from all aspects.

Further work on supplementation of sal seed meal on milk producing cows is still in progress. However, with the available information it shows that there is depression of milk yield without affecting its composition when sal seed meal is used at 20 per cent level of the concentrate mixture, while substitution of sal fruits up to 20 per cent in the ration is found to be most economical for milk production.

Sal seed and sal seed cake can be used in growing chick ration up to 5 per cent and in laying up to 10 per cent level. The use of greater percentage in chick shows growth depressing effect and in layers lower egg production. Further discolouration of yolk (greenish) is also evidenced.

Verma and Panda (1972) determined ME value of sal seed and sal seed meal which are found to be 2,718 and 2,653 Kcal/kg respectively when the oil content was 16.10 per cent and 8.58 per cent for sal seed and seed meal respectively. Sarkar and Banerjee, however, found 2,64 and 2.34 Kcal/gm when the oil content was 13.64 per cent and 1.31 per cent respectively for sal seed and sal seed cake.

D.C.P. was 1.52 per cent and T.D.N. 65.34 per cent with pigs at 10 months of age and D.C.P. 1.55 per cent and T.D.N. 58.96 per cent at 14 months of age.

Growth studies on pigs by replacing 50, 75 and 10 per cent ragi in the concentrate mixture by deoiled sal seed meal for 8 months indicated progressive decrease in growth rate with the increase in the percentage of deoiled sal seed meal in the concentrate mixture.

Research works are in progress to remove tannins from sal seed meal. Panda et al (1968) showed that washing sal seed cake overnight in cold water could remove 60 per cent tannic acid. Boiling for half an hour also had the same result. Patel et al. (1972) found that 65 per cent of tannins could be removed by decinormal caustic soda. Treatments with calcium hydroxide at 0, 1, 1.5 and 2.0 per cent level have been tried without any significant improvement. Passing of steam at 15 lbs pressure for 1 hour, however, eliminated tannic acid to the extent of about 70 per cent as found by Sarkar and Banerjee (1973) at Bidhan Chandra Krishi Viswavidyalaya. Studies with such processed sal seed meal have shown very encouraging results and much greater percentage could be used.

**2. Cassava (Tapioca) Root**

It is a very good source of energy and rich in carbohydrates. Tapioca roots contain a glucoside, linamarin, which when acted upon by an enzyme liberates HCN (0.03 per cent in the flesh). Varieties considered poisonous contain much higher HCN. It is low in protein (2 per cent) and rich in NFE (85 per cent). Reports from Philippines suggest the possibility of making cassava silage from chopped, freshly dug tubers.

In India, dried tapioca roots are sold in the name of tapioca chips, and the meal in the name of tapisoca flour. This can be used safely upto 10 per cent level in chick and broiler feeds. In laying, ration upto a maximum of 20 per cent can be included with supplementation of methionine (0.15 per cent) or when proper care is taken of protein quality due to replacement of cereals from the diet. In ruminants this may be used in higher percentage with economic advantage provided it is mixed with other palatable feed stuffs.

**3. Tapioca Starch Waste**

This is a by-product obtained during the manufacture of starch from tapioca roots. Like chips it is also low in protein and fat. It is, however, rich in fibre, about 10-12 per cent. This is mostly used in the ration for cattle and buffaloes. It has 2.00 per cent D.C.P. and 64 per cent T.D.N. on DM basis for ruminants. Tapioca waste can be used safely upto 30 per cent level of the concentrate mixture with a considerable economy for maintaining body-weight, milk yield and butterfat production. Tapioca waste can replace at least 50 per cent of maize as a source of energy for growing pigs without affecting the carcass characteristics.

**4. Tapioca Thippi**

During manufacture of sago, first the tapioca roots/tubers are deskinned and soaked in water. The tubers are then fed into the crusher adding equal amount of water for extraction of milk. The milk thus obtained is allowed to pass through a sieve to remove the fibrous material. This fibrous material in pulp form when dried is known as Tapioca thippi.

Studies in chicks at Bidhan Chandra Krishi Viswa Vidyalaya by Sarkar and Banerjee showed that it contained low protein and fat but fibre content was 8-9 per cent. This could replace unaffected. The use of 15 per cent level in a 4 week trial showed that the gain in body weight was lower by only 19.8 gm and FER higher by 0.28 when compared with the control ration. The ME as determined by Sarker and Banerjee was 2.45 Kcal/gm. Tapioca thippi can be used in cattle and pigs in the same way as tapioca starch waste.

### 5. Tapioca Milk Residue

Tapioca tubers after deskinning and soaking in water are fed into the crusher and milk is obtained. The heavier starch particles are collected for sago preparation while the lighter starch particles which cannot get together to form the crystals of sago are collected by a different process and dried. This dried second grade starch is known at tapioca milk residue.

It is a by-product of tapioca root in preparation of sago. It contains about 3-4 per cent protein, 3–4 per cent fat, about 2.5 per cent fibre and 66-70 per cent starch. This material can be used at a maximum level of 20 per cent in chick without any adverse effect on growth and feed efficiency. The ME value is 8.99 Kcal/gm. This can also be used in cattle in the same way as tapicca chips.

### 6. Palm Flour

Palm flour of good quality is obtained when the trees are cut before flowering, usually at the age of sixty years. The pith of the tree is cut into small pieces, dried and powdered to get the palm flour. This is low in protein and very rich in NFE. Fibre content is about 8.0 per cent. This can be used as a source of energy and can be used at a level of 17.5 per cent in chick ration in complete replacement of rice polish. In layer's ration it can be included upto 11.5 per cent replacing rice polish completely without affecting production and feed consumption.

Not much studies have been done with palm flour in cattle, but the proximate composition suggests that this can be used in cattle also for growth and production with economic advantage.

### 7. Tamarind Seed Powder

This is mostly used in textile and paper industry. It is a fairly good source of protein and energy. About 0 5 million tonnes of Tamarind seed are available in India. It is not very much palatable. It contains 15-20 per cent protein and about 5 per cent fibre. This has 13 per cent D.C.P. and 64 per cent T.D.N. It can be used in cattle as a component of concentrate mixture.

Tamarind seeds contain tannin, but overnight soaking in cold water reduces the tannin content. Increasing level of tamarind seed in chick ration from 10 to 30 per cent have revealed progressive decline in the growth ratio and FER.

### 8. Triticale

This is a cross between wheat and rye. This can be used favourably for egg and meat type growing chicks replacing maize to the extent of 50 per cent and 100 per cent respectively, in terms of weight gain and FER. In broiler chicks, triticale effected a better weight gain compared to that in laying strain. ME is 2043-3357 Kcal/kg for different varieties.

### 9. Mango Seed Kernel

This is a by-product available after extraction of juices from mangoes or from the leftovers of fruits after the same has been consumed by human beings. The availability of this by-product can be grossly estimated to be more than 1 million tonnes per year. It contains about 8 per cent protein. It is very rich in NFE, about 75-80 per cent, and low in fibre, about 3 per cent. This has 6 per cent D.C.P. and 70 per cent T.D.N.

This can be used as one of the ingredients of concentrate mixture upto a level of 40 per cent in bullocks, 20 per cent level for growing cattle and 10 per cent level to cows without affecting growth, milk production and fat content.

This can also be used in poultry in more or less the same way as sal seed meal. The tannin content, however, is less (5-7 per cent) than sal seed meal (9-13 per cent).

**10. Oak Kernel**

Large quantities of oak kernels are available from the oak forests. Experiments conducted so far have pointed out that this material cannot be used in either poultry or cattle ration exclusively or in appreciable amount. Oak kernels contain tannin which may be the factor for lower D.C.P. intake on higher level of oak kernel in cattle ration. Results suggest that oak kernel may be used to replace maize in cattle ration with only two thirds efficiency.

Oak kernel was used in starter's mash at levels 0, 2, 5 and 10 per cent replacing equal quantity of maize. There was no significant difference in growth rate of chicks on 0, 2 and 5 per cent levels of oak kernel. Higher (10 per cent) level showed adverse effect such as poor growth, low feed efficiency and low nitrogen retention probably due to high content of tannin.

## D. OTHER MISCELLANEOUS UNCONVENTIONAL FEED

**1. Sea Weed Meal**

India has got a long coastal belt—where different varieties of sea weeds are available in plenty. Experiments indicated that some weeds are rich in protein while others are in minerals. Experiments so far suggest that it could be used at 15 per cent level in concentrate mixture without any adverse effect on growth and milk production. The nutritive value of sea weed meals has a wide variation, being 9 to 19.93 per cent crude protein and 23 to 44.62 per cent total ash; while the extracted variety of sea weed meal contains more protein but less minerals. Observations revealed the possibilities of utilising sea weeds as cattle feed.

**2. Babul Pods** (*Acacia arabica*)

It grows extensively over a wide area in India. Babul was tried on growing calves and milch animals to effect economy in feed cost. It contains about 14 per cent protein, 10.0 per cent D.C.P. and 74 per cent T.D.N. It can be used as a component of concentrate mixture in cattle ration.

**3. Rain Tree Pods**

It is found in Bengal, Assam, Orissa, Bombay, Southern India as shed tree. The pods are palatable. As a component of concentrate mixture it can be included in the cattle ration. It contains about 8-9 per cent D.C.P. and 64 per cent T.D.N.

**4. Jack Fruit Waste**

The waste from ripe fruits is more palatable than the waste from raw fruits. It contains 7.9 per cent protein, 14.1 per cent crude fibre, 0 80 per cent calcium and 0.10 per cent phosphorus. This is a rich source of energy, being 65.3 per cent nitrogen-free extract. The nutritive value of jack fruit waste has been estimated in cattle, the T.D.N. value being 19.9 per cent. The material is very poor in D.C.P. content which is only 1.2 per cent.

**5. African Payal (*Salvinia molesta*, Mitchell)**

This material as such is not relished by cattle and hence affects the feed consumption. The chemical composition of african payal shows crude protein 13.2 per cent, nitrogen-free extract 46.9 per cent; while the crude fibre content is very high, being 23.5 per cent. Among the minerals, calcium is 1 35 per cent with low phosphorus content (0.35 per cent).

**6. Sugar Cane Bagasse**

Sugar cane bagasse is the fibrous residue of sugar cane stalks after the juice has been pressed out in factories and mainly two varieties are available viz., (1) fine bagasse and (2) coarse bagasse. The chemical compositions of fine and coarse varieties depend on the place of production being crude protein 2.23–4.74 per cent and 1.76–3.32 per cent, crude fibre 36.52–42.1 per cent and 40.49–43.22 per cent, ether extract 0.52–1.68 per cent and 0.53–0.87 per cent, ash 2.60–3.49 per cent and 1.81–2.58, per cent nitrogen-free extract 51.95–54.8 per cent 50.39–54.54 per cent. The in-vitro dry matter digestibility of various samples of sugar cane bagasse range between 19-40 per cent.

**7. Sugar Beet Pulp**

It is a by-product of cane sugar. Its chemical composition reveals that it cannot be considered as a concentrate because of its high ADF (44.37 per cent), CF (25.98 per cent) and lignin (6.69 per cent) contents. It might be better classified as a good roughage as its D.C.P. is 3.46 per cent and T.D.N. is 58.11 per cent.

**8. Sugar Cane Tops**

These include the growing point of the cane, a few of the upper nodes, and accompanying leaves. On large farms the tops and dry leaves are burned off before the cane is processed for disposal, while on small farms the tops are cut for livestock feed. The feeding value of fresh cane tops is not very promising: 0.5 to 1.5 per cent crude protein, 0.5 per cent fat, and 9 per cent crude fibre. The material serves as a roughage in conjunction with concentrates. In South Africa, cattle fed 6 to 7 kg of sugar cane tops per 100 kg live weight, along with groundnut meal, gained 0.6 kg per day.

Sugar cane tops as worked out by Bharatiya Agro-industries Foundation, can be very well ensiled alone as well as with 0.5 per cent urea. The silage is well acceptable to cross-bred cattle and contain 4.0 per cent D.C.P. and 47.8 per cent T.D.N.

**9. Petro-Protein**

It is high in protein which is about 52.37 per cent. It contains 11.7 per cent ether extract, 26.48 per cent NFE, 9.45 per cent ash, 0.41 per cent calcium and 1.81 per cent phosphorus. The digestibility co-efficients of crude protein and ether extract range from 89.9-99 per cent (average 95.7 per cent) and 58.6-69.0 per cent (average 61.9 per cent), respectively. Petro-protein is estimated to contain a significant amount of T.D.N. on dry matter basis. Calcium balance is found to be negative. It seems to be very good source of protein and phosphorus and thus it can replace groundnut.

**Table 10**

**Chemical composition and nutritive value of agro-industrial by-products as livestock feed**

| Common name | Botanical name | *Chemical composition (%) DM basis* | | | | | | | | *Incriminating factors* | *Remarks* |
|---|---|---|---|---|---|---|---|---|---|---|---|
| | | *CP* | *EE* | *CF* | *NFE* | *Ash* | *AIA* | *Ca* | *P* | | |
| 1 | 2 | 3 | 4 | 5 | 6 | 7 | 8 | 9 | 10 | 11 | 12 |
| | | A. *Crop residues & grasses* | | | | | | | | | |
| 1. Arali grass | *Leearsia hexandra* | 6.2 | 1.0 | 23.8 | 51.1 | 17.9 | — | 0.2 | 0.1 | — | — |
| 2. Aruna grass | *Setana palmofolia* | 14.0 | 3.8 | 19.1 | 52.8 | 10.2 | — | 1.2 | 0.6 | | |
| 3. Dal grass | *Hymonaehne amoleyicaulis* | 5.10 | 1.6 | 23.7 | 62.2 | 7.3 | — | 0.8 | 0 2 | — | — |
| 4. Dush grass | *Erianthus longisetus* | 5.3 | 0.6 | 28.0 | 58.9 | 7.2 | — | 0.3 | 0.2 | — | — |
| 5. Ganja refuse | *Cannabis sativa* | 17.2 | 12.3 | 9.1 | 41.4 | 20.0 | — | — | — | May be present | Poor |
| 6. Hadapoda | *Richardia brazalensis* | 11.4 | 2.8 | 21.0 | 51.2 | 13.6 | — | 0.4 | 0.2 | — | — |
| 7. Kharika grass | *Microstigium ciliatum* | 5.5 | 1.0 | 33.7 | 49.9 | 9.9 | — | 0.4 | 0.2 | — | — |
| 8. Kodo husk | *Paspalum scorbiculatum* | 4.1 | 1.5 | 32.1 | 46.8 | 15.5 | — | — | — | — | — |
| 9. Nal grass | *Arundo donax* | 8.9 | 2.4 | 15.5 | 58.2 | 15.0 | 0.2 | 0.1 | — | | — |
| 10. Popy husk | *Opium* spp. | 1.1 | — | 11.2 | 72.7 | 15.1 | — | — | — | May be present | — |
| 11. Paddy straw | *Oryza sativa* | 4.0 | 1.0 | 35.7 | 48.7 | 11.4 | — | — | — | Oxalates, selenium | — |
| 12. Paddy husk | *Oryza sativa* | 2.1 | 1.0 | 42.9 | 32.3 | 21.8 | — | — | — | Silica, oxalates | — |
| 13. Sugarcane tops | *Saccharum officinarum* | 8.1 | 1.9 | 31.7 | 53.2 | 6.1 | — | — | — | — | — |
| 14. Sorghum straw | *Sorghum vulgare* | | | | | | | | | | |
| a. Untreated | | 4.4 | 1.2 | 32.1 | 52.7 | 9.7 | — | — | — | — | |
| b. Steam treated | | 5.1 | 1.0 | 29.6 | 53.7 | 10.6 | — | — | — | — | Palatability & digestibility improves |
| 15. Ulu grass | *Temporates arundimacae* | 5.9 | 1.9 | 34.5 | 50 9 | 7.8 | — | 0.3 | 0.2 | — | — |
| 16. Wheat straw | *Triticum vulgare* | 3.1 | 1.1 | 35.7 | 48.7 | 11.4 | — | — | — | Major roughate | — |

| 1 | 2 | 3 | 4 | 5 | 6 | 7 | 8 | 9 | 10 | 11 | 12 |
|---|---|---|---|---|---|---|---|---|---|---|---|
| 17. Spent wheat straw | — | 4.7 | 1.3 | 31.3 | 45.5 | 17.2 | — | — | — | | — |
| 18. Urea treated straw | — | 6.4 | 0.9 | 52.5 | 28.5 | 11.6 | — | — | — | — | N. content digestibility & palatability improves |
| | | | | *B. Agro-Industrial By-Products* | | | | | | | |
| 1. Brewery waste | | 28.9 | 5.9 | 4.2 | 35.6 | 25.4 | 0 7 | 5.7 | 3.4 | — | Palatable |
| 2. Cocoa h· sk | *Theobroma cacao* | 14.2 | 7.5 | 14.2 | 55 3 | 8.5 | — | — | — | — | — |
| 3. Cornsteep concentrate | *Zea mays* | 51.5 | 2.7 | — | 22.0 | 23.8 | — | 0.3 | 4.2 | — | — |
| 4. Petro protein | *Candida tropi‹alis* | 53.3 | 2.4 | 0.9 | 35 0 | 8 4 | 0.2 | 0.5 | 1.4 | — | — |
| 5. Rale Seeds | *Sataria helica* | 9.9 | 2.2 | 8.6 | 75.8 | — | — | — | — | — | — |
| 6. Sugarcane bagasse | | | | | | | | | | | |
| Untreated | | 2.9 | 0.9 | 41.7 | 49.6 | 4.9 | — | — | — | — | Low intake |
| Stem treated | | 3.2 | 0.9 | 39.2 | 52.3 | 4.4 | — | — | — | — | Palatability improves |
| 7. Tapioca leaf meal | *Manihot utilissima* | 4.9 | 1.0 | 19.2 | 69.3 | 5.6 | — | 0.5 | 0.2 | HCN 17.6 mg/ 100 g | — |
| 8. Tapioca starch waste | | 4.9 | 1.0 | 19.2 | 69.3 | 5.6 | — | — | — | — | — |
| 9. Tea waste | *Camellia sineusis* | 28.7 | 3.6 | 18.3 | 43.8 | 5.6 | — | — | — | Tannins 1.9% Caffene 3.1% | — |
| 10. Decaffeinated tea waste | *Camellia assamica* | 18.1 | 0.3 | 12.6 | 60.0 | 9.1 | 1.2 | 5.6 | 0.8 | Tannins 0.8% | In growing new Hampshire piglets |

| | | | | | | | | | | | | |
|---|---|---|---|---|---|---|---|---|---|---|---|---|
| 11. | Tomato waste | *Lyeopersicon esculentum* | 23.9 | 17.7 | 21.2 | 27.7 | 9.5 | 5.0 | 0.4 | 0.4 | — | Palatable |
| 12. | Warai bran | *Panicum milliaeam* | 6.2 | 4.8 | 18.7 | 58.2 | 12.1 | — | — | — | — | — |
| | | | C. *Forest and Plantation By-Products* | | | | | | | | | |
| 1. | Ajar seed | *Lagerstroemia flosreginae* | 10.1 | 0.8 | 12.0 | 72.9 | 4.1 | 0.6 | 0.9 | 0.5 | — | — |
| 2. | Anatta seeds (spent) | *Bixa orellana* | 11.8 | 4.9 | 15.8 | 62.4 | 5.1 | — | — | — | Tannins 1.0% | — |
| 3. | Arjun fruit | *Termindia arjuna* | 9.8 | 1.7 | 47.7 | 34.0 | 6.8 | — | — | — | — | — |
| 4. | Ambadi cake | *Hibiscus cannabinus* | 23.4 | 6.3 | 19.7 | 40.2 | 10.4 | — | — | — | — | — |
| 5. | Babul seed chuni | *Acacia nilotica* | 16.6 | 6.0 | 12.3 | 60.7 | 4.4 | 0.1 | 0.9 | 0.3 | Tannins 2.7% | — |
| 6. | Banana rhyzome | *Musa sapientum* | 6.1 | 1.8 | 7.2 | 77.0 | 7.9 | — | — | — | Tannins 1.1% | — |
| 7. | Fallen bamboo leaves | *Bambusa vulgaris* | 18.3 | 2.7 | 25.7 | 36.2 | 17.1 | — | — | — | — | — |
| 8. | Cashew apple waste | *Anacordium occidentale* | 10.6 | 4.4 | 6.8 | 74.4 | 3.9 | — | — | — | — | — |
| 9. | Cashew bran | *A. occidentale* | 16.9 | 29.0 | 6.5 | 43.9 | 3.7 | — | 0.6 | 0.3 | — | — |
| 10. | Cocoa husk | *Theobroma cacao* | 7.8 | 2.3 | 35.1 | 47.6 | 7.2 | — | — | — | — | — |
| 11. | Coconut meal (deoiled) | *Cocos nucifera* | 27.2 | 1.2 | 8.9 | 55.2 | 7.5 | — | — | — | — | — |
| 12. | Coconut Pith | *Cocos nucifera* | 1.8 | 2.9 | 19.3 | 70.6 | 5.4 | — | 0.3 | 0.1 | — | — |
| 13. | Coconut oil residue | *C. nucifera* | 28.9 | 44.5 | 0.4 | 17.9 | 8.3 | 2.6 | 0.2 | 0.7 | — | — |
| 14. | Coffee husk | *Coffea arabica* | 7.7 | 2.5 | 26.5 | 57.9 | 5.4 | — | — | — | Tannins 2.8% | — |
| 15. | Damaged apple | *Malus sylvestris* | 12.0 | 2.8 | — | 78.5 | 3.2 | — | 0.2 | 0.1 | — | — |
| 16. | Dhupa cake | *Veteria indica* | 6.7 | 7.0 | 8.9 | 70.5 | 6.9 | 3.7 | 0.3 | 0.8 | — | — |
| 17. | Jack fruit waste | *Artocarpus heterophyllus* | 24.5 | 3.5 | 9.3 | 73.7 | 5.0 | 0.8 | 0.4 | 0.1 | — | — |
| 18. | Karanj cake (expeller) | *Pongamia glabra* | 27.2 | 9.0 | 4.9 | 55.6 | 3.2 | 0.8 | — | — | May be present | Unpalatable |
| 19. | Solvent extracted karanj cake | | 34.1 | 0.2 | 4.1 | 58.2 | 3.3 | 0.8 | — | — | May be present | Palatable |

| 1 | 2 | 3 | 4 | 5 | 6 | 7 | 8 | 9 | 10 | 11 | 12 |
|---|---|---|---|---|---|---|---|---|---|---|---|
| 20. Kasai leaves | *Bridelia retuja* | 18.1 | 2.8 | 22.2 | 49.1 | 7.9 | — | — | — | — | — |
| 21. Kokam cake | *Garninia indica* | 16.6 | 1.6 | 4.4 | 70.9 | 7.4 | — | — | — | — | Palatable |
| 22. Kosum cake | *Scheiohera pleasa* | 19.1 | 12.0 | 9.9 | 53.8 | 5.3 | 3.1 | — | — | — | — |
| 23. Kuvadia seeds Chakunda | *Cassia tora* | 18.6 | 7.9 | 9.9 | 54.2 | 9.4 | 2.6 | 0.9 | 0 6 | Tannin 0.8% chrysophanic acid (0.08%) | — |
| 24. Madhu leaves (fallen) | *Madhuca indica* | 12.7 | 2.8 | 16.7 | 01.5 | 6.4 | — | — | — | — | — |
| 25. Madhu seed cake | *Madhuca indica* | 20.4 | 2.7 | 13.3 | 57.2 | 6.5 | 0.7 | 0.4 | 0.2 | Mawrin tannin 1.5% Saponin 21.4% Sapogenol 8.4% | Palatable with other feeds |
| 26. Mango seed kernels | *Mangifera indica* | 6.7 | 12.8 | 0.1 | 76.8 | 3.6 | 1.3 | 0.3 | 0.3 | Tannin 5.4% | Palatable |
| 27. Mango leaves | *Mangifera indica* | 8.9 | 4.1 | 24.0 | 55.4 | 6.7 | — | — | — | — | — |
| 28. Nahar seed | *Mesua ferrea* | 12.8 | 25.3 | 7.1 | 50.0 | 4.8 | — | 2.2 | 1.0 | — | — |
| 29. Neem seed cake | *Azadirachta indica* | 13.3 | 19.9 | 5.5 | 51.2 | 10.1 | — | 1.6 | 0.3 | Tannin 1.5% bitter principles | Poor palatability |
| 30. Niger seed cake | *Guizotia abyssinica* | 33.2 | 5.7 | 13.6 | 38.0 | 9.5 | 3.4 | — | — | — | Palatable |
| 31. Palas seeds | *Butea manosperma* | 27.7 | 18.9 | 5.9 | 37.8 | 7.8 | — | — | — | May present | Poor palatability |
| 32. Palm male flower (Spadix) | *Bonassus flabellifer* | 10.4 | 1.9 | 13.9 | 67.8 | 6.0 | 0.5 | 3.3 | 0.3 | Tannins 8.7% | Palatable with other fodders |
| 33. Pilludi cake | *Salvadora persica* | 23.9 | 0.9 | 6.0 | 49.3 | 20.0 | 3.0 | 3.8 | 0.6 | Oxalate 4% | Not palatable |
| 34. Pine apple bran | *Ananas sativus* | 4.3 | 2.0 | 16.5 | 72.6 | 4.6 | — | 0.4 | 0.2 | — | — |

| | | | | | | | | | | | |
|---|---|---|---|---|---|---|---|---|---|---|---|
| 35. | Rain tree fruit meal | *Enterolobium saman* | 15.5 | 1.8 | 13.5 | 65.5 | 3.7 | — | — | — | — | — |
| 36. | Rubber seed cake | *Ficus elastica* | 35.1 | 12.5 | 7.1 | 34.8 | 10.5 | 0.8 | 1.0 | 0.8 | HCn-9 mg/ 100 g | Palatable with other feeds |
| 37. | Sal seed cake | *Shorea robusta* | 8.6 | 2.5 | 1.3 | 84.4 | 3.1 | 0.8 | 0.2 | 0.2 | Tannins 8.2% | Palatable with other feeds |
| 38. | Silk cotton seed cake | *Bombax malabaricum* | 24.7 | 10.0 | 16.9 | 40.6 | 7.8 | — | 1.1 | 0.9 | — | — |
| 39. | Tamarind leaves | *Tamarindus indica* | 12.6 | 4.4 | 20.9 | 53.6 | 8.6 | — | — | — | — | — |
| 40. | Tamarind seed | *Tamarindus indica* | 19.8 | 4.7 | 2.1 | 70.3 | 3.1 | — | — | — | — | — |
| 41. | Teak leaves (Fallen) | *Tictona grindis* | 7.0 | 2.6 | 17.4 | 55.9 | 17.1 | — | — | — | May present | Poor palatability |
| 42. | Teak seed | *Tictona grindis* | 7.4 | 1.9 | 58.9 | 28.1 | 3.8 | — | — | — | May present | |
| 43. | Tender leaves cutting | *Dispinos melaxylon* | 10.1 | 1.6 | 23.5 | 53.8 | 11.1 | — | — | — | ,, | |
| 44. | Tumba cake | *Citrullus colocynthis* | 16.0 | 0.4 | 46.5 | 29.2 | 7.9 | — | — | — | — | |
| 45. | Vilayati babul | *Prosopsis juliflora* | 12.5 | 3.6 | 25.6 | 53.3 | 5.1 | 0.3 | 0.4 | 0.2 | Tannins 1.5% | Palatable |
| | | | D. *Aquatic and Marine By-Products* | | | | | | | | | |
| 1. | Crabwaste | | 29.7 | 2.5 | 16.1 | 0.5 | 51.2 | 0.5 | 17.1 | 1.4 | — | — |
| 2. | Fish protein concentrate | | 67.3 | 1.0 | — | 19.5 | 11.4 | 1.0 | 3.9 | 1.6 | — | — |
| 3. | Fish silage | | 48.4 | 11.5 | — | 26.5 | 13.6 | — | 5.0 | 2.1 | — | — |
| 4. | Frog meal | | 66.8 | 4.8 | 2.3 | 2.6 | 23.5 | — | 11.8 | 5.4 | — | — |
| 5. | Prawn waste | | 32.1 | 5.6 | 6.0 | 15.4 | 40.9 | 17.4 | 9.3 | 1.3 | — | — |
| 6. | Sea weed | *Sargassum* sp. | 9.5 | 3.8 | 8.1 | 59.5 | 19.4 | 2.5 | 4.1 | — | — | — |
| 7. | Squille meal | | 37.6 | 3.01 | 1.9 | 9.1 | 38.4 | 4.1 | 10.0 | 2.0 | — | — |
| 8. | Water hyacinth | *Eichhornia crassipes* | | | | | | | | | | |
| | a) Raw | | 11.4 | 1.4 | 19.9 | 52.4 | 15.1 | — | 1.6 | 0.6 | Oxalates 3.0% | — |
| | b) Extracted | | 9.0 | 1.0 | 20.1 | 62.0 | 7.9 | — | 1.3 | 0.4 | ,, | — |

| 1 | 2 | 3 | 4 | 5 | 6 | 7 | 8 | 9 | 10 | 11 | 12 |
|---|---|---|---|---|---|---|---|---|---|---|---|
| 9. African payal | *Salvinia molesta* | 13.2 | 3.7 | 23.5 | 46.9 | 12.7 | — | — | — | — | — |
| | | E. *Animal Organic Wastes* | | | | | | | | | |
| 1. Cattle dung | | 8-18 | 1-3 | 23-52 | 14-48 | 3-21 | — | 0-9-5.3 | 1.6-4.5 | — | Composition varies with type of diet |
| 2. Cattle manure solids | | 6-7 | — | — | — | 10-13 | — | — | — | — | Liquid solid separated |
| 3. Poultry litter | | 21-30 | — | 17-20 | 30-35 | 15-25 | — | 2.1 | 1.8 | — | Varies with litter type |
| 4. Dehydrated poultry excreta | | 30-40 | 2-3 | 13-15 | 29-28 | 21-28 | — | 6.9 | 1.6-2.5 | — | Composition varies with type of birds/age etc. |
| 5. Swine excreta | | 19-24 | 4-6 | 15-20 | 30-40 | 18-22 | — | 3.2 | 2.5 | — | Composition varies with the diet, age etc. |
| 6. Digested dung slurry | | 14.4 | 1.2 | 22.5 | 32.0 | 29.1 | — | 1.5 | 1.0 | — | — |

*Source* : Data compiled by Dr. M. L. Punj, Project Coordinator, AICRP—Agricultural By-Products and published in *Dairy Guide*, Volume 8, No. 6, 1986.

# 7

# IDENTIFYING FEEDS FROM THEIR COMPOSITION

**Students of feeds and feeding very often talk about the proximate composition and nutritive value of innumerable feed stuffs. This might seem initially to be due to extra-ordinary callibre. But actually they relate individual feeds to a certain general feed group on the basis of distinguishing chemical composition characters.**

**It should be realised that in many instances there is considerable overlapping of different feed groups with respect to their content of the various nutritive fractions. Even so, information such as is presented in Table ? will surely guide a student to identify feeds from their composition.**

**The first criterion of putting the feeds in two categories on is the basis of their respective moisture content, (1) Air-dry and (2) High moisture feed.**

**I. If a feed contains over 80% dry matter (DM), it should be regarded as an air-dry feed, e.g.,**

| | |
|---|---|
| **Mineral products** | **Energy rich concentrates** |
| **Hays** | **Protein rich concentrates** |
| **Straws** | **(both plant and animal** |
| **Other dry roughages** | **origin)** |

**II. On the otherhand, if a feed contains less than 80% DM, it should be regarded as a high moisture feed e.g.,**

| | |
|---|---|
| **High moisture grains** | **Fresh forages** |
| **Molasseses** | **Wet by-products** |
| **Haylages** | **Root crops** |
| **Silages** | **Fresh whole or skimmed milk.** |

**I. Air-dry roughages vs. Air-dry concentrates**

**1. An air-dry non-mineral feed may be grouped either as roughages or as concentrates based on the crude fiber and/or TDN content. Generally all air-dry roughages will contain over 18% CF and less than 60% TDN. On the other hand air-dry concentrates will usually contain less than 18% CF and over 60% TDN.**

**2. Air-dry roughages may further be divided on the basis of their composition as (i) Legume hays, (ii) Non-legume hays and (iii) Low-quality air-dry forages.**

**The hays are characterised by having CF from 18-34%, TDN from 40-60% and a significant amount of carotene whereas the low-quality dry roughages are higher in fiber and lower in**

TDN with little or no carotene and a protein value under 6.0% except for groundnut hulls which is about 6.6%.

The legume hays contain over 10.5% CP and over 0.9% calcium while non-legume hay have values for CP and calcium less than the former.

**Energy rich concentrates vs. Protein rich concentrates**

Air-dry concentrates having more than 18% CP are classed as protein rich concentrates and those with less than 18% CP as energy feeds.

The protein rich concentrates may be either of animal or plant origin. When the amount of protein content, is above 47% then it is of animal origin and if it is less than 47% then it is of plant origin. The latter may be either deoiled meals which will run under 1.0% EE or expeller type where the ether extract will usually be more than 4.0%

**II. High Moisture Feeds**

**A. High moisture grains**

Among high moisture feeds, if the composition of a feed shows that it contains DM between 60-80%, the feed in that case may be either high moisture grain or molasses. Protein and crude fiber values in this case will help to identify the feed. High moisture grains will have more than 7% CP and some fibers but molasses has got less than (3% cane 6% beet) 7% CP and no CF.

In recent years in developed countries like U.S.A., Canada a considerable quantity of some grains mostly maize (corn) and Jowar (sorghum) are harvested when the moisture content varies between 22-40% and it is commonly referred to high moisture grains—not that it is extremely high in moisture content, but that it is simply somewhat higher than that normally harvested for air-dry preservation.

High moisture grains have been found to be equal to and in some instances superior to air-dry grains as a feed for most classes of livestock on a dry matter basis. The improvement in efficiency is believed to be due to the fact that in early harvested grain, the starch and protein components are not in the crystalline states as with dry grains. Another factor is that early harvested grain would require considerably less wetting in the rumen for microbial digestion. Other advantages of the use of high moisture grain are as below :

1. Harvesting of such grains can begun 2-3 weeks earlier than usual harvesting time thus decreases the risk of potential losses caused by poor weather and bird eating.
2. Harvesting losses are 5-10% less than regular practice.
3. Handling costs for high moisture grains are reduced because they are ready for feeding when they come from special silo meant for preservation of grains. For best results, the silo should be as nearly airtight as it can be made. The acid preservation of high moisture grain involves the addition of 1-1.5% propionic acid (or a mixture of propionic acid with either acetic or formic acid) to high moisture cereal grain to inhibit mould or spoilage, thereby alleviating artificial drying or the necessity to store in an airtight silo.

**B. Haylages**

Haylage, sometimes called low-moisture silage, is a form of preserved forage with characteristics between those of hay and silage. It is made from grass and/or legume to a moisture level of about 45-55% when harvested or wilted to this level if the harvested forage is having higher moisture percent before ensiling. It must be preserved by processes somewhat different from those for wilted or unwilted silage. The silos should be well constructed and as airtight as possible so that the oxygen present is soon used up, the $CO_2$ that is produced is trapped and held within the silo. These conditions prevent the forage from spoiling by moulding, oxidising, heating etc. *Air exclusion is the key to the success or failure of making low moisture silage.*

*Advantages*

1. Properly made haylage has a pleasant aroma and is a palatable high quality feed. Animals usually receive more DM and net feed value than silage made from the same cut.

2. If forage is mowed with the intention of making hay and the weather becomes unfavourable for drying, the partially dried forage can be made into haylage.

*Disadvantages*

1. With haylage, fine chopping, good packing and complete sealing against air entrance inside the silo is a must and more critical than with silage.

2. The danger of excessive heating which lowers protein digestibility is more acute in haylages than silages.

However, being easy to prepare and preserve in a gas type silo or other special silos as mentioned above, and capped with plastic until feeding is initiated, haylage is gaining popularity as a dairy feed. Nutritive value depends on the stage of the growth of the crop when cut and on the percentage or dry matter in it.

**C. Wet by-product feeds**

Wet by-product feeds might be confused with fresh forages on the one hand, and root crops, on the other, based on their content of DM. However, the fresh forages can usually be differentiated from the wet by-products on the basis of carotene content. Root crops likewise be differentiated from wet by-products in that the latter will contain over 3% crude fibre on a wet basis while the root crops will have lower values.

**D. Root crops**

Occassionally root crops might be confused with fresh milk on the basis of DM content, but when crude fibre content is taken into consideration (root crops always have some amount of CF) the confusion can be cleared out.

**III. Identifying Individual Feeds**

With more experience it is possible to distinguish between two feed ingredients of the same feed

Table 11

Identifying feeds from their Composition (figures are on as fed basis)

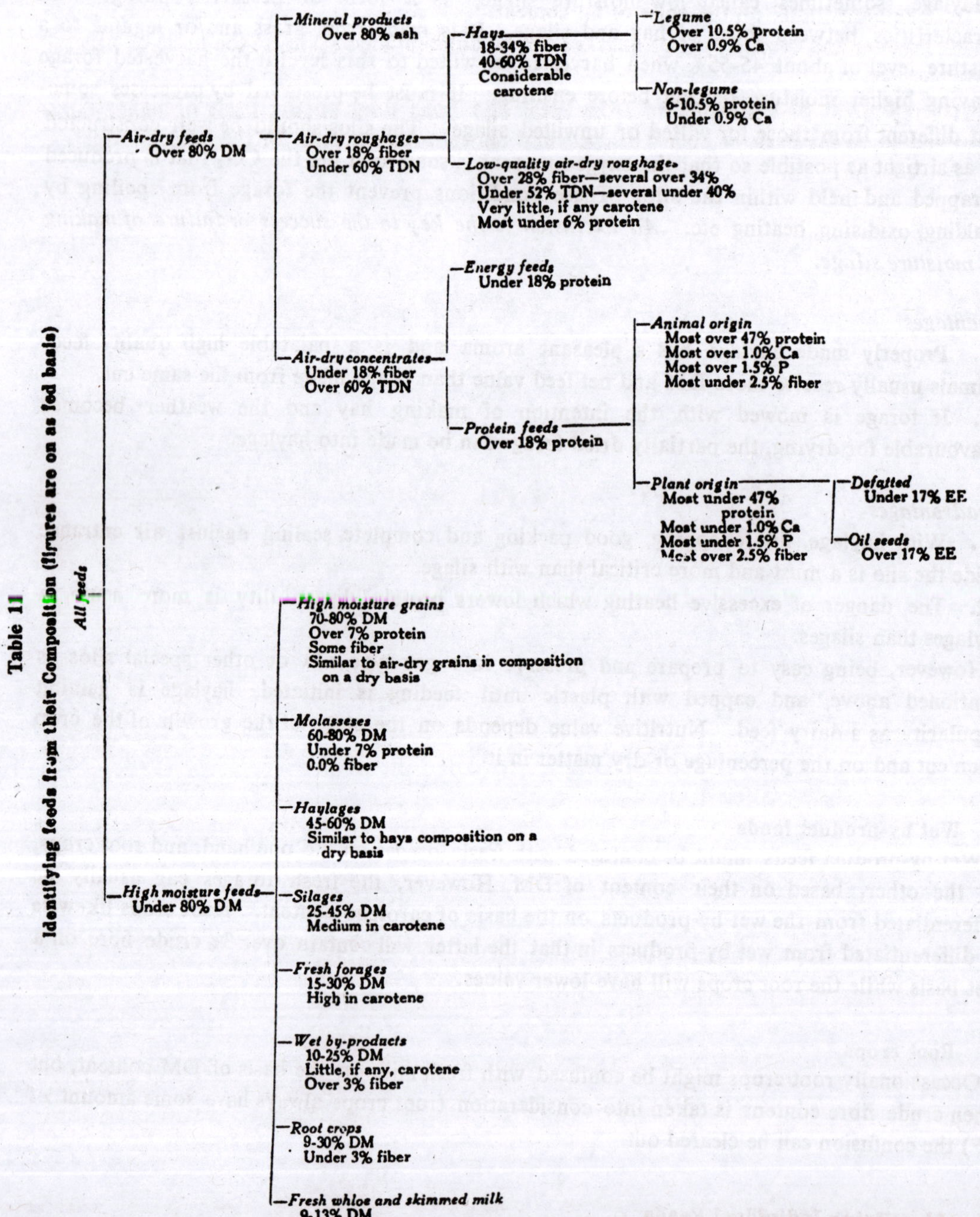


Source : Feeds and Feeding by Arthur E. Cullison ; Prentice-Hall of India Pvt. Ltd. New Delhi—110 001 (1978).

**group on the basis of their composition. For example fresh whole milk can be distinguished from fresh skimmed milk on the basis of fat content.**

**Ghani, expeller and deoiled type of oilcakes can be differentiated again on the basis of oil and protein content.**

**Meat scrap might be distinguished from meat and bone meal on the basis of higher bone content and so on the basis of higher calcium and phosphorus contents for the latter product.**

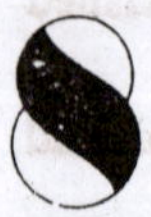

# ANIMAL FEED PREPARATION AND PROCESSING FOR MAXIMUM ECONOMY

Feed represents the major cost in animal production. Even with sheep, which typically consume more forage than other domestic species, feed may represent 55 per cent or higher of the total production costs; with poultry, a value of 74-80 per cent might be more appropriate; for pork it varies between 65 and 75 per cent; and for finishing cattle it may represent 55 per cent of the total production cost and 70 per cent for milk. Hence, it is important that feed be processed economically in such a manner as to make for maximum efficiency.

Feed processing refers to performing all the operations necessary to achieve the maximum potential nutritional value of a feedstuff. The process involves changing ingredients in such a manner as to maximise their natural value and the net returns from their use.

Feed processing may be accomplished by physical, chemical, thermal, bacterial or other alterations of a feed ingredient before it is fed. The primary reasons for processing feeds are:

1. To make more profit: Feed efficiency can be routinely improved by as much as 10-15 per cent by changing the method of feed processing. Thus profits may be enhanced by either reducing costs, or increasing production or both.

2. To change moisture content: Moisture content of a feedstuff may need to be changed to make it safer to store, made more palatable and more digestible, or to process it otherwise. Grains are generally stored below 14 per cent moisture.

On the other hand it may also be desirable to add water to a finely ground meal mixture at the time of feeding in order to lessen dustiness and to increase palatability.

3. To alter particle size: Some feeds need to be reduced in size so that they can be consumed and are more digestible. In some cases particle size is increased (agglomerated) by pelleting or cubing.

4. To change density of feed: The weight per unit volume or the bulk of the ration affects total intake. For this reason, very bulky feeds are sometimes pelleted or cubed in order to increase energy density and feed consumption. On the other hand, horsemen favour flaked grains rather than ground or pelleted to minimise digestive disturbances.

5. To change palatability: In most instances, feeds are processed in such a manner as to increase palatability.

6. To increase nutrient availability.

7. To detoxify or remove undesirable components: Some feeds may contain toxic substances, the excess consumption of which may cause decreased nutritive value of the feeds or may injure some vital organs or even cause death. The following information may be helpful in this connection:

8. To lessen moulds, salmonella and other harmful substances: Moulds on feeds have long been a problem. Aflatoxin is a common term used for a group of toxins produced by fungi and is common in the expeller variety of groundnut cakes. Proper harvesting, drying and storage are important factors in lessening aflatoxin contamination and toxic production. Propionic and acetic acids will inhibit mould growth. Treatment with ammonia or ammonium hydroxide will detoxify feeds.

Salmonella, rod shaped bacteria, is of importance from two distinct aspects; (a) food poisoning in man, and (b) disease in domestic animals. In meat meal it is invariably present and is destroyed by pelleting.

**Table 12**

**Natural inhibitors in feedstuffs**

| Feedstuff | Inhibitor(s)/Toxins | Deactivation process |
|---|---|---|
| Cottonseed meal | Gossypol: cyclopropene fatty acids | Adding iron salts; rupturing pigment gland |
| Soybean meal | Trypsin inhibitor: an unidentified factor | Heat; autoclaving |
| Linseed meal | Crystalline water soluble substance | Water treatment |
| Raw fish | Thiaminase | Heat |
| Lucerne meal | Saponins: pectin methyl esterase | Limit amount feed |
| Rapeseed | Isothiocyanate: thyroactive materials | |
| Groundnut meal | Aflatoxin | Treatment with ammonia or ammonium hydroxide |

9. To reduce storage, transportation space and cost: Sometimes forages are processed in a certain way in order to reduce storage and transportation space.

10. To improve keeping qualities: Since feeds are seasonally produced, some of them must be stored for use in the non-growing season.

Forages may either be dried to safe storage levels, ranging from 25 per cent moisture in loose hay to 16-17 per cent for cube or preserved by ensiling at 60-70 per cent moisture content. (Cubing refers to the practice of compressing long or coarsely cut hay in cubes about 1.25 inches square and 2 inches long with a bulk density of about 15 kg per cubic foot.)

## PROCESSING METHODS

### I. Grain processing methods

Grain processing methods are divided conveniently into dry and wet processes. The primary objective is to improve the availability and digestibility of starch which is present at about 70-80 per cent in grains. However, the method of accomplishing this is complicated because: (1) the type of starch varies among grains in its digestibility; and (2) availability of starch even varies from one grain variety to another, particularly in milo.

Grain Processings

A. *Dry Processings*
1. Grinding
2. Dry rolling or Cracking
3. Popping
4. Extruding
5. Micronising
6. Roasting
7. Pelleting
8. Dehulling

B. *Wet Processings*
1. Soaking
2. Steam rolling
3. Steam flaking
4. Pressure cooking
5. Exploding
6. Reconstitution
7. Ensiling at high moisture content

## A. DRY PROCESSING

**Grinding**

Grinding is that process by which a feedstuff is reduced to a particle size by impact, shearing or attrition. The process is most common, economical and simple, other than soaking. A wide variety of equipment is available and all of it allows some control of particle size. Coarsely ground grains are preferred for ruminants while finer ground grains are more common for poultry and swine.

**Dry rolling or cracking**

The method refers to passing grain without steam between a closely fitted set of steel rollers which are usually grooved on the surface. It breaks the hull and/or seed coat and results in an end product of coarsely ground grain sometimes referred to as flaking. Cattle seem to prefer flaked grain to finely ground grain, and are usually better for it.

**Popping**

Most readers are familiar with popped rice (*khai*) and popped maize which is produced by action of the rapid application of dry heat, causing a sudden expansion of the grain which ruptures the endosperm. For increasing digestibility all grains may be processed by this method, but it appears that it is specially effective in processing sorghum or other milo grains.

Popped milo requires more storage space due to its light density.

**Extruding**

Extruding usually involves grinding the grain, followed by heating with steam in order to soften it, then forcing the softened steamed ground grain through a machine with a spiral screw which expels the grain through a tapered head to produce a ribbon like product. Extruding animal feeds is generally confined to pet foods.

**Micronising**

Micronising is essentially the same as popping, except that heat is provided in the form of infra-red energy.

**Roasting**

Roasting is accomplished by passing the grain through a flame or heating it to the desired temperature in some form of an oven for a period of time, resulting in some expansion of the grain, which produces a palatable product. The method may be used with whole soybeans to destroy heat labile inhibitors and thus improve nutritive value for poultry and swine.

**Pelleting**

Pelleting is accomplished by grinding the material and then forcing it through die openings by a mechanical process. Feedstuff usually is, but not always, steamed to some extent prior to pelleting. Pellets can be made into small chunks, or cylinders of different diameters, length and degrees of hardness. The advantages of pelleting feeds are as follows:

1. Feeds to be pelleted are usually ground first—the pellets so formed being appreciated by the consumer.
2. Pelleting feed to a free flowing form, facilitates its handling and use in a self feeder.
3. Pelleted feeds are usually less dusty and more palatable.
4. The feed reduces storage space requirement.

The process involves about 10 per cent more cost than non-pelleted concentrates.

**Dehulling (Corticated form)**

Dehulling is the process of removing the outer coat of grain, nuts and some fruits as the hulls are high in fibres and low in digestibility in swine, poultry and other monogastric animals. The best known outer covering of cereal grains are barley hulls, oat hulls and rice hulls. Today hulls are combined with other residue from the milling of these cereal grains and are marketed as by-products.

The protein content of such unhulled (undecorticated) oilseeds as soybeans, cottonseeds, groundnuts, sunflowers, and safflowers is relatively low.

B. WET PROCESSING

**Soaking**

Hard grains soaked for 12 to 24 hours in water is a practice long in use by livestock feeders (which are not mechanically processed) for feeding of sore mouthed horses and mules. Benefits are also obtained by soaking oilseed by-products like mustard cake in water and thereby alleviating the toxicity factors like HCN.

**Steam rolling**

Rolling refers to a process by which grain is compressed into flat particles by passing it between rollers. Steam rolling is also called crimping, and steam crimping refers to exposing grain to steam for a short period of time, usually one to eight minutes, followed by rolling. The steam softens the kernel, producing a more intact, crimped-appearing product than that produced by dry rolling. Steam rolling offers little or no advantage in feed efficiency over grinding or dry rolling. However, the product may be useful for very young animals before their teeth are fully developed or for very old animals with badly worn teeth.

**Steam flaking**

Steam flaking grains are prepared in a similar manner but with relatively rigid quality controls. Grain is subjected to high moisture steam for a sufficient time to raise the water content to 18-20 per cent and the grain is then rolled to produce a rather flat flake. Thin flakes are better as they allow more efficient rupture of starch granules whereby a more desirable texture is produced.

**Pressure cooking**

The product is very similar to steam processed flaked grain. In the case of pressure flaking, the grain is subjected to steam under pressure for a short time, such as 50 psi (pounds per square inch) for one to two minutes. Steam is injected into the cooker till the grain in the chamber reaches a temperature approaching 300° F. The grain is then expelled from the cooker at a temperature below 200° F and with 20 per cent moisture these are flaked. In comparison with steam flaking, flakes produced by pressure are less brittle.

**Exploding**

Exploding is the swelling of grain, produced by steaming under pressure followed by releasing to the air. Steam is injected into high-tensile strength steel 'bottles' to raise pressure to 250 psi. After about 20 seconds, a valve opens to let the grain escape as expanded balls with the hulls removed. Under high pressure, moisture is forced into the kernels, which when released into the air swell to several times the original size.

**Reconstitution**

Reconstituted grain is mature grain that is harvested at the normal moisture level (10-14 per cent), following which water is added to bring the moisture level to 25-30 per cent and the wet product is stored in an upright silo (for required compaction) for 15 to 21 days prior to feeding. The grains are rolled and ground at the time of removal.

Properly reconstituted milo (sorghum) and steam processed flaked milo give similar results with fattening cattle.

**Ensiling at high moisture content**

High moisture grain refers to grain harvested at a moisture level of 20 to 35 per cent and stored without drying in a silo. It may be ground before ensiling or ground and rolled stored in either of the two ways.

1. It may be ensiled (fermented) in an oxygen limiting (anaerobic type) silo.
2. It may be preserved by the addition of 1-1.5 per cent propionic acid (or a mixture of propionic acid with either acetic or formic acid) to inhibit mould on storage.

This is a particularly useful procedure when weather conditions do not allow normal drying in the field and it obviates the need to dry the grain artificially.

**II. Roughage processing methods**

Before discussing each of the common methods of roughage preparation, the following points may be noted at the beginning:

1. The preparation of forages normally does not increase the nutritive value of the initial product.

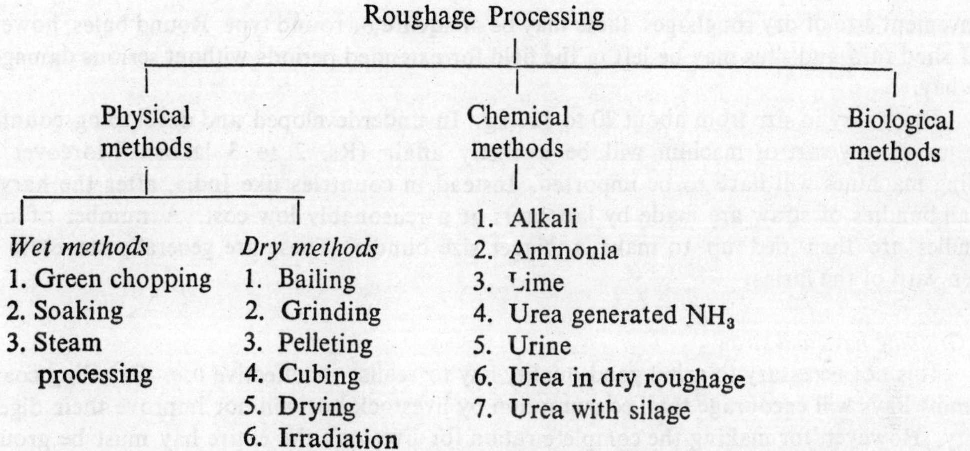


2. In preparing roughages, avoid processing those (a) with high moisture, which may lead to spontaneous combustion, and (b) in which there are foreign materials (wire, nail, etc.).

## PHYSICAL METHODS

### A. Wet methods

1. *Green chopping*

This refers to converting the green crop residues into 1 to 4 cm length pieces by chaff cutters. The main advantage is due to less wastage of unpalatable parts. By mixing poor quality roughages in chopped green materials, it will mask the effects of the former.

2. *Soaking*

This method is not considered to be practical except possibly with chopped straw.

3. *Steam processing*

The steam treatment of forage particularly of low quality roughages like *bagasse* has been reported to cause increased voluntary intake and higher digestibility in cattle. Chemical studies indicated extensive degradation of cellulose and hemicellulose and the production of undesirable poly-phenolic compounds when *bagasse* was steam processed. Apart from this the method involves extra expenditure.

### B. Dry methods

1. *Bailing*

Baling is probably the most common method used in developed countries to harvest roughage. Forage is cut and allowed to dry in the field. In areas of high humidity, a hay conditioner may be used at the time the hay is cut. For proper baling the moisture level must be sufficiently low (15 to 20 per cent) at the time of baling. Since bales are packages or bundles of convenient size of dry roughages, these may be of square or round type. Round bales, however, will shed rain and thus may be left in the field for extended periods without serious damage to the hay.

Bales vary in size from about 20 to 120 kg. In underdeveloped and developing countries the use of any sort of machine will be a costly affair (Rs. 2 to 3 lakhs). Moreover the baling machines will have to be imported. Instead in countries like India, after the harvest, small bundles of straw are made by labourers at a reasonably low cost. A number of small bundles are then tied up to make a bigger size bundle. These are generally stored in the open yard of the farms.

2. *Grinding hays and straw*

It is not necessary to grind good quality hay to realise its effective use. Grinding coarse, stemmy hays will encourage total consumption by livestock but will not improve their digestibility. However, for making the complete ration for livestock the entire hay must be ground. The coarser the hay that is ground, the more it will retain its bulk value. In general, grinding hay causes a drop in the milk fat in dairy cows due to low production of acetic acid in rumen.

In the conduct of digestion trials, it has been the practice to chop roughages and sometimes grind the entire ration to insure uniformity and prevent selective consumption of the feeds offered. When a research worker does this, he should be aware of the possible differences that will occur in the data. He should know if his results will be applicable to practical conditions in which they may be used.

3. *Pelleting of roughages*

Hays and straws must be ground prior to pelleting—thus, pelleting embraces most of the advantages and disadvantages of grinding. The method reduces the space requirement for storage by as much as 75 per cent. Pelleting of hay and straws increases consumption and performances in beef cattle. It also reduces dustiness. The process when applied to roughages, will cost twice as much as pelleting concentrates.

Pelleted roughages are metabolised somewhat differently; as a result of more rapid passage out of the rumen, less cellulose is digested and relatively less acetic acid is produced. Utilisation of metabolisable energy usually is more efficient. Pelleted high quality roughages will produce performance (gain in weight) in young cattle or lambs almost comparable to high grain feeding.

4. *Cubing*

"Cubes" are nothing more than large pellets. These may be of square or round shape having the diameter and length between 2 to 3 inches and 1 to 4 inches respectively. Grinding before cubing is not required, but usually water is sprayed on the dry hay and straw as they are cubed.

Although cubes have an advantage, as they can be fed on the ground in clean pastures, and no troughs are needed, it is difficult to detect (visually) low quality roughages in them, and besides the method is costly.

### 5. *Drying of roughages*

Drying entails removal of excess moisture of green crop residues to 14-15 per cent level either by natural or by artificial heat. In tropical countries like India, sun drying is the only feasible method. However, in some developed countries where sunshine is not plentiful, artificial drying is resorted to which involves a process, in which forage is cut by a hay chopper or silage cutter immediately after harvest and dried in large drum driers of different sizes.

The process is helpful to save utilisation of green forages in scarcity periods. Large amounts of fodders can thus be stored in a comparatively smaller storage spaces.

However, there are usually losses of some of the leaves and other finer and more nutritious parts while drying is taking place. Also more energy is required to chew dry hay and have it pass through the digestive tract than with green forages.

### 6. *Irradiation*

Improvement of digestibility of wheat straw by high voltage X-rays has been found to be due to the breaking of the cellulose and hemicellulose bonds, resulting in formation of oligosaccharides, which can be utilised by the rumen organisms. Forage lignin on the other hand resists irradiation. Upon irradiation, ergosterol, a plant sterol, yields calciferol, commonly known as vitamin $D_2$. The method involves high cost and technology.

## CHEMICAL METHODS

### 1. *Alkali treatment*

Treating straw with alkali can give a product of considerable nutritive value. The process of alkali soaking was first used on straw in Germany in 1919, during World War I when there was a critical shortage of livestock feed. The mode of action of alkali is not completely understood. It reduces the strength of the intermolecular hydrogen bonds which bind the cellulose fibre without affecting much of the cell wall. Further, it has been suggested that alkali saponifies uronic acid and acetic acid esters and neutralises are thus hydrolysed. This would perhaps account for the solubilisation of silica and hemicelluloses. Amorphous silica may be converted to soluble silicates. The hydrolysis of uronic acid and acetic acid esters could account for most of the alkali which cannot be recovered by washing the treated straw.

The usual method requires large quantities of water and is impracticable in areas where water supplies are limited. The process consists of soaking the straw in 10 times its weight of 1.5 per cent NaOH solution for about 24 hours. The liquid is then drained off and can be used for succeeding batches of straw. The straw is washed after treatment until freed from the alkali. The treatment will in case of wheat straw increase organic matter digestibility from 46 per cent to more than 70 per cent. Unfortunately the total yield of the organic matter is reduced due to heavy leaching of 20 per cent organic matter. Moreover the method is tiresome as well as costly.

To eliminate leaching losses, the Canadian workers preferred to use low concentration alkali sprayed on the chopped straw (4 kg NaOH per 160 kg of straw). In this method only 30 per cent of water was used when compared to the earlier method, but there remained a high amount of residual alkali in the straw.

According to another method the straw is treated for 15 minutes in a hot (80-90°C) solution of NaOH. The liquid is pressed out and the treated straw dried in a grass drier. The hot gases ($CO_2$ and $SO_2$) in the drier neutralise the excess residual alkali in the straw.

2. *Ammonia treatment*

Treatment of straw with anhydrous ammonia will add $N_2$ to the straw which can be used by rumen microorganisms; in addition, the ammoniation of straw will improve significantly the degradability of its fibrous constituents which will result in the production of more energy in the form of VFA. The crude protein content ($N \times 6.25$) of wheat straw has been shown to increase from 2.71 to 8.85 per cent on 3 per cent ammonia treatment along with an increase of degradability of cellulose from 48.07 to 60 per cent.

The ammonia method requires that a stack of straw be covered so that the ammonia does not escape.

3. *Lime treatment*

Calcium hydroxide generated from lime may prove to be the cheapest alkali available for the effective treatment of coarse roughages. Both wet and dry methods of treatment have been used. In the wet method, 1.25 per cent of commercial grade lime is used and the straw is soaked in the lime solution for several days and the digestibility has been shown to increase by 24 to 30 per cent. In the dry method, 4 per cent lime is dusted on the moist straw and stacked for reaction. The higher concentration of lime in this method is used to compensate the slow reaction and low solubility of lime. Firstly, although the dry method of treatment is equally good in terms of increased digestibility the dry matter intake reduced from 86 g/kg 0.75 (in the wet method) to 48 g/kg 0.75 (in dry method). Secondly, the excess calcium is likely to affect the utilisation of other minerals particularly phosphorus, when such lime is a potential cheap source of alkali for treatment of straws particularly the paddy straw.

4. *Urea-generated $NH_3$ treatment of roughages*

Although scientifically very sound, the method of treatment of straws with anhydrous or liquid $NH_3$ directly is also full of practical difficulties particularly the handling problems at farmers' level. Thus an entirely new approach is being experimented upon in various countries including India, Bangladesh, Srilanka, Malaysia, Philippines and Thailand wherein urea treated (3 to 5 per cent) straw is stored for about four weeks to allow the release of $NH_3$ which attacks the ligno cellulosic bonds in a similar manner as anhydrous or aquous ammonia does in the direct treatment. Obviously, the approach is full of tremendous possibilities because of its simplicity on one hand and easy availability of urea with the farmers on the other.

It has been reported that such urea treated (5 per cent stacked wheat straw) diet was as good as the green sorghum and could support a growth rate of 300 g/day in cross breed heifers with only 1 kg/day of concentrate. It has been further reported that the replacement of untreated wheat straw with urea treated stacked wheat straw in diets consisting of napier grass-wheat straw or berseem-wheat straw resulted in an increase of 2 to 3 litres of milk/day in cross breed cows, despite a decrease in the daily allowance of concentrate.

Recently, it has been realised that the milk production in buffaloes up to five kg/day could be sustained on feeding urea generated ammonia treated wheat straw. However, in this experiment while the percentage of milk fat and protein increased, those of total solids and SNF decreased slightly. Thus, under normal village conditions, it is expected that simple urea treatment with stacking can be the cheapest and more practicable way of enhancing the nutritive value of coarse fodders.

5. *Urine treatment*

Animal urine can also be used as a source of urea which can generate ammonia to have a similar effect on improving the degradability of fibrous constituents on the coarse fodders. Although the urine treatment can also have an added advantage of minerals like calcium and phosphorus to some extent, it adds a very small amount of urea in relation to water content. If the moisture in the treated straw has to be kept at a low level, urine should be essentially fortified with urea to have optimum results.

6. *Urea added to dry roughages*

An addition of urea molasses to straw has become popular for increasing nutritive value. A solution of 10 kg molasses and 2 kg urea in 10 kg of water is spread by a sprayer on straws in 100 kg lots and spread evenly under the sun over an area of 20 × 20 ft. The treated straws can form maintenance ration when supplied along with the proper amount of 2 per cent mineral and 1 per cent salt and vitamin $AD_3$ mixture. About 8 kg of this enriched paddy straw per animal per day will supply sufficient nitrogen for the animals to synthesise the required amount of protein for maintenance.

7. *Urea mixed with silage*

Another way of feeding urea to cattle—especially dairy cattle—is through the addition of urea to crops which are being ensiled. If chopped, the whole maize plant is being ensiled at 35 per cent to 40 per cent dry matter, urea is then added at a level of 0.5 per cent of wet material. This level should increase the crude protein level of the silage on a dry matter basis about five points.

## BIOLOGICAL TREATMENTS

Use of selected bacterial and fungal culture in roughages has been considered during the past few years to increase the nutritive value of roughages over the chemical treatments.

1. Since plant residues constitute a good quantity of cellulosic materials including cellulose, hemicellulose and lignin, the biological treatment causes simplification of these compounds by releasing appropriate enzymes from microbes so that the materials ultimately become easily digestible upon intake by the ruminants.

Before selecting appropriate species for biodegradation of lignin in straws and hays one must be careful, so that the species degrades only lignin and not hollocelluloses, can be grown in unsterilised condition and finally it should not produce any toxins.

2. The fast growth rate of these microbes result in enriching the roughages with protein values also.

In one study it has been observed that a maximum of 30 per cent crude protein in the biomass obtained within four days of fermentation from an initial value of 3 per cent crude protein in the alkali treated (1.0 per cent NaOH) sugar cane bagasse when the cellulolytic mould *Aspergillus terreus* GN-1 was grown on it.

However, at this stage the large scale adoption of this method should wait till sufficient research results are obtained to have a standard procedure.

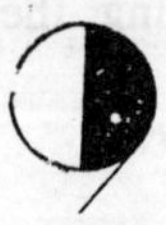

# ANTI-NUTRITIVE FACTORS IN ANIMAL FEEDSTUFFS

Anti-nutritive substances are defined as 'those generated in natural feedstuffs by the normal metabolism of the species from which the material originates and by different mechanisms exerting effects contrary to optimum nutrition".

These anti-nutritive substances are often referred to as *"toxic factors"* because of the deleterious effects they produce when eaten by animals. The term "toxic factor", however, is misleading, because there is an implication that the substances are lethal beyond a certain level of intake. In fact, for most animals they are not and produce less effects such as reduced growth, poor feed conversion, hormonal changes and occasional organ damage.

### Types of anti-nutritive substances

On the basis of the type of nutrients affected and the biological response produced in the animal the toxic factors can be classified into five major groups as follows:

1) Substances depressing digestion or metabolic utilisation of proteins:
   (a) Protease inhibitors.
   (b) Lectins, or Ricin (hemagglutinins).
   (c) Saponins.
   (d) Polyphenolic compounds. (TANNINS)
2) Substances reducing the solubility or interfering with the utilisation of mineral elements :
   (a) Phytic acid
   (b) Oxalic acid.
   (c) Glucosinolates.
   (d) Gossypol.
3) Substances inactivating or increasing the requirements of certain vitamins and hormones:
   (a) anti-vitamins. A, D, E, K and anti-pyridoxine, (b) Mimosine (anti hormone).
4) Cyanogens. 5) Nitrate and Nitrite
6) Moulds and mycotoxins in animal feedstuffs.

### Substances depressing digestion or metabolic utilisation of proteins

**a) Protease inhibitors**

Substances that inhibit proteolytic enzymes and thereby growth of non-ruminants are distributed throughout the plant kingdom but are particularly abundant in seeds of legumes.

In the case of soybeans identification of two main groups of protease inhibitors have recently been made namely: (1) *Kunitz* inhibitors have few disulphide bonds and a specificity towards trypsin. (2) *Bowman-Brik* inhibitors have a high proportion of disulphide bonds, inhibiting both trypsin and chymotrypsin.

Feeding raw soybeans to pigs, chicks and rats have resulted in reduced growth rate, pancreatic hyperplasia and low production. Although ruminants are capable of utilising raw soybeans without suffering any deleterious effects, a better response in milk production and growth rate is obtained on diets containing treated soybean.

The inhibitory substances are mostly heat labile and thus before feeding any leguminous grain to non-ruminants, the situation is generally corrected by proper heat treatment. Since overheating can damage some nutrients, such as amino acids and vitamins, quality control tests have been developed to assess the adequacy of heat treatment. These include trypsin inhibitor and urease assays, cresol red absorption, protein dispersibility index (PDI) and nitrogen solubility index (NSI).

**b) Lectins or ricin (hemagglutinins)**

This important group of anti-nutritional factors are found in both plant and animal tissue. At first, while studying the toxicity of castor bean cakes (after the oil had been extracted) a toxic fraction capable of agglutinating human red blood cells was noted as "*ricin*". Subsequently, similar active extracts from other edible legume seeds were obtained.

Lectins are protein in nature, resistant to digestion by pancreatic juice. Although very resistant to destruction by dry heat, lectins are destroyed by the same conditions as those used to inactivate protease inhibitors.

**c) Saponins**

Saponins are widely distributed in the plant kingdom and have been identified in 500 species belonging to more than 80 different families. The important common forages which have caused saponin poisoning of livestock are lucerne (*Medicago sativa*), white clover (*Trifolium repens*), red clover (*T. prateuse*) and soyabean (*Glycine max*).

*Chemical Structure and General Properties*

Saponins are plant glycosides which yield on hydrolysis sugars (pentoses, hexoses and uronic acids) and *aglycones* derived from polycyclic ring systems and are known as *sapogenins*. The saponins are divided into two main groups from the point of view of chemical nature of sapogenins: Steroids ($C_{27}$) or triterpenoides ($C_{30}$), with the triterpenoid sapogenins further divided into three classes based on the compounds ursane, oleanane or lupane.

They have three significant characteristics: (i) a bitter taste, (ii) foaming in aqueous solution, and (iii) hemolysis of red blood cells.

Poultry are much more sensitive than pigs. A 20 per cent lucerne meal in a poultry diet (equivalent to 0.3 per cent saponin) produces a significant growth depression attributable solely to the saponin whereas the same level is harmless for pigs.

Due to the bitter taste of saponins, it has been suggested that the reduced feed intake is due to unpalatability.

Much of the biological activity of saponins can be related to the following characteristic properties.

Saponin
(Acid hydrolysis)
Sugar — Sapogenin
Steroid — Triterpenoid

Structure of a lucerne saponin

1. Structurally saponins have a lipid-soluble aglycone and a water-soluble glycone parts which jointly confers lower surface tension and thus form stable foam when dissolved in water.
2. Most of the saponins readily combine with cholesterol resulting minimisation of the activity of original saponin.
3. Saponins possess the ability to haemolyse red blood cells.
4. They tend to alter the permeability of the cell wall and thereby exert a general toxicity on many organised tissues.

*Distribution of Saponins in Plants*

Saponins are present in all parts of the plant, i.e., leaves, stems, roots and blossoms of the plant. The amount varies from 2-3 per cent. The content varies with cutting, the first cutting averaged lower than the second and third. Saponin content is highly correlated with protein ash, fat and N-free extract and significantly negatively correlated with crude fibre and hay yield. It was further suggested that average saponin contents of the leaves are twice as much as those of the stems and that the saponin content declines as the plant becomes older. Roots of lucerne are known to be richer source of saponins than its top.

Among common livestock forages, soybean and lucerne contain a significant amount of saponins.

*Adverse Actions upon Excessive Eating*

1. In ruminant saponins have been suggested as being involved in formation of bloat by altering the surface tension of the ruminant contents due to entrapment of countless bubbles of fermentation gases throughout the ingesta.
2. It also increases the respiratory rate which later on becomes irregular.
3. Saponins also have found to inhibit the actions of certain enzymes, e.g., α-chymotrypsin.
4. The compound has got the ability to lyse red blood cells.
5. Levels of lucerne meal in poultry mash, in excess of 5 per cent decrease the weight gain chickens and also depress egg production in layers when the levels rises more than 7 per cent. The effect can partly be reversed by feeding of cholesterol and cotton seed oil in the diet with which saponins get binded.
6. In general the effects of ingestion of saponins include excessive salivation, increased respiratory tract secreti n, gastroenteritis, vomiting, diarrhoea, haemolysis, haematuria, damage to livers and kidney tissues, cystitis, bloating, reduction of gastric motility, reduction of cholesterol absorption from the gut, lowering of blood and liver cholesterol levels, reduction of food intake, reduction of growth rate.

**d) Polyphenolic compounds (tannins)**

The term tannin was introduced by Seguin in 1796 to describe the substances present in a number of vegetable extracts which are responsible for converting putrescible animal skins into the stable product leather by the tanning process.

*Definition*

Also known as tannic acid, gallotannin and gallotannic acid. It is now defined to include those naturally occurring compounds having high molecular weight (500–3000) and containing a sufficiently large number of phenolic hydroxyl groups (1 to 2 per 100 molecular weight) to enable them to form effective cross-links between proteins and other macromolecules.

The substances in general also termed as group of phenolic non-nitrogenous plant toxins that are frequently glycosides with astringent properties.

*Types of Tannins*

Chemically tannins may be grouped into two broad categories; 1. Hydrolysable tannins and 2. Condensed tannins. Most tannin extracts appear to contain mixtures of both the types of tannins but generally one or the other predominates at least in any given part of the plant.

A. HYDROLYSABLE TANNINS. The more important group compounds can be readily hydrolysed by water, acids, bases or enzymes (tannin acyl-hydrolases). The hydrolysable tannins are those in which *gallic acid* and its related compounds like *hexahydroxydiphenic* acid are linked in sufficient proportion to a sugar by glycosidic linkages to provide polyphenolic compounds of relatively high molecular weight. Such compounds are also known as *gallotannins* because of the presence of gallic acid.

On hydrolysis such compounds yield glucose or some other polyhydric alcohol together with gallic acid or other phenolic acids related to it. Chinese gallotannins for example, on hydrolysis yield gallic acid and glucose in a ratio of 7 to 10 moles of the former to 1 mole of the latter.

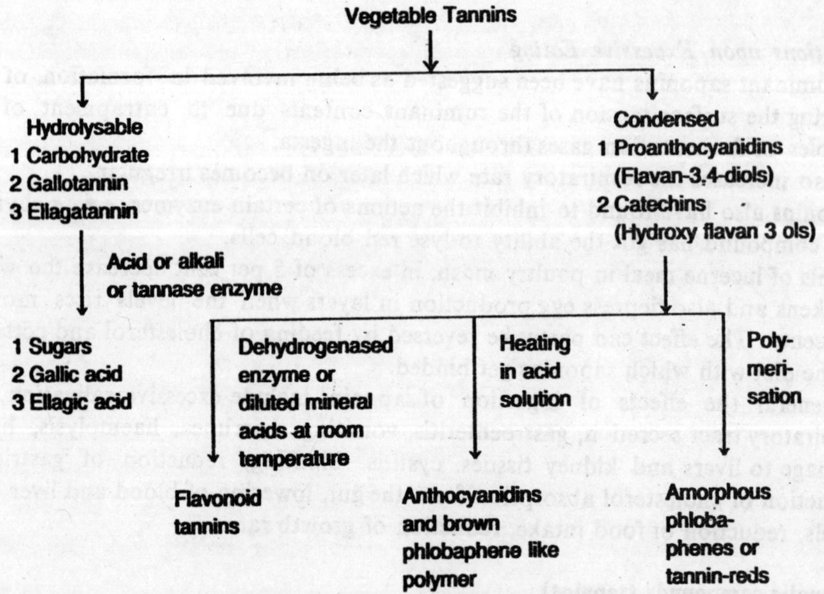


**Fig. 11** – *Types of vegetable tannins.*

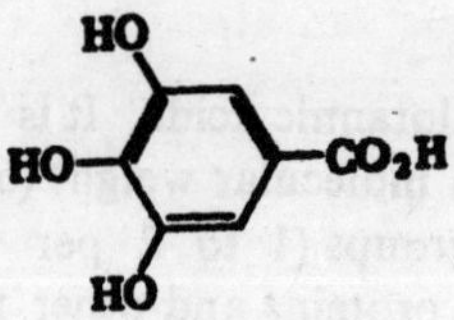

Gallic acid

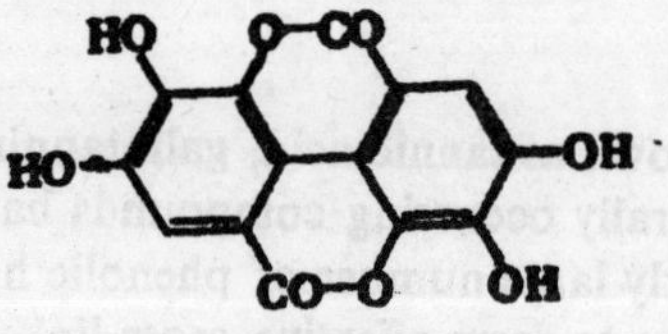

Ellagic acid

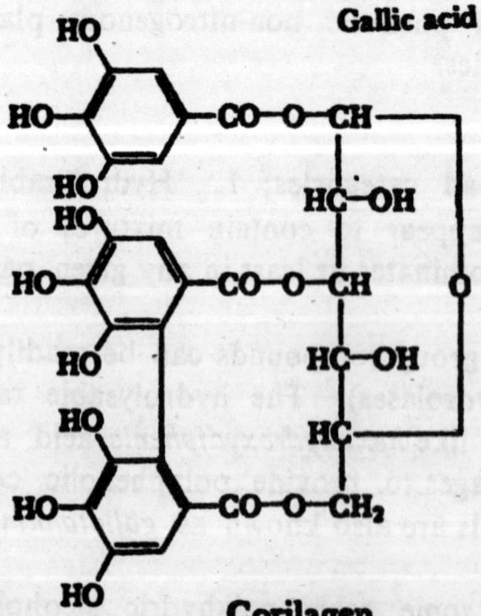

**Corilagen.**
($C_{27}H_{24}O_{18}$)

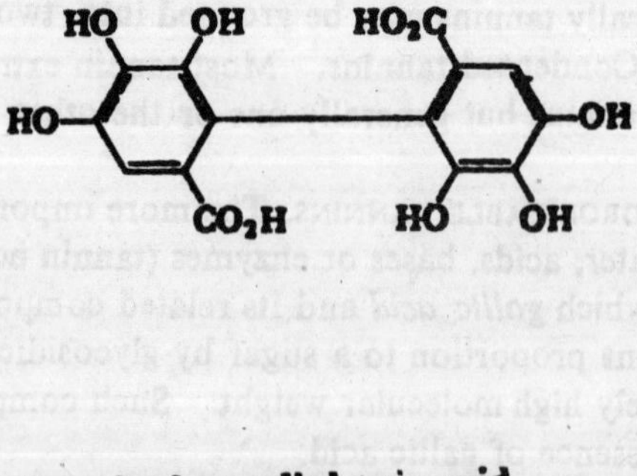

**hexahydroxydiphenic acid**

Until 1950, only other phenolic compound of proved structure which had been isolated from hydrolysable tannins was *ellagic acid* in place of gallic acid. Such hydrolysable tannins are known as *ellagitannins*. It is very difficult to separate such closely related substances by classical organic chemical techniques.

The simplest example of ellagitannin is *corilagen*, the tannin which occur in divi-divi (*Caesalpinia coriaria*) and also in *Eucalyptus sieberiana* has the structure as given above with an emperical formula $C_{27}H_{24}O_{18}$.

B. CONDENSED TANNIN. Compounds contain only phenolic nuclei, although polysaccharides or proteins may be irreversibly linked to them *in vivo* or during the course of isolation. On treatment with hydrolytic reagents, tannins of this class give no significant yields of lower molecular weight compounds, but instead tend to polymerise, especially in acid solution, to yield insoluble amorphous often red coloured products known as phlobaphenes (Greek dye). Most tannins of this type are formed by the condensation of two or more molecules of flavan-3-ols, such as catechin or flavan-3, 4-diols such as leucocyanidin or mixture of the two. Tannins of this type are usually termed *non-hydrolysable* or more commonly *condensed*. Since the majority of these tannins appear to be formed by the polymerisation of flavans, it is convenient to refer to this group specifically as *flavolans* and to use the term condensed tannin in its wider sense.

*Properties of Tannins*

1. The most important property of tannins is undoubtedly their capacity to bind proteins; they are thus inhibitors of enzymes. It is considered likely that this property is shown in the living cell as tannins are assumed to be separated from the cytoplasm in the cell.
2. Plant protein-tannin interactions may be important in relation to pasture quality and also in consumption of certain grain (salseed, sorghum, milo, etc.), in terms of feed utilisation by the domestic livestock.
3. The low palatability of some herbage plants such as cotton grass (*Imperata cylindrica*) and of some grains as has already mentioned have been attributed to their high tannin content.
4. They are also markedly astringent—that is, they cause a dry or puckery sensation in the mouth, probably by reducing the lubricant action of the glycoproteins in the saliva.

5. The presence of tannins in a feedstuff has been assumed to affect voluntary intake as it causes a dry or puckery sensation in the mouth, probably by reducing the lubricant action of the glycoproteins in the saliva. High tannin content also depresses cellulose activity and thereby affects digestion of crude fibre. Besides, tannins may cause loss of mucus, epithelial edema, irritation and damage to alimentary canal tissue, which, in turn facilitate greater tannin absorption, thus causing toxicity.

*Distribution of Tannins*

Both hydrolysable and condensed tannins are widely distributed in nature. In many species both classes are present together but generally one or the other predominates. Hydrolysable tannins being usually extracted from leaves or fruit and condensed ones from bark or heartwood.

Table 13

**Distribution of tannins in livestock feeds and fodders**

| *Name of the Feed Stuff* | *Approximate percentage (%)* |
|---|---|
| Sorghum | 0.004—10.50 |
| Milo | 2.00 — 3.00 |
| Salseed Meal | 9.00 —12.00 |
| Mango seed Kernal | 5.00 — 7.00 |
| Mustard oil cake | 2.80 — 3.20 |
| Rape seed cake | 3.00 — 3.50 |
| Lucerne meal | 0.10 — 3.50 |
| Tamarind seed | ? |
| Oak kernel | ? |
| Dhaincha | ? |

## Methods of detannification

A huge production of 5.5 million tonnes deoiled *sal* seed meal per year in India spurred work on the detannification of deoiled *sal* seed meal in the hope that it would be more nutritious for feeding cattle. Similarly, sorghums which contain high tannin will have more feeding value upon detannification. The methods available for removal/inactivation of tannins can be divided into two main catogories: (1) Physical, and (2) Chemical.

### 1. Physical treatments

(a) Soaking and cooking of tannin containing feed stuffs have been found very effective in decreasing the tannin content. However, these treatments cause a substantial loss of dry matter between 20-70 per cent.

(b) Anaerobic storage of moist sorghum grains for two and nine days at 25°C resulted in 40 per cent and 92 per cent reduction in tannins respectively. The nutritive value of the treated grains was found to be higher.

### 2. Chemical treatments

a) Addition of tannin complexing agents like polyethylene glycol (PEG) and polyvinylpyroldone (PVP) prevent formation of complex(es) between tannin and protein as well as break the already formed complex(es), thus liberating protein. The addition of PVP and PEG also

**Table 14**

*General histopathological implications of feeding tannin in different species*

| Source/mode of feeding tannins | species | level | symptoms |
|---|---|---|---|
| Tea, banana or plums, stomach tube | rats | 0.5 mg /kg W* | Primary cell degeneration in liver. Decrease in total protein and increase in total lipid content of liver and serum |
| Tannic acid and coffee powder | rats | 0.25 – 1.0 % in DM | Lesions in small intestine and kidney |
| Sal seed meal | chicks | 1.5 % in DM | Decrease in hemoglobin concentration and white and red blood cells. Swelling and hydropic generation of hepatic cells. Coagulation necrosis in renal tubules of kidney |
| Tannic acid | chicks | 0.5 % in CM | Hydropic degeneration of Islets cells of pancreas. |
| | | 1.0 % in CM | Hydropic degeneration of tips of Intestinal villi. |
| | | 2 – 3 % in CM | Mucinous and catarrhal degeneration in Intestinal glands |
| Sal seed meal | cattle | 2.66 % in CM | Mucous threads in urine and irritation of the urethra |
| Sal seed meal | cattle | 3.09 % in CM | Toxic degenerative changes in kidney, liver, spleen and intestines |
| Quercus incana 3 % in CM | cattle | 0.16 % in DM | Albumin in urine |

* W = Boby weight; CM = Concentrate Mixture.

alleviated the deleterious effects of tannins in chicks and rats, respectively.

b) Treatment with alkalies like NaOH, $Ca(OH)_2$ and lime water of *sal* seed meal was found to be very effective in removing tannins (74-100 per cent), but treatments with $Na_2CO_3$ and $NaHCO_3$ were comparatively less effective (about 50 per cent removal). A loss of 20-70 per cent dry matter was also observed in these studies. A 100 per cent inactivation of tannins was observed in both *sal* seed meal and soybean grains on CaO treatment. The treatment with $NH_4OH$ appears to be advantageous as it increases the NPN content besides reducing tannins. In addition, excess $NH_4OH$ can be removed from feedstuffs by secretion.

c) Formaldehyde treatment of sorghum grains to inactivate their tannins has been found to be quite successful.

d) Treatment with organic solvents like acetone and methanol have been used. Acetone was found to be more effective and reduced tannin up to 72 per cent while methanol reduces 37 per cent tannin. High cost of organic solvents discourages their application.

e) Treatments with $H_2O_2$ and HCl have also been tried. $H_2O_2$ tιeatment was fouud to reduce tannic acid in *sal* seed meal by only 17 per cent. The boiling of *sal* seed meal with 0.1N HCl reduces 64 per cent tannin. A much higher reduction with HCl was obtained for sorghum grains. The inactivtaion by HCl appears to be due to polymerisation of tannins to higher oligomeric polymers.

## Substances reducing the solubility or interfering with the utilisation of mineral elements

### a) *Phytic acid*

**Phytates are the salts of phytic acid. Phytic acid is formed due to combination of six phosphate molecules with Inositol, a cyclic alcohol with six hydroxy radicals like that of hexose sugar.**

**Inositol**

**Phytic acid**

**1 ml cyclic alcohol + 6 phosphate molecule = Phytic acid**
**(Inositol)**

**Unlike animal protein supplements, phytate occurs naturally in all foods of plant origin in association with vegetable protein. Thus the vegetable feed ingredients which are rich in**

protein, also are generally found rich in phytate content as in soybean, sesame, rapeseed meal, cotton seed meal, etc.

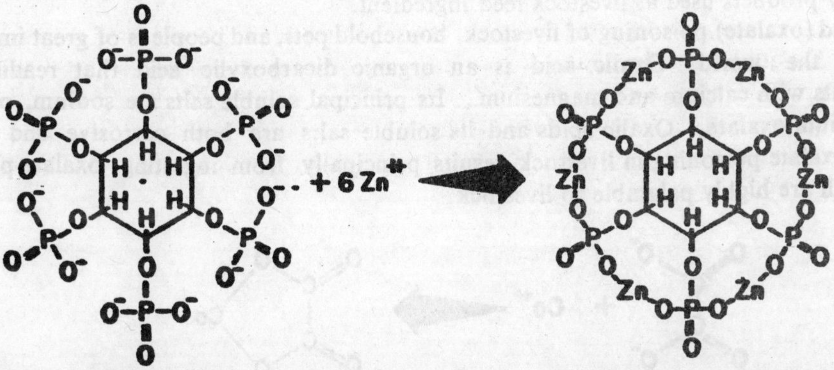

Phytic acid + 6 $Zn^{++}$ → Insoluble zinc phytate

The anionic character of phytate makes it ideal for forming complexes with mineral elements, particularly the transitional element such as zinc, iron and manganese resulting the minerals insoluble in the intestinal tract.

Solubility of these complexes mainly varies with pH, and calcium ion concentration, e.g., calcium enhances the formation of Zn–phytate complex. The effect of pH on solubility is particularly significant as because pH 6 is the approximate pH of the duodenum and upper jejunum the site of absorption of heavy elements including zinc. Neither phytate nor the zinc-phytate or calcium-Zn-phytate complex are absorbed under this pH range.

About half or more of the phosphorus in cereal grains is in the form of phytin. The availability of phytin phosphorus to all non-ruminants is influenced by the level of vitamin D, calcium, the calcium to phosphorus ratio, amount of zinc in the feed, alimentary tract pH and other factors. How Vitamin D specifically acts in improving the utilisation of phytin phosphorus is not clear.

A good guide to assume that no more than 50 per cent of the phosphorus in plant feeds is available to non-ruminants. By contrast, the phosphorus, in inorganic mineral supplements and of animal origins are usually available at the rate of more than 80 per cent.

Thus, it should be stressed that the calcium, phosphorus, zinc, and manganese levels determined by a chemical analysis of a feed gives an idea of only total content but does not indicate about the amount of these elements which will be available to the animal.

In ruminants, the selected ruminal microbes are in a position to hydrolyse phytates by secreting the enzyme *phytases* so that it no longer binds the minerals as mentioned. Thus ruminants can utilise phytin phosphorus satisfactorily.

For non-ruminants supplementation with adequate minerals (which are affected by phytates) is the usual practice followed to-day in livestock feeding to overcome the adverse effect of phytates.

b) *Oxalic acid*

In both the vegetable and animal kingdoms oxalic acid is found as free and in salt forms. Plants which are particularly rich in oxalates include beet, spinach and a number of agro-industrial by-products used as livestock feed ingredient.

Oxalic acid (oxalate) poisoning of livestock, household pets, and people is of great importance throughout the world. Oxalic acid is an organic dicarboxylic acid that readily forms insoluble salts with calcium and magnesium. Its principal soluble salts are sodium, potassium and ammonium oxalate. Oxalic acids and its soluble salts are both corrosive and systemic poisons. Oxalate poisoning in livestock results principally from ingesting oxalate-producing plants, which are highly palatable to livestock.

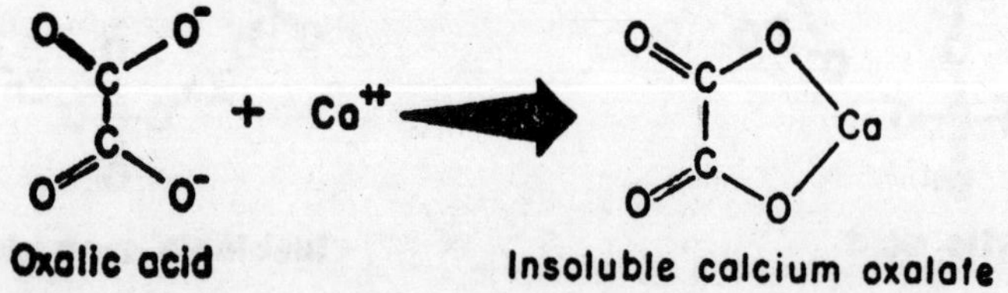

Oxalic acid + $Ca^{++}$ → Insoluble calcium oxalate

Animal response to oxalate poisoning varies with species of animal and species of plant (kind of oxalate differs in different plant species) consumed. Thus cattle, sheep and horses differ in their responses to oxalate. Cattle fed on paddy straw or on certain other grasses containing 2 per cent oxalate develop a negative calcium balance but sheep do not develop at this level. There is good evidence that ruminants fed gradually increasing quantities of high oxalate plant acquire the ability to tolerate the large quantities of dietary oxalic acid and further this tolerance depends upon the increased degradation of oxalic acid by ruminal microbes.

Oxalate is apparently split to carbon dioxide and formate, and the hydrogen from formic acid is used to synthesise methane. Oxalate degrading aerobic bacteria have been isolated from rumen content. Bacterial degradation of oxalate to a non-toxic form and thus tolerance for oxalate are acquired by gradually increasing the quantity of oxalate-containing plant material. Increased degradation rates were also induced by intra-ruminal infusion of sodium oxalate. When the dietary amount exceeds certain level, normal degradation is interrupted and the excess oxalates combine with feed calcium to form insoluble calcium oxalate and thus become unavailable for absorption or the excess oxalate (20-30 mg per cent) may be absorbed from the rumen into the blood stream where it can combine with calcium to produce hypocalcemia. The insoluble calcium oxalate may then crystalise in various tissues, specially kidneys and rumen wall.

Oxalate poisoning in sheep and cattle are characterised by rapid and laboured respiration, depressions, weakness, coma and death. A hypocelcemia occuring in animals result in convulsions and tetany. The marked hypocalcemia is accompanied by an increase in plasma phosphorus, magnesium and sodium. Motility of the gastrointestinal tract becomes greatly depressed shortly after the initiation of intoxication.

Its anti-nutritive effect is mainly through complexing with calcium. The acid precipitates calcium and renders it less available for absorption. The magnitude of the problem is debatable as certain species of livestock have been shown to metabolise oxalic acid in such a way as to render it harmless. With cattle and sheep there is evidence that the rumen micro-organisms can split the calcium as well as decompose the oxalic acid.

In pigs and poultry, diets containing oxalic acid cause depression in growth and a reduction in calcium retention.

c) *Glucosinolates* (*Thioglucosides*)

Glucosinolates are responsible for the pungent flavours found in some cultivated plants belonging to the *Cruciferae*, specially the genus *Brassica*, which includes cabbage, turnips, rapeseed, mustard seed. Their main biological effect is to depress the synthesis of the *thyroid hormone* (Thyroxine and Triiodothyronine), thus producing goitre, although the latter is not caused by the glucosinolates *per se* but by their products of hydrolysis.

The glucosinolates occur in the root, stem, leaf and seed, and are always accompanied by the enzyme *thioglucosidase*, which is capable of hydrolysing them to glucose, acid sulphate and either thiocyanates, isothiocyanates or nitriles. Some of the isothiocyanates are subsequently cyclised to *oxazolidine-2-thiones* (OZT). It is interesting to note that thioglucosidase is also present in some intestinal bacteria and is important when intact glucosinolates are fed to animals.

**Table 15**

DISTRIBUTION OF GLUCOSINOLATES IN BRASSICAS

Number identified: 70
Number present in plant: 1–7
Occurrence: root, stem, leaf, seed
Chemistry:

$$R-C\begin{cases}S-C_6H_{11}O_5\\ NOSO_3^-\end{cases} \xrightarrow[H_2O]{\text{Thioglucosidase}} \text{D-glucose plus } HSO_4$$

$R-N=C=S$ Isothiocyanate; $R-C\equiv N$ Nitrile; $R-S-C\equiv N$ Thiocyanate

R = methyl, benzyl, 3-butenyl, etc.

| | *R group* | *Common name* | *Amount*[a] ($\mu$g/g) |
|---|---|---|---|
| *Brassica campestris* (Polish rape) | 3-Butenyl<br>(R)-2-hydroxy-3-butenyl | Gluconapin<br>Progoitrin | 18 000–44 000<br>2 000–20 000 |
| *Brassica napus* (Argentine rape) | 3Butenyl<br>(R)-2-hydroxy-3-butenyl | Gluconapin<br>Progoitrin | 10 000–22 000<br>18 000–50 000 |
| *Brassica napus* (Bronowski var.) | | Gluconapin<br>Progoitrin | 1 000– 4 000<br>1 000–23 000 |

[a] Air-dried.

Progoitrin and epiprogoitrin are the glucosinolate precursors of the anti-thyroid compound *goitrin* (5-vinyl-OZT) as well as precursors of nitriles and epithionitriles. Oxazolidine-2-thiones (OZT) other than those formed from progoitrin and epigoitrin are also goitrogenic.

The thyroid-supressing effect of these substances is due to their reducing the incorporation of iodine into the precursors of thyroxine as well as interfering with its secretion.

It has been noted that 0.15 per cent 5-vinyl-OZT in the diet of young chickens causes depression of growth rate, hyperplasia and hypertrophy of the thyroid. In growing pigs, 10-20 per cent rapeseed meal in the diet produces growth depression, hyperplasia of the thyroids and enlargement of the liver and kidneys. Protein bound iodine in the blood serum is reduced and difficulty in conception of gilts can occur. Furthermore, litter size and weight of the pigs at weaning are reduced.

In contrast, ruminants appear to be less susceptible to the toxic effect of glucosinolates compared with pigs and poultry. This is probably the result of the glucosinolates being relatively unhydrolysed in the rumen.

When feed containing goitrogenic substances are fed in excessive quantities but are soaked or cooked in water, the disease (goiter) is much less likely to develop as the cooking process eliminates the enzyme. An adequate supply of iodized salt is another preventive measure specially in areas where non-ruminants consume goitrogenic substances in a large dose. For treatment a daily injection of thyroxine @ 0.1 to 0.3 mg is advocated.

d) *Gossypol*

Gossypoi pigments are polyphenolic compounds found exclusively in the pigment glands of cottonseed. At least 15 such pigments have been identified in extracts of both cottonseed meal and oil, but the most predominant is the yellow ($C_{30}H_{30}O_8$). These pigments can exist either in a free form or as a gossypol-protein complex. Whole seeds contain a total of 1.09-1.53 g/100 g, of which an average of 0.19 g/100 g exists in the free form. Decorticated seeds contain a total of approximately 2 g/100 g, of which 0.15 g/100 g is in the free form.

The physiological effects of free gossypol, in addition to reduced appetite and loss of body weight, include accumulation of fluid in the body cavities, cardiac irregularity, reduced oxygen carrying capacity of the blood and an adverse effect on certain liver enzymes.

Pigs and rabbits appear to be more sensitive than poultry where 0.06 per cent free gossypol in the diet can depress growth in young chickens. In laying birds, 0.15 per cent of free gossypol reduces egg production. In the case of pigs a dietary level of 0.01 per cent reduces growth rate. The toxic effects of gossypol can be overcome by supplementing the diet with iron in the form of ferrous sulphate.

**Table 16**

**Utilisation of cottonseed meal gossypol pigments**

| Species | Maximum level in diet |
|---|---|
| Broilers | 60 ppm free form |
| | 300 ppm with 600 ppm ferrous sulphate |
| Laying hen | 400 ppm with 1600 ,, ,, ,, |
| Breeding hen | 120 ppm free form |
| Pigs | 100 ppm free form |
| | 400 ppm with 400 ,, ,, ,, |

Horses and ruminants appear to be more resistant.

Although heat treatment as in the commercial production of the meal decreases the proportion of free gossypol in favour of the combined form, the availability of lysine in the protein complex is reduced because of the interaction of the aldehyde groups of gossypol with the amino group of lysine.

Varieties with seeds containing less than 0.01 per cent total gossypol (0.002 per cent in the free form) are now available abroad.

**Substances inactivating or increasing the requirements of certain vitamins**

(a) *Anti-vitamin A*

Raw soybeans contain an enzyme *Lipoxygenase*, which catalyses oxidation of carotene, the precursor of vitamin-A. It has been noted that 30 per cent of ground, raw soybeans in the diet of dairy calves produces a sharp lowering of vitamin A and carotene in blood plasma. The enzyme can be destroyed by heating soybeans for 15 minutes with steam at atmospheric pressure.

(b) *Anti-vitamin D*

Rachitogenic activity of isolated soya protein (unheated) has been found with chicks and pigs. The effect could be partially eliminated by increasing the vitamin D in the diet by 8-10 fold. Autoclaving eliminates this rachitogenic activity.

(c) *Anti-vitamin E*

The author while working for his Ph. D. programme at Cornell University in the U.S.A. observed that diets containing raw kidney beans (*Phaseolus vulgaris*) produce muscular dystrophy in lambs by reducing plasma vitamin E. Alcohol extraction of the beans reveals two factors with anti-vitamin E activity, one being alcohol soluble and heat-stable, the other being heat-labile and alcohol-insoluble. By autoclaving beans the anti-vitamin activity is eliminated.

(d) *Anti-vitamin K*

"Sweet clover disease" is characterised by a fatal haemorrhagic condition in cattle and has been known for over 20 years. The active principle responsible for this disease is dicoumarol, which reduces the prothrombin level of the blood, thus interfering with the blood clotting mechanism. The effect is due to reducing vitamin K utilisation in the production of thrombin by the liver.

(e) *Anti-pyridoxine*

It has been demonstrated that the nutritive value of linseed meal for chicks can be considerably improved after extracting the meal with water and autoclaving. An antagonist of pyridoxine, (a member of B vitamins) from linseed which has been identified as 1-amino-D-proline, and occurs naturally in combination with glutamic acid as a peptide is known as *linatine*.

(f) *Mimosine* (*Leucaena leucocephala*)

The plant *Subabul* and some other legumes contain a toxic substance known as *Mimosine* which is a free amino acid, present at about 3 to 5 per cent of the dry matter. The young leaves are comparatively richer in mimosine content.

Livestock grow without any bad effect when fed subabul plant for short durations. On prolong feeding or when it is the sole feed, the animals become the victim of mimosine content.

Among various domestic animals, horses, sheep, pigs and even rabbit are highly sensitive to mimosine and thus they should never be fed with subabul. The main symptoms of mimosine toxicity are reduced growth rate and weight loss, excessive salivation, loss of hair, eroded gum, lesions on tongue, enlarged thyroid gland and poor reproductive efficiency. In adult cattle and buffaloes the mimosine is degreded to 3, 4 dihydroxy pyridone (DPH) by the rumen microbes. Excess DPH is absorbed into the blood stream whereby it reaches to the thyroid gland and thus inhibits further biosynthesis of the hormone thyroxine.

It has been observed that ferrous sulphate in the ration decreases the absorption of DPH. Drying of subabul leaves at high temperature reduces mimosine by 50 per cent.

**Cyanogens**

Cyanide in trace amounts is fairly widespread in the form of glucosides and relatively high levels can be found in certain grasses such as *'jowar* (sorghum) and sudan grass, linseed, maize and cassava root. These plants generally contain cyanogenetic glycosides, which can be hydrolysed to prussic acid by the enzyme usually present in the same plant under a number of conditions during their growing period, or as they are being digested by animals. Maize, linseed, *jowar*, sudan grass may develop toxic levels of prussic acid also known as hydrocyanic acid (HCN) in the new growth that follows either a period of drought, or a period of heavy trampling or physical damage by frost etc. Heavy nitrate fertilisation of the soil followed by an abundant irrigation or rainfall may increase the prussic acid poisoning potential of these crops. Note that the grasses mentioned so far are not abused in any way if growing conditions are favourable.

**Table 17**

MAIN TYPES OF CYANOGENS

| *Glucoside* | *Compounds* | *Source* |
|---|---|---|
| Amygdalin | Glucoside of benzaldehyde cyanohydrin | Almonds |
| Dhurrin | Glucoside of β-hydroxy-benzaldehyde cyanohydrin | Sorghum Grasses |
| Linamarin | Glucoside of acetone cyanohydrin | Cassava |

In plants the glucoside is non-toxic in the intact issues and as stated earlier, when the plants are damaged or begin to decay, hydrolytic enzyme from the same plant is released, liberating HCN. This reaction can take place in the rumen by microbial activity. The HCN is rapidly absorbed and some is eliminated through the lungs, but the greater part is rapidly detoxified in the liver by conversion to thiocyanate. Excess cyanide ion can quickly produce anoxia of the central nervous system through inactivating the cytochrome oxidase system, and death can result within a few seconds. Based on the intensity animals show nervousness, abnormal breathing, trembling or jerking muscles, blue colouration of the lining of the mouth, spasms or convulsions and respiratory failure.

Animals which have not shown much evidence of toxicity may be injected intravenously with 3 g of sodium nitrate and 15 g sodium thiosulphate in 200 ml $H_2O$ for cattle; for sheep, 1 g sodium nitrate and 2.5 g sodium thiosulphate in 50 ml $H_2O$.

Ruminants are more susceptible to HCl poisoning than are horses and pigs, because in the latter two species the enzyme concerned in the release of HCN is destroyed by the gastric HCl.

**Nitrates and nitrites**

Animal forages and drinking water when contaminated with inorganic nitrates and nitrites cause an acute toxicosis in cattle resulting from formation of *methemoglobin* (a true oxidation product of haemoglobin) which is unable to transport oxygen because the iron is in the ferric ($Fe^{+++}$) rather than the usual ferrous ($Fe^{++}$) state. The situation is more common in forages where either nitrogenous fertilizers have been used at a very high dose or the forages have been harvested at a very early stage of their growth. It appears to be a more serious problem in the ruminant since nitrates are reduced to the more toxic nitrites in the rumen. If the amount is not much, nitrite is reduced to ammonia. When excess nitrate is ingested, the toxic nitrite may accumulate and absorbed from the rumen because the activity of nitrate reductase exceeds that of nitrite reductase. The rates of nitrate and nitrite reduction by a given population of ruminal microbes appears to depend upon the supply of fermentable energy sources which supply hydrogen for the reduction. A high dose of concentrates in the daily ration and adequate feeding of Vitamin A have a protective effect.

Symptoms seen in acute toxicity include laboured breathing (dyspena), grinding of the teeth, uneasiness and excessive salivation.

**Moulds and mycotoxins in animal feedstuffs**

A mycotoxin is a fungal metabolite causing pathological or physiological changes in man or animals. Mycotoxin poisoning is well known to affect many farm animals. Symptoms depend on the amount of toxin in the feed, the period for which the feed is ingested, the nutritional status of the feed and the susceptibility of the animal.

Mycotoxins can be produced at any stage from the growing crop to the formulated feed. The greatest potential for mould spoilage and mycotoxin production is in the growing crop or stored raw material. The stressing of plants by drought often results in cracked seeds favouring insect infestation. Thus the protective outer layer of the grains gets damaged and endogenous mould spores present within the grains or kernels are given access to oxygen, moisture and nutrients leading to mould growth. A wet period around harvest may result in the crop being harvested at a high moisture favouring mould growth and thereby toxin production. One of the greatest potentials for mould growth and mycotoxin production is the storage of inadequately dried products and rewelting of dried and stored products. Rewelting may occur by rain during shipment of finished products to the consumers place.

To prevent or minimise the exposure of animals to mycotoxins good quality fungus-free viable seed should be used, with the minimal mechanical damage during planting and harvesting. Insecticides and fungicides should be applied correctly and when necessary. The harvested crop must be adequately dried and correctly stored, with preservatives applied carefully. Special precautions should be taken to prevent welting from rain leakage during shipment.

The three most important types of mycotoxins are: (1) aflatoxins, (2) ochratoxin A and (3) zearalenone.

## Aflatoxin

Aflatoxins are common term used for a group of toxins which differ in their chemical structure and in intensity of producing toxic effects. As the various compounds of this group are produced by the fungi *Aspergillus flavus* and *A. parasiticus* they resemble very much to each other and are commonly termed Aflatoxins. The structures of similar compounds named as $B_1$, $M_1$, $B_2$, $G_1$, $G_2$ are given in the next page.

The production of toxins by the above two fungi depends on the following conditions:

1. The strain of the fungus,
2. The nature of the substrate,
3. The temperature and humidity of the environment immediately surrounding the area of mould growth.

A toxin producing strain of Aspergillus will produce one or more member of the aflatoxins when moisture content of a suitable substrate is in equilibrium with a relative humidity of greater than 85 per cent and the temperature is between 12° to 42°C. The optimum temperature of the aflatoxins is around 27°C.

Some aflatoxins are acutely toxic to a wide range of animals. About 25 µg of aflatoxin $B_1$ will almost certainly kill a day old duckling.

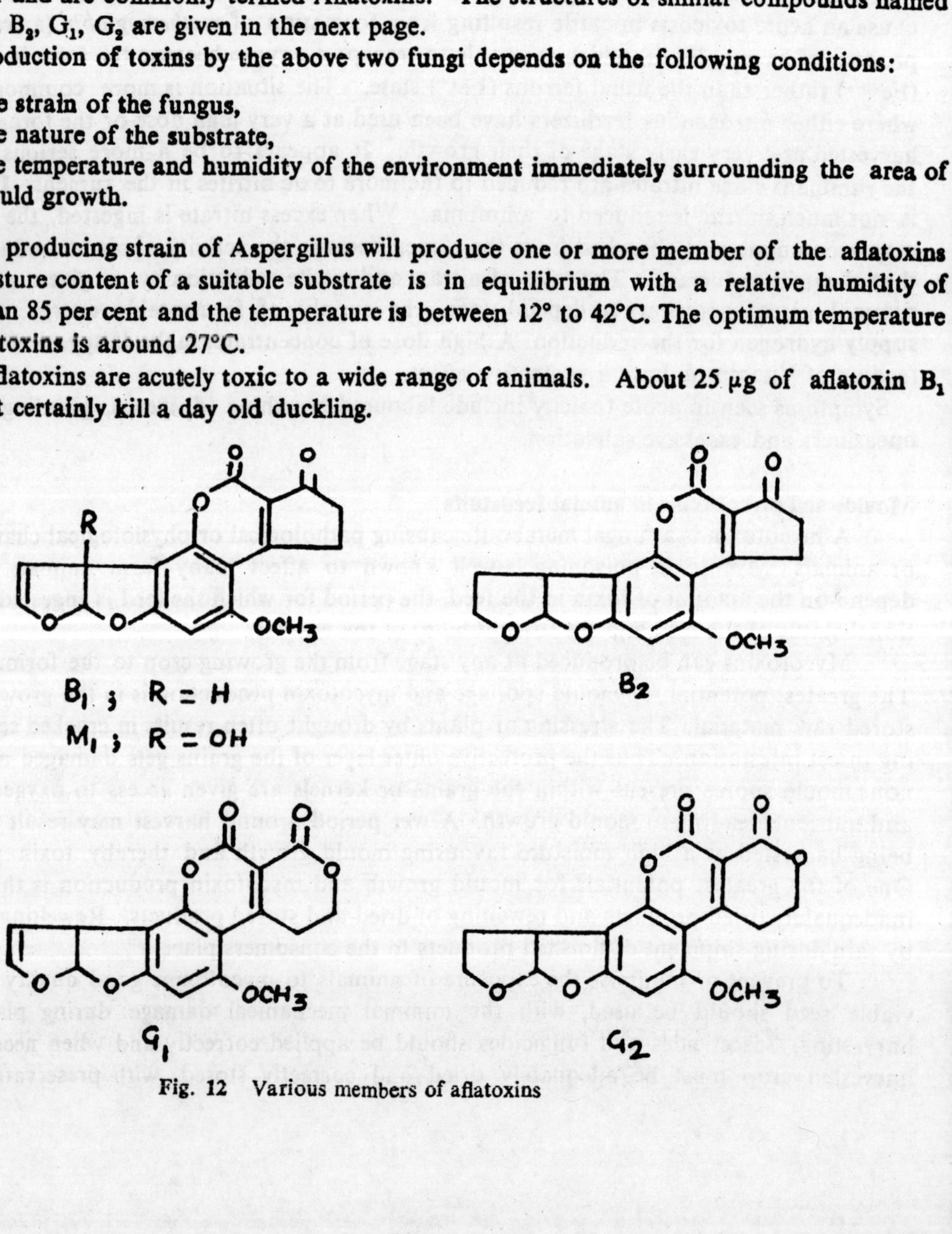

$B_1$ ; R = H
$M_1$ ; R = OH

$B_2$

$G_1$

$G_2$

Fig. 12 Various members of aflatoxins

**The aflatoxins $B_1$, $B_2$ and $G_1$ produce liver cell carcinomas in experimental animals. Aflatoxin $B_1$ is the most potent hepatocarcinogen and can produce liver cancer in rats. Malignant tumours have also been produced by $B_1$ in non-human primates. Although chickens appear to be fairly insensitive to acute toxic effects of the aflatoxins, outbreaks of *aflatoxicosis* have been reported where large amounts of aflatoxins have accidentally been fed to chickens. In general, the consumption of contaminated feed by an animal may result in an unhealthy situation comprising liver damage with marked bile duct proliferation and a decrease production or even in its death. However, the presence of the aflatoxins in feed can also result in deposition of these toxins or their metabolites in the animal meat or in their products (egg, milk etc). If these are consumed as human food, the presence of toxins could represent a human health problem.**

**Table 18**

FEED INGREDIENTS WITH DEMONSTRATED NATURAL CONTAMINATION BY AFLATOXIN

| | |
|---|---|
| Corn (stored and field) | Malt sprouts |
| Peanut meal | Soyabean meal |
| Cottonseed (processed and field) | Sunflower seed meal |
| Copra | Safflower meal |
| Rye | Rapeseed |
| Oats | Rice bran |
| Sorghum | Linseed meal |
| Wheat | Alfalfa |
| Barley | Cocoa cake |
| Millet | Sugar scrap |
| Sesame cake | Palm kernel |
| Cassava | Pumpkin seeds |
| | Sheanut |

**Table 19**

SOME EXAMPLES OF DIETARY AFLATOXIN CONCENTRATIONS WHICH HAVE CAUSED TOXICOSIS IN FARM ANIMALS

| *Species* | *Age* | *Aflatoxin content* (mg/kg; ppm) | *Duration of feeding* | *Effects* |
|---|---|---|---|---|
| Calf | Weanling | 0.2–2.2 | 16 weeks | Stunting, death, liver damage |
| Steer | 2 years | 0.2–0.7 | 20 weeks | Liver damage |
| Cow | 2 years | 2.4 | 7 months | Liver damage |
| Pig | Newborn | 0.23 | 4 days | Stunting |
| Pig | 2 weeks | 0.17 | 23 days | Anorexia, stunting, jaundice |
| Pig | 4–6 weeks | 0.4–0.7 | 3–6 months | Stunting, liver damage |
| Chicken | 1+ weeks | 0.8 | 10 weeks | Stunting, liver damage |
| Duck | Unknown | 0.3 | 6 weeks | Liver damage, death |

## Ochratoxin A

Ochratoxin A is a mycotoxin produced by species of the genera *Aspergillus* and *Penicillium.* The toxin affects the proximal kidney tubules, causing nephropathy in pigs and poultry. On slaughter, the kidneys are larger, lighter in colour and firmer than normal.

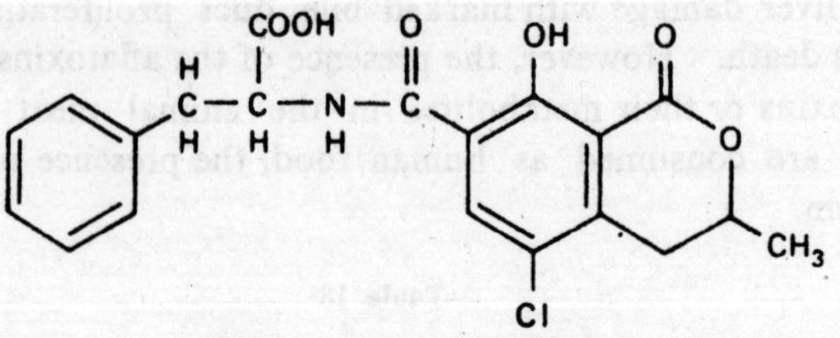

**Fig. 13** Structure of ochratoxin A

**Table 20**

**Feed ingredient found contaminated with ochratoxin A**

| | |
|---|---|
| Barley grains | Linseed meal |
| Oats grains | Soybean meal |
| Wheat grains | Rice bran |
| Maize grains | |

**Table 21**

**Symptoms of ochratoxin a toxicosis in chicken**

| Level in the feed (mg/kg) | Symptoms observed |
|---|---|
| <0.5 | Diarrhoea, soiled eggs |
| 0.5 | Decreased egg production |
| 1.0 | Decreased egg size |
| | Decreased growth rate |
| 2.0 | Body weight reduced |
| 4.0 | High morbidity |

## Zearalenone

Zearalenone is an oestrogenic mycotoxin produced by several *Fusarium* species and occurs frequently on many agricultural commodities. Pigs, in particular, are sensitive to the oestrogenic effects of zearalenone. The consumption of a ration containing 1-5 mg/kg of zearalenone rapidly results in a whole host of oestrogenic symptoms as below:

(1) Swollen and enlarged vulva.
(2) Vaginal and rectal prolapse.

(3) Precocious enlargement of mammary glands.
(4) Reduced testis size in young males.
(5) Shrunken ovaries in young females.

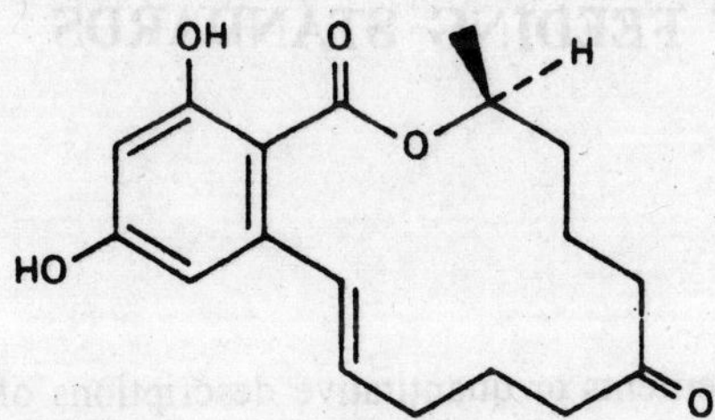


Fig. 14 Structure of zearalenone

(6) Enlarged, oedematus and tortuous uterus.
(7) Infertility and abortion.
(8) Reduced litter size.
(9) Stillborn, weak and splayleg piglets.

# 10

# DEVELOPMENT OF FEEDING STANDARDS

Feeding standards are statements or quantitative descriptions of the amounts of one or more nutrients needed by animals.

Since the beginning of the nineteeth century, the scientists of the world started formulating some standards for feeding livestock, and as such with the advancement of science the standards were developed from time to time. For convenience all such standards are grouped under major headings on the basis of the principles of the standards. They are: (a) comparative type; (b) digestible nutrient system; and (c) production value type, which are discussed below.

Feeding standards usually are expressed in quantities of nutrients required/day or as a percentage of diet, the former being used for animals given exact quantities of a diet and the latter more commonly when rations are fed ad libitum.

## A. COMPARATIVE TYPE

### 1. Hay standard

In 1810 German scientist Thaer suggested that different feeds should be compared using meadow hay as a unit. This standard provided that 100 lbs. of meadow hay was equal in nutritive value to 91 lbs. of clover hay or 200 lbs. of potatoes, 625 lbs. of mangels. Nothing was known of the chemical value of these feeds and the physiological requirements of the animals. The only measure was the practical feeding experience.

### 2. Scandinavian "feed unit" standard

In 1884, Professor Fjord formulated the Scandinavian feeding standard. In this system only one factor, namely, the feed unit was taken into account. The value of one pound of common grain such as corn, barley, or wheat, is given as one unit value and the value of all other foods is based upon this. According to this standard one feed unit is required for each 150 lbs. of body weight and an additional unit for every three pounds of milk production.

Later on it was suggested that in the food unit the ration should also include 0.065 lb. of digestible protein for every 100 lbs. of body weight and 0.05 lb. digestible protein for each pound of milk produced.

This system is somewhat similar to the feeding value of Thaer where he used meadow hays instead of grains.

As the grains are of different types in different countries, the feed units should also be different. Hence the Scandinavian units are not applicable in our country unless experiments are conducted here with our own grains.

## B. DIGESTIBLE NUTRIENT SYSTEM

**1. Grouven's feeding standard**

In 1859 Grouven, a German chemist published his feeding standard with crude protein, carbohydrates and fat contained in the feed as the basis of the standard. According to this standard a cow weighing 1,000 lbs. should be fed 28.7 lbs. of dry matter containing 2.67 lbs. of crude protein, 0.6 lb. of crude fat and 14.55 lbs. of crude carbohydrates.

Very soon after the standard of Grouven, Henneberg and Stohaan found that the total

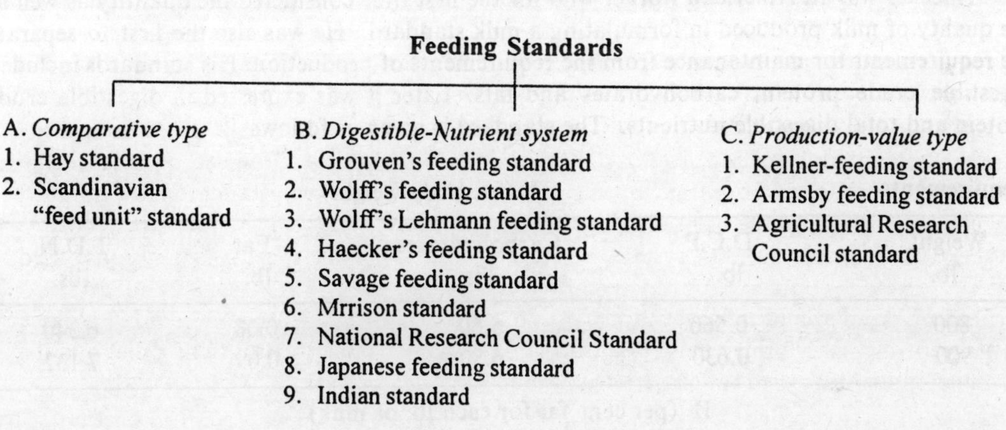


nutrients contained in a feed did not form an accurate guide to its value. The proportion of digestible parts varied with different feeds and hence the digestible nutrients would be more valuable. So due to this defect Grouven's feeding standard is now abandoned.

Feeding Standards
A. *Comparative type*
1. Hay standard
2. Scandinavian "feed unit" standard
B. *Digestible-Nutrient system*
1. Grouven's feeding standard
2. Wolff's feeding standard
3. Wolff's Lehmann feeding standard
4. Haecker's feeding standard
5. Savage feeding standard
6. Mrrison standard
7. National Research Council Standard
8. Japanese feeding standard
9. Indian standard
C. *Production-value type*
1. Kellner-feeding standard
2. Armsby feeding standard
3. Agricultural Research Council standard

**2. Wolff's feeding standard**

In 1864 Dr. Emil Von Wolff proposed a standard on digestible protein, digestible carbohydrates and digestible fats contained in a feeding stuff. His standard for dairy cows weighing 1,000 lbs. was 24.5 lbs. of dry matter containing 2.5 lbs. of digestible carbohydrates and 0.4 lb. of digestible fats. This has a nutritive ratio of 1 : 5.4. This standard though an improvement over the standard of Grouven, yet it does not consider the quantity and quality of milk produced.

**3. Wolff's Lehmann feeding standard**

Dr. G. Lehmann of Berlin modified Wolff's standard in 1896. Till then Wolff's standard was in use. He took into account the quantity of milk produced, but he failed to take into account the quality of milk. The requirements of a cow with a body weight of 1,000 lbs. as fixed by this standard, for maintenance and maintenance-cum-milk production are given separately below·

| *For maintenance only* | | *For production and maintenance* (A 1,000 pound cow giving 11 lbs. of milk daily) | |
|---|---|---|---|
| 1. Dry matter | 18 lb. | 1. Dry matter | 25 lb. |
| 2. Crude protein | 0.7 " | 2. Crude protein | 1.6 " |
| 3. Fat | 0.1 " | 3. Fat | 0.3 " |
| 4. Carbohydrates | 8.0 " | 4. Carbohydrates | 10.0 " |

**4. Haecker's feeding standard**

Haecker was an American worker who for the first time considered the quantity as well as the quality of milk produced in formulating a milk standard. He was also the first to separate the requirements for maintenance from the requirements of production. His standards included digestible crude protein, carbohydrates and fats. Later it was expressed in digestible crude protein and total digestible nutrients. The standard is given as follows:

| Requirements | | I (for body weight) | | |
|---|---|---|---|---|
| Weight lb. | D.C.P lb. | Carbohydrates lbs. | Fat lb. | T.D.N. lbs. |
| 800 | 0.560 | 5.60 | 0.08 | 6.340 |
| 900 | 0.630 | 6.30 | 0.09 | 7.132 |
| | | II (per cent fat for each lb. of milk) | | |
| Fat% | | | | |
| 3.0 | 0.047 | 0.20 | 0.017 | 0.285 |
| 4.0 | 0.054 | 0.24 | 0.021 | 0.341 |

**5. Savage feeding standard**

Another American scientist Savage came to the conclusion that the Haecker standard was too low especially in protein. He suggested that in case of milking cows at least 24 lbs. of dry matter should be provided for an average cow. The nutritive ratio should not be wider than 1 : 6 or narrower than 1 : 4.5. About two-thirds of the dry matter should be from the roughages and one-third from the concentrates. Therefore, the protein requirement was increased about 20 per cent above the standard of Haecker. According to this standard for maintenance of 1,000 lbs. cow the requirement of D.C.P. and T.D.N. was 0.700 and 7.925 lb. respectively. In addition for every pound of milk having different fat percentages each had specific recommendations.

**6. Morrison feeding standard**

Morrison F.B. observed stockmen spending large sums of money for entirely unnecessary amounts on protein supplement, thus considerably reducing their profits. He therefore, endeavoured to combine in one set of standards what seem in the judgement to be the best guide available in computation of rations for the various classes of stock. These standards were first persented in the 15th edition of "Feeds and Feeding" published in 1915 and were then called "Modified Wolff and Lehmann standard". They soon came to be known as the Morrison Feeding standard". These standards have expressed in terms of Dry Matter (D.M.), Digestible Proteins (D.P.) and Total Digestibile Nutrients (T.D.N.)

In 1936 the standards were revised. For those who desired to use net energy values instead of T.D.N. in computing rations, net energy allowances in therms were also included.

Again in 1948 with further addition to the knowledge, more changes were made in the standards.

In the year 1956, Morrison included in the standard the allowances for Calcium, Phosphorus and Carotene besides digestible carbohydrates, digestible proteins and net energy in therms. The average of Morrison's standards has been accepted for Indian livestock which are given ahead under the heading "*Feeding Standards for Cattle*" (see page 140 – 141 ).

**7. National Research Council (N.R.C.) standard**

A sub-committee of the committee on animal nutrition of the National Research Council recommended a nutrient allowance for dairy cattle which was first published in 1945 with the latest revision in 1971. The requirements are quite similar to those of the Morrison standard and are based on the size of the animal.

The standard includes digestible protein and total digestible nutrients and also includes the recommended requirements for calcium, phosphorus, carotene and vitamin D for dairy cattle, beef cattle, pigs, poultry, sheep, dogs, horses, laboratory animals etc. It is believed that these N.R.C. reports representing in each case the pooled judgement of a group of experts in the field of species in question. Today in a number of countries N.R.C. standards are followed where they use ME for poultry, DE for swine and horses, DE, ME and TDN for sheep, ME, TDN and $NE_m$ and $NE_g$ for beef cattle and, for dairy cattle, values are given for DE, ME, TDN, $NE_m$ and $NE_g$ for growing animals with additional values as $NE_l$ for lactating cows. From time to time, the NRC revises these feeding standards in keeping with new information and changing feeding practices.

**Table 22**

**MANNER IN WHICH ENERGY REQUIREMENTS ARE EXPRESSED IN THE NRC FEEDING STANDARD**

| Livestock | Total Digestible Energy (TDN) | Gross Energy (GE) | Digestible Energy (DE) | Metabolizable Energy (ME) | Net Energy Maintenance ($NE_m$) | Net Energy Growth ($NE_g$) | Net Energy Lactation ($NE_{lac}$) |
|---|---|---|---|---|---|---|---|
| Beef cattle ......... | Yes | No | No | Yes | Yes | Yes | No |
| Dairy cattle ........ | Yes | No | Yes | Yes | Yes | Yes | Yes |
| Sheep ............ | Yes | No | Yes | Yes | No | No | No |
| Swine ............ | No | No | Yes | Yes | No | No | No |
| Poultry ........... | No | No | No | Yes | No | No | No |
| Horses ........... | No | No | Yes | No | No | No | No |
| Rabbits ........... | Yes | No | No | No | No | No | No |
| Mink and foxes .... | No | Yes | No | No | No | No | No |
| Fish[1] (trout, salmon, and catfish) ...... | No | No | No | No | No | No | No |

[1]No energy requirements have been established for fish by the NRC.

**8. Japanese feeding standards for dairy cattle**

The recently revised standard is presented below:

**Table 23**

| Fat content of milk % | Digestible protein gm | TDN gm | DE Mcal | ME Mcal | Energy in milk | Milk ME % Util. |
|---|---|---|---|---|---|---|
| Nutrients/kg milk[2] | | | | | | |
| 3.0 | 42.8 | 242 | 1.06 | 0.87 | 0.605 | |
| 3.5 | 44.5 | 263 | 1.15 | 0.95 | 0.660 | |
| 4.0 | 46.4 | 268 | 1.25 | 1.03 | 0.716 | 69.2 |
| 4 5 | 50 2 | 308 | 1.35 | 1.11 | 0.771 | |
| 5.0 | 53.0 | 330 | 1.44 | 1.19 | 0.826 | |
| 5.5 | 55.9 | 352 | 1.54 | 1.27 | 0.181 | |
| 6.0 | 58.7 | 373 | 1.63 | 1.35 | 0.935 | |

1. Maintenance requirements based on live weight raised to the 0.75 power. Maintenance=37.37 g TDN/kg or 116.3 kcal ME/kg (equivalent to 0.58 lb dig. protein. 8.1 lb TDN or 11.4 Mcal ME per 1,000 lb cow).
2. For milk production, nutrient requirements were calculated on the basis of 154 parts dig. protein per 100 parts milk protein, and 1,444 kcal ME per 1,000 kcal milk energy. The same factors for converting ME to DE and TDN as used by the NRC were used in the calculations, i.e. 1.640 kcal ME/lb TDN or 3.61 Mcal ME/kg TDN, and 2,000 kcal DE/lb TDN.

**9. Indian standards**

India has been almost entirely dependent on standards drawn up by Late F.B. Morrison of Cornell University in U.S.A. Dr. K.C. Sen, the first Director, National Dairy Research Institute, Bangalore and Karnal has compiled the feeding standards based on Morrison's recommendation where he adopted the average of maximum and minimum values recommended by Morrison. Standards have been presented in Tables, 24 – 29.

These modified values are still functioning in many of our established dairy farms.

Considering the fact that nutrient needs of livestock and poultry breeds under tropical environments are different from those developed in temperate climate, the Indian Council of Agricultural Research realising the necessity of setting up suitable feeding standards for the Indian livestock and poultry, assigned this task to the Late Dr. N.D. Kehar, the then Chairman, I.C.A.R. Scientific Panel on Animal Nutrition and Physiology, as he had been associated with this type of research activities for about two decades. The Scientific Panel set up sub-committees for each species by inviting experts from various institutes of the country. On the basis of the scientific information arising from experimental work carried out in India over the past two decades, nutrient requirements of Indian livestock and poultry ultimately been published by I.C.A.R. in January 1985 under the able Chairmanship of the Panel Dr. K. Prodhan, Hariana Agricultural University, which will no doubt form a strong basis for judicious feeding of our livestock and poultry with a scope for further revision wherever newer data on nutritional requirements become available.

Standards have been presented in the Table 30 – 42.

## C. PRODUCTION VALUE TYPE

### 1. Kellner feeding standard

In 1907 Kellner, a German scientist, investigated a feeding standard based upon "Starch" as the unit of measurement. He took into account not only the digestibility of the feeds as calculated from the amount lost in faeces and urine but also the entire loss from the body including energy expended in digestion and passing the food inside the body (chewing, etc.). For measuring the amount of energy lost from the body as heat, Kellner devised a respiration apparatus. Here heat is determined indirectly by finding the amount of carbon dioxide gas liberated or by measuring the amount of oxygen gas used up in oxidation which take place in the body. The animal breathes through an airtight mask placed over its nose and mouth.

According to this system, a 1,000 lbs animal needs 0.6 lb of digestible protein and 6.35 lbs of starch equivalent. This starch equivalent in turn can be converted into heat energy by a method worked out by Armsby and Kellner.

Any of the feeds the composition of which is known may be converted to starch equivalent by using the following factors:

| | | |
|---|---|---|
| Dig. protein | × 0.94 | = S.E. |
| Fat from coarse fodder | × 2.1 | = S.E. |
| Fat from cereal grain | × 2.1 | = S.E. |
| Fat from oil seeds | × 2.4 | = S.E. |
| Dig. carbohydrates and fibre | × 1.0 | = S.E. |

### 2. Armsby feeding standard

Armsby standard is based on true protein and net energy values. By means of the respiration calorimeter, Armsby determined the net energy required for mastication, digestion, assimilation and also the amount of heat and gases given off through the excretory channels. Thus after considering the various losses of energy such as in urine, faeces, gases and in the work of digestion, he was able to estimate the amount of net energy available for productive purposes. Armsby expresses his standard in two factors, that is true protein and therms of net energy.

A common criticism of the Armsby standard is that the expense of determining requirements of the animals and the net energy in the various feeds is excessively high. The net energy values of only a very few feeds has actually been determined, and most of the values have been computed from the Table of Morrison's digestible nutrients. Armsby standard is not as widely used as are the standards based on digestible nutrients.

### 3. Agricultural Research Council (A.R.C.) standard

The nutritive requirement of various livestock in the United Kingdom have been presented in Ministry of Agriculture's Bulletins. These are prepared by the Technical Committee of the Agricultural Research Council of Britain. Requirements are set forth in three separate reports dealing with poultry, ruminants and pigs, each of these reports extensive summaries of the literature upon which the requirements are based. The most attractive feature of the British Feeding Standards is that the unit of energy requirements has been expressed in terms of Starch equivalent instead of T.D.N. or ME or NE as are in Morrison and in N.R.C. Standards.

# FEEDING STANDARDS FOR CATTLE

## Modified Morrison's Standard

**Table 24**

**Daily nutrient requirements of a calf growing at the rate of 0.5 kg per day during first two years and reaching adult body weight at the age of approximately 3 years**

| *Body wt. (kg)* | *DCP (kg)* | *Energy* | | *Ca (g)* | *P (g)* | *Vitamin A (I.U.)* |
|---|---|---|---|---|---|---|
| | | *T.D.N. (kg)* | *ME (kcal)* | | | |
| 45 | 0.17 | 0.9 | 3290 | 7 | 6 | 2000 |
| 70 | 0.22 | 1.3 | 4680 | 12 | 10 | 3000 |
| 100 | 0.28 | 1.9 | 6900 | 13 | 10 | 4000 |
| 150 | 0.35 | 2.6 | 9360 | 13 | 12 | 6500 |
| 200 | 0.40 | 3.0 | 11500 | 13 | 12 | 8500 |
| 300 | 0.47 | 4.0 | 12600 | 13 | 12 | 12,500 |
| 450 | 0.48 | 5.0 | 13600 | 12 | 12 | 17,000 |

**Table 25**

**Daily maintenance requirement of dairy stock**

| *Body wt. (kg)* | *DCP (kg)* | *Energy* | | *Ca (g)* | *P (g)* | *Carotene (mg)* |
|---|---|---|---|---|---|---|
| | | *TDN (kg)* | *ME (kcal)* | | | |
| 250 | 0.168 | 2.02 | 7.27 | 6 | 6 | 27 |
| 300 | 0.197 | 2.36 | 8.50 | 7 | 7 | 32 |
| 350 | 0.277 | 2.70 | 9.72 | 8 | 8 | 37 |
| 400 | 0.254 | 3.03 | 10.91 | 9 | 9 | 42 |
| 450 | 0.282 | 3.37 | 12.13 | 10 | 10 | 47 |
| 500 | 0.296 | 3.64 | 13.28 | 11 | 11 | 52 |
| 550 | 0.336 | 4.00 | 14.40 | 12 | 12 | 57 |

**Table 26**

**Requirement for production of 1 kg of milk (to be added to requirement for maintenance and also for growth if any).**

| *Fat content of milk %* | *DCP (kg)* | *Energy* | | *Ca (g)* | *P (g)* |
|---|---|---|---|---|---|
| | | *TDN (kg)* | *ME (kcal)* | | |
| 3.0 | 0.040 | 0.27 | 0.97 | 2.0 | 1.4 |
| 3.5 | 0.042 | 0.29 | 1.04 | 2.0 | 1.4 |
| 4.0 | 0.045 | 0.32 | 1.15 | 2.0 | 1.4 |
| 4.5 | 0.048 | 0.34 | 1.22 | 2.0 | 1.4 |
| 5.5 | 0.051 | 0.36 | 1.30 | 2.0 | 1.4 |
| 6.0 | 0.057 | 0.41 | 1.41 | 2.0 | 1.4 |
| 7.5 | 0.063 | 0.46 | 1.66 | 2.0 | 1.4 |

**Table 27**

**Nutrients required for working bullocks per head per day**

| *Body wt. (kg)* | *Normal work* | | | *Heavy work* | | |
|---|---|---|---|---|---|---|
| | *DCP (kg)* | *TDN (kg)* | *M.E. (Mcal)* | *DCP (kg)* | *TDN (kg)* | *M.E. (Mcal)* |
| 300 | 0.33 | 3.1 | 11.2 | 0.42 | 4.0 | 14.4 |
| 400 | 0.45 | 4.0 | 14.4 | 0.52 | 4.8 | 17.2 |
| 500 | 0.56 | 4.9 | 17.6 | 0.71 | 6.4 | 23.1 |

**Table 28**

**Feeding standards for a bull in service**

| *Body wt. (kg)* | *DCP (kg)* | *TDN (kg)* | *ME (kcal)* | *Ca (g)* | *P (g)* | *Vit. A (I.U.)* |
|---|---|---|---|---|---|---|
| 500 | 0.43 | 4.5 | 16.2 | 12 | 12 | 21200 |
| 600 | 0.48 | 5.1 | 18.2 | 14 | 14 | 25400 |
| 700 | 0.54 | 5.7 | 20.5 | 15 | 15 | 29600 |
| 800 | 0.60 | 6.3 | 22.5 | 18 | 18 | 33800 |

**Table 29**

**Additional requirement from 5th month of pregnancy (to be added with maintenance allowances)**

DCP (kg): 0.14 TDN (kg): 0.70

# Indian standards

## Nutrient Requirements of Cattle and Buffaloes

**Members of the sub-committee**

1. Dr. S.P. Arora, NDRI
2. Dr. V.N. Murty, IVRI
3. Dr. S.S. Negi, IVRI
4. Dr. G.V. Raghavan, APAU, Hyderabad.

**Table 30**

**Nutrient requirements of growing cattle**
**(Growth rate 550 g/day)**

| Live Weight (kg) | DM (kg) | DCP (g) | TDN (kg) | Ca (g) | P (g) |
|---|---|---|---|---|---|
| 70 | 2.10 | 259 | 1.39 | 8 | 5 |
| 80 | 2.33 | 282 | 1.53 | 9 | 6 |
| 100 | 2.78 | 328 | 1.80 | 12 | 9 |
| 120 | 3.23 | 373 | 2.07 | 15 | 11 |
| 140 | 3.67 | 419 | 2.34 | 17 | 12 |
| 150 | 3.90 | 442 | 2.47 | 20 | 13 |
| 160 | 4.12 | 463 | 2.61 | 20 | 13 |
| 180 | 4.57 | 510 | 2.88 | 20 | 13 |
| 200 | 5.02 | 556 | 3.14 | 20 | 13 |
| 220 | 5.47 | 601 | 3.41 | 22 | 15 |
| 240 | 5.97 | 647 | 3.68 | 25 | 17 |

**Table 31**

**Nutrient requirements of growing buffaloes**
**(Growth rate 450 g/day)**

| Live Weight (kg) | DM (kg) | TDN (kg) |
|---|---|---|
| 70 | 1.97 | 1.24 |
| 80 | 2.20 | 1.38 |
| 100 | 2.65 | 1.64 |
| 120 | 3.10 | 1.91 |
| 140 | 3.56 | 2.18 |
| 160 | 4.01 | 2.45 |
| 180 | 4.46 | 2.72 |
| 200 | 4.21 | 2.98 |
| 220 | 5.36 | 3.25 |

Table 32

**Nutrient Requirements for maintenance of cattle and buffaloes**

| Live Weight (kg) | DM (kg) | DCP (g) | TDN (kg) | Ca (g) | P (g) |
|---|---|---|---|---|---|
| 250 | 4-5 | 140 | 2.20 | 25 | 17 |
| 300 | 5-6 | 168 | 2.65 | 25 | 17 |
| 350 | 6-7 | 195 | 3.10 | 25 | 17 |
| 400 | 7-8 | 223 | 3.55 | 28 | 20 |
| 450 | 8-9 | 250 | 4.00 | 31 | 23 |
| 500 | 9-10 | 278 | 4.45 | 31 | 23 |
| 550 | 10-11 | 310 | 4.90 | 31 | 23 |
| 600 | 11-12 | 336 | 5.35 | 31 | 23 |

Table 33

**Nutrient requirements per kg of milk production**

| Fat (%) | DCP (g) | TDN (g) |
|---|---|---|
| 3.0 | 48 | 275 |
| 3.5 | 51 | 300 |
| 4.0 | 55 | 325 |
| 4.5 | 58 | 350 |
| 5.0 | 62 | 375 |
| 5.5 | 65 | 400 |
| 6.0 | 68 | 425 |
| 6.7 | 72 | 450 |
| 7.0 | 75 | 475 |
| 7.5 | 79 | 500 |

*Note*: 2.8 g calcium and 2 g phosphorus should be provided per kg of milk produced.

## Nutrient Requirements of Sheep

**Members of the sub-committee**

1. Dr. B.C. Patnayak, CSWRI
2. Dr. C.S. Mathur, University of Udaipur, Bikaner
3. Dr. P.T. Rakshi

**Table 34**

**Nutrient requirements for growing lambs**

| Live Weight (kg) | Rate of gain (g/day) | DM (g) | DCP (g) | TDN (g) | Ca (g) | P (g) |
|---|---|---|---|---|---|---|
| 10 | 50 | 400 | 35 | 220 | 2.0 | 1.5 |
| | 100 | 450 | 45 | 280 | 2.5 | 1.5 |
| | 150 | 500 | 55 | 340 | 3.0 | 2.0 |
| 15 | 50 | 500 | 45 | 300 | 2.8 | 2.0 |
| | 100 | 600 | 55 | 360 | 3.5 | 2.5 |
| | 150 | 700 | 65 | 450 | 4.5 | 3.0 |
| 20 | 50 | 700 | 50 | 400 | 3.5 | 2.5 |
| | 100 | 800 | 70 | 520 | 4.5 | 3.0 |
| | 150 | 1,000 | 80 | 640 | 5.5 | 3.6 |
| 25 | 50 | 800 | 65 | 500 | 4.0 | 3.0 |
| | 100 | 1,100 | 85 | 700 | 5.0 | 3.5 |
| | 150 | 1,200 | 100 | 800 | 6.0 | 4.0 |

**Table 35**

**Nutrient requirements for maintenance of adult sheep**

| Live Weight (kg) | DM (g) | DCP (g) | TDN (g) | Ca (g) | P (g) |
|---|---|---|---|---|---|
| 20 | 500 | 25 | 240 | 3.0 | 1.8 |
| 25 | 625 | 30 | 300 | 3.2 | 2.0 |
| 30 | 750 | 32 | 360 | 3.5 | 2.5 |
| 35 | 875 | 35 | 420 | 4.0 | 2.8 |
| 40 | 1000 | 40 | 480 | 4.5 | 3.0 |
| 45 | 1125 | 42 | 500 | 5.0 | 3.5 |
| 50 | 1250 | 45 | 540 | 5.5 | 3.8 |
| 55 | 1375 | 50 | 600 | 6.0 | 4.0 |
| 60 | 1450 | 54 | 640 | 6.5 | 4.5 |

## Nutrient Requirements of Goat

**Members of the sub-committee**

1. Dr. S.N. Singh, RBSC, Agra
2. Dr. Kedar Nath, IVRI
3. Dr. M. Shivaraman, KAU

Table 36

**Nutrient requirements of kids**
**(Growth rate 50 g/day)**

| Live weight (kg) | DM (g) | DCP (g) | TDN (g) | Ca (g) | P (g) |
|---|---|---|---|---|---|
| 10 | 425 | 25 | 275 | 1.8 | 1.1 |
| 15 | 600 | 30 | 350 | 2.0 | 1.2 |
| 20 | 700 | 35 | 400 | 2.4 | 1.4 |
| 25 | 800 | 40 | 450 | 2.6 | 1.5 |
| 30 | 950 | 45 | 500 | 2.9 | 1.6 |

Table 37

**Nutrient requirements for maintenance of goats**

| Live weight (kg) | DM (g) | DCP (g) | TDN (g) | Ca (g) | P (g) |
|---|---|---|---|---|---|
| 30 | 900 | 35 | 400 | 2 0 | 1.0 |
| 40 | 1200 | 40 | 500 | 2.5 | 1.2 |
| 50 | 1400 | 45 | 560 | 2.7 | 1.4 |
| 60 | 1600 | 55 | 670 | 3.0 | 1.6 |
| 70 | 1800 | 60 | 760 | 3.5 | 1.8 |

## Nutrient Requirements of Camels

**Member of the sub-committee**
Dr. C.S. Mathur, Bikaner

Table 38

**Nutrient requirements of growing camels**
**(Growth rate 100 g/day)**

| Live weight (kg) | DM (kg) | DCP (g) | TDN (g) | Ca (g) | P (g) |
|---|---|---|---|---|---|
| 200 | 5.0 | 250 | 2,000 | 80 | 30 |
| 250 | 6.0 | 325 | 2,500 | 100 | 35 |
| 300 | 7.5 | 350 | 3,000 | 120 | 50 |
| 350 | 9.0 | 470 | 3,800 | 145 | 60 |
| 400 | 10.0 | 600 | 4,700 | 185 | 80 |
| 450 | 10.5 | 650 | 5,000 | 200 | 100 |

Table 39

Nutrient requirements for maintenance of camels

| Live weight (kg) | DM (kg) | DCP (g) | TDN (g) | Ca (g) | P (g) |
|---|---|---|---|---|---|
| 500 | 12.0 | 500 | 5,500 | 300 | 100 |
| 550 | 13.0 | 525 | 6,000 | 225 | 120 |
| 600 | 14.0 | 550 | 6,500 | 250 | 150 |
| 650 | 15.0 | 600 | 7,000 | 250 | 150 |
| 700 | 16.5 | 650 | 7,500 | 250 | 150 |

## Nutrient Requirements of Poultry

**Members of the sub-committee**

1. Dr. P.V. Rao, APAU
2. Dr. R.C. Khera
3. Dr. C.V. Reddy, APAU
4. Dr. S.P. Netke, JNKVV
5. Dr. B. Panda, CARI

Table 40

Nutrient content of diets for broiler, layer and breeder

| Nutrient | Broiler | | Layer | | | Breeder |
|---|---|---|---|---|---|---|
| | Starter | Finisher | Starter | Finisher | Laying | |
| Metabolizable energy (kcal/kg) | 2,900 | 2,900 | 2,700 | 2,500 | 2,850 | 2,850 |
| C.P. (%) | 24 | 19 | 20 | 16 | 17 | 17 |
| Linoleic acid (%) | 1 | 1 | 1 | 1 | 1 | 1 |
| *Minerals* | | | | | | |
| Calcium (%) | 1.0 | 1.0 | 1.0 | 1.0 | 3.5 | 3.5 |
| Available P (%) | 0.45 | 0.45 | 0.45 | 0.45 | 0.5 | 0.5 |
| Sodium (%) | 0.2 | 0.2 | 0.2 | 0.2 | 0.2 | 0.2 |
| Potassium (%) | 0.4 | 0.4 | 0.4 | 0.4 | 0.4 | 0.4 |
| Manganese (%) | 70 | 70 | 70 | 70 | 70 | 70 |
| Iron (mg/kg) | 80 | 80 | 80 | 80 | 80 | 50 |
| Copper (mg/kg) | 8 | 8 | 8 | 8 | 8 | 8 |
| Zinc (mg/kg) | 40 | 40 | 40 | 40 | 60 | 60 |
| *Vitamin (per kg)* | 0.6 | 0.6 | 0.6 | 0.6 | 0.5 | 0.5 |
| Vitamin A, IU | 2,000 | 2,000 | 3,000 | 3,000 | 5,000 | 5,000 |
| Vitamin D3, IU | 600 | 600 | 600 | 600 | 1,000 | 1,000 |
| Vitamin E (mg) | 20 | 20 | 20 | 10 | 10 | 20 |

**Table** 40 (Continued)

| Nutrient | Broiler | | Layer | | | Breeder |
|---|---|---|---|---|---|---|
| | Starter | Finisher | Starter | Finisher | Laying | |
| Vitamin K (mg) | 2 | 2 | 2 | 2 | 2 | 2 |
| Thiamin (mg) | 4 | 4 | 4 | 2 | 2 | 2 |
| Riboflavin (mg) | 5 | 5 | 5 | 5 | 5 | 8 |
| Pantothenic acid (mg) | 15 | 15 | 15 | 15 | 15 | 15 |
| Nicotinic acid (mg) | 40 | 40 | 40 | 20 | 20 | 20 |
| Pyridoxine (mg) | 6 | 6 | 6 | 6 | 6 | 9 |
| Biotin (mg) | 0.2 | 0.2 | 0.1 | 0.1 | 0.1 | 0.15 |
| Folic acid (mg) | 2 | 2 | 1 | 1 | 0.5 | 0.5 |
| Vitamin $B_{12}$ (mg) | 0.02 | 0.02 | 0.009 | 0.005 | 0.003 | 0.005 |
| Choline (mg) | 1,500 | 1,500 | 1,300 | — | — | — |

**Table 41**

**Dietary amino acid levels for poultry**
**(Per cent of diet)**

| Amino acid | Broiler starter | Broiler finisher and chick starter | Grower | Layer and breeder |
|---|---|---|---|---|
| Arginine | 1.33 | 1.16 | 0.93 | 0.79 |
| Glycine and/or serine | 1.10 | 0.96 | 0.77 | |
| Histidine | 0.44 | 0.38 | 0.30 | 0.31 |
| Isoleucine | 0.83 | 0.72 | 0.58 | 0.50 |
| Leucine | 1.54 | 1.34 | 1.07 | 1.21 |
| Lysine | 1.22 | 1.06 | 0.85 | 0.50 |
| Methionine+Cystine | 0.83 | 0.72 | 0.58 | 0.54 |
| Methionine | 0.44 | 0.38 | 0.31 | 0.29 |
| Cystine | 0.39 | 0.34 | 0.27 | 0.25 |
| Phenylalanine+Tyrosine | 1.45 | 1.26 | 1.00 | 0.99 |
| Phenylalanine | 0.78 | 0.68 | 0.54 | 0.54 |
| Tyrosine | 0.67 | 0.58 | 0.46 | 0.45 |
| Threonine | 0.78 | 0.68 | 0.54 | 0.41 |
| Tryptophan | 0.23 | 0.20 | 0.16 | 0.13 |
| Valine | 0.94 | 0.82 | 0.66 | 0.65 |
| Protein | 24.0 | 19.0 | 16.0 | 17.0 |

## Nutrient Requirements of Swine

**Members of the sub-committee**

1. Dr. K. Prodhan, HAU
2. Dr. D.P. Sharda, HAU

**Table 4[illegible]**

**Nutrient content of diets for growing and 'Finishing' pigs**

| Nutrients | Live weight class (kg) | | | | | |
|---|---|---|---|---|---|---|
| | 5-10 | 10-20 | 20-30 | 30-40 | 40-50 | 50-60 |
| CP (%) | 18 | 16 | 16 | 16 | 14 | 14 |
| TDN (%) | 70 | 68 | 68 | 68 | 68 | 68 |
| DE (kcal/kg) | 3,100 | 3,000 | 3,000 | 3,000 | 3,000 | 3,000 |
| Ca (%) | 0.8 | 0.6 | 0.6 | 0.6 | 0.5 | 0.5 |
| P (%) | 0.6 | 0.5 | 0.5 | 0.5 | 0.4 | 0.4 |
| Common salt (%) | 0.6 | 0.5 | 0.5 | 0.5 | 0.5 | 0.5 |

# 11

# BALANCED RATION, ITS CHARACTERISTICS AND COMPUTATION FOR CATTLE AND BUFFALOES

**Ration**

A ration is the feed allowed for a given animal during a day of 24 hours. The feed may be given at a time or in portions at intervals.

**Balanced ration**

A balanced ration is a ration which provides the essential nutrients to the animal in such proportion and amounts that are required for the proper nourishment of the particular animal for 24 hours.

## DESIRABLE CHARACTERISTIC OF A RATION

**1. Liberal Feeding**

Milk cows produce plenty of milk just after calving not necessarily because they are properly fed, but because they inherently do so. This inherent quality of the cow can be made use of for increasing the milk production by providing food liberally. Liberal feeding should on no account be mistaken for overfeeding. Overfeeding is doubly wasteful because it wastes food and it also injures the animal's system. By liberal feeding, one means that the animal should be provided in plenty with all the requirements which are necessary for full milk production and maintenance of her body. There should also be some allowance made for what goes as a waste in preparation and serving the food to the cow.

**2. Individual Feeding**

Cows of the same breed and age and receiving practically the same food and care vary widely in their productive ability. In order to obtain maximum profits, cows must be fed individually according to the individual production and requirements instead of allowing the same ration to each animal in the herd.

**3. The Ration Should Be Properly Balanced**

With a correct and balanced ration a cow can get the best out of all the constituents present in her food and production of milk is frequently cheaper per unit in consequence. With an improperly balanced ration much of it is wasted. What matters is not what the cow eats but what she digests; because the amount digested alone goes for milk production and maintenance of her body. A balanced ration is thus more purposeful and beneficial.

**4. The Food Must Be Palatable**

Digestive power and appetite are not the same in cattle at all times and under all circumstances. Much depends upon the availability of foodstuffs, force of habits and usages in a certain locality. Whatever food be given to an animal it must be to its liking. Evil smelling, mouldy, musty, spoiled and inferior foods are unpalatable and must not be given to the animals. If some excellent food is not good in taste, they should be improved by special preparations like addition of salt, or other feed additives.

**5. Variety of Feed in the Ration**

By combining many feeds in a ration a better and balanced mixture of proteins, vitamins and other nutrients are furnished than by depending on only a few. Variety of feeds in the ration makes it more palatable.

**6. The Feeds Composing the Ration Should Be Good and Sound**

It is self-evident that the addition of unsound, mouldy, musty and poor quality feeds in a ration reduces the feeding value of the mixture. Apart from this, the low quality may contain poisonous or unwholesome ingredients. Cleanliness is an important condition in quality.

**7. The Ration Should Contain Enough of Mineral Matter**

Every litre of milk yielded by a cow contains a little more than 0.70% of mineral matter. If the amount of mineral matter in the ration is not sufficient to meet the demand in milk yield, the cow shall have to draw upon her own body supplies or fall down in milk yield. At the end of her lactation she will be left as an extremely weak animal and her milk yield in subsequent lactation will go down considerably.

**8. The Ration Should Be Fairly Laxative**

This is important, otherwise the food will be incompletely digested. Constipation is often the cause of most of the digestive troubles. It is, therefore, necessary to give such foods which are laxative in character.

**9. The Ration Should Be Fairly Bulky**

The stomach of cattles are very capacious and they do not feel satisfied unless their bellies are properly filled up. From the point of providing energy and heat generated values, indigestible fibre is not of any great importance but it pays an important role in giving a feeling of fullness to cattle. If the bulk of the ration supplied is small, however rich it might be in its nourishing constituents, cattle may fall a victim to the depraved habits of eating earth, rags, dirty refuses, etc., for filling up stomachs.

**10. Allow Much of Green Fodder**

Green succulent fodders are of great importance in the feeding of milch animals because of their cooling and slightly laxative action. They aid the appetite and keep the animal in good condition. Green fodders are bulky, easily digestible, laxative and contain enough of necessary vitamins. Leguminous green fodders are very rich in proteins. It should be borne in mind that at the cost of the optimum dose of concentrates, too much green fodder alone may not supply sufficient dry matter requirements.

**11. Avoid Sudden Changes in the Diet**

Sudden changes are often the cause of many digestive troubles, the more notable being the "*Tympanitis*", "*Impaction*", etc. These diseases reduce the milk yield and have depressing influences on the general constitution of the body of the animal. All changes of the food must be gradual and slow. An animal system receiving a certain food or a mixture of foods gets accustomed to it. It gets upset by sudden changes.

**12. Maintain Regularity in Feeding**

Cattle like other animals are creatures of habits and get so much used to routine that marked changes may lead to restlessness. As the feeding hour approaches, their glandular secretions become active in anticipation of the meal. Irregularity in milking and feeding tells very badly on the productive powers of an animal. The time of feeding should be evenly distributed so that the animals are not kept too long without food.

**13. The Feed Must Be Properly Prepared**

The feed must be well prepared. Some feeds require special preparations before administration in order to render them more digestible and palatable. Hard grains like gram, barley, wheat, maize, etc., should be grounded before feeding so that their mastication may become easy. Coarse fodders like dry jowar, bajra and green fodders of these crops should be chaffed before feeding. Some dry fodders, such as *bhusa* of cereals and legumes should be moistened. Soaking of feeds like various types of cakes and cotton seed softens them and makes them more palatable.

**14. A Ration Should Not Be Too Bulky**

If the ration is too bulky, the animal will fail to get all its nutrient requirements.

**15. Economy in Labour and Cost**

The ultimate object of rearing animals is to make profits. The cost of the feeds and the labour in feeding should be minimised to an extent that economic efficiency is not affected.

## COMPUTATION OF RATION FOR CATTLE AND BUFFALOES

In the computation of ration for cattle and buffaloes, the prime consideration is to ascertain and to meet up the total requirement in terms of (i) dry matter, (ii) digestible protein, i.e. DCP and (iii) energy i.e., TDN for 24 hours.

**Requirement of Dry Matter (DM)**

The requirement of the quantity of dry matter depends on the body weight of the animal and also with the nature of its production. Cattle will generally eat daily 2.0 to 2.5 kg dry matter for every 100 kg of live weight. Buffaloes and crossbred animals are slightly heavy eaters and their dry matter comsumption varies from 2.5 to 3 kg daily per 100 kg body weight. This means that the animal in question should consume only so much. Naturally, all its requirements whether organic nutrients like carbohydrate, protein and fat or minerals or vitamins should come from the total dry matter that has to be allotted. Under Indian conditions, while computation of ration is made, the amount of grazing, is neglected as it is extremely poor. Since the bulk is essential, the dry matter allowance should be divided as follows:

Total dry matter (DM)—
- $\frac{2}{3}$ (as roughages)
  - $\frac{2}{3}$ dry roughages or 3/4 if sufficient legume is available
  - $\frac{1}{3}$ green roughages (If the green fodder is legume, this proportion may be only 1/4 of the total roughage ration.)
- $\frac{1}{3}$ (as concentrates)

*Illustration 1*

For a cross-bred cow weighing 400 kg, the dry matter requirement will be provided as indicated below:

| | |
|---|---|
| Total DM requirement (kg)<br>(@ 2.5 kg per 100 kg body weight) | =(4×2.5)=10 |
| DM as concentrates (kg) | =(10×1/3)=3.33 or say 3.5 |
| DM as roughages (kg) | =(10×2/3) = 6.66 or say 6.5 |
| DM as dry roughages (kg) | =(6.6×3/4)=4.95 or say 4.9 |
| DM as green roughages (kg)<br>(When legume will be available) | =(6.6×1/4)=1.65 or say 1.6 |

**Requirement of Digestible Protein & Energy (DCP & TDN)**

While calculating the total requirements of DCP and TDN one has to consider the physiological needs, or say, the purpose for which the animal has to be fed, i.e. whether the animal is just to maintain itself or in addition to carry out the advanced stage of pregnancy or whether the animal is under production. In later case it is also necessary to consider the quantity and quality of milk. The requirement of DCP and TDN requirement for all these purposes separately may be obtained from the appropriate Tables. What one has to do is to add up the additional requirements on top of maintenance requirement as per physiological coniditon.

*Illustration 2*

Find out the total requirements of DCP and TDN for a cow weighing 400 kg and yielding 10 litres of milk having 4.5% fat.

**Computing Ration As Per Requirement**

The average DCP and TDN contents of variety of feeds and fodders are already calculated by various scientists and the average values are given in appropriate Tables. From these feeds, one has to select suitable concentrates and roughages as available in the locality at a suitable rate.

| | DCP (kg) | TDN (kg) |
|---|---|---|
| For maintenance | 0.254 | 3.03 |
| For 10 litres of milk (having 4.5% fat) | 0.480 | 3.40 |
| Total amount given: | 0.734 | 6.43 |

*Illustration 3*

Computer a ration for a cow weighing 400 kg, giving 10 litres of milk having 4.5 percent fat. The locally available feedstuff are as follows:

1. Wheat srat
2. Cowpea fodder
3. Oasts (flowering) fodder
4. Maize (crushed)
5. Groundnut cake
6. Gram chuni

STEP I: Find out the requirements of DM, DCP and TDN (already worked out in previous two illustrations)

DM requirement (kg)=10
Total DCP (kg)=0.734
Total TDN (kg)=6.43

STEP II: Find out the amount of DCP and TDN that are consumed through roughages:

| *Ingredients* | *Digestible Nutrients per 100 kg DM* | | | *Amount of DM (kg) to be given (Already worked out)* | *Amount of DCP & TDN given through dry matter* | | *Actual amount of ingredients on fresh* basis (kg)* |
|---|---|---|---|---|---|---|---|
| | *DCP (kg)* | *TDN (kg)* | | | *DCP* | *TDN* | |
| (4.9 kg) Dry roughage | | | | | | | |
| Wheat straw | 0 | 48.9 | | 4.9 | — | 2.396 | 5.4 |
| (1.6 kg) Green roughage | | | | | | | |
| Oats (flowering) | 7.7 | 72.0 | — | 1.0 | 0.077 | 0.720 | 3.3 |
| Cowpea | 20.3 | 62.2 | | 0.6 | 0.122 | 0.373 | 2.0 |
| Total amount given: | | | | 6.5 | 1.199 | 3.489 | |

*The dry matter per cent of dry and green roughages have been calculated on 90 and 30% respectively.

Amount of DCP and TDN given through roughages are 0.199 and 3.489 respectively. This amount is now to be subtracted from the total requirements. The balance, i.e., (.734 – .199)=

0.535 kg of DCP and (6.430—3.489)=2.941 kg of TDN to be given through concentrates. The quantity of concentrate mixture to be given is 3.5 kg as dry matter.

STEP III: Distribute 3.5 kg dry matter among the various ingredients of the concentrate group in such a proportion that the balance 0.535 kg DCP and 2.941 kg TDN are supplied.

It is natural that while balancing the DCP and TDN requirement several trials may have to run to reach the closest figure. This might initially seem to be tiresome but little practice will make it easier.

To this amount of concentrate always add common salt and mineral mixture @ 1 percent each.

| *Ingredients* | *Digestible Nutrients per 100 kg. dry matter* | | *Amount of DM (kg) alloted now* | *Amount of DCP and TDN given through dry matter* | | *Actual amount of ingredients on fresh basis** |
|---|---|---|---|---|---|---|
| | *DCP* | *TDN* | | *DCP* | *TDN* | |
| 1. Maize | 7.0 | 87.1 | 1.5 | 0.105 | 1.306 | 1.66 kg. |
| 2. GNC cake | 49.1 | 77.0 | 0.5 | 0.5 | 0.385 | 0.55 ,, |
| 3. Gram chuni | 13.6 | 87.5 | 1.5 | 0.204 | 1.312 | 1.66 ,, |
| Total given | | | 3.5 | 0.554 | 3.003 | |
| Required | | | 3.5 | 0.535 | 2.941 | |

*The dry matter per cent of all sorts of concentrates have been calculated on 90% basis.

*Summary of the Calculations Made So Far:*

For a cow weighing 400 kg. and yielding 10 litres of milk having 4.5% fat, the following ingredients may be given for 24 hours.

1. Wheat straw 5.4 kg.
2. Oat fodder 3.3 kg. (flowering stage)
3. Cowpea 2.0 kg.
4. Maize 1.66 kg.
5. Groundnut cake 0.55 kg.
6. Gram chuni 1.66 kg.

Salt and mineral mix each @ 1% of the concentrate mixture.

***Illustration 4***

Compute a ration for a cow weighing 450 kg. yielding 7.0 litres of milk having 4.5 percent fat. The cow is in advanced stage of pregnancy. The locally available feedstuffs are as follows:

1. Wheat straw
2. Oat (flowering stage)
3. Lucerne
4. Maize (crushed)
5. Sesame cake
6. Gram chuni
7. Rice bran

*A. Requirement of DM*

| | |
|---|---|
| (@ 2.5 kg. per 100 kg. live wt.) | =( 4.5 ×2.5)=11.25 kg. |
| DM as total roughages | =(11.25×2/3) = 7.5 ,, |
| DM as concentrate | =(11.25×1/3) = 3.75 ,, |
| DM as dry roughages | =( 7.5 ×3/4) = 5.6 ,, |
| DM as green roughages | =( 7.5 ×1/4) = 1.9 ,, |

### B. *Requirement of DCP and TDN*

| | DCP (kg) | TDN (kg) |
|---|---|---|
| For maintenance | 0.282 | 3.37 |
| For 7 litres of milk having 4.5% fat | 0.336 | 2.38 |
| Pregnancy allowance | 0.140 | 0.70 |
| Total | 0.758 | 6.45 |

### C. *Amount of DCP and TDN that are consumed through roughages*

| *Ingredients* | *Digestible Nutrients per 100 kg DM* | | *Amount of DM (kg) to be given* | *Amount of DCP and TDN given through DM* | | *Actual amount of ingredients on fresh basis (kg)* |
|---|---|---|---|---|---|---|
| | *DCP (kg)* | *TDN (kg)* | | *DCP* | *TDN* | |
| *Dry Roughages* | 5.6 kg | | | | | |
| Wheat straw | — | 48.9 | 5.6 | — | 2.738 | 6.33 |
| *Green Roughages* | 1.9 kg | | | | | |
| Oats (flowering) | 7.7 | 72.0 | 1.0 | 0.077 | 0.720 | 3.33 |
| Lucerne | 16.2 | 60.2 | 0.9 | 0.146 | 0.122 | 3.00 |
| | | | 7.5 | 0.223 | 3.580 | |

### D. *Balance of DCP and TDN to be given through concentrate mixture of 3.75 kg dry matter.*

D.C.P. (0.758—0.223)=0.535 kg

T.D.N. (6 45—3.58)=2.87 kg

| *Ingredients* | *Digestible nutrient per 100 kg DM* | | *Amount of DM (kg) alloted now** | *Amount of DCP and TDN given through DM* | | *Actual amount of ingredients on fresh basis (kg)* |
|---|---|---|---|---|---|---|
| | *DCP (kg)* | *TDN (kg)* | | *DCP (kg)* | *TDN (kg)* | |
| 1. Maize | 7.0 | 87.1 | 0.5 | 0.035 | 0.435 | 0.55 |
| 2. Gram chuni | 13.6 | 87.5 | 1.0 | 0.136 | 0.875 | 1.11 |
| 3. Rice bran | 9.1 | 76.1 | 1.5 | 1.136 | 1.121 | 2.22 |
| 4. Sesame cake | 34.0 | 80.0 | 0.75 | 0.255 | 0.600 | 0.28 |
| | | | Given=3.75 | 0.582 | 3.033 | |
| | | | Required=3.75 | 0.535 | 2.870 | |

N.B.: To this amount of concentrate mixture add common salt and mineral mixture @ 1% each.

*In case you find it difficult to fulfil the requirements of DCP and TDN after giving a certain proportion of ingredients, further trials should be made.

***If carotene (or green feed) is supplied, the amount of the provitamin has to be given in international units at four times the above rates (1 mg of carotene=1600 I.U.). In other words, 1 mg of carotene can replace only 400 I. U. of vitamin A.**

## FEEDING CATTLE AND BUFFALOES BY THUMB RULE METHOD

So far the conventional, or say, orthodox method of computation of ration for dairy cattle has been discussed. Although the method described is founded on scientific and rational basis, the common farmer of our country, may at times, be confounded with a labyrinth of calculation which may seem to be very simple to technical personnel. The following thumb rule may guide them to feed their livestock satisfactorily with particular reference to cases where individual attention and computation on body weight basis seem to be rather impractical.

While considering the feeding schedule of an adult dairy-cattle, proper considerations should first be made for the purpose for which the animal has to be fed. These are (1) maintenance ration, (2) gestation ration and (3) production ration. The approach here is based on practical experiences rather than scientific basis as in conventional method discussed earlier.

### 1. Maintenance Ration

This is the minimum amount of feed required to maintain the essential body processes at their optimum rate without gain or loss in body weight or change in body composition. The discussion on this aspect will remain limited to the concentrate part of the ration as in most parts of India, green is seldom available. In urban areas of our land, straw is considered to be the only basic roughage.

Under such circumstances, the object should be to compound concentrate mixture which will provide at least 20 per cent protein (14–16 per cent DCP) and 68–72 per cent TDN. Reasonable varieties of feed should be included so that when compounded, the mixture should be quite palatable and slightly laxative and balanced with minerals and vitamins. Variety of feed also offers other advantages, e.g., the imbalance of protein or minerals of one feed can be corrected by the other feed.

The amount of concentrate mixture and straw that will provide optimum maintenance requirement for an adult dairy cattle without any computation whatsoever are given below:

| *Item* | *For zebu cattle* | *For cross-breed/pure breed Indian cows/buffaloes* |
|---|---|---|
| 1. Straw | 4 kg | 4–6 kg |
| 2. Concentrate mixture (with straw only or with little greens) | 1–1.25 kg | 2.00 kg |

Let us, however, see how far in reality the above quantity satisfies the maintenance requirement of an adult dairy cattle.

*Example I*

As per nutrition standard it will be observed that the maintenance requirement of an adult *deshi* cow weighing 250 kg will be DCP 0.168 kg and TDN 2.02 kg. According to thumb rule method the amount of DCP and TDN supplied as per quantities alloted will be:

| Item | DCP | TDN |
|---|---|---|
| 1. Straw 4 kg (DCP=0.0; TDN=42.0) | 0.000 | 1.68 |
| 2. Concentrate mix. 1.25 kg (DCP=14.0 and TDN=68.0 minimum) | 0.175 | 0.85 |
| | 0.175 | 2.53=Given |
| | 0.168 | 2.02=Recommended |

*Example* 2.

The nutritional requirement for an adult cow weighing 450 kg will be 0.28 kg DCP and 3.37 kg TDN (same table as for above cow). To be satisfied by thumb rule method as below:

| Item | DCP | TDN |
|---|---|---|
| 1. Straw 5 kg or more (DCP=0.0; TDN=42.0) | 0.00 | 2.10 |
| 2. Concentrate mixture 2 kg (DCP=14.0 and TDN=68.0 minimum) | 0.28 | 1.36 |
| | 0.28 | 3.46=Given |
| | 0.28 | 3.37=Recommended |

Now the question remains as to how to formulate the concentrate mixture that will provide 14–16% DCP and a minimum of 68% TDN without taking recourse to computation. For this the following assumptions may be made.

| | | |
|---|---|---|
| Oil cakes | 25–35 parts | To be fortified with 1% mineral mixture, 1-2% Salt and 20-30 gm vit $AD_3$/100 kg, containing 50,000 I.U. Vit. A and 5,000 I.U. Vit $D_3$ per gram |
| Millets/cereals | 25–35 parts | |
| Cereal by-products | 10–25 parts | |
| Pulse cnuni | 5–20 parts | |

The computation of the above mixture will reveal that if quality ingredients are chosen then the above concentrate mixture will provide a minimum of 15% DCP and 70% TDN and for that a farmer need not know necessarily the computation of ration in terms of DCP and TDN. Where the principal roughage is straw, limestone powder @ 1—2% (able to pass through 150 mesh) should also be given.

Let us now take a concrete example of a type of concentrate mixture to prove that the above assumption is correct.

From the above, it will be clear that the assumption made earlier holds good and therefore a farmer need not necessarily go into details of DCP and TDN for his computation work.

A farmer desirous of producing concentrate mixture of his own should know the various types of ingredients required for making concentrate mixture ideal for livestock feeding. If he is not well conversant with the quality of raw feed ingredients and unconventional feedstuffs available in the region, he may not be able to compute an ideal concentrate mixture for his stock economically. The various types of feed ingredients generally used for computing concentrate mixture have already been discussed at the beginning of this chapter but for ready reference the names of the commonly found ingredients are mentioned here again.

1. *Protein Supplements* (Primary sources of protein)

(a) Vegetable protein supplements—oil cakes, e.g., groundnut cake, sesame cake, cotton seed cake, mustard cake, linseed cake etc.

**Table 43**

| *Feed stuffs* (*1*) | *Parts* (*2*) | *DCP* | | *TDN* | |
|---|---|---|---|---|---|
| | | *Per qnt.* | *As Per column 2* | *Per qnt.* | *As per column 2* |
| *Oil Cakes* | | | | | |
| Groundnut caks | 10 | 38 | 3.80 | 73 | 7.30 |
| Sesame cake | 8 | 32 | 2.56 | 72 | 5.76 |
| Mustard cake | 5 | 28 | 1.40 | 72 | 3.60 |
| Linseed cake | 5 | 28 | 1.40 | 72 | 3.60 |
| *Cereals* | | | | | |
| Maize | 20 | 7 | 1.40 | 80 | 16.00 |
| Barley | 10 | 8 | 0.80 | 76 | 7.60 |
| *Bran* | | | | | |
| Wheat bran | 15 | 10 | 1.50 | 65 | 9.75 |
| Rice bran | 10 | 8 | 0.80 | 66 | 6.60 |
| *Pulse Chuni* | | | | | |
| Gram chuni/Arhar chuni | 14 | 11 | 1.54 | 68 | 9.52 |
| *Others* | | | | | |
| Salt | 1 | | | | |
| Mineral Mixture | 1 | | | | |
| Limestone Powder | 1 | | | | |
| GIVEN | | | 15.20 | | 69.73 |
| RECOMMENDED (minimum) | | | 14.00 | | 68.00 |

(b) Animal protein supplement—fish meal, skim milk powder etc. (used chiefly in compounding concentrate mixture for calves in early months).

2. *Grain supplement* (primary source of energy)—cereal grains like maize, wheat etc., millet grains like jowar, milo etc.
3. *Cereal by products* (diluents—medium energy content, and source of minerals)—wheat bran, rice bran, maize etc.
4. *Pulse chunis* (medium protein, energy source)—mung chuni, arhar chuni, massoor chuni, kalai chuni etc.
5. *Salt*
6. *Minerals*
7. *Vitamins*

In the formulation of any concentrate mixture, primary consideration is given to protein and energy content of the ration which are satisfied by selecting suitable protein supplements and grain supplements respectively as indicated in Table 43. In general, cereal by-products are palatable and laxative; they furnish good amount of minerals, particularly phosphorus excepting maize and bran which are mostly used as diluents to protein and energy supplements. Pulse chunies are also palatable and supply medium energy depending on the amount of husk present in them. If a good amount of broken pulses are present then the nutritive value of these chunies is much better than brans both in protein and energy content. The addition of salt (1-2 per cent) to the concentrate mixture increases palatability and supplies sodium and chlorine to the animal. Minerals are vitally important particularly when good quality greens are not available. When straw is used as a major source of roughage, mineral and vitamin supplements are essential. Commercial mineral mixtures are available for use in cattle ration and may be used at 1-2 per cent level. Vitamin mixture (Vit. A and $D_3$; Vit. A—50,000 I.U., Vit. $D_3$ 5,000 I.U., per gram) is also commercially available in suitable packs and its use @ 20-30 gm per 100 kg of concentrates will be sufficient. This amount of vitamin mixture is a must particularly when no or little greens are available to the stock. When straw is used as the sole source of roughage, the addition of 1—2 per cent limestone powder (should pass through 150 mesh) will be very beneficial.

## 2. Gestation Ration

In the case of pregnancy, further allowance from the fifth month of pregnancy onwards must be made for proper growth of the foetus and to keep the mother fit for optimum milk production on calving. For this, in addition to maintenance ration, a further amonut of 1.25 and 1.75 kg concentrate mixture is recommended for zebu and cross bred cow/buffaloes respectively.

Let us now examine whether in reality the above quantity satisfies the gestation requirement as recommended in the conventional method.

*Example 1:* The nutritional requirement for an adult cow weighing 250 kg and at an advanced stage of gestation is as follows:

| Requirement: | DCP | TDN |
|---|---|---|
| For maintenance | 0.17 | 2.02 |
| For pregnancy | 0.14 | 0.70 |
| Total | 0.31 | 2.72 |

To be satisfied by:

| Items | DCP | TDN |
|---|---|---|
| 1. Straw 4 kg or more | 0.00 | 1.68 |
| 2. Concentrate mix 2.5 kg (1.25 for maintenance+1.25 kg for pregnancy allowance) | 0.35 | 1.70 |
| Given— | 0.35 | 3.38 |
| Recommended— | 0.31 | 2.72 |

*Example 2:* The nutritional requirement for a cross-bred cow/Indian milch breed weighing 450 kg and at an advanced stage of pregnancy will be as follows:

| Requirement: | DCP | TDN |
|---|---|---|
| For maintenance | 0.28 | 3.37 |
| For pregnancy | 0.14 | 0.70 |
| Total | 0.42 | 4.07 |

To be satisfied by:

| Items | DCP | TDN |
|---|---|---|
| 1. Straw 5.0 kg or more | 0.00 | 2.10 |
| 2. Concentrate mixture 3.75 kg (2.00 kg for maintenance+1.75 kg for pregnancy allowance) | 0.52 | 2.55 |
| Given— | 0.52 | 4.65 |
| Recommended— | 0.42 | 4.07 |

For high yielder, it is desirable to go for liberal feeding of pregnant dams particularly cross-bred cows/buffaloes from 8th month of pregnancy of 6 weeks before calving with the object of securing full development of mammary glands for optimum milk production. For this 2.0 to 3.0 kg of concentrate for Zebu and between 4.0—5.0 kg for cross-bred/pure bred Indian cattle/buffaloes over and above maintenance requirements are recommended.

**3. Production Ration**

Production ration is the additional allowance of ration for milk production over and above the maintenance requirement. For Zebu 1 kg additional amount of concentrate is required for every 2.5 kg of milk over and above the maintenance requirement while the same amount of concentrate is required for every 2.0 kg of milk for cross-bred/Indian milch breed/buffaloes.

As before, let us now examine whether in reality the above quantity satisfies the requirement for a milk producing cow or not by comparing the amount derived by conventional method.

*Example 1;* Requirement for Zebu weighing 250 kg and producing 4 kg of milk of 4.5% fat will be (by conventional method) as follows:

| Requirement: | DCP | TDN |
|---|---|---|
| For maintenance | 0.168 | 2.02 |
| For production | 0.192 | 1.36 |
| Total | 0.360 | 3.38 |

To be satisfied by:

| Items | DCP | TDN |
|---|---|---|
| 1. Straw 4 kg or more | 0.00 | 1.68 |
| 2. Concentrate mixture 2.85 kg (1.25 kg for maintenance+1.60 kg for production) | 0.40 | 1.94 |
| Given— | 0.40 | 3.62 |
| Recommended— | 0.36 | 3.38 |

*Example 2:* Requirement for a cow weighing 450 kg and producing 10 kg milk of 4% fat will be as follows:

| Requirement | DCP | TDN |
|---|---|---|
| For maintenance | 0.28 | 3.37 |
| For production | 0.45 | 3.16 |
| Total requirement— | 0.73 | 6.53 |

To be satisfied by:

| Items | DCP | TDN |
|---|---|---|
| 1. Straw 5 kg or more | 0.00 | 2.10 |
| 2. Concentrate mixture 7 kg (2.0 kg for maintenance+5.0 kg for production) | 0.98 | 4.76 |
| Given— | 0.98 | 6.86 |
| Recommended— | 0.73 | 6.53 |

The above two examples are sufficient to prove that the requirement of dairy cattle can be met easily by using the thumb rule method. But for buffaloes where milk is extremely rich in energy due to high fat percentage, thumb rule method does not work as efficiently as for low yielders with moderate fat percentage. An example of this situation may be studied as below:

*Example 3:* Requirement of a buffalo weighing 450 kg and producing 10 kg milk of 8% fat will be

| | DCP | TDN |
|---|---|---|
| For maintenance | 0.28 | 3.37 |
| For production | 0.69 | 5.06 |
| Total requirement | 0.97 | 8.43 |

To be satisfied by:

| Items | DCP | TDN |
|---|---|---|
| 1. Straw 6 kg | 0.00 | 2.52 |
| 2. Concentrate mixture 7 kg (5 kg for production+2 kg for maintenance) | 0.98 | 4.76 |
| Given | 0.98 | 7.28 |
| Recommended | 0.97 | 8.43 |

Therefore, the energy requirement of the buffalo is not satisfied.

In this example, it has been shown that by using thumb rule method, the requirement of energy (TDN) could not be fulfilled. For high yielders with high fat percentage, this kind of situation is very common. To overcome this sort of critical situation generally observed in the case of buffaloes, at least, 10 kg extra amount of green fodders like Paragrass, Maize, Guinea grass etc., should be supplied to meet the demands of energy requirement. An attempt to increase the quantum of straw to fulfill the energy requirement is likely to fail since the buffaloes will not consume 9 kg of straw for reasons of unpalatability. Therefore, in the above example, inclusion of further 10 kg of commonly found paragrass (1.4 DCP and 12.0 TDN) will add additional amount of 0.14 kg of DCP and 1.20 kg of TDN, to fulfill the energy requirement of the baffaloe ration.

If can be concluded, however, that the requirement of a crossbred cow producing more than 15 litres of milk per day or a buffaloe producing 10 litres of milk or more per day may not be met by thumb rule feeding with straw only as the roughage part of the ration unless supplemented with greens like maize, fodder, paragrass of good quality hay etc. Alternatively, TDN content of the concentrate mixture should be increased enormously (beyond 80 per cent).

So long the quantity of concentrate mixture containing 20% crude protein or 14-16 per cent DCP and 68% TDN with straw as the sole roughage are available to fulfill the energy requirements of the high yielders, there will be no problem. In rainy seasons, however, or in areas where greens are available for stock feeding, the crude protein percentage of the concentrate mixture may be reduced in line with the quantity of greens that farmer can provide to his stock, e.g., with good quality legumes like lucerne, berseem or cowpea or their hay as the roughage, the protein content of the concentrate mixture can be safely reduced to 14-16 per cent; with mixed legumes and grass or good quality paragrass, guinea grass, maize fodder, etc., as the roughage, the protein content may be reduced to 17-18 per cent protein only. Further, depending on the amount of greens/hay that a livestock owner can provide to his stock, the amount of concentrate mixture should be determined, e.g., if he can provide, say 20 kg greens like paragrass, guinea grass, dub grass etc., to his stock, this will furnish approximately 0.24—0.28 kg DCP and 2.4 kg TDN and consequently the quantum of concentrate mixture will be automatically reduced to provide the rest of the nutrients required. *Roughly speaking, for every 10 kg of good quality greens, 1 kg concentrate can be cut from the concentrate quota with the additional advantage of dry matter, TDN, minerals and vitamins in favour of greens.* A farmer feeding his cross bred cow with 7 kg concentrate with paddy straw as the roughage for production of 10 kg milk may safely reduce his feeding chart to 5 kg concentrates and 20 kg greens like paragrass/dub grass etc., plus straw. The resultant effect on milk production by this change will be much better since it provides better nutrition by way of increased TDN minerals, vitamin etc., coupled with unidentified factor (?) present in grass juices. Further this change is also economically advantageous. At the present market rate, the cost of 2 kg concentrates having minimum 20% protein and 68% TDN will be Rs. 2.50 or more whereas the cost of 20 kg greens will be no more than Rs. 1.50 and in country side, particularly in rainy seasons, dub grass will be readily available at practically no cost. This is the reason why during the rainy season when grass grows abundantly, emaciated country cattle pick up conditions easily. It should be noted, however, that grass allowed to become over-ripe loses much of its nutritive value while it has the maximum value in the prime stage of growth.

**Table 44**

**Some recommended feed formulae***

**I**

| | |
|---|---|
| Wheat bran | 50 |
| Mustard and rape oilcake | 30 |
| Gram chuni | 20 |
| | 100 |

**II**

| | |
|---|---|
| Cotton seed oilcake (decorticated) | 20 |
| Groundnut oilcake | 15 |
| Gram husk | 15 |
| Gram chuni | 35 |
| Wheat bran | 15 |
| | 100 |

**III**

| | |
|---|---|
| Gram chuni | 35 |
| Guar | 15 |
| Rice bran | 15 |
| Cotton seed oilcake | 35 |
| | 100 |

**IV**

| | |
|---|---|
| Linseed oilcake | 35 |
| Gram chuni | 40 |
| Wheat bran | 25 |
| | 100 |

**V**

| | |
|---|---|
| Wheat bran | 35 |
| Sesamum oilcake | 25 |
| Gram chuni | 20 |
| Barley | 20 |
| | 100 |

**VI**

| | |
|---|---|
| Oat | 30 |
| Gram | 40 |
| Groundnut oilcake | 20 |
| Wheat bran | 10 |
| | 100 |

**VII**

| | |
|---|---|
| Gram | 35 |
| Maize | 40 |
| Groundnut oilcake | 20 |
| Gram husk | 5 |
| | 100 |

**VIII**

| | |
|---|---|
| Sesamum oilcake | 20 |
| Horse gram | 40 |
| Jowar | 20 |
| Rice bran | 10 |
| Gram husk | 10 |
| | 100 |

| IX | |
|---|---|
| Coconut oilcake | 25 |
| Tapioca flour | 25 |
| Groundnut oilcake | 20 |
| Gram chuni | 30 |
| | 100 |

| X | |
|---|---|
| Tapioca flour | 25 |
| Horse gram | 25 |
| Groundnut oilcake | 25 |
| Wheat bran | 25 |
| | 100 |

| XI | |
|---|---|
| Maize | 25 |
| Maize gluten feed | 25 |
| Maize bran | 25 |
| Wheat bran | 25 |
| | 100 |

| XII | |
|---|---|
| Cotton seed oilcake | 30 |
| Wheat bran | 20 |
| Maize | 50 |
| | 100 |

| XIII | |
|---|---|
| Mustard and rape oilcake | 25 |
| Cotton seed oilcake | 25 |
| Wheat bran | 20 |
| Barley | 30 |
| | 100 |

| XIV | |
|---|---|
| Mustard and rape oilcake | 40 |
| Barley | 40 |
| Oat | 20 |
| | 100 |

| XV | |
|---|---|
| Groundnut oilcake | 20 |
| Gram | 40 |
| Maize | 35 |
| Gram husk | 5 |
| | 100 |

| XVI | |
|---|---|
| Sesamum oilcake | 20 |
| Gram | 40 |
| Barley | 35 |
| Rice bran | 5 |
| | 100 |

| XVII | |
|---|---|
| Groundnut oilcake | 10 |
| Cotton seed oilcake | 20 |
| Rice bran | 10 |
| Maize | 30 |
| Gram | 30 |
| | 100 |

| XVIII | |
|---|---|
| Gram chuni | 35 |
| Guar meal | 15 |
| Wheat bran | 30 |
| Groundnut oilcake | 10 |
| Gram husk | 10 |
| | 100 |

| XIX | |
|---|---|
| Mustard and rape oilcake | 40 |
| Barley | 40 |
| Wheat bran | 20 |
| | 100 |

| XX | |
|---|---|
| Groundnut oilcake | 20 |
| Wheat bran | 30 |
| Barley | 30 |
| Gram | 20 |
| | 100 |

| XXI | |
|---|---|
| Groundnut oilcake | 25 |
| Wheat bran | 30 |
| Maize | 25 |

| | |
|---|---|
| Gram | 20 |
| | 100 |

XXII

| | |
|---|---|
| Berseem or lucerne meal | 30 |
| Moth chuni | 30 |
| Ground oats | 20 |
| Molasses | 10 |
| Wheat bran | 10 |
| | 100 |

XXIII

| | |
|---|---|
| Brewer's yeast | 20 |
| Wheat or rice bran | 30 |
| Maize or tapioca flour | 20 |
| Gram or horse gram | 30 |
| | 100 |

XXIV

| | |
|---|---|
| Maize | 35 |
| Distillery waste (dried) | 35 |
| Groundnut oilcake | 15 |
| Wheat bran | 15 |
| | 100 |

XXV

| | |
|---|---|
| Distillery waste (dried) | 35 |
| Fish or meat meal | 15 |
| Tapioca | 30 |
| Molasses | 10 |
| Gram | 10 |
| | 100 |

XXVI

| | |
|---|---|
| Maize | 40 |
| Blood meal | 20 |
| Wheat bran | 30 |
| Molasses | 10 |
| | 100 |

XXVII

| | |
|---|---|
| Coconut oilcake | 20 |
| Groundnut oilcake | 20 |
| Gram chuni | 20 |
| Tapioca flour | 20 |
| Wheat bran | 20 |
| | 100 |

XXVIII

| | |
|---|---|
| Sesamum oilcake | 30 |
| Gram chuni | 20 |
| Jowar | 25 |
| Mango seed kernel (dried) | 15 |
| Rice bran | 10 |
| | 100 |

*Formulated by Indian Standard Institution to constitute at least 15% digestible crude protein and 70% total digestible nutrients. (First revision of I.S. 2052—1962-1968).

Table 45

**Average rates of feeding of concentrates, green and dry fodder assumed for different categories of livestock and poultry**

(in kg)

| *Categories of Livestock* | *Rates of feeding per day* | | |
|---|---|---|---|
| | *Concentrates* | *Green fodder* | *Dry fodder* |
| **A. Cattle** | | | |
| 1. crossbred (milch) ... | 2.75 | 20.00 | 6.00 |
| 2. females over 3 years of age: | | | |
| (i) improved cows (milch) | 1.20 | 10.00 | 6.00 |
| (ii) other milch cows and not calved even once ... | 0.125 | 3.5 | 3.16 |
| 3. males over 3 years of age ... | 0.17 | 4.96 | 5.65 |
| 4. males less than 3 years of age: | | | |
| (i) crossbred (young stock) | 1.50 | 10.00 | 2.00 |
| (ii) other young stock ... | 0.016 | 1.58 | 1.47 |
| **B. Buffaloes** | | | |
| 1. females over 3 years of age: | | | |
| (i) improved buffaloes ... | 1.50 | 10.00 | 6.00 |
| (ii) other milch buffaloes and those not calved even once ... | 0.41 | 5.72 | 5.08 |
| 2. males over 3 years of age | 0.109 | 6.51 | 5.43 |
| 3. less than 3 years of age ... | 0.01 | 1.59 | 1.64 |
| **C. Poultry** | | | |
| (i) improved layers ... | 0.123 | 0.020 | ... |
| (ii) growing stock ... | 0.041 | 0.007 | ... |
| **D. Other Livestock** | | | |
| (i) improved sheep ... | 0.274 | ... | 0.40 |
| (ii) improved pigs ... | 2.50 | 1.00 | ... |
| (iii) horses and ponies ... | 0.50 | ... | ... |

# APPENDIX

## Chemical composition and nutritive value of Indian feeding stuffs

| Sl. No. | Name | Chemical composition on DM basis | | | | | kg/100 kg DM-basis** | | Mcal/kg dry matter | |
|---|---|---|---|---|---|---|---|---|---|---|
| | | CP | CF | NFE | EE | TA | DCP | TDN | DE | ME |
| | | | | | | | kg per 100 kg raw material | | | |
| 1 | 2 | 3 | 4 | 5 | 6 | 7 | 8 | 9 | 10 | 11 |
| | *Roughages* | | | | | | | | | |
| 1. | Pearl-millet (*Pennisetum typhoides*) | | | | | | | | | |
| | Just before flowering | 16.2 | 28.2 | 38.8 | 2.0 | 14.7 | — | — | — | — |
| | Milk stage | 10.6 | 28.0 | 50.2 | 2.1 | 9.2 | — | — | — | — |
| | Dough stage | 8.8 | 24.9 | 56.2 | 1.9 | 8.2 | — | — | — | — |
| | Ripe stage | 8.9 | 24.0 | 57.7 | 1.7 | 7.7 | — | — | — | — |
| | Mature stage | 3.8 | 32.7 | 51.6 | 1.4 | 10.6 | — | — | — | — |
| | All analysis | 6.9 | 31.8 | 48.9 | 1.5 | 10.9 | 4.3 | 59.2 | 2.6 | 2.1 |
| 2. | Barley (*Hordeum vulgare*) | 11.5 | 31.8 | 43.4 | 1.9 | 11.4 | 8.2 | 60.5 | — | — |
| | One month | 15.8 | 19.1 | 45.4 | 3.1 | 16.6 | — | — | — | — |
| | Two months | 6.6 | 31.1 | 49.4 | 2.4 | 10.6 | — | — | — | — |
| | Three months | 5.4 | 27.0 | 57.3 | 2.5 | 7.8 | — | — | — | — |
| 3. | Berseem (*Trifolium alexandrinum*) | | | | | | | | | |
| | Average (all analysis) | 17.4 | 25.9 | 40.7 | 1.9 | 14.2 | 12.5 | 59.2 | 2.6 | 2.1 |
| | 9-week old | 26.7 | 14.9 | 39.8 | 3.0 | 15.6 | — | — | — | — |
| | 12-week old | 21.5 | 20.6 | 41.0 | 2.6 | 14.3 | — | — | — | — |
| | 15-week old | 17.3 | 24.2 | 43.9 | 1.8 | 12.9 | — | — | — | — |
| | 18-week old | 16.9 | 22.7 | 43.7 | 1.8 | 14.9 | — | — | — | — |
| | 24-week old | 15.8 | 28.5 | 38.3 | 1.4 | 16.0 | — | — | — | — |
| 4. | Black-gram (*Vigna mungo*) | 13.0 | 2.9 | 51.0 | 3.7 | 11.4 | — | — | — | — |
| 5. | Cowpea (*Vigna unguiculata*) | | | | | | | | | |
| | Average | 18.2 | 25.3 | 39.6 | 2.6 | 14.2 | — | — | — | — |
| | Large variety | 28.1 | 26.7 | 33.1 | 3.0 | 9.2 | 20.3 | 62.2 | 2.7 | 2.2 |
| | Small variety | 16.5 | 30.9 | 39.4 | 3.0 | 10.3 | 12.4 | 58.9 | 2.6 | 2.1 |

| 1 | 2 | 3 | 4 | 5 | 6 | 7 | 8 | 9 | 10 | 11 |
|---|---|---|---|---|---|---|---|---|---|---|
| 6. | *Crotalaria medica*, pre-flowering | 19.7 | — | — | — | — | — | — | — | — |
| | Seed formation | 16.9 | — | — | — | — | — | — | — | — |
| | Height 28.8 cm | 18.2 | — | — | — | — | — | — | — | — |
| | Height 43.2 cm | 19.4 | — | — | — | — | — | — | — | — |
| 7. | Gram (*Cicer arietinum*) | | | | | | | | | |
| | Podding stage | 8.6 | 36.8 | 43.0 | 0.8 | 10.8 | — | — | — | — |
| | Green fodder | 10.9 | 33.1 | 44.9 | 2.1 | 9.1 | — | — | — | — |
| | Whole plant | 11.3 | 27.2 | 48.0 | 2.2 | 11.4 | — | — | — | — |
| 8. | Bermuda grass (*Cynodon dactylon*) | | | | | | | | | |
| | Young | 21.9 | 18.6 | 44.1 | 2.7 | 12.6 | — | — | — | — |
| | Prime | 10.0 | 31.9 | 44.0 | 1.4 | 12.6 | — | — | — | — |
| | Ripe | 4.9 | 39.7 | 46.1 | 1.2 | 8.1 | — | — | — | — |
| | Average | 10.5 | 28.2 | 47.8 | 1.8 | 11.8 | — | — | — | — |
| 9. | *Cyperus rotundus* | 8.9 | 26.7 | 49.4 | 2.4 | 13.0 | — | — | — | — |
| 10. | Green panic grass | 10.8 | 44.1 | 34.2 | 1.3 | 9.6 | — | — | — | — |
| 11. | Guinea grass (*Panicum maximum*) | | | | | | | | | |
| | Maximum | 14.0 | 41.8 | 50.0 | 2.7 | 16.1 | — | — | — | — |
| | Minimum | 4.7 | 31.6 | 35.6 | 0.7 | 11.4 | — | — | — | — |
| | Average | 7.7 | 37.3 | 39.4 | 1.7 | 13.9 | 3.0* | 51.5* | 2.3 | 1.9 |
| | Young (average) | 7.9 | 38.4 | 37.0 | 1.2 | 15.5 | 4.4 | 55.0 | 2.4 | 2.0 |
| 12. | Napier, Elephant grass (*Peninsetum purpureum*) | 6.2 | 28.1 | 47.5 | 2.3 | 16.0 | 55.4 | 44.0 | 2.4 | 2.0 |
| | Vegetative | 15.6 | 27.4 | 36.7 | 1.2 | 19.1 | — | — | — | — |
| | October cut | 14.5 | 27.9 | 38.2 | 2.2 | 17.1 | — | — | — | — |
| | November cut | 9.2 | 29.2 | 43.2 | 1.9 | 16.6 | — | — | — | — |
| 13. | *Pennisetum polystahyon* | | | | | | | | | |
| | October cut | 11.2 | 28.4 | 41.5 | 2.6 | 16.3 | — | — | — | — |
| | November cut | 10.2 | 38.5 | 37.4 | 1.8 | 11.7 | — | — | — | — |

| | | | | | | | | | |
|---|---|---|---|---|---|---|---|---|---|
| 1st cut | 17.4 | 23.0 | 42.3 | 1.4 | 15.9 | — | — | — | — |
| In seed | 2.8 | 34.5 | 49.8 | 1.1 | 11.8 | — | — | — | — |
| 2nd cut | 12.2 | 31.4 | 44.2 | 1.7 | 10.4 | — | — | — | — |
| 4th week | 6.4 | 28.6 | 46.2 | 1.1 | 17.6 | — | — | — | — |
| 6 weeks | 4.9 | 29.9 | 49.7 | 0.9 | 14.6 | — | — | — | — |
| 8 weeks | 5.4 | 33.0 | 47.2 | 0.8 | 13.5 | — | — | — | — |
| 14. Napier hybrid | 10.2 | 30.5 | 41.0 | 2.1 | 16.2 | — | — | — | — |
| 15. Para grass (*Brachiaria mutica*) | 12 0 | 28.2 | 45.7 | 2.9 | 11.2 | 67.9 | 59.5 | — | — |
| In running water | 6.9 | 35.4 | 46.1 | 0.8 | 10.8 | — | — | — | — |
| Waterlogged | 15.4 | 32.3 | 38.0 | 1.2 | 13.1 | — | — | — | — |
| 16. *Peninsetum pedicellatum* | 7.4 | 22.2 | 49.0 | 2.8 | 18.6 | — | — | — | — |
| 17. Pusa Giant Napier grass | 2.9 | 37.2 | 52.5 | 1.8 | 7.0 | — | — | — | — |
| 18. Sudan grass (*Sorghum sudandse*) | 5.7 | 27.0 | 51.0 | 1.9 | 14.4 | 1.6 | 44.4 | 2.0 | 1.6 |
| 19. Groundnut (*Arachis hypogaea*), Average | 9.8 | 34.1 | 48.1 | 0.7 | 7.3 | — | — | — | — |
| 20. Guar (*Cyamopsis tetragonoloba*) | 8.6 | 30.0 | 47.6 | 1.7 | 12.7 | 6.1 | 48.8 | 2.2 | 1.8 |
| 2 month old | 18.1 | 31.9 | 37.6 | 1.9 | 10.4 | — | — | — | — |
| 3 month old | 12.8 | 29.5 | 49.2 | 1.5 | 6.9 | — | — | — | — |
| 21. Lucerne (*Medicago sativa*) | | | | | | | | | |
| Maximum | 25.8 | 35.2 | 39.9 | 3.1 | 11.8 | — | — | — | — |
| Minimum | 16.8 | 27.0 | 30.2 | 1.3 | 9.4 | — | — | — | — |
| Average | 20.2 | 30.1 | 36 6 | 2.3 | 10.7 | 13.5 | 58.8 | 2.6 | 2.1 |
| 1st cut | 20.8 | 22.9 | 40.6 | 3.4 | 12.3 | — | — | — | — |
| 2nd cut | 18.1 | 24.9 | 43.5 | 2.6 | 10.9 | — | — | — | — |
| 3rd cut | 20.4 | 22.8 | 44.2 | 2.7 | 9.7 | — | — | — | — |
| 4th cut | 20.7 | 18.4 | 47.5 | 3.2 | 10.3 | — | — | — | — |
| Flowering | 16.9 | 29.0 | 41.8 | 3.5 | 8.8 | — | — | — | — |
| 1st month | 24.5 | 16.2 | 41.0 | 2.6 | 15.7 | — | — | — | — |
| 2nd month | 20.3 | 25.7 | 36.1 | 3.1 | 14.8 | — | — | — | — |
| 3rd month | 16.0 | 29.7 | 40.1 | 3.5 | 10.7 | — | — | — | — |

| 1 | 2 | 3 | 4 | 5 | 6 | 7 | 8 | 9 | 10 | 11 |
|---|---|---|---|---|---|---|---|---|---|---|
| 22. | Maize (*Zea mays*) Average | 7.2 | 30.8 | 51.6 | 1.8 | 8.6 | 4.2 | 67.8 | 3.0 | 2.5 |
| | January | 12.1 | 29.6 | 44.2 | 1.1 | 13.0 | — | — | — | — |
| | February | 8.2 | 27.2 | 51.9 | 0.9 | 11.8 | — | — | — | — |
| | March | 6.4 | 29.9 | 51.2 | 0.9 | 11.6 | — | — | — | — |
| | Dough stage | 5.1 | 26.9 | 59.3 | 1.5 | 7.3 | — | — | — | — |
| 23. | Oat (*Avena sativa*) | | | | | | | | | |
| | Young | 14.6 | 32.9 | 36.4 | 2.1 | 13.9 | — | — | — | — |
| | Milk stage | 6.4 | 28.7 | 53.2 | 2.3 | 9.3 | — | — | — | — |
| | Ripe | 9.2 | 34.8 | 44.8 | 1.8 | 9.4 | — | — | — | — |
| | Flowering | 10.8 | 31.0 | 45.9 | 1.8 | 10.4 | — | — | — | — |
| | Green | 5.3 | 34.2 | 47.1 | 2.5 | 10.9 | 10.5 | 66.7 | 2.9 | 2.4 |
| | 1st month | 18.8 | 18.0 | 37.5 | 3.6 | 22.1 | — | — | — | — |
| | 3rd month | 5.3 | 27.3 | 55.9 | 3.5 | 8.1 | — | — | — | — |
| 24. | Pea (*Pisum sativum*) | | | | | | | | | |
| | Podding | 11.8 | 29.8 | 48.7 | 1.0 | 8.7 | 7.8* | 72.9* | 3.2 | 2.6 |
| | 11½ weeks | 16.7 | 22.6 | 54.4 | 2.4 | 3.9 | — | — | — | — |
| 25. | *Pennisetum polystachyon* | 5.3 | 34.6 | 45.7 | 2.0 | 12.1 | — | — | — | — |
| 26. | Soyabean (*Glycine max*, syn. *G. hispida*), average | 13.0 | 31.3 | 45.3 | 1.7 | 8.8 | — | — | — | — |
| | Soyabean (*Glycine javanica*) | 10.1 | 32.7 | 47.9 | 0.7 | 8.6 | — | — | — | — |
| 27. | Water hyacinth (*Eichhornia crassipes*), average | 9.8 | 21.6 | 51.2 | 1.5 | 15.9 | — | — | — | — |
| | | | *Silages* | | | | | | | |
| 28. | Guinea grass (*Panicum maximum*) | 5.2 | 38.7 | 44.6 | 1.5 | 9.9 | — | — | — | — |
| 29. | Sorghum (*Sorghum bicolor*), average | 5.9 | 37.3 | 44.4 | 1.8 | 10.6 | 2.4 | 51.1 | 2.3 | 1.9 |
| 30. | Maize (*Zea mays*) | 7.9 | 24.6 | 55.1 | 1.1 | 11.3 | 3.4 | 61.1 | 2.7 | 2.2 |
| 31. | Oat (*Avena sativa*). | — | — | — | — | — | 4.1 | 62.2 | 2.7 | 2.3 |
| | Acid brown | 7.3 | 40.8 | 40.6 | 1.6 | 9.7 | — | — | — | — |

| | | | | | | | | | |
|---|---|---|---|---|---|---|---|---|---|
| Fruity green | 8.1 | 39.8 | 39.6 | 3.0 | 9.5 | — | — | — | — |
| 32. Ragi straw (*Eleusine coracana*) | 3.6 | 38.8 | 46.7 | 1.5 | 9.6 | 0.3 | 52.8 | 2.3 | 1.9 |
| 33. Rice straw (*Oryza sativa*) | 5.9 | 30.0 | 47.5 | 1.7 | 11.4 | — | — | — | — |
| 34. Spear grass (*Heteropogon contortus*) | — | — | — | — | — | 1.7 | 50.2 | — | — |
| Young | 6.6 | 36.8 | 43.1 | 1.3 | 12.2 | — | — | — | — |
| Prime | 6.6 | 32.6 | 43.6 | 1.6 | 15.5 | — | — | — | — |
| 35. Water hyacinth silage | 7.3 | 5.4 | 25.9 | 1.2 | 60.3 | — | — | — | — |
| | | | *Hays* | | | | | | |
| 36. Alfalfa hay | 14.1 | 31.7 | 41 6 | 1.8 | 10.8 | — | 12.0 | 2.5 | 2.0 |
| 37. Bermuda grass (Cynodon dactylon), average | 8.4 | 20.2 | 56.5 | 1.4 | 11.6 | 4.0 | 48.8* | 2.1 | 1.8 |
| 38. Guinea grass (*Panicum maximum*) | | | | | | | | | |
| Hay, pre-flowering stage | 7.6 | 38.1 | 37.1 | 1.2 | 16.0 | 4.1 | 47.3 | 2.1 | 1.7 |
| Hay, flowering stage | 4.8 | 42.1 | 39.7 | 1.2 | 12.3 | 2.1 | 46.7 | 2.1 | 1.7 |
| 39. Sorghum (*Sorghum bicolor*) hay | 6.9 | 40.7 | 41.3 | 1.4 | 9.8 | 2.8 | 51.4 | 2.3 | 1.9 |
| Prime | 4.3 | 38.9 | 47.1 | 1.2 | 8.5 | 0.6 | 51.6 | 2.3 | 1.9 |
| Ripe | 4.4 | 42.1 | 44.8 | 1.1 | 7.6 | 2.2 | 5[illegible].0 | 2.2 | 1.8 |
| 40. Oat (*Avena sativa*) | 5.6 | 35.9 | 48.4 | 1.7 | 8.3 | 2.6 | 60.1 | 2.8 | 2.3 |
| 41. Para grass hay | 5.3 | 34.6 | 45.7 | 2.0 | 12.4 | 2.1* | 46.2* | 2 0 | 1.7 |
| | | | *Legume hays* | | | | | | |
| 41. Berseem (*Trifolium alexandrinum*) | 14.7 | 30.6 | 41.0 | 1.6 | 12.1 | 10.3 | 65.8 | 2.9 | 2.4 |
| 42. Cowpea (*Vigna unguiculata*) hay | 15.3 | 34.8 | 35.4 | 1.1 | 13.3 | 10.3 | 50.5 | 2.2 | 1.8 |
| Large variety without pods | 11.4 | 32.8 | 45.9 | 1.4 | 8.6 | 7.5 | 55.6 | 2.4 | 2.0 |
| Small variety | 11.7 | 41.4 | 35.4 | 1.4 | 10.1 | 7.7 | 48.0 | 2.1 | 1.7 |
| 43. Gram hay, average | 12.2 | 33.0 | 41.8 | 2.3 | 10.2 | — | — | — | — |
| 44. Groundnut hay | 21.5 | 24.5 | 38.2 | 1.0 | 14.8 | 14.9 | 48.9 | 2.2 | 1.8 |
| 45. Kudzu vine (*Pueraria lobata*) | 17.7 | 23.4 | 24.3 | 0.6 | 34.1 | 11.7 | 32.6 | 1.4 | 1.2 |
| 46. Lucerne hay | 21.3 | 29.4 | 35.2 | 1.4 | 12.7 | 16.4 | 55.9 | 2.5 | 2.0 |
| 47. Soyabean hay | 15.0 | 29.1 | 42.6 | 1.3 | 12.0 | 10.9* | 54.0* | 2.4 | 1.9 |

| 1 | 2 | 3 | 4 | 5 | 6 | 7 | 8 | 9 | 10 | 11 |
|---|---|---|---|---|---|---|---|---|---|---|
| | | | *Straws* | | | | | | | |
| 48. | Pearl-millet straw, average | 3.5 | 37.8 | 47.7 | 1.1 | 9.8 | 0.9 | 53.4 | 2.4 | 1.9 |
| 49. | Barley straw | 2.2 | 47.4 | 41.4 | 0.9 | 8.1 | 0.8* | 46.9* | 2.0 | 1.7 |
| 50. | Groundnut straw | 8.1 | 40.6 | 39.4 | 1.0 | 10.9 | — | — | — | — |
| 51. | Sorghum (*Sorghum bicolor*) straw, average | 3.8 | 35.6 | 51.0 | 1.3 | 8.3 | 1.2 | 56.4 | 2.5 | 2.0 |
| 52. | Maize kadbi (straw) | 3.6 | 33.2 | 51.9 | 0.8 | 10.5 | — | — | — | — |
| 53. | Paddy straw, average | 3.4 | 33.6 | 42.6 | 1.2 | 18.4 | 0.2 | 45.9 | 1.9 | 1.5 |
| | IR 8 | 3.6 | 42.2 | 32.1 | 1.5 | 20.6 | 0.3 | 40.5 | 1.6 | 1.4 |
| | IR 20 | 3.7 | 39.2 | 35.6 | 1.6 | 19.9 | 0.5 | 41.2 | 1.8 | 1.5 |
| 54. | Wheat bhoosa, average | 3.6 | 34.0 | 1.5 | 13.7 | — | — | — | — | — |
| 55. | Wheat straw, average | 3.2 | 34.9 | 43.8 | 1.5 | 11.6 | 0.0 | 48.4 | 2.1 | 1.7 |
| | | | *Concentrates, Grains and Seeds* | | | | | | | |
| 56. | Pearl-millet grains, average | 11.7 | 1.1 | 78.9 | 5.5 | 2.8 | 5.1 | 60.6 | 2.7 | 2.2 |
| 57. | Barley | 10.1 | 5.0 | 79.4 | 2.0 | 3.5 | 7.4 | 86.0 | 3.4 | 2.8 |
| | Heads | 9.9 | 20.0 | 64.0 | 1.1 | 4.7 | — | — | — | — |
| 58. | Black-gram average | 26.1 | 5.8 | 62.7 | 0.9 | 5.1 | 13.5 | 63.4 | 2.8 | 2.3 |
| | With pods, average | 10.8 | 30.5 | 42.6 | 1.7 | 14.2 | — | — | — | — |
| 59. | Babool pods (*Acacia nilotica*) | 11.0 | 13.8 | 68.5 | 1.0 | 5.7 | 5.8 | 62.3 | 2.7 | 2.2 |
| 60. | Arhar, tur (*Cajanus cajan*), Average | 20.3 | 16.2 | 64.0 | 1.9 | 10.8 | 14.4 | 74.1 | 3.3 | 2.7 |
| | With pods | 9.7 | 27.3 | 46.5 | 2.6 | 13.7 | — | — | — | — |
| | Chuni, average | 14.8 | 20.6 | 54.8 | 2.6 | 7.2 | 7.8 | 64.3 | — | — |
| | Grain with pods | 13.9 | 28.8 | 46.8 | 3.1 | 7.4 | — | — | — | — |
| 61. | Gram | | | | | | | | | |
| | Average | 20.0 | 9.8 | 62.6 | 4.1 | 3.5 | 13.5 | 87.2 | 3.8 | 3.1 |
| | With pods | 16.2 | 23.8 | 43.2 | 2.8 | 9.1 | — | — | — | — |
| | *Chuni*, average | 17.4 | 11.4 | 61.7 | 4.3 | 5.3 | — | — | — | — |
| | Crushed | 25.9 | 9.8 | 57.9 | 2.0 | 4.2 | — | — | — | — |

| | | | | | | | | | |
|---|---|---|---|---|---|---|---|---|---|
| 62. Groundnut, kernel | 31.3 | 1.4 | 13.6 | 51.6 | 2.2 | — | — | — | — |
| 63. Horse-gram (*Dolichos biflorus*) | | | | | | | | | |
| Average | 24.0 | 5.7 | 63.3 | 1.0 | 5.5 | — | — | — | — |
| With pods | 7.2 | 37.7 | 42.4 | 1.2 | 11.5 | — | — | — | — |
| 64. Sorghum (*Sorghum bicolor*) | 15.2 | — | 79.5 | 2.5 | 2.8 | 7.3 | 85.7 | 3.1 | 10.2 |
| 65. Linseed | 19.2 | 6.8 | 32.6 | 36.1 | 7.8 | 15.6 | 117.6 | 5.2 | 4.3 |
| 66. Maize | 11.1 | 1.9 | 80.7 | 4.4 | 1.9 | 8.2 | 94.3 | 3.5 | 2.9 |
| 67. Oat, average | 9.3 | 15.5 | 69.4 | 5.8 | 5.1 | — | — | 3.5 | 2.8 |
| 68. Paddy crushed, average | 7.5 | 10.1 | 72.9 | 1.5 | 8.4 | — | — | — | — |
| 69. Ragi grains (*Eleusine coracana*) grains | 10.3 | 3.7 | 81.0 | 1.2 | 3.9 | — | — | — | — |
| 70. Rice | 8.3 | 0.4 | 89.1 | 10.9 | 1.3 | — | — | — | — |
| Broken | 7.0 | 0.6 | 87.4 | 0.4 | 4.6 | — | — | — | — |
| 71. *Sesamum indicum* seeds | 19.9 | 1.6 | 21.3 | 51.3 | 5.8 | — | — | — | — |
| 72. Soyabean seeds | 41.6 | 6.6 | 28.8 | 17.4 | 6.1 | 37.5 | 87.5 | 3.9 | 3.2 |
| 73. Sunhemp seeds | 35.0 | 10.0 | 46.0 | 3.7 | 5.3 | 30.8 | 70.3 | 3.1 | 2.5 |
| 74. Tamarind (*Tamarindus indica*) | | | | | | | | | |
| Seeds | 18.3 | 26.4 | 44.4 | 7.4 | 3.5 | 5.3 | 60.1 | 2.6 | 2.2 |
| *Cakes and meals* | | | | | | | | | |
| 75. Ambadi cake (*Hibiscus cannabinus*) | 26.7 | 16.6 | 40.9 | 7.1 | 0.87 | 5.7 | 62.4 | 2.38 | 1.93 |
| 76. Coconut-cake | | | | | | | | | |
| (country-mill pressed) | 23.4 | 12.9 | 42.3 | 13.0 | 8.4 | 21.1 | 90.1 | 4.0 | 3.2 |
| Expeller pressed, average | 23.5 | 10.2 | 49.9 | 9.6 | 6.8 | 22.8 | 83.86 | 3.7 | 3.0 |
| 77. Cotton-seed-cake, average | 27.5 | 18.4 | 38.4 | 9.4 | 6.4 | 19.4 | 79.6 | 3.5 | 2.9 |
| 78. Cotton-meal | — | — | — | — | — | 31.6 | 86.0 | 3.8 | 3.1 |
| 79. Groundnut-cake, average | 47.0 | 6.1 | 33.1 | 6.6 | 7.5 | 46.4 | 78.9 | 2.9 | 0.7 |
| 80. Linseed-cake, average | 28.2 | 9.5 | 47.4 | 5.1 | 9.7 | 25.9 | 71.8 | 3.2 | 2.6 |
| 81. Linseed-meal | 29.9 | 9.8 | 49.4 | 4.1 | 6.8 | — | — | — | — |

| 1 | 2 | 3 | 4 | 5 | 6 | 7 | 8 | 9 | 10 | 11 |
|---|---|---|---|---|---|---|---|---|---|---|
| 82. | Mahua-cake (*Madhuca butyracea*) | 17.9 | 5.6 | 50.2 | 17.2 | 9.0 | 8.0 | 60.0 | 2.6 | 2.2 |
| 83. | Niger-cake | 33.2 | 16.7 | 38.4 | 1.3 | 10.4 | 18.9 | 58.7 | 2.5 | 2.1 |
| 84. | Rape-cake (*Brassica campestris*), average | 35.0 | 7.9 | 38.0 | 10.0 | 9.0 | 39.0 | 86.8 | 3.8 | 3.1 |
| 85. | Safflower-cake | 42.8 | 15.2 | 26.6 | 8.5 | 6.8 | 32.2* | 69.3* | 3.0 | 2.5 |
| 86. | Sesame-cake (*Sesamum indicum*) Average | 42.7 | 5.1 | 33.1 | 6.5 | 12.6 | 42.6 | 86 9 | 3.8 | 3.1 |
| 87. | Ghani pressed | 36.4 | 10.7 | 35.7 | 11.2 | 15.9 | — | — | — | — |
| 87. | Sesame-cake, Sunflower-seed-cake | 26.2 | 22.9 | 23.6 | 20.5 | 6.8 | 22.7 | 71.0 | 3.1 | 2.6 |
| 88. | Soyabean-cake | 40.9 | 6.1 | 31.3 | 14.4 | 7.3 | — | — | — | — |

* As no digestibility figures have been reported by Indian workers, foreign digestibility coefficients have been used to calculate the nutritive values of these feeds. These figures are therefore approximate. Where not available, the values of DE and ME are calculated from the TDN values as follows:

1 kg TDN = 4.4 Mcal of DE
1 kg TDN = 3.4 Mcal of ME

** For converting the values expressed on dry matter to those on raw-matter basis, the following *ad hoc* figures for dry matter content of different category of feeding stuffs may be employed :

(a) All air-dry-materials, such as dry roughages, cake, grain etc. 90%
(b) Succulent silage 30%
(c) Green pasture, green forages 25%
(d) Jowar (Prime) 30%
Sorghum (ripe) 40%
(e) Green legume 20%

*Source* : K. C. Sen, S. N. Ray and S. K. Ranjhan, "Nutritive values of Indian cattle feeds and the feeding of animals. Pub. ICAR.

# APPENDIX

## Macro- and Micro-elements in the feeding stuffs on dry-matter basis

| | Per cent | | | | | | Parts per million | | |
|---|---|---|---|---|---|---|---|---|---|
| | Total ash | Ca | P | Mg | Na | K | Cu | Co | Mn |
| 1 | 2 | 3 | 4 | 5 | 6 | 7 | 8 | 9 | 10 |
| *Alysicarpus rugosus* | 9.60- | 1.00- | 0.11- | — | — | — | — | — | — |
| | 10.39 | 1.52 | 0.35 | | | | | | |
| Pearl-millet (*Pennisetum typhoides*) | | | | | | | | | |
| Flowering stage | 11.30- | 0.50- | 0.21- | 0.29 | 0.05 | 3.98 | — | — | — |
| | 12.63 | 0.64 | 0.38 | | | | | | |
| Milk stage | 9.21 | 0.52 | 0.21 | 0.25 | 0.10 | 2.81 | — | — | — |
| Dough stage | 7.68- | 0.43- | 0.12- | — | — | — | — | — | — |
| | 11.00 | 0.52 | 0.45 | | | | | | |
| Ripe stage | 7.68- | 0.36- | 0.19- | 0.20 | 0.10 | 2.46 | — | — | — |
| | 10.56 | 0.39 | 0.20 | | | | | | |
| Barley (*Hordeum vulgare*) | | | | | | | | | |
| | 11.37- | 0.51- | 0.25- | 0.18 | 0.70 | 3.30 | — | — | — |
| One month | 16.62 | 0.84 | 0.37 | — | — | — | — | — | — |
| Two months | 10.55 | 0 52 | 0.24 | — | — | — | — | — | — |
| Three months | 7.75 | 0.47 | 0.18 | — | — | — | — | — | — |
| Berseem (*Trifolium alexandrinum*) | 8.49- | 1.44- | 0.14- | 0.19- | 0.27- | 1.11- | 10.5- | 0.36- | 37.5- |
| | 20.25 | 2.89 | 0.40 | 0.47 | 1.91 | 4.22 | 21.0 | 1.06 | 286.7 |
| 9 weeks | 15.63 | 1.48 | 0.31 | — | — | — | — | — | — |
| 12 weeks | 14.30 | 1.54 | 0.24 | — | — | — | — | — | — |
| 15 weeks | 12.90 | 1.94 | 0.20 | — | — | — | — | — | — |
| 18 weeks | 14.90 | 2.58 | 0.18 | — | — | — | — | — | — |
| 24 weeks | 16.00- | 1.50- | 0.20- | — | — | — | — | — | — |
| | 18.00 | 2.01 | 0.42 | | | | | | |

| 1 | 2 | 3 | 4 | 5 | 6 | 7 | 8 | 9 | 10 |
|---|---|---|---|---|---|---|---|---|---|
| 1 month | 18.85 | 1.85 | 0.40 | — | — | — | — | — | — |
| 2 months | 21.80 | 2.18 | 0.52 | — | — | — | — | — | — |
| 3 months | 12.99 | 1.80 | 0.30 | — | — | — | — | — | — |
| 1st cut | 14.80 | 1.62 | 0.36 | — | — | — | — | — | — |
| 2nd cut | 12.07-14.40 | 1.46-1.73 | 0.33-0.35 | — | — | — | — | — | — |
| 3rd cut | 11.16-14.20 | 1.44-1.83 | 0.32-0.37 | | | | | | |
| 4th cut | 8.92-13.20 | 1.43-1.99 | 0.32-0.35 | — | — | — | — | — | — |
| 5th cut | 7.56-12.64 | 1.32-1.46 | 0.32-0.39 | — | — | — | — | — | — |
| Blackgram (*Vigna mungo*) | 9.72-11.36 | 1.02-2.55 | 0.33-0.39 | — | — | — | — | — | — |
| Cowpea (*Vigna unguiculata*) | 10.86-17.45 | 1.40-2.13 | 0.30-0.45 | — | — | — | 8.4 | — | — |
| Large variety | 9.17 | 1.43 | 0.30 | — | — | — | — | — | — |
| Small variety | 17.27 | 1.47 | 0.31 | — | — | — | — | — | — |
| Gram (*Cicer arietenum*) | | | | | | | | | |
| Podding stage | 10.84 | 1.25 | 0.33 | — | — | — | — | — | — |
| Green fodder | 9.07 | 1.28 | 0.23 | 0.27 | 0.64 | 2.30 | — | — | — |
| Whole plant | 11.38 | 1.41 | 0.25 | 0.28 | 0.26 | 2.16 | — | — | — |
| Bermuda grass (*Cynodon dactylon*) | 7.97-13.97 | 0.36-0.70 | 0.10-0.36 | 0.12-0.36 | 0.05-0.42 | 0.70-3.20 | 7.1-18.7 | 0.10 | |
| Young | 12.58-13.51 | 0.58-0.76 | 0.18-0.36 | 0.23-0.27 | 0.11-0.38 | 1.96-4.28 | — | — | |
| Prime | 11.91-13.10 | 0.50-0.64 | 0.19-0.28 | 0.19-0.25 | 0.21-0.59 | 1.04-1.94 | — | — | |

|  |  |  |  |  |  |  |  |  |  |
|---|---|---|---|---|---|---|---|---|---|
| Ripe | 8.08-15.67 | 0.39-0.91 | 0.10-0.31 | 0.12-0.21 | 0.13-0.64 | 0.70-1.66 | — | — |  |
| October | 16.83 | 0.34 | 0.24 | — | — | — | — | — |  |
| November | 9.82-16.16 | 0.24-0.94 | 0.14-0.25 | — | — | — | — | — |  |
| Bengal variety | 13.51 | 0.66 | 0.21 | — | — | — | — | — |  |
| Blue panic grass (*Panicum antidotale*) | 7.97-9.51 | 0.37-0.39 | 0.09-0.31 | 0.21 | 0.25 | 1.62 | — | — |  |
| 1st cut | 12.23 | 0.38 | 0.38 | — | — | — | — | — |  |
| 2rd cut | 13.31 | 0.48 | 0.24 | — | — | — | — | — |  |
| Guinea grass (*Panicnm maximum*) | 11.39-16.07 | 0.39-0.61 | 0.16-0.39 | 0.23-0.34 | 0.17-0.55 | 0.85-3.14 | 7.2 | 0.16 |  |
| Young | 15.54 | 0.51 | 0.39 | 0.23 | 0.48 | 3.14 | — | — |  |
| Prime | 12.15-13.94 | 0.39-1.81 | 0.24-0.31 | 0.27-0.44 | 0.32-0.42 | 1.20-2.13 | — | — |  |
| September cut | 10.45 | 0.44 | 0.20 | — | — | — | — | — |  |
| October cut | 11.62 | 0.46 | 0.44 | — | — | — | — | — |  |
| November cut | 11.39 | 0.42 | 0.34 | — | — | — | — | — |  |
| Napier (elephant) grass (*Pennisetum purpureum*) | 16.70 | 0.50 | 0.68 | 0.22 | 0.50 | 3.99 | 15.4 | 0.42 | 38 2 |
| Vegetative | 19.09 | 0.45 | 0.69 | — | — | — | — | — | — |
| October cut | 17.14 | 0.34 | 0.21 | — | — | — | — | — | — |
| November cut | 16.59 | 0.22 | 0.30 | — | — | — | — | — | — |
| Thin | 16.52 | 0.17 | 0.48 | — | — | — | — | — | — |
| Napier hybrid | 16.17 | 0.46 | 0.37 | — | — | — | — | — | — |
| Para grass (*Brachiaria mutica*) | 9.53-15.16 | 0.28-0.37 | 0.16-0.35 | — | — | — | — | — | — |
| In running water | 10.77 | 0.23 | 0.11 | — | — | — | — | — | — |
| Water logged | 13.08 | 0.35 | 0.28 | — | — | — | — | — | — |
| Rye (*Lolium perenne*) | 7.77 | 0.36 | 0.32 | — | — | — | 11.6 | — | — |

| 1 | 2 | 3 | 4 | 5 | 6 | 7 | 8 | 9 | 10 |
|---|---|---|---|---|---|---|---|---|---|
| Sudan grass (*Sorghum sudanense*) | 14.39-18.85 | 0.46-0.85 | 0.49-0.58 | 0.30 | 0.06 | 1.65 | 7.1 | — | — |
| | | *Cultivated fodders* | | | | | | | |
| Lucerne (*Medicago sativa*) | 9.27-17.66 | 1.39-2.60 | 0.17-0.49 | 0.16-0.48 | 0.05-0.39 | 1.83-4.09 | 9.8-15.5 | 0.17-0.37 | 23.2-76.0 |
| 1st cut | 12.33 | 1.57 | 0.43 | — | — | — | — | — | — |
| 2nd cut | 10.89 | 1.56 | 0.40 | — | — | — | — | — | — |
| 3rd cut | 9.74 | 1.61 | 0.45 | — | — | — | — | — | — |
| 4th cut | 10.26 | 1.38 | 0.41 | — | — | — | — | — | — |
| Flowering | 8.83 | 1.66 | 0.41 | — | — | — | — | — | — |
| 1st month | 15.71 | 1.96 | 0.42 | — | — | — | — | — | — |
| 2nd month | 14.83 | 2.24 | 0.35 | — | — | — | — | — | — |
| 3rd month | 10.69 | 1.89 | 0.24 | — | — | — | — | — | — |
| Maize (*Zea mays*) | 8.15-9.98 | 0.52 | 0.28 | 0.45 | — | 1.34 | 6.1-21.0 | 0.28 | 49.7-331.5 |
| January | 13.02 | 0.68 | 0.21 | — | — | — | — | — | — |
| February | 11.81 | 0.54 | 0.23 | — | — | — | — | — | — |
| March | 11.64 | 0.61 | 0.19 | — | — | — | — | — | — |
| Dough stage | 7.29 | 0.49 | 0 19 | — | — | — | — | — | — |
| Oat (*Avena sativa*) | | | | | | | | | |
| Young | 13.91 | 0.48 | — | 0.33 | 0.22 | 0.81 | 4.38 | — | — |
| Pea (*Pisum sativum*) | | | | | | | | | |
| Podding | 8.69 | 0.99 | 0.27 | — | — | — | — | — | — |
| 11 weeks | 3.89 | 1.16 | 0.26 | 0.19 | — | 0.76 | — | — | — |

| | | | | | | | | | |
|---|---|---|---|---|---|---|---|---|---|
| Soybean | | | | | | | | | |
| *Glycine max* (syn. G. *hispida*) | 8.29-9.40 | 0.92-1.34 | 0.25-0.43 | 0.84 | — | 1.95 | — | — | — |
| Teosinte (*Euchlaena mexicana*) | 10.80 | 0.76 | 0.16 | 0.30 | — | 1.86 | — | — | — |
| | | | *Silages* | | | | | | |
| Sorghum (*Sorghum bicolor*) | | | | | | | | | |
| Young | 8.04 | — | — | — | — | — | — | — | — |
| Prime maximum | 14.98 | — | — | — | — | — | — | — | — |
| Prime minimum | 6.80 | — | — | — | — | — | — | — | — |
| Average | 10.63 | 0.46 | 0.18 | 0.25 | — | 2.06 | — | — | — |
| Ripe | 6.49 | — | — | — | — | — | — | — | — |
| Maize (*Zea mays*) | 11.33 | — | — | — | — | — | — | — | — |
| Oat (*Avena sativa*) | | | | | | | | | |
| Acid brown | 9.70 | — | — | — | — | — | — | — | — |
| Fruity green | 9.50 | — | — | — | — | — | — | — | — |
| Rice straw (Oryza sativa) | 11.40 | — | — | — | — | — | — | — | — |
| Spear grass (*Heteropogon contortus*) | | | | | | | | | |
| Young | 12.22 | — | — | — | — | — | — | — | — |
| Prime | 15.33 | — | — | — | — | — | — | — | — |
| Wheat straw (*Triticum aestivum*) | 14.62 | — | — | — | — | — | — | — | — |
| | | | *Hays* | | | | | | |
| African fox-tail (*Cenchrus ciliaris*) | 10.18-11.91 | 0.26-0.31 | 0.18-0.31 | 0.17-0.19 | 0.07-1.01 | 0.34-1.74 | — | — | — |
| Young | 12.70 | — | — | — | — | — | — | — | — |
| Prime | 10.90 | — | — | — | — | — | — | — | — |
| Ripe | 9.93 | — | — | — | — | — | — | — | — |
| Post-flowering | 12.69 | 0.44 | 0.41 | — | — | — | — | — | — |

| 1 | 2 | 3 | 4 | 5 | 6 | 7 | 8 | 9 | 10 |
|---|---|---|---|---|---|---|---|---|---|
| Bermuda grass (*Cynodon dactylon*), average | 10.07-14.97 | 0.35-0.51 | 0.19-0.26 | 0.14-0.28 | 0.19-0.73 | 0.86-2.10 | — | — | |
| Giant star grass hay (*Cynodon plectostachys*) | 10.82 | 0.37 | 0.11 | — | — | — | — | — | — |
| Pre-flowering | 6.78 | 0.31 | 0.37 | — | — | — | — | — | — |
| Guinea grass (*Panicum maximum*) | | | | | | | | | |
| Hay, pre-flowering stage | 16.00 | — | — | — | — | — | — | — | — |
| Hay, flowering stage | 12.30 | — | — | — | — | — | — | — | — |
| Jowar hay | 9.77 | 0.27 | 0.24 | 0.27 | 0.19 | 2.21 | — | — | — |
| Prime | 8.51 | 0.27 | 0.24 | 0.27 | 0.19 | 1.39 | — | — | — |
| Ripe | 7.62-10.23 | 0.23-0.37 | 0.04-0.24 | 0.13 | 0.23 | 1.58 | — | — | — |
| Kudzu vine hay (*Pueraria lobata*) | 34.10 | 1.61 | 0.47 | — | — | — | — | — | — |
| Oat (*Avena sativa*) | 0.34 | 0.33 | 0.17 | 0.13 | 0.52 | 0.03 | — | — | — |
| Sugarcane (*Saccharum officinarum*) leaves | 6.09 | 0.39 | 0.06 | 2.22 | 0.34 | 0.83 | — | — | — |
| | | | *Legume hays* | | | | | | |
| Berseem (*Trifolium alexandrinum*) | 12.13 | 1.48 | 0.28 | 0.37 | 0.43 | 3.23 | — | — | — |
| Cowpea (*Vigna unguiculata*) hay | | | | | | | | | |
| Large variety, without pods | 8.56 | 1.00 | 0.23 | — | — | — | — | — | — |
| Small variety | 10.09 | 1.10 | 0.27 | — | — | — | — | — | — |
| Groundnut hay | 14.81 | 1.89 | 0.26 | 0.75 | 0.13 | 2.71 | — | — | — |
| Lucerne hay | 12.74 | — | — | — | — | — | — | — | — |
| Soyabean hay | 12.04 | 2.04 | 0.26 | 0.72 | 0.22 | 1.68 | — | — | — |
| | | | *Straws* | | | | | | |
| Pearl-millet (*Pennisetum typhoides*) straw | 5.89-17.51 | 0.30-0.56 | 0.03-0.36 | — | — | — | 4.50 | — | — |

| | | | | | | | | | |
|---|---|---|---|---|---|---|---|---|---|
| Barley stalks | 6.08 | 0.33 | 0.08 | 0.21 | 0.20 | 1.31 | — | — | — |
| Barley straw | 8.05 | 0.31 | 0.07 | 0.09 | 0.22 | 2.23 | 3.90 | — | — |
| Black gram *bhoosa* | 14.25 | 1.74 | 0.16 | — | — | — | — | — | — |
| Gram stalk (*Cicer arietinum*) | 6.17 | 0.34 | 0.12 | 0.22 | 0.06 | 2.42 | — | — | — |
| Groundnut straw | 10.86 | 1.19 | 0.12 | — | — | — | — | — | — |
| Sorghum (*Sorghum bicolor*) straw | 6.50-<br>9.82 | 0.33-<br>0.52 | 0.05-<br>0.32 | — | — | — | 4.4-<br>8.9 | 0.15 | 43.2 |
| Small red grain variety | 8.07 | 0.37 | 0.30 | — | — | — | — | — | — |
| White large grain variety | 7.33 | 0.29 | 0.05 | — | — | — | — | — | — |
| Maize *kadbi* straw | 10.54 | 0.56 | 0.11 | — | — | — | — | — | — |
| Oat straw | — | — | — | — | — | — | 3.6-<br>8.7 | 0.24 | 36.5-<br>81.0 |
| Paddy straw | 12.84-<br>22.19 | 0.14-<br>0.70 | 0.05-<br>0.30 | — | — | — | 4.3-<br>12.1 | 0.06 | 61.3-<br>155.5 |
| Wheat bhoosa | 13.29-<br>14.07 | 0.30-<br>0.48 | 0.07-<br>7.16 | 0.07 | 0.21 | 4.1-<br>7.5 | 0.07-<br>0.26 | 28.6-<br>48.7 | 176.7-<br>185.0 |
| *Concentrates: Grains and Seeds* | | | | | | | | | |
| Bajra (*Pennisetum typhoides*) grain | 2.68-<br>3.30 | 0.12 | 0.38-<br>0.46 | — | — | — | 12.4-<br>14.0 | 0.28 | 10.9 |
| Barley | 2.69-<br>4.53 | 0.06-<br>0.16 | 0.14-<br>0.39 | 0.13 | 0.04 | 0.47 | 4.1 | 0.15 | — |
| Black-gram (*Vigna mungo*) | 4.29-<br>5.66 | 0.14-<br>0.24 | 0.33-<br>0.43 | — | — | — | — | — | — |
| Cassia tora seeds | 9.08 | 0.72 | 0.20 | — | — | — | — | — | — |
| Cotton seed | 4.15-<br>5.59 | 0.17-<br>0.33 | 0.45-<br>0.65 | — | — | — | — | — | — |
| Gram (*Cicer arietinum*) | 2.63-<br>3.59 | 0.31 | 0.43 | — | — | — | — | — | — |
| Groundnut kernel | 2.15 | — | — | — | — | — | — | — | — |

| 1 | 2 | 3 | 4 | 5 | 6 | 7 | 8 | 9 | 10 |
|---|---|---|---|---|---|---|---|---|---|
| Horse-gram (*Dolichos biflorus*) | 0.65-1.26 | 0.31-0.40 | 0.23-0.39 | — | — | — | — | — | — |
| With pods | 11.51 | 1.66 | 0.13 | — | — | — | — | — | — |
| Sorghum (*Sorghum bicolor*) | 2.80 | — | — | — | — | — | 9.8 | — | — |
| Sorghum with cobs | 9.25 | 0.37 | 0.07 | — | — | — | — | — | — |
| Linseed | 7.77 | 0.26 | 0.62 | — | — | — | — | — | — |
| Maize | 1.85-1.94 | 0.01-0.07 | 0.40-0.41 | — | — | — | 3.8-10.9 | 0.04 | — |
| Oat | 4.79-5.80 | 0.11 | 0.41 | — | — | — | 5.3 | 0.10 | — |
| Ragi (*Eleusine coracana*) grains | 3.89 | 0.61 | 0.45 | — | — | — | — | — | — |
| Rape (*Brassica campestris*) grains | 5.42-6.02 | 0.49-0.51 | 0.65-0.71 | — | — | — | — | — | — |
| Rice | 1.28 | 0.16 | 0.21 | 0.11 | — | 0.27 | 9.8 | — | — |
| Rice broken | 4.64 | 0.16 | 0.16 | — | — | — | — | — | — |
| *Sesamum indicum* seeds | 5.82 | 0.81 | 0.50 | — | — | — | — | — | — |
| *Sesbania bispinosa* seeds | 4.95 | 0.37 | 0.59 | — | — | — | — | — | — |
| Soyabean seeds | 6.11 | 0.41 | 0.77 | — | — | — | — | — | — |
| Tamarind (*Tamarindus indica*) seeds | 3.49 | 0.14 | 0.30 | — | — | — | — | — | — |
| Coconut-cake | | | | | | | | | |
| Country mill pressed | 8.37 | 0.40 | 0.74 | — | — | — | — | — | — |
| Expeller pressed | 6.25-8.34 | 0.09-0.14 | 0.54-0.59 | — | — | — | — | — | — |
| Cotton seed-cake | 4.78-7.96 | 0.28 | 1.28 | — | — | — | 9.8-17.8 | 0.23-0.49 | 11.2-41.2 |
| Guar-meal | — | — | — | — | — | — | 16.2 | 0.48 | 18.9 |

| | | | | | | | | | |
|---|---|---|---|---|---|---|---|---|---|
| Groundnut-cake | 5.61-12.26 | 0.12-0.51 | 0.48 0.82 | 0.33 — | 0.24 — | 1.19 — | 16.6-50.4 | 0.33-0.56 | 26.9 |
| Linseed-cake | 7.85-11.19 | 0.37-0.51 | 0.77-0.96 | 0.59 | 0.35 | 0.76 | 11.6-22.2 | 0.15-0.82 | — |
| Linseed-meal | 6.78 | — | — | — | — | — | 1 | — | — |
| Maize-cake | 2.52-3.45 | 0.23 | 0.52 | — | — | — | — | — | — |
| Mahua (*Madhuca indica*) cake | 9.03 | — | — | — | — | — | — | — | — |
| Mustard-cake | — | — | — | — | — | — | 13.3-29.1 | — | — |
| Rape (*Brassica campestris*) cake | 7.96-9.99 | 0.66-0.84 | 1.07-1.17 | — | — | — | 10.6 | — | — |
| Safflower-cake | 6.80 | — | — | — | — | — | — | — | — |
| Sesame-cake (*Sesamum indicum*) | 11.02-14.87 | 1.11-3.00 | 0.62-0.98 | — | — | — | 9.2 | — | — |
| Ghani pressed | 11.62-17.11 | 2.07-3.00 | 1.07-1.19 | — | — | — | — | — | — |
| Soybean-cake | 7.26 | 0.36 | 0:93 | — | — | — | — | — | — |

# APPENDIX

## Carotene content of the Indian feeding stuffs on dry-matter basis

| Name of material | Age in weeks | DM % | Carotene content (ppm) |
|---|---|---|---|
| 1 | 2 | 3 | 4 |
| | *Grass (Green)* | | |
| Napier grars | 2 | — | 233.3 |
| | 3 | — | 208.7 |
| | 4 | — | 167.6 |
| | 5 | — | 153.9 |
| | 6 | — | 150 0 |
| | 7 | — | 114.1 |
| | 13 | 26.8 | 106.2 |
| Guinea grass | 2 | — | 260.9 |
| | 3 | — | 247.9 |
| | 4 | — | 200.0 |
| | 5 | — | 147.1 |
| | 6 | — | 123.8 |
| | 7 | — | 107.8 |
| | 13 | 23.8 | 118.1 |
| Rhodes grass | 12 | 29.6 | 163.5 |
| Sudan grais | 2 | — | 121.7 |
| | 3 | — | 173.4 |
| | 4 | — | 151.7 |
| | 5 | — | 111.8 |
| | 6 | — | 112.0 |
| | 7 | — | 111.4 |
| | 14 | 33.0 | 97.0 |
| Spear grass | 7 | 37.2 | 137.3 |
| Anjan grass | 14 | 28.2 | 178.9 |
| Dub grass | 4 | 21.4 | 397.5 |
| | *Legumes (Green)* | | |
| Berseem | 3 | 32.3 | 210.6 |
| | 4 | — | 323.1 |
| | 5 | — | 300.1 |
| | 6 | — | 256.4 |
| | 7 | — | 284.4 |
| | 8 | — | 254.6 |
| | 9 | 11.5 | 254.6 |
| Lucerne | 2 | — | 231.1 |
| | 3 | — | 250.0 |
| | 4 | — | 333.5 |
| | 5 | — | 329.7 |
| | 6 | 13.3 | 256.3 |
| | 7 | — | 227.4 |

| 1 | 2 | 3 | 4 |
|---|---|---|---|
| Cowpea | 12 | 23.5 | 231.9 |
| Groundnut plant | — | 21.4 | 237.1 |
| Linseed plant | — | 25.0 | 142.2 |
| Khesari plant | — | 18.2 | 356.6 |
| Pea plant | — | 15.5 | 388.5 |
| Rape-seed plant | — | 19.7 | 380.8 |
| Moong plant | — | 23.9 | 213.4 |
| Guar plant | — | 25.0 | 183.8 |
| *Cereals and Millets (Green)* | | | |
| Barley | 3 | — | 428.6 |
| | 4 | — | 363.2 |
| | 5 | — | 311.1 |
| | 6 | — | 279.4 |
| | 7 | — | 257.8 |
| | 8 | 12.0 | 279.4 |
| Oat | 3 | — | 288.9 |
| | 4 | — | 336 0 |
| | 5 | — | 272.4 |
| | 6 | — | 279.3 |
| | 7 | — | 246.2 |
| | 8 | 12.3 | 228.6 |
| Bajra | 14 | 19.3 | 350.0 |
| Maize | 12 | 18.3 | 285.0 |
| Jowar | 15 | 33.0 | 276.0 |
| *Hays, Straws and By-products* | | | |
| Hay (mixed ripe grasses) | — | — | 0.6 |
| Berseem hay | — | 85.3 | 74.0 |
| Shaftal hay | — | 90.0 | 175.0 |
| Wheat hay (old) | — | 90.0 | 7.0 |
| Oat hay (old) | — | 94.0 | 7.2 |
| Rice straw | — | — | Nil |
| Cane tops | — | 35.9 | 165.0 |
| Wheat bran | — | — | 0.1 |

### Table 46

**Chemical composition (in per cent of dry matter) of different legume and non-legume forages harvested* at pre-flowering (I), flowering (II) and post-flowering (III) stages, as per detergent systems of feed analysis**

| *Forage* | *Stage* | *DM* | *CP* | *NDF* | *Cell content* | *ADF* | *Cellu-lose* | *HC* | *Lignin* | *Silica* | *Ash* |
|---|---|---|---|---|---|---|---|---|---|---|---|
| 1 | 2 | 3 | 4 | 5 | 6 | 7 | 8 | 9 | 10 | 11 | 12 |
| | | | | | *Legumes* | | | | | | |
| Berseem | I | 11.86 | 22.58 | 42.47 | 57.53 | 35.16 | 24.31 | 7.31 | 10.23 | 0.66 | 12.32 |
| (*Trifolium alexandrinum* | II | 16.23 | 17.67 | 49.58 | 50.42 | 38.64 | 25.68 | 10.94 | 11.79 | 1.26 | 11.24 |
| | III | 32.17 | 15.54 | 53.31 | 46.69 | 41.72 | 26.87 | 11.59 | 13.11 | 1.76 | 9.56 |
| Cowpea | I | 11.67 | 24.23 | 43.24 | 56.76 | 34.49 | 23.79 | 8.75 | 9.85 | 0.83 | 13.04 |
| (*Vigna unguiculata*) | II | 14.34 | 20.24 | 49.78 | 50.22 | 37.29 | 25.31 | 12.49 | 11.11 | 1.07 | 11.56 |
| | III | 17.03 | 17.09 | 54.03 | 45.97 | 40.79 | 27.81 | 13.24 | 14.23 | 1.19 | 11.15 |
| Guar | I | 15.18 | 20.23 | 42.34 | 57.66 | 37.27 | 26.48 | 5.07 | 10.03 | 0.83 | 12.55 |
| (*Cyamopsis* | II | 16.98 | 17.46 | 48.44 | 51.56 | 42.46 | 30.10 | 5.98 | 11.59 | 0.92 | 10.63 |
| *tetragonoloba*) | III | 22.71 | 15.34 | 55.07 | 44.93 | 47.65 | 33.08 | 8.42 | 12.51 | 1.07 | 9.28 |
| Lucerne | I | 20.46 | 23.41 | 37.29 | 62.71 | 30.55 | 21.39 | 7.14 | 8.23 | 0.99 | 11.96 |
| *Medicago sativa* | II | 25.37 | 20.00 | 43.64 | 56.36 | 35.83 | 24.56 | 7.77 | 9.45 | 1.30 | 10.58 |
| | III | 29.91 | 15.93 | 50.69 | 49.31 | 39.82 | 26.10 | 10.87 | 11.09 | 1.84 | 10.31 |
| | | | | | *Non-legumes* | | | | | | |
| Anjan grass | II | 33.23 | 4.73 | 71.95 | 28.05 | 37.42 | 27.62 | 34.53 | 8.30 | 1.50 | — |
| Pearl-millet | I | 19.53 | 11.76 | 56.66 | 43.34 | 38.59 | 33.28 | 18.07 | 4.42 | 1.09 | 12.19 |
| (*Pennisetum typhoides*) | II | 24.20 | 7.67 | 64.25 | 35.75 | 40.99 | 34.13 | 23.26 | 4.94 | 1.65 | 9.54 |
| | III | 33.87 | 6.13 | 69.78 | 30.22 | 43.37 | 34.31 | 26.41 | 7.05 | 2.00 | 8.53 |
| Sorghum | I | 17.96 | 12.48 | 55.93 | 44.07 | 37.85 | 30.21 | 18.08 | 5.77 | 1.86 | 9.53 |
| (*Sorghum bicolor*) | II | 29.93 | 9.01 | 65.67 | 34.33 | 41.90 | 32.56 | 23.77 | 6.68 | 2.54 | 8.36 |
| | III | 38.88 | 7.22 | 70.35 | 29.65 | 46.02 | 34.32 | 24.33 | 7.92 | 3.48 | 7.58 |

| | | | | | | | | | | | |
|---|---|---|---|---|---|---|---|---|---|---|---|
| **Maize** | I | 19.46 | 11.05 | 55.07 | 44.93 | 33.92 | 26.72 | 21.15 | 5.66 | 1.55 | 10.22 |
| (*Zea mays*) | II | 25.77 | 8.98 | 62.32 | 37.68 | 38.28 | 29.46 | 24.04 | 6.75 | 2.01 | 8.91 |
| | III | 35.43 | 7.58 | 66.45 | 33.55 | 41.64 | 31.03 | 24.81 | 8.07 | 2.41 | 6.91 |
| **Mustard** | II | 22.10 | 8.50 | 59.90 | 40.10 | 36.70 | 27.20 | 23.20 | 7.70 | 1.80 | — |
| (*Brassica juncea*) | | | | | | | | | | | |
| **Oat** | I | 13.11 | 11.69 | 47.24 | 52.76 | 29.96 | 22.28 | 17.28 | 5.54 | 1.76 | 9.05 |
| (*Avena sativa*) | II | 17.63 | 10.21 | 52.21 | 47.69 | 32.18 | 23.24 | 20.08 | 7.14 | 1.82 | 7.51 |
| | III | 29.10 | 7.98 | 69.63 | 30.37 | 37.58 | 26.87 | 32.05 | 8.04 | 2.31 | 9.12 |
| **Sudan grass** | I | 17.33 | 13.06 | 56.02 | 43.98 | 37.27 | 29.40 | 18.75 | 5.29 | 1.91 | 10.07 |
| (*Sorghum sudanense*) | II | 27.61 | 8.80 | 62.87 | 37.13 | 42.84 | 33.24 | 20.03 | 7.06 | 2.52 | 8.93 |
| | III | 35.04 | 6.88 | 67.77 | 32.23 | 46.16 | 34.10 | 21.61 | 7.97 | 3.54 | 7.76 |
| **Teosinte** | I | 14.27 | 7.03 | 61.56 | 38.44 | 39.33 | 29.52 | 22.23 | 8.05 | 1.63 | 10.60 |
| (*Euchlaenea mexicana*) | II | 25.87 | 6.19 | 67.22 | 32.78 | 41.72 | 31.11 | 25.50 | 8.46 | 1.87 | 8.89 |
| | III | 34.28 | 4.81 | 71.69 | 28.31 | 45.11 | 33.18 | 26.58 | 9.33 | 2.26 | 7.13 |

Table 47

Chemical composition (in per cent of dry matter) of straws/stovers as per detergent systems of feed analysis

| | *CP* | *NDF* | *Cell content* | *ADF* | *Cellulose* | *Hemicellulose* | *Lignin* | *Silica* |
|---|---|---|---|---|---|---|---|---|
| Bajra karbi | 3.15 | 79.50 | 20.50 | 55.60 | 39.40 | 23.90 | 12.80 | 3.40 |
| Gram bhoosa | 6.55 | 65.40 | 34.60 | 48.30 | 32.60 | 17.10 | 13.10 | 2.60 |
| Jowar karbi | 4.25 | 79.70 | 20.30 | 54.20 | 41.00 | 25.50 | 9.00 | 4.20 |
| Moong bhoosa | 10.30 | 45.10 | 54.90 | 33.90 | 20.10 | 11.20 | 5.50 | 8.30 |
| Oat hulls | 3.10 | 69.40 | 30.60 | 38.00 | 26.80 | 31.40 | 7.40 | 3.80 |
| Rice straw | 2.10 | 74.70 | 25.30 | 53.60 | 37.00 | 21.10 | 8.20 | 8.40 |
| Oat straw | 3.40 | 70.40 | 29.60 | 48.60 | 36.52 | 31.80 | 8.50 | 3.60 |
| Sarsan straw | 4.30 | 71.40 | 28.60 | 42.30 | 30.60 | 29.10 | 9.00 | 2.70 |
| Sugarcane tops | 6.30 | 67.00 | 33.00 | 38.20 | 25.70 | 28.80 | 7.50 | 5.00 |
| Urd bhoosa | 10.06 | 46.10 | 53.90 | 30.99 | 19.20 | 15.11 | 5.99 | 5.10 |
| Wheat bhoosa | 2.60 | 76.20 | 23.80 | 51.80 | 36.30 | 24.40 | 9.70 | 5.80 |

*Source* : K.C. Sen, S.N. Ray and S.K. Ranjhan. Nutritive values of Indian cattle feeds and the feeding of animals. Published by ICAR, New Delhi.

# Part II : PRINCIPLES OF ANIMAL NUTRITION

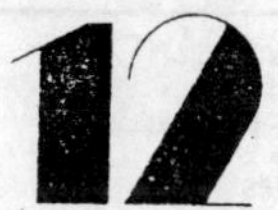

# NUTRIENTS OF FEEDING STUFF AND ANIMAL BODY

A nutrient is a substance that promotes the growth, maintenance, function, and reproduction of a cell or an organism. The principal nutrients of all feeding stuffs are water, organic and mineral matters. The organic in turn is composed of crude protein, ether extract, crude fibre and nitrogen free extract. The occurrence of these nutrients in feeds and their role as constituents of feed in the nutrition of animal body may briefly be stated as follows.

**Table 48**

Nutrient contributions of major feedstuff groups.[a]

| Feedstuff | Relative value | | | | | | |
|---|---|---|---|---|---|---|---|
| | | | Minerals | | Vitamins | | |
| | Protein | Energy | Macro | Trace | Fat-sol. | B-complex | Bulk |
| High quality roughage | ++ | ++ | ++ | ++ | +++ | + | +++ |
| Low quality roughage | + | + | + | + | – | – | ++++ |
| Cereal grains | ++ | +++ | + | + | + | + | + |
| Grain millfeeds | ++ | ++ | ++ | ++ | + | ++ | ++ |
| Feeding fats | – | ++++ | – | – | – | – | – |
| Molasses | + | +++ | ++ | ++ | – | + | – |
| Fermentation products | +++ | ++ | + | ++ | – | ++++ | ± |
| Oil seed proteins | +++ | +++ | ++ | ++ | + | ++ | ++ |
| Animal proteins | ++++ | +++ | +++ | +++ | ++ | +++ | + |

[a] Relative values are indicated by number of +. Feeding values (nutrient content and availability) of any product depends on many different factors which are discussed in the text.

## WATER

It may seem strange to speak of water as a food. but in view of the fact that the body is composed of about two-thirds water and that a food is any substance used by the body for building tissue it is obvious that water is a very important food. Experiments have shown that animals may live for more than 100 days without organic food but they die in 5 to 10 days when deprived of water. Water is lost in the urine, faeces, expired air and from the skin. Water is obtained by drinking, from the feed (green succulent fodder contains on an average 70 per cent moisture while dry roughage and concentrates contain about 10 per cent moisture), and from metabolic water, that is, water formed from oxidation of nutrients.

## Table 49 CLASSIFICATION OF NUTRIENTS BY ANALYSIS

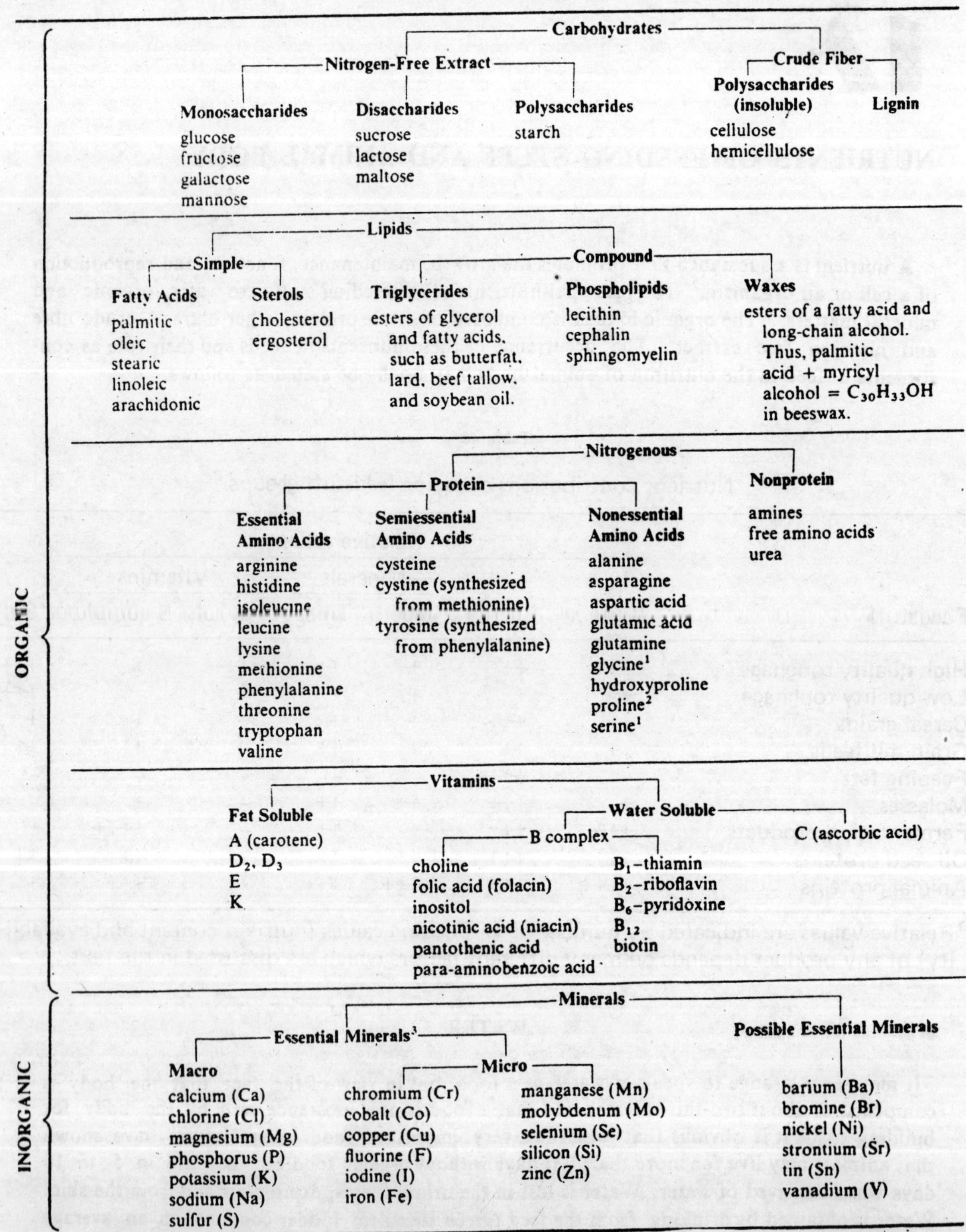

**ORGANIC**

- **Carbohydrates**
  - **Nitrogen-Free Extract**
    - **Monosaccharides**: glucose, fructose, galactose, mannose
    - **Disaccharides**: sucrose, lactose, maltose
    - **Polysaccharides**: starch
  - **Crude Fiber**
    - **Polysaccharides (insoluble)**: cellulose, hemicellulose
    - **Lignin**
- **Lipids**
  - **Simple**
    - **Fatty Acids**: palmitic, oleic, stearic, linoleic, arachidonic
    - **Sterols**: cholesterol, ergosterol
  - **Compound**
    - **Triglycerides**: esters of glycerol and fatty acids, such as butterfat, lard, beef tallow, and soybean oil.
    - **Phospholipids**: lecithin, cephalin, sphingomyelin
    - **Waxes**: esters of a fatty acid and long-chain alcohol. Thus, palmitic acid + myricyl alcohol = $C_{30}H_{33}OH$ in beeswax.
- **Nitrogenous**
  - **Protein**
    - **Essential Amino Acids**: arginine, histidine, isoleucine, leucine, lysine, methionine, phenylalanine, threonine, tryptophan, valine
    - **Semiessential Amino Acids**: cysteine, cystine (synthesized from methionine), tyrosine (synthesized from phenylalanine)
    - **Nonessential Amino Acids**: alanine, asparagine, aspartic acid, glutamic acid, glutamine, glycine[1], hydroxyproline, proline[2], serine[1]
  - **Nonprotein**: amines, free amino acids, urea
- **Vitamins**
  - **Fat Soluble**: A (carotene), $D_2$, $D_3$, E, K
  - **Water Soluble**
    - **B complex**: choline, folic acid (folacin), inositol, nicotinic acid (niacin), pantothenic acid, para-aminobenzoic acid, $B_1$–thiamin, $B_2$–riboflavin, $B_6$–pyridoxine, $B_{12}$, biotin
    - **C (ascorbic acid)**

**INORGANIC**

- **Minerals**
  - **Essential Minerals**[3]
    - **Macro**: calcium (Ca), chlorine (Cl), magnesium (Mg), phosphorus (P), potassium (K), sodium (Na), sulfur (S)
    - **Micro**: chromium (Cr), cobalt (Co), copper (Cu), fluorine (F), iodine (I), iron (Fe), manganese (Mn), molybdenum (Mo), selenium (Se), silicon (Si), zinc (Zn)
  - **Possible Essential Minerals**: barium (Ba), bromine (Br), nickel (Ni), strontium (Sr), tin (Sn), vanadium (V)

[1]Under some conditions, glycine or serine synthesis may not be sufficient for most rapid growth; either glycine or serine may need to be supplied in the diet.

[2]When diets composed of crystalline amino acids are used, proline may be necessary to achieve maximum growth.

[3]Required by at least one animal species.

All water contained in the organism belongs to one of the two main fractions: extracellular and intracellular. The former fraction is represented by the water in the blood plasma, interstilial fluids (the fluid between the cells or body parts) and lymph (the watery fluid in the lymph vessels collected from the tissue fluids). In the body of the adult animal intracellular (within a cell) water represents about 70 per cent and extracellular fluid (fluid within the body but outside the cells) accounts for 30 per cent of total amount of water.

**Table 50**

**Distribution of body water**

| Water fraction | % of body weight | % of total water |
|---|---|---|
| Total | 65 | 100 |
| Extracellular | 20 | 30 |
| Intracellular | 45 | 70 |
| Plasma water | 5 | 7.5 |
| Interstitial | 15 | 22.5 |

Cell membranes separate the intracellular from the interstitial fluid. The latter, in turn, is separated from blood plasma and from the lymph by capillary walls acting as a dialysing membrane, which is permeable to electrolytes and crystalloids, but impermeable to suspended proteins and to the configurational elements of the blood, except for leucocytes.

The bulk of the water in extracellular and intracellular fluids, which acts as solvent for inorganic and organic compounds is known as free water.

### Metabolic Water

**When organic compounds such as fats, proteins and carbohydrates are oxidised in the animal body, one of the end products is water. Similary, when proteins, carbohydrates and fats are synthesised liberation of water takes place. The water which is available to the animal body by such biochemical reaction is known as *metabolic water*. One molecule of glucose on**

**Table 51**

**Production of metabolic water**

**(Yield in gm Water from 1 gm of substance oxidised)**

| *Substance* | | | *Water* |
|---|---|---|---|
| Glucose | ... | ... | 0.60 |
| Starch | ... | ... | 0.56 |
| Tributyrin | ... | ... | 0.77 |
| Tristearin | ... | ... | 1.11 |
| Protein (average) | ... | ... | 0.42 |

oxidation gives six molecules of water. It has been estimated that a person producing 2,400 calories per day obtain about 300 ml of water as a result of oxidation of food. The metabolic water is just useful to the animal as that from any other source.

In certain circumstances this water may form the major, if not the only source of supply; for example, in the incubating chick and in hibernating animals.

A study of the manner in which water exists in protoplasm has revealed that it may exist either in the free state or in combination with certain of the constituents of protoplasm, usually proteins, in the form of bound water.

**Bound water**

Bound water differs from free water in that it is bound with proteins in colloidal system or water present inside cells as hydrated ions, as well as the water enclosed between fibrous molecules. Therefore, bound water does not separate easily from protoplasm by freezing at low temperature or by evaporation at high temperature or under dry conditions.

**Table 52**

**Composition of an enfire adult mammalian animal**

| | |
|---|---|
| Water | 60% |
| Protein | 16% |
| Fat | 20% |
| Ash | 4% |

**Table 53**

**Average water content of bovine and human body at various ages**

| Bovine | % Water | Human | % Water |
|---|---|---|---|
| Embryo | 90 | Embryo | 93 |
| New born calf | 80 | New born infant | 72 |
| 6-12 m calf | 65 | 2 m infant | 70 |
| Mature steer | 55 | Adult | 60 |

**Table 54**

**Average content of water in organs and tissue of animals**

| Organ or tissue | $H_2O$% | Organ or tissue | $H_2O$% |
|---|---|---|---|
| Fatty tissue | 7 | | |
| Dentine | 10 | Kidneys | 81 |
| | | Whole blood | 82 |
| Bone | 28 | Brain (Grey matter) | 86 |
| Skin | 58 | Elastic tissue | 90 |
| Liver | 70 | Lymph | 95 |
| Muscles | 75 | Gastric juices | 97 |
| Heart, lungs | 80 | Spinal fluid | 99 |

Bound water is of special interest in connection with the ability of plants and animals to resist low temperature and drought.

## FUNCTIONS OF WATER IN ANIMAL BODY

1. CELL RIGIDITY AND ELASTICITY. **The body must have a definite form which it can retain and yet, within limits, it must be able to change its shape by confirming to some extent to the force applied at any particular point. This is made possible by the liquid contents of the cell. In particular, the cerebrospinal fluid acts as cushion for the nerves.**

2. SOLVENT ACTION. By its solvent action it serves as a universal medium in which the intra- and extra-cellular chemical reaction take place. Probably no chemical reaction inside the body can take place without water.

3. HYDROLYTIC REACTIONS. Hydrolysis is an important chemical process involved in digestion and other metabolism. In this process the H and OH ions of water are introduced into bigger molecules and the latter is broken down into smaller units.

4. IONIC AND OTHER REACTIONS. The process of living depends upon a continuous series of chemical reactions and many of these reactions require a medium in which to act; in the animal body this medium is water. The dielectric constant of water being very high, oppositely charged ions can co-exist in water without much interference.

5. LUBRICATION. Water acts as a lubricant to prevent friction and drying. In joints, pleura, conjunctiva, etc., the aqueous solution practically free from fat acts as a lubricant against rubbing and drying.

6. TRANSPORT. Water acts as a vehicle for various physiological processes, such as:

(a) For absorption of food material from intestine.
(b) For reabsorption from kidney tubules.
(c) For the transport of various foodstuffs from place to place.
(d) For the drainage and excretion of the end products of metabolism.
(e) For the manufacture of various secretions, such as digestive juices, etc.
(f) For carrying the hormones (water soluble) to their places of activity.

7. HEAT REGULATION. Body temperature is regulated by water in following ways:

(*a*) *Heat absorption*. Due to high specific heat of water more heat is required to raise the temperature of 1 gm. of water to 1°C than most of the known solids and liquids. By virtue of this property water can absorb large quantity of heat.

(*b*) *Heat conduction and distribution*. Heat conducting power of water being very high, it acts as a very good agent in carrying away heat from the site of production and distributing it throughout the body. By the above two properties water acts as an important buffer.

(*c*) *Heat loss*. Water helps heat loss through urine and stool and by evaporation from skin, lungs, etc. Water has got the highest latent heat of evaporation, 589 cal. per gm which means that to change 1 gm of liquid water to 1 gm of water vapour without any change in temperature, 589 cal. are required. By this means the body is able to rid itself of 589 cal. of heat for every gm of water it evaporates.

8. RESPIRATORY FUNCTION. Although $CO_2$ and $O_2$ are only slightly soluble in water, yet this solubility is of immense importance for the gaseous exchange in the tissues and lungs. The fishes derive oxygen almost exclusively from dissolved oxygen in water.

9. REFRACTIVE MEDIUM. The aqueous humour helps to keep up the shape and tension of the eye ball and acts as a refractive medium for light.

It is, therefore, apparent that the animal should be given liberal quantities of water. Deficiency of water on the other hand, delays digestion, assimilation and excretion of waste products through urine. If the deficiency of water in an animal be continued long then its blood tends to thicken with a rise in temperature. Animals, like men, can stand lack of food much longer than lack of water.

**Water migration and water balance in the body**

The animal obtains water for satisfying all physiological needs from various sources. Drinking of fresh water partly fulfils the requirement, the water content of concentrate and dry roughages varies between 12 to 16 per cent, while the green forages may contain as high as 70 per cent moisture.

In a body the water received through drinking and from the feed during fermentation is known as exogenous water which is absorbed by the intestinal wall, enters the blood stream and participates in metabolic processes.

During metabolism of various body nutrients either in the liver or in other tissues, oxidation is a very common physiological phenomenon that takes place with concomitant release of water molecules. In quantitative terms the oxidation of 1 kg of fat, carbohydrate or protein theoretically yields 1,070 g, 550 g, 400 g of water respectively. In the case of birds, the amount of metabolic water may be readily calculated, since the conversion of one kcal is accompanied by the liberation of 0.135 g water. If a bird utilises, for example, 300 kcal per day, the amount of metabolic water formed is 40 g or 15 per cent of the amount of water required in 24 hours. Thus the metabolic water contributes a significant share of water input of the body.

**Table 55**

**Routes of input and output of body water**

| Input into the body | Output from the body |
|---|---|
| 1. In drinking water | 1. Through urine |
| 2. Water content of feed | 2. Through faeces |
| 3. As metabolic water derived either from oxidation of nutrients or from polymerisation of compounds such as amino acids into peptides. | 3. Through respiration |
| | 4. As in sweat |
| | 5. Through milk |
| | 6. Through saliva,—most of which will be absorbed lower down the G.I. tract and thus a temporary loss. |

Elimination of water from the body proceeds mainly via the urine, faeces, respiration, via the skin (sweat) and through milk and other products. Elimination of water by the kidneys cannot fall below a certain critical level, which is determined by the amount of electrolytes and nitrogenous substances excreted (urea in mammals, uric acid in birds).

**Table 56**

**Average volume of urine excreted by animal**

| Animal species | Average amount (litre) | Range (litre) | ml/kg body weight |
|---|---|---|---|
| Horse | 5 | 2-11 | 4-18 |
| Cow during lactation | 7 | 5-14 | 17-45 |
| Sheep, Goat | 1 | 0.5-2 | 10-40 |
| Pig | 4 | 2-6 | 5-30 |
| Dog | 0.6 | 0.4-1 | 20-100 |
| Hen | 0.1 | 0.5-0.2 | 25-120 |

The average percentage water contents of animal faeces are: Sheep 68, horses, dogs and birds 75, pig 80, cattle 84.

At a comfortable temperature (20 to 25°C) heat formation and dissipation through the lungs and skin are more or less constant, and regulated by physical factors. When the temperature increases, the loss of water through the skin and lungs becomes important. Evaporation of one gram of water at 22°C is accompanied by the loss of 0.584 kcal, and at 39°C by the loss of 0.578 kcal. Accordingly, thermal stress brings about intensification of blood circulation in skin capillaries, more rapid respiration, and increased exudation of water by the sweat glands and respiratory organs. Water loss via perspiration (sweating) does not occur in birds, goats, rabbits and dogs. In cattle a temperature near about 30°C will cause evaporation losses equal to 25 per cent of the total water losses.

Study of the water balance in animals involves on one side the amount of water entering the body with feed, drink and metabolic water, while on the other side loss of water through faeces, urine, by evaporation and milk.

**Table 57**

**Daily water balance of Holstein cow fed lucerne hay**

| | Non-lactating (litres) | Lactating (litres) |
|---|---|---|
| **Intake:** | | |
| Drinking water | 26 | 51 |
| Water in feed | 1 | 2 |
| Metabolic water | 2 | 3 |
| Total | 29 | 56 |
| **Output:** | | |
| In faeces | 12 | 19 |
| In urine | 7 | 11 |
| By evaporation | 10 | 14 |
| In milk | 0 | 12 |
| Total | 29 | 56 |

## Factors Controlling Water Input and Output

The body has a remarkable ability to regulate its retention and excretion of water. If water is withheld the following compensator mechanisms are initiated to provide enough water for maintenance.

1) Urine excretion is reduced as is the water content of the faeces.

2) Animals become sedentary, seeking shade whenever possible to reduce the loss of water from surface evaporation and sweating.

3) There is reduction in feed consumption except from feeds that are high in moisture.

4) Hormonal control.

a) During water scarcity, the antidiuretic (ADH) hormone is secreted by the pituitary gland following stimulation of osmoreceptors in the hypothalamus. ADH stimulates resorption of water in the kidney tubules.

b) Adrenal corticosteroids which affect sodium metabolism indirectly affects water excretion.

c) Also in certain circumstances the six hormones may have an effect because animals tend to become alternately hydrated and then dehydrated during the oestrus cycle.

5) Neurological mechanism: Intake of drinking water is also controlled by a neurological mechanism and a thirst centre has been identified in the hypothalamus. Thus in the ruminant the thirst centre has a double function, not only does it stimulate drinking to replace body fluids, but it also serves to maintain ruminal flora and fauna which require a constant proportion of water for utilising feed intake. It is not surprising therefore that one of the first signs of water deprivation in the ruminant is a decline in appetite. There is thus an interdependency between dry matter intake and water. Whenever the intake of one is reduced the voluntary intake of the other is affected.

6) Individual variation: This is a most important factor governing water intake. Conditions remaining the same, one animal may require as high as 50 per cent or more than the average requirement. That is why a general recommendation is made for providing unrestricted amount of water to all domestic animals.

7) Species variation: Variability between species has also been noted. European cattle (*Bos taurus*) drink more than Indian cattle (*Bos indicus*).

8) Physiological conditions: Pregnancy and lactation impose additional demands in common livestock but the same has not been noted for sheep.

9) Temperature: Environmental temperature is another important factor. In one information it has been shown that at an environmental temperature of 40°F the water intake of cattle is 3.09 kg/kg dry matter consumed; at 60°F it is 3.84 kg/kg; at 80°F it is 5.17 kg/kg of dry matter consumption.

10) Age: Young calves, because of the high content of water in their liquid diet, necessarily consume more water than older animals on dry matter diets. The total consumption of water by calves varies from 5.4 to 7.5 kg/kg dry matter, and small additional amounts of water may be consumed as drinking water.

11) The type and composition of the diet: Grass may contain over 80 per cent water, especially after rain, but dry diets given to housed animals may contain only 5.7 per cent water. Cows on pasture, eating lush grass may consume 150 per cent more water than housed indoors.

High protein diets may impose extra requirement for water presumably because much of the protein is converted into urea which is then excreted in urine via the kidneys. In general it has been found that high protein diets require 26-30 per cent more water than those on low protein diets.

Salt in ration may increase water consumption from 22-100 per cent and thus care should be taken to provide adequate water supplies for cattle receiving salt blocks containing urea additives. If adequate water supplies are not made available to the animal, the blood eventually thickens, resulting in a decreased ability to transport nutrients and waste products. Animal body composition varies between 40 and 65 per cent water depending on age, condition (fatness), species and breed. On a fat-free basis, muscle tissue comprises 70 to 75 per cent water. It has been suggested that the body of an animal may lose virtually all its fat and about one-half of its protein and still survive, but a loss that exceeds approximately 10 per cent of its water may result in death.

**Effects of water restriction**

Depending upon the degree of water restrictions the following observations have been noted:

1). Food intake is drastically reduced. Research carried out on European cattle breeds has shown that a one-day deprival of water coupled with the feeding of roughages leads to a depression of feed intake of 24 per cent and a two-day deprival of water to a depression of 62 per cent.

2) Increase in pulse rate and in rectal temperature.

3) Increase in respiration.

4) Tingling and numbness of fingers and feet.

5) Low production.

6) Decrease in fertility rate—it has been reported that heifers kept on a restricted water supply following mating had a conception rate of 57.9 per cent as compared to 78.3 per cent in controls.

7) During dehydration the animal gives priority to maintaining blood volume and composition. In the early stages blood volume is maintained by transfer of water from the connective tissue spaces into the blood plasma. This leads to loss of skin elasticity and mobility which is a characteristic sign of a moderate degree of dehydration. When no further compensation is possible by this means plasma volume begins to fall and the blood becomes increasingly concentrated, the proportion of cells and total solid rising steadily as the dehydration progresses. The degree of dehydration can be assessed most readily by the rising concentration of haemoglobin and haematocrit.

Due to haemoconcentration large increase in blood urea results from reduced filtration rate in the kidneys. Increases in serum sodium and in serum osmolarity may also develop. The final stages of dehydration involve severe curtailment of blood volume and increase in blood viscosity which lead to circulatory failure, coupled with uremia and metabolic acidosis—presumably due to failure of the kidney to adjust the acid/base balance.

Clinical signs of dehydration in an adult cow are said to occur when there is an 8-10 per cent loss of body weight.

**Characteristics of water balance in camels**

Camels, that is *Camelus dromedarius* and *C. bactrianus*, have developed a special adaptibility to their environment as regards to their water requirements. Whereas most mammals suffer physical disorders when there is a water loss of 12-15 per cent of their body weight.

camels can support a water loss of 25 per cent. Even a shortage of water lasting for several weeks does not harm the camel physically. When there is a lack of water, an increasingly concentrated urine is formed in the course of time, and urine excretion falls from 5-10 litres (with adequate water supplies) to 0.5 litres.

Camels are able to re-absorb the urea in the kidney tubuli to a large extent, and can return it to the rumen where it is utilised by the microbes for protein synthesis. It is a remarkable fact that the camel's body temperature can rise during the day with increasing ambient temperatures to 40.5°C without any significant increase in sweat formation. During the night the body temperature can fall with sinking ambient temperatures to 34°C.

Under favourable feeding conditions, camels store deposits of fat which can be drawn upon in periods of short supply and the oxidation of which produces small quantities of water (approx. 1-3 litres/day). Water requirements in non-lactating camels amount on an average at a temperature of 41°C to 61 ml/kg/day. Merino sheep kept under the same climatic conditions have a water requirement of 110 ml/kg/day, whereas cattle have 148 ml/kg/day.

After long periods of water shortage, camels can drink up to 80 litres of water within 10 minutes. A certain amount of water is stored in the rumen, the water content of which is reduced in the course of long periods of lack of water.

## Water requirements

The many factors that influence water requirements make it difficult to recommend specific allowances, For instance, new tissue growth in young animals contains approximately 75 per cent water; and it has been suggested that *non-lactating adult cattle need between 3 and 8.5 kg water for each kg of dry matter consumed.* These amounts should be increased by approximately 50 per cent for pregnant animals during the last part of the gestation period. Lactation requires an additional 0.87 kg water for each kg of milk produced. These amounts are for temperate zones and must be modified for arid and tropical regions. There is an interdependency between water and dry matter intakes. Whenever the intake of one is reduced, the voluntary intake of the others is affected. Sheep and cattle respond quickly to a reduced water intake. Camels as has been covered, and to a lesser extent goats,tolerate longer periods of water deprivation without adverse affects on dry matter intake. Ultimately, however, the need for water becomes apparent in all species as a reduction of dry matter intake (DMI). Each area having its own unique environment, breeds of animals, and feed resources must determine the optimum requirements compatible with the available supply. Ambient temperature affects an animal's requirement of water. In cool weather the water intake for cattle (*Bos taurus*) may be as low as 3 kg/kg DMI. There is some evidence that Indian breeds (*Bos indicus*), on an average consume less water than the amounts consumed by European breeds.

Water containing nitrates, alkalines, salts or other contaminants may be unsuitable for animal use. Water containing 10,000 ppm of soluble salts for example, may be toxic to some animals. Whenever possible, the water supply should be clean, free from toxic substances and available *ad libitum* to animals at all times.

## CARBOHYDRATES

Carbohydrates literally means *hydrate of Carbon.* When sugars are heated for a long time in a test tube, a black residue (Carbon) and droplets of water condensed on the sides of the tube will be obtained.

Carbohydrates are all compounds of carbon, hydrogen and oxygen. Generally but not always the hydrogen and oxygen in carbohydrates are present in the proportion of two hydrogen atoms to one oxygen atom as in $H_2O$, from which fact the term "carbohydrates" (carbon hydrate) was derived and thus carbohydrates were originally represented with an empirical formula $C_x(H_2O)_n$. Glucose has the molecular formula $C_6H_{12}O_6$ and can be written as carbon hydrate, $C_6(H_2O)_6$.

Today we retain the name but are not bound to the empirical formula. Many substances not carbohydrates contain hydrogen and oxygen in the proportion of $H_2O$ such as acetate ($C_2H_4O_2$) and lactic acids ($C_3H_6O_3$). Also some carbohydrates, such as deoxyribose ($C_5H_{10}O_4$), rhamnose ($C_6H_{12}O_5$) do not contain hydrogen and oxygen in the proportion of $H_2O$.

*Carbohydrate thus may well be defined as polyhydroxy (more than one OH group) aldehyde or polyhydroxy ketone as in monosaccharides*; their polymers as oligo and polysaccharides; their reduction products as polyhydric alcohols; oxidation products as aldonic, uronic and saccharic acid; substitution products as amino sugars.

In plants carbohydrates are produced by means of photosynthesis. Solar energy from the sun is captured by chloroplasts and changed to chemical energy in the form of carbohydrates using atmospheric $CO_2$ and water from the soil.

$$6CO_2 + 6H_2O + \overset{\text{Solar}}{\text{energy}} = 6O_2 + C_6H_{12}O_6$$

Carbohydrates constitute by far the greatest proportion of organic material on the face of the earth, and the most abundant carbohydrate is cellulose which not only forms the principal diet of ruminants but is also found in all woods.

The starches are abundant and widespread, specially in grains, tubers and roots where they serve as reserve food material for plants and are utilised as the chief carbohydrate food of man.

Cane sugar or sucrose is present in the nectar of flowers, in fruits and in the juices of various plants. Large quantities of pentosans are found in plants, specially in seed husks, maize cobs, in other fibrous structures, plant gums and mucilages.

The glucosides are a class of carbohydrate derivatives which are frequent constituents of plants. A number of these substances are important drugs, among which are the glucosides of digitalis used in the treatment of heart disease.

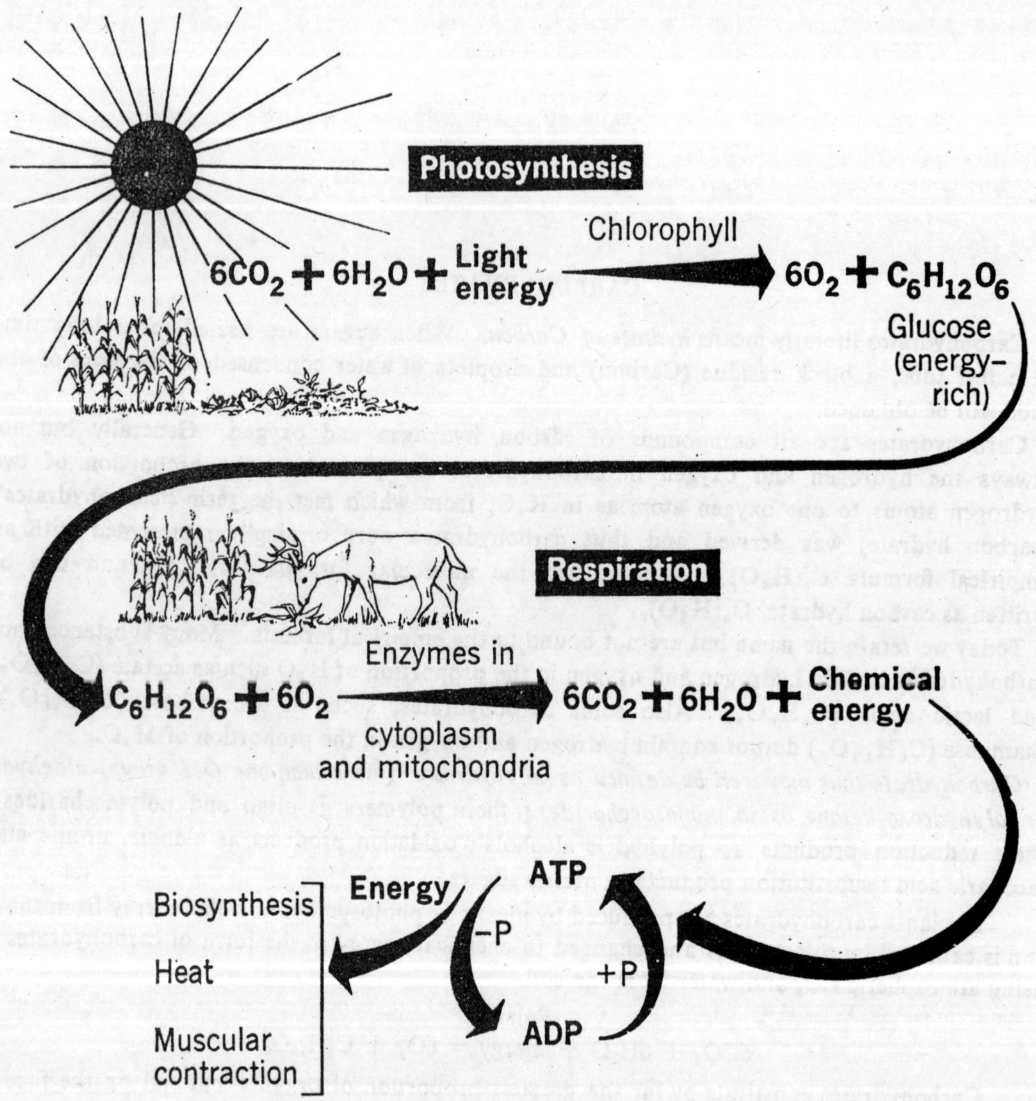


**Fig. 15** Energy relationships in life.

Carbohydrates are the major constituents of most plants comprising from 60—90 percent of their dry mass (mostly as cellulose). They form the woody framework of plants as well as the chief reserve food stored in seeds. In contrast, animal tissue contains very small (less than 1%) amount but without which life will be at stake. Humans, the special animals not only utilise carbohydrates for their food (about 60-75% by mass of the average diet), but also for their clothing (cotton, linen, rayon), shelter (wood), fuel (wood), and paper (wood).

The amount of carbohydrate present in an adult human body is about 300-350 gm. Of this

110 gm is stored as glycogen in the liver. Another 200-250 gm is present as glycogen in cardiac smooth and skeletal muscle and about 15 gm makes up the glucose in the blood and extracellular fluid.

Glucose is the sugar of blood and other body fluids. Human blood normally contains 80 to 120 mg glucose in each 100 ml. Glucose is oxidised preferentially by most of the tissues of the body to provide energy. Ordinarily more than half of the energy of the body is provided by the oxidation of glucose, except converted to fats and stored in fat depots in human and other non-ruminants.

**Is Carbohydrate a Dietary Essential?**

Although carbohydrates are essential components of the nucleic acids and of structural compounds such as hyaluronic acid and although they are required as energy producing substrate for certain organs such as the central nervous system, all the necessary sugar units can be manufactured in the body from precursors derived from the amino acids and the glycerol of various fats. As a result, no carbohydrate is required in the diet, and it has been shown experimentally that human beings can survive in good health for months on a diet of meat and fats which provide only a very small amount of sugar.

In spite of this, ration of our livestock as well as of the Indian population consists of a considerable amount of carbohydrates. It may be noted that although carbohydrate is not a dietary essential, it is definitely metabolically essential. All organic compounds namely fat protein etc. are oxidised only in the presence of carbohydrates. DNA, RNA and some other vital organic molecules cannot be formed without carbohydrate components. Although less than 1 per cent is present in a human body, yet without this carbohydrate presence the existence of living creatures is at stake.

## BIOLOGICAL IMPORTANCE

**1. Energy**

The principal function of carbohydrate in the form of glucose and glycogen is to furnish energy for the body. More than 50 per cent of the energy value of the diet is provided by the carbohydrates.

Glucose + 2 ATP (or glycogen + 1 ATP) $\rightarrow$ 2 Lactic acid + 4 ATP

Glucose + 2 ATP (or glycogen + 1 ATP) $\rightarrow$ $6CO_2 + 6H_2O$ + 40 ATP.

Thus each gram of carbohydrate when oxidised yields on an average four kilocalories. Excess glycogen in the blood is stored in the liver and muscles, as glycogen apart from conversion of body fat in non-ruminants which is also utilised as a source of energy needs when glycogen stores are depleted.

**2. Protein-sparing action**

The body will use carbohydrate preferentially as a source of energy when it is adequately supplied in the diet, thus sparing protein for tissue building. Since meeting energy needs of the body takes priority over other functions, any deficiency of calories in the diet will be made up by using adipose and protein tissues.

### 3. Oxidation of protein and fat

It is said that proteins and fats are burnt (oxidised) in the flame of carbohydrate. It means that certain intermediary compounds of glucose oxidation through Kreb cycle are absolutely necessary for oxidation of proteins and fats. When the glucose content of the body is severely restricted, fats and proteins will be metabolised faster than the body can take care of the intermediate products. The accumulation of these incompletely oxidised products of protein and mainly of fats will lead to ketosis.

### 4. Carbohydrate in body compounds

Structurally, carbohydrate accounts for a very small part of the weight of the body. Nevertheless, monosaccharides are vitally important constituents of numerous compounds that regulate metabolism. Among these are:

i) Deoxyribonucleic acid (DNA) and ribonucleic acid (RNA), the compounds that possess and transfer the genetic characteristics of the cell, contain deoxy-ribose and ribose respectively.

ii) Glucuronic acid (is formed from glucose by oxidation of UDP-glucose) which occurs in the liver and is also a constituent of a number of mucopoly-saccharides. Glucuronic acid in the liver when combines with toxic chemicals and bacterial by-products acts as a detoxifying agent.

iii) Hyaluronic acid, the disaccharide composed of glucosamine and glucuronic acid is a viscous substance that forms the matrix of connective tissue.

HYALURONIC ACID

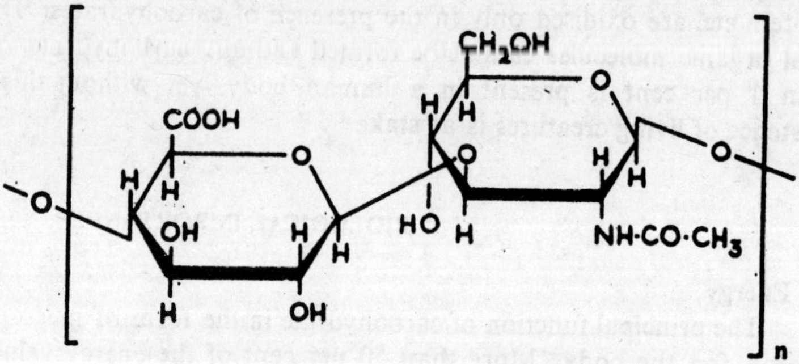

β-Glucuronic acid N-Acetylglucosamine

iv) Heparin, a mucopolysaccharide consists of chains of glucuronic acid and glucosamine, containing sulphate ester groups. Molecular weight is about 20,000 and its exact structure is still in doubt. The compound is exceptionally noted for its anticoagulant property.

HEPARIN

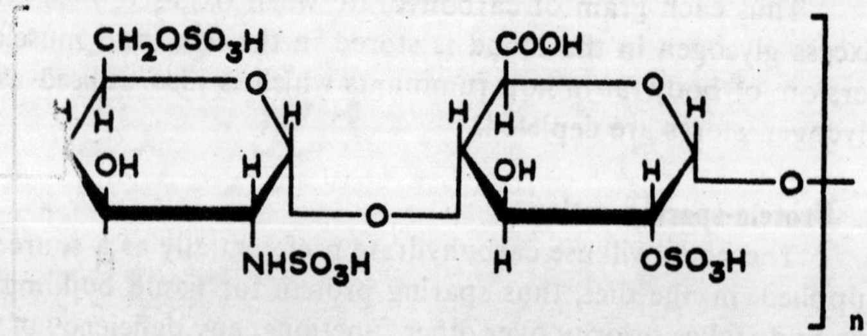

Sulfated glucosamine Sulfated glucuronic acid

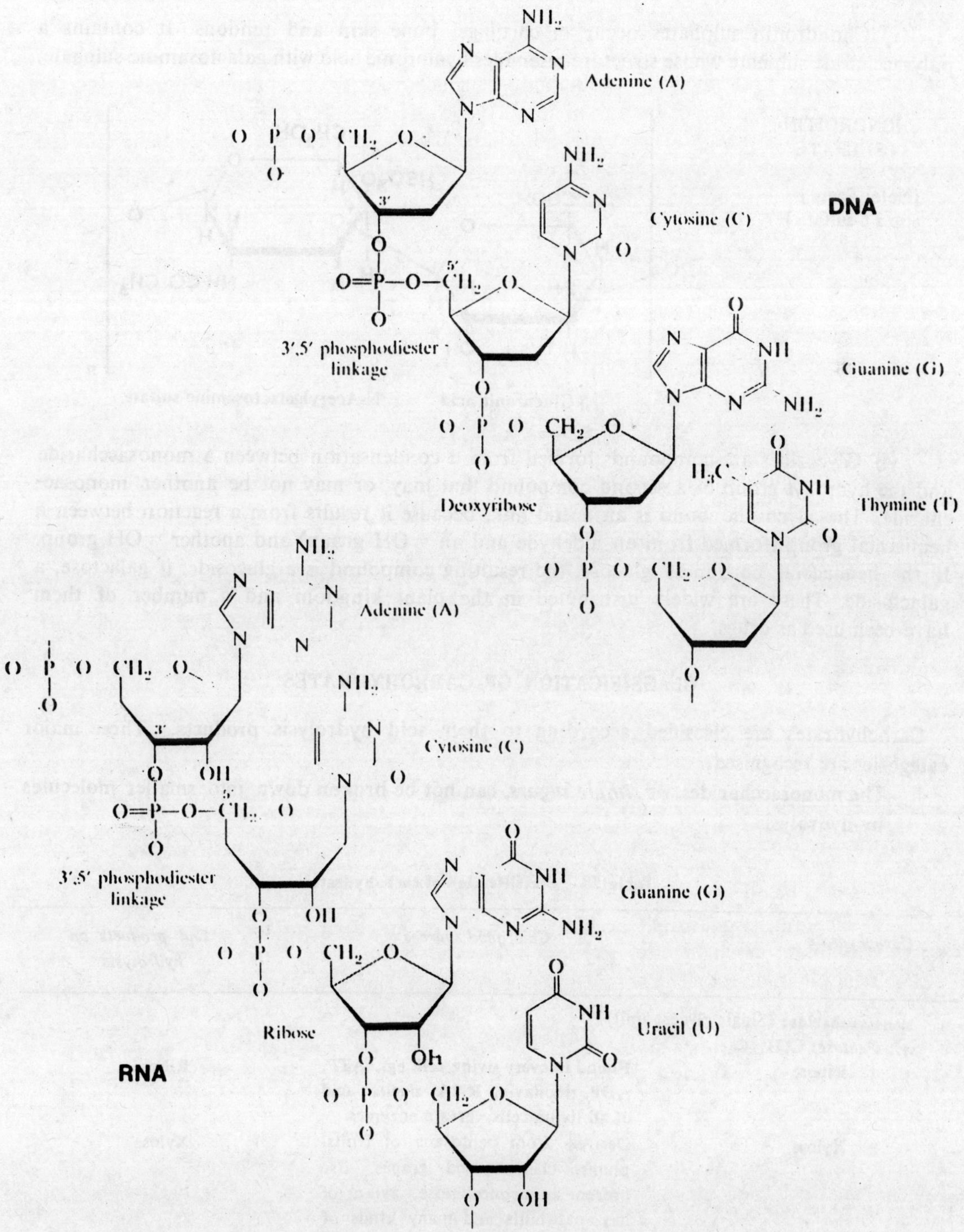

**Fig. 16** Partial chemical structures of the strands of DNA and RNA. The sequence of nucleotides differs for each naturally occurring type of DNA or RNA.

v) Chondroitin sulphates occur in cartilage, bone skin and tendons. It contains a polysaccharide sulphate whose structure resembles hyaluronic acid with galactosamine sulphate.

**CHONDROITIN-4-SULFATE**

[Note: There is also a 6-sulfate.]

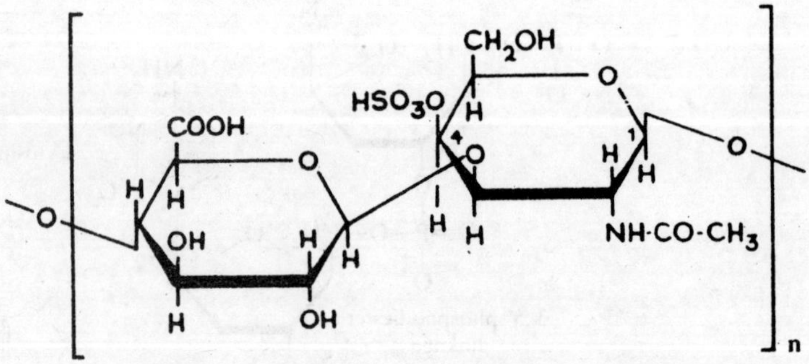

β-Glucuronic acid    N-Acetylgalactosamine sulfate

vi) Glycosides are compounds formed from a condensation between a monosaccharide and the hydroxyl group of a second compound that may, or may not be another monosaccharide. The glycosidic bond is an acetal link, because it results from a reaction between a hemiacetal group (formed from an aldehyde and an —OH group) and another —OH group. If the hemiacetal portion is glucose, the resulting compound is a glucoside; if galactose, a galactoside. These are widely distributed in the plant kingdom and a number of them have been used as drugs.

## CLASSIFICATION OF CARBOHYDRATES

Carbohydrates are classified according to their acid hydrolysis products. Three major categories are recognised.

1. The monosaccharides, or *simple sugars*, can not be broken down into smaller molecules by hydrolysis.

**Table 58 Classification of carbohydrates**

| *Carbohydrate* | *Chief food sources* | *End products on hydrolysis* |
|---|---|---|
| 1 **Monosaccharides** (Single glycose unit) | | |
| *A. Pentoses* $C_5H_{10}O_5$ | | |
| 1. Ribose | Found in every living cell, eg., ATP, ADP, riboflavin, RNA, nucleic acid of all living cells, certain enzymes. | Ribose |
| 2. Xylose | Derived from pentosans of fruits-plums, cherries and grapes, also present in hemicellulose, xylan of hay, oat hulls and many kinds of wood. | Xylose |
| 3. Arabinose | Acids of meat products and seafood, in gums as gum-arabic. | Arabinose |

Table 58 (*Contd.*)

| *Carbohydrate* | *Chief food sources* | *End products on hydrolysis* |
|---|---|---|
| *B. Hexoses*, $C_6H_{12}O_6$ | | |
| 1. Glucose | Majority of the carbohydrates taken in by the body are present in fruits & honey, eventually converted tc glucose in free from. | Glucose |
| 2. Fructose | Fruits, honey, with glucose in sugar. | Fructose |
| 3. Galactose | Lactose, galactosides of brain and nervous tissue and lactose of milk. | Galactose |
| 4. Mannose | Present in mannans, a group of polysaccharides, widely distributed in plants, also found in blood serum globulins and certain egg proteins. | Mannose |
| **2. Oligosaccharides (2 to 10 glucose units)** | | |
| *A. Disaccharides* $C_{12}H_{22}O_{11}$ | | |
| 1. Sucrose | Cane and beet sugar, molasses | Glucose + Fructose |
| 2. Lactose | Milk and milk products | Glucose + Galactose |
| 3. Maltose | Malt products | Glucose + Glucose |
| *B. Trisaccharides* $C_{18}H_{32}O_{16}$ | | |
| 1. Raffinose | Sugar beets | Glucose + Fructose + Galactose |
| **3. Polysaccharides** | | |
| *A. Homopolysaccharides* | | |
| (a) Glucans | | |
| Starch | Present in many plants as a reserve carbohydrate | Glucose |
| Dextrins | Intermediates resulting from the hydrolysis & digestion of starch | Glucose |
| Glycogen | Main carbohydrate storage product in animal body | Glucose |
| Cellulose | Major structural component of all plant cell walls, also present in outer covering of seeds. | Glucose |
| (b) Fructans | | |
| Inulin | Occurs in some plants | Fructose |
| Levan | Occurs in some plants | Fructose |
| *B. Heteropolysaccharides* | | |
| Hemicellulose | Stalks and leaves of vegetables outer covering of seeds | Xylose, Arabinose, Galactose, Glucose, Mannose and frequently Uronic acid (End products varies.) |
| Pectin | Inside plant cell walls (middle lamella) | Galacturonic acid + Rhamnose units |
| Gum | Bark and leaves | Monosaccharides + Uronic acid |
| Mucilage | In certain plants and seed | Monosaccharides + Disaccharides + Uronic acid (highly variable composition) |

2. The disaccharides yield two monosaccharide molecules upon hydrolysis.
3. The polysaccharides yield many monosaccharide molecules upon hydrolysis.

For the most part, the mono and disaccharides are sweet tasting, crystalline solids, readily soluble in water and insoluble in non-polar or organic solvents.

Another way of classifying carbohydrates is on the basis of sugar and non-sugar groups. The term 'sugar' is applied to those carbohydrates which contain less than 10 monosaccharide units, while non-sugar comprise members of the carbohydrate family having more than 10 monosaccharide units.

*1. Monosaccharides*

Monosaccharides or simple sugars are those that can not be hydrolysed into simpler form, seldom found free in nature. Rather, they constitute the building block of more-complex carbohydrate molecules. They may be subdivided into trioses, tetroses, pentoses, hexoses or heptoses, depending upon the number of carbon atom they possess ; and as aldoses or ketoses, depending upon whether the aldehyde or ketone group is present. Examples are :

| | *Aldoses* | *Ketoses* |
|---|---|---|
| Trioses ($C_3H_6O_3$) | Glyceraldehyde | Dihydroxyacetone |
| Tetroses ($C_4H_8O_4$) | Erythrose | Erythrulose |
| Pentoses ($C_5H_{10}O_5$) | Ribose | Ribulose |
| Hexoses ($C_6H_{12}O_6$) | Glucose | Fructose |

(a) *Trioses*

H O
C
H C OH
$CH_2OH$
Glyceraldehyde

$CH_2OH$
C=O
$CH_2OH$
Dihydroxyacetone

Both of these compounds are found in plant and animal cells and play an important role in carbohydrate metabolism.

(b) *Pentoses*

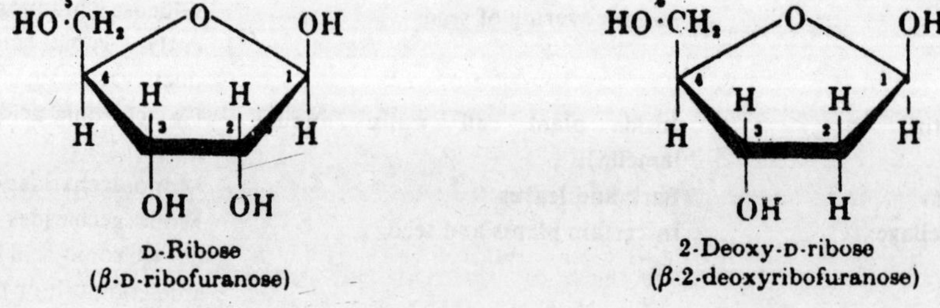


D-Ribose
(β-D-ribofuranose)

2-Deoxy-D-ribose
(β-2-deoxyribofuranose)

Both sugars are found in the nucleic acid of all living cells. Ribose is also an intermediate in the pathway of carbohydrate metabolism and is a constituent of several of the coenzymes.

**Table 59**

Examples of pentoses.

| Sugar | Source | Importance | Reactions |
|---|---|---|---|
| D-Ribose | Nucleic acids. | Structural elements of nucleic acids and co-enzymes, eg, ATP, NAD, NADP (DPN, TPN), flavoproteins. | Reduce Benedict's, Fehling's, Barfoed's, and Haynes' solutions. Forms distinctive osazones with phenylhydrazine. |
| D-Ribulose | Formed in metabolic processes. | Intermediates in hexose monophosphate shunt. | Those of keto sugars. |
| D-Arabinose | Gum arabic. Plum and cherry gums. | These sugars are used in studies of bacterial metabolism, as in fermentation tests for identification of bacteria. They have no known physiologic function in man. | With orcinol-HCl reagent gives colors: violet, blue, red, and green. |
| D-Xylose | Wood gums. | | With phloroglucinol-HCl gives a red color. |
| D-Lyxose | Heart muscle. | A constituent of a lyxoflavin isolated from human heart muscle. | |

(c) *Hexoses*

**Table 60**

Hexoses of physiologic importance.

| Sugar | Source | Importance | Reactions |
|---|---|---|---|
| D-Glucose | Fruit juices. Hydrolysis of starch, cane sugar, maltose, and lactose. | The "sugar" of the body. The sugar carried by the blood, and the principal one used by the tissues. Glucose is usually the "sugar" of the urine when glycosuria occurs. | Reduces Benedict's, Haynes', Barfoed's reagents (a reducing sugar). Gives osazone with phenylhydrazine. Fermented by yeast. With $HNO_3$, forms soluble saccharic acid. |
| D-Fructose | Fruit juices. Honey. Hydrolysis of cane sugar and of inulin (from the Jerusalem artichoke). | Can be changed to glucose in the liver and intestine and so used in the body. | Reduces Benedict's, Haynes', Barfoed's reagents (a reducing sugar). Forms osazone identical with that of glucose. Fermented by yeast. Cherry-red color with Seliwanoff's resorcinol-HCl reagent. |
| D-Galactose | Hydrolysis of lactose. | Can be changed to glucose in the liver and metabolized. Synthesized in the mammary gland to make the lactose of milk. A constituent of glycolipids and glycoproteins. | Reduces Benedict's, Haynes', Barfoed's reagents (a reducing sugar). Forms osazone, distinct from above. Phloroglucinol-HCl reagent gives red color. With $HNO_3$, forms insoluble mucic acid. Not fermented by yeast. |
| D-Mannose | Hydrolysis of plant mannosans and gums. | A constituent of prosthetic polysaccharide of albumins, globulins, mucoproteins. A sugar frequently occurring in glycoproteins. | Reduces Benedict's, Haynes', Barfoed's reagents (a reducing sugar). Forms same osazone as glucose. |

1. GLUCOSE. The majority of carbohydrates taken in by the body are eventually converted to a glucose in series of a metabolic pathways. Glucose is the circulating carbohydrate of animals ; the blood of cow, sheep, goat, pig and laying chicken contain, 40-70 ; 30-50 ; 46-60 ; 80-120 and 130-290 mg per 100 ml respectively.

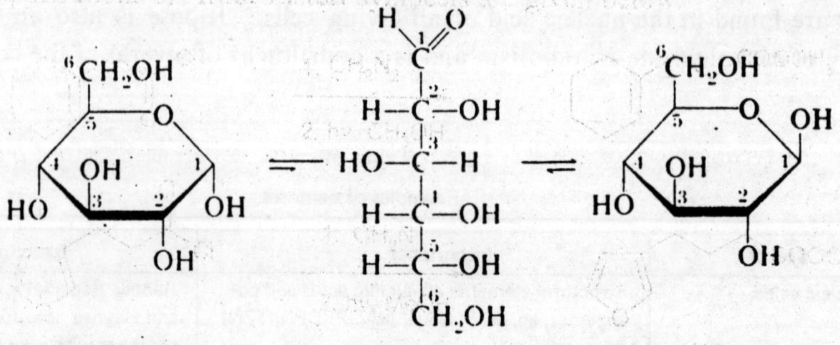

α-D(+)-Glucose ⇌ D(+)-Glucose ⇌ β-D(+)-Glucose

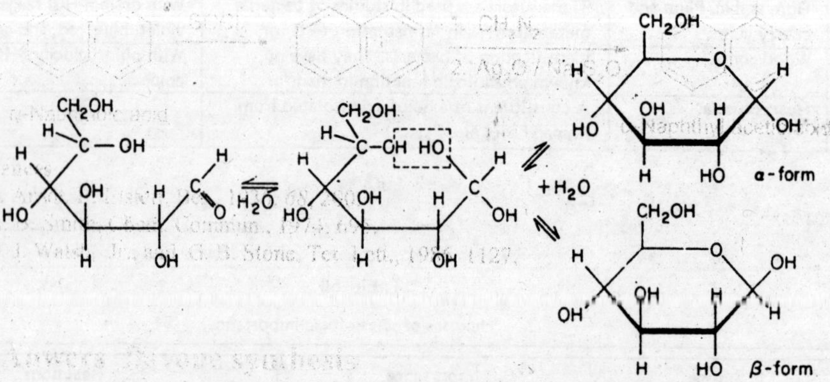

α-form

β-form

Formation of a hemi-acetal bond and the cyclization of glucose.

Glucose is the most abundant sugar found in nature. It is commonly found in fruits, especially in ripe grapes, and for this reason it is often referred to as *grape sugar*. It is also known as *dextrose*, a name that derives from the fact that the sugar is dextrorotatory. Commercially, glucose is made by the hydrolysis of starch. Glucose is only 75 per cent as sweet as table sugar (sucrose) but it has the same caloric value.

2. GALACTOSE. It is formed by the hydrolysis of lactose (milk sugar), a disaccharide composed of a glucose unit and a galactose unit. It does not occur in nature in the uncombined

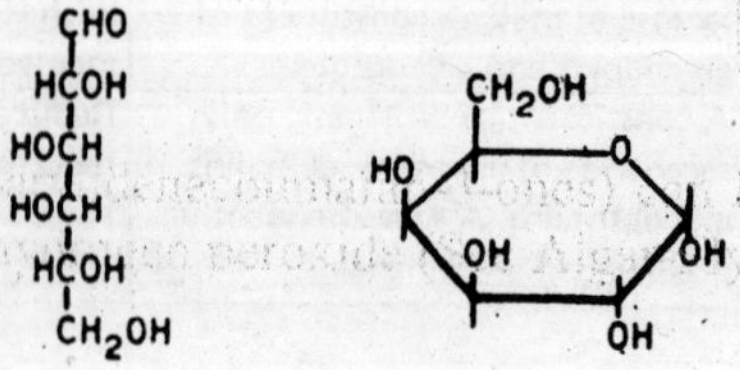

D-GALACTOSE

state. The galactose needed by the human body for the synthesis of lactose (in the mammary glands) is obtained by the conversion of D-glucose into D-galactose. In addition, galactose is an important constituent of the glycolipids which occur in the brain and in the Myelin sheath of nerves.

3. **FRUCTOSE.** Fructose is the only naturally occurring ketohexose. In the free state it occurs predominantly in the pyranose form whereas in nature the furanose form predominates (as in sucrose and insulin). This sugar is also referred to as *levulose* because it has an optical rotation which is strongly levorotatory (–92°). It is the sweetest sugar, and it is found, together with glucose and sucrose, in sweeter fruits and honey.

$CH_2OH$
C=O
HOCH
HCOH
HCOH
$CH_2OH$

$HOCH_2$ O OH HO $CH_2OH$ OH

D-FRUCTOSE

Table 61

**Relative sweetness in water of some compounds**

| *Less sweet that sucrose* | | *More sweet than sucrose* | |
|---|---|---|---|
| Lactose | 0.16 | Fructose | 1.1 |
| Liquid glucose | 0.23 | Cyclamate | 30.0 |
| Sorbitol | 0.54 | Saccharin | 350.0 |
| Glucose (dextrose) | 0.75 | | |

Sucrose (Household sugar) = 1

## *II. Disaccharides*

Disaccharides are compound sugars composed of two monosaccharides. The manner in which two monosaccharide molecules are joined together is of particular interest, e.g., both cellobiose and maltose contain two molecules of glucose, but they differ in the manner in which the glucose units are joined. In maltose it is alpha 1, 4-Glucosidic linkage while in cellobiose it is beta 1, 4-Glucosidic linkage. Humans lack necessary enzyme to hydrolyse beta glucosidic enzyme and so cannot utilise cellulose as a source of glucose. The microbes present in ruminants can secrete necessary enzymes and thus can utilise cellulose materials. The termite also contains such microbes whose enzymes (*Cellulase*) catalyse cellulose hydrolysis of the wood or straw.

1. *Sucrose* : Sucrose is known as beet sugar, cane sugar, table sugar or simply as sugar. It is probably the largest selling pure organic compound in the world. As its names apply, sucrose is obtained from sugar canes and sugar beets (whose juice contain 14-20% sugar) by evaporation of the water and recrystallisation. The dark brown liquid that remains after crystallisation of the sugar is sold as molasses.

The presence of the 1, 2-glucosidic linkage makes it impossible for sucrose to exist in the alpha or beta configuration or in the open chain form. This is a direct result of the fact that the potential aldehyde group of the glucose moity and the ketone group of the fructose moity have been tied up in the formation of the 1, 2 (head-to-head) linkage. As long as the sucrose molecule remains in tact, it can not uncyclise to form the open chain structure. Sucrose, therefore, does not undergo reactions that are typical of aldehydes and ketones, and it is said to be a *non-reducing* sugar.

2. *Maltose* : It does not occur in free state but occurs in animals as the principal sugar formed by the enzymatic (ptyalin) hydrolysis of starch. It is fairly abundant in germinating



grain where it is formed by the enzyme (diastase) breakdown of starch. In the manufacture of beer, maltose is liberated by the action of malt (germinating barley) on starch, and for this reason it is often referred to as *malt sugar*.

3. *Cellobiose* : Cellobiose is obtained by the partial hydrolysis of cellulose. It may be

β-1,4-Glucosidic linkage

Cellobiose → (H⁺ or emulsin) 2 D-Glucose

further hydrolysed to yield two molecules of glucose by the action of the enzyme *cellobiase* (which is specific for beta glucosidic linkage).

**4.** *Lactose* : It is known as milk sugar as it occurs only in milk (human milk contains 7.5% lactose whereas cows milk, which is not as sweet, contains about 4.5% lacotose). Lactose is

β-1,4-Galactosidic linkage

Lactose → (H⁺ or lactase) D-Galactose + D-Glucose

composed of one molecule of D-glucose and one nolecule of D-galactose which are obtained upon hydrolysis of lactose by the enzyme *lactuse.*

**Table 62** Disaccharides.

| Sugar | Source | Reactions |
|---|---|---|
| Maltose | Digestion by amylase or hydrolysis of starch. Germinating cereals and malt. | Reducing sugar. Forms osazone with phenylhydrazine. Fermentable. Hydrolyzed to D-glucose. |
| Lactose | Milk. May occur in urine during pregnancy. | Reducing sugar. Forms osazone with phenylhydrazine. Not fermentable by yeasts. Hydrolyzed to glucose and galactose. |
| Sucrose | Cane and beet sugar. Sorghum. Pineapple. Carrot roots. | Nonreducing sugar. Does not form osazone. Fermentable Hydrolyzed to fructose and glucose. |
| Trehalose | Fungi and yeasts. The major sugar of insect hemolymph. | Nonreducing sugar. Does not form an osazone. Hydrolyzed to glucose. |

### *III Polysaccharides*

These are the most abundant carbohydrates found in nature. They serve as reserve food substances and as structural components of plants. The members of this group are condensation products joined together by glycosidic linkages. Biochemically the three most important members are starch, glycogen and cellulose. These are homopolysaccharides since each of them yields only one type of monosaccharide (glucose) upon complete hydrolysis.

Heteropolysaccharides on the other hand yield more than one particular type of components (sugar acids, amino sugars or non-carbohydrates) etc. as in hemicelluloses, gums, mucilages etc.

1. *Starch:* This is the most important source of carbohydrates in the human diet. We often think of potatoes as a "starchy" food, yet other plants contain a much greater percentage of starch (e.g., potatoes 15%, wheat 55%, maize 65% and rice 75%).

Repeating unit: $n = 100\text{-}1000$

Amylose

$\alpha$-1,6-Glucosidic linkage

Amylopectin

Starch is a mixture of two polymers, *amylose* (10-20 percent) and *amylopectin* (80-90 percent). Amylose is a straight chain polysaccharide composed entirely of D-glucose units joined by an $\alpha$-1, 4-glucosidic linkage, as in maltose. Thus amylose might be thought of as polymaltose. Amylopectin is a branched chain polysaccharide composed of glucose units which are linked primarily by $\alpha-1,\ 4$—glucosidic bonds, but that have an occasional $\alpha-1,\ 6$-glucosidic linkage responsible for the branching. It has been estimated that there are over 1,000 glucose units in amylopectin, and that branching occurs about one over 25 units.

Glucose molecules

Polysaccharide chain

The unbranched amylose molecules have a helical structure. A corkscrew is a familiar item that also has a helical structure.

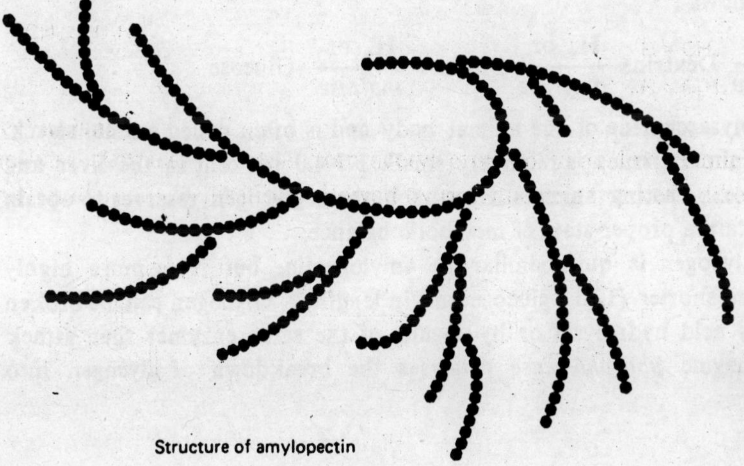

Structure of amylopectin

Amylopectin is a highly branched polysaccharide. The principal chain is bonded with $\alpha$-1,4-glycosidic linkages. The branches off of the chain result from $\alpha$-1,6-glycosidic linkages.

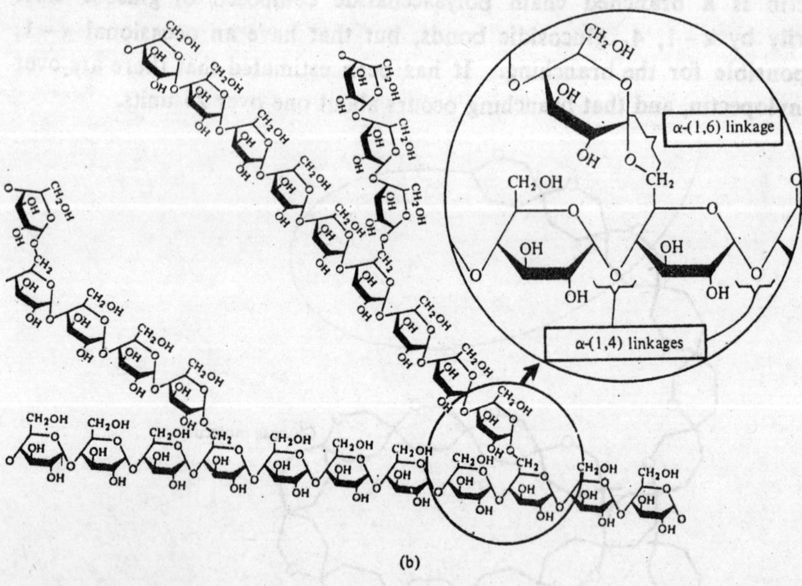


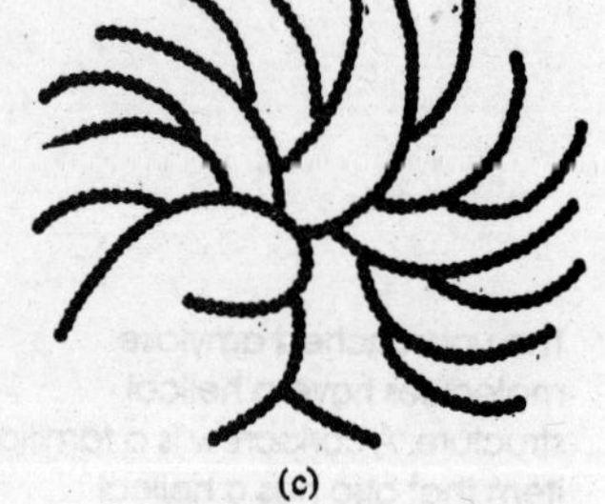


(a) The conformation of the amylose chain. (b) Branch points of amylopectin. (c) Branched array of glucose units in amylopectin or glycogen.

**The complete hydrolysis of starch (amylose and amylopectin) yields glucose, in three sucesive stages, which is as follows :**

$$\text{Starch} \xrightarrow[\textit{amylase}]{H_+ \text{ or}} \text{Dextrins} \xrightarrow[\textit{amylase}]{H_+ \text{ or}} \text{Maltose} \xrightarrow[\textit{maltase}]{H_+ \text{ or}} \text{Glucose}$$

**2. *Glycogen :* It is the polysaccharide of the animal body and is often called animal starch. The amount of glycogen in animal tissues is relatively small, 1.5-4.0 per cent in the liver and 0.5-1.0 per cent in the muscle. Fasting animals draw upon these glycogen reserves to obtain that glucose needed to maintain a proper state of metabolic balance.**

**In terms of structure, glycogen is quite similar to amylopectin, but it is more highly branched and its branches are shorter (12-18 glucose unit in length). Glycogen can be broken down into its D-glucose by acid hydrolysis or by means of the same enzymes that attack starch. In animals, the enzyme *phosphorylase* catalyses the breakdown of glycogen into phosphate esters of glucose.**

**CELLULOSE**

Subunits: D-glucose
Linkages: β–(1-4) glycosidic bonds
Branching: none; linear chains
Molecular weight: 50,000 to 2,000,000
Function: structural element of plant cell walls; forms microfibrils several hundred angstroms in length

**CHITIN**

Subunits: 2-acetamido-2-deoxy-D-glucose
Linkages: β-(1-4) glycosidic bonds
Branching: none; linear chains
Molecular weight: difficult to estimate because of tightly-bound noncarbohydrate material, especially proteins and inorganic salts.
Function: structural element in lower plants (e.g., fungi) and in invertebrates, especially arthropods where it serves as exoskeletal material

**GLYCOGEN**

Subunits: D-glucose
Linkages: α-(1-4) glycosidic bonds
α-(1-6) glycosidic bonds
Branching: about 9%
Molecular weight: from several hundred thousand to about 100,000,000.
Function: nutritional glucose reservoir in animals.

**STARCH (AMYLOSES AND AMYLOPECTINS)**

| | AMYLOSES | AMYLOPECTINS |
|---|---|---|
| Subunits: | D-glucose | D-glucose |
| Linkages: | α-(1-4) glycosidic bonds | α-(1-4) and α-(1-6) glycosidic bonds |
| Branching: | None: linear chains | About 4% |
| Molecular weight: | 4000 to 40,000 | 50,000 to 1,000,000 |
| Function: | Nutritional reservoir for glucose in plants | Nutritional reservoir for glucose in plants |

Some major polysaccharides.

**3. *Cellulose :* Cellulose is a fibrous carbohydrate found in all plants where it serves as a structural component of the plant's cell wall. Cotton fibre and filter paper are almost entirely cellulose. Wood is about 50% cellulose. Most of straw contains 20—40% cellulose.**

Repeating unit

Cellulose

Complete hydrolysis of cellulose yields only D-glucose, whereas partial hydrolysis of cellulose yields the disaccharide cellobiose. Thus cellulose must be composed of chains of D-glucose units (about 2,000—3,000) joined by β 1. 4-glucosidic linkages. The chains are almost exclusively linear, unlike those of starch, which are highly branched. The linear nature of the cellulose chain allows a great deal of hydrogen bonding between hydroxyl groups on adjacent chains. As a result, the chains are closely packed into fibres, and there is little interaction with water or with any other solvent.

Cellulose yields, D-glucose upon complete acid hydrolysis, yet human and the carnivorous animals cannot utilise cellulose as a source of glucose. Our digestive juices lack the enzymes that hydrolyse beta glucosidic linkages. Ruminants can do so as they contain microorganisms in the digestive tracts whose enzyme *(Cellulose)* catalyse cellulose hydrolysis.

4. *Hemicelluloses*: These are the most complex plant carbohydrates which are present not only in the cell walls of all plants and trees but also found in certain seeds. Hemicellulose and lignin together form the incrusting material of the secondary wall thickening of plant cells, thus the cell walls gets strengthened.

Hemicellulose is much less resistant to chemical degradation than cellulose, soluble in mild alkali as well as in mild acid.

Basically it is a polymer of D-xylose made up of β 1, 4 linked xylose units (a pentose sugar) with side chains of other sugars or compounds derived from sugars. Hemicelluloses obtained from leaves and stems of most plants have main chain of xylose units linked with side chains of arabinose and uronic acids like glucuronic and galacturonic acids. (These acids are formed form glucose and galactose respectively upon oxidation. The sugar acids contains their aldehyde group). In many plant seeds the xylose chain is linked up directly with glucose or mannose. The composition of hemicelluloses thus are found variable among plant parts and with species. Hemicellulose *A* is less bonded, often higher in xylan and relatively richer in stems than leaves. Hemicellulose *B* contains more branched fractions often high in arabinose or in various urononic acids.

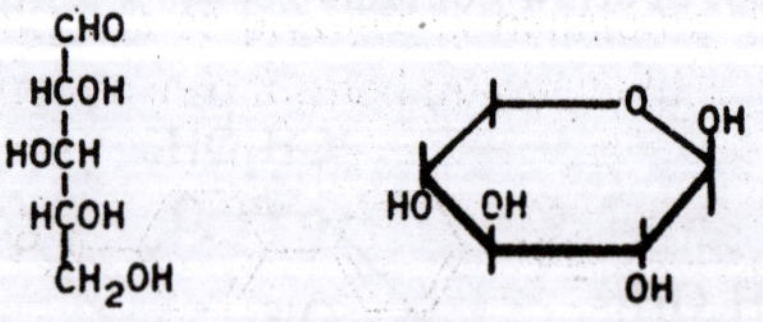

D-XYLOSE

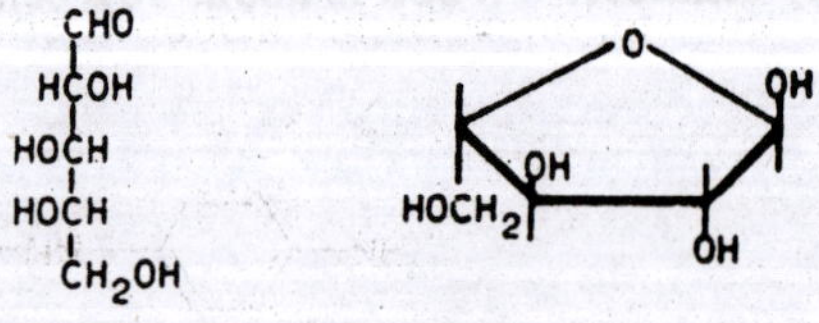

L-ARABINOSE

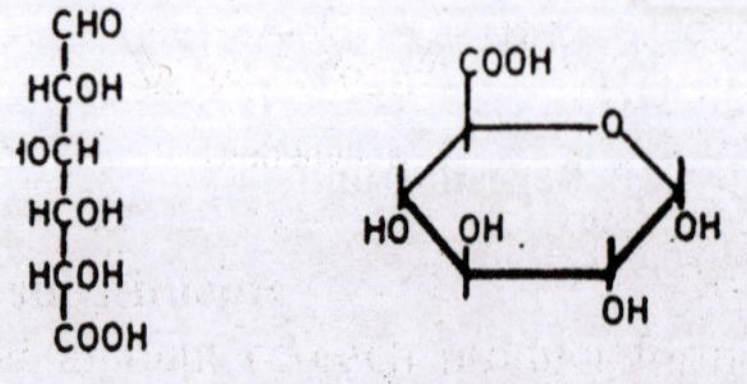

D-GLUCURONIC ACID

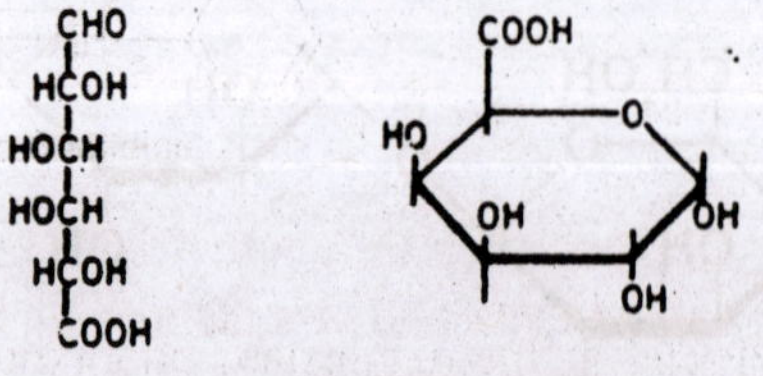

D-GALACTURONIC ACID

The compound may constitute up to 20% of the crude fibre in diets of herbivorous animals. The enzyme *hemicellulases* are produced by some rumen bacteria and ciliate protozoa. All enzymes so far identified appear to be of the endo type which randomly attack the glycosidic chain.

Cellulose and hemicellulose are not digested to sugars but to VFA and gases. These are absorbed at the site of their formation ; that is, they are absorbed through the walls of the rumen and colon in ruminants. In pig, rabbit, guinea pig, dog and poultry through caicum. In human through small and large intestine. In horse VFA's are absorbed through caecum and colon.

Non-ruminants digest relatively more hemicellulose than cellulose as compared to ruminants that digest about equal amounts of both carbohydrates.

**Table 63**

**Comparative Digestibilities of fiber fractions by various non-ruminants**

| *Species* | *Body wt.* kg | *Feed* | *Hemicellulose* % | *Cellulose* % |
|---|---|---|---|---|
| Elephant | 1930—3400 | Lucerne | 49—68 | 56 |
| Horse | 388— 460 | Lucerne | 55—72 | 45—66 |
| Zebra | 340— 386 | Timothy | 54—58 | 39—48 |
| Ass | 136— 277 | Timothy | 53—59 | 39—45 |
| Pig | 48— 89 | Lucerne | 22—54 | 9—59 |
| Man | 64— 89 | Veg + fruit | 94—98 | 15—55 |
| Dog | 11— 12 | Cereal | 30—54 | 7—22 |

Source : Nutritional Ecology of the Ruminants by Van Soest, 1982. O & B Books, Inc. Corvallis, Oregon 97330. U.S.A.

A relatively better utlisation of legume compared to grass hemicellulose is made by non-ruminants.

## CRUDE FIBER AND NITROGEN-FREE EXTRACT

The chemical classification of carbohydrates has already been discussed. In the case of ruminant animals, a more relevant classification of the carbohydrates is to divide most of the broad family into nitrogen-free extract (NFE) and crude fiber.

### Crude Fiber (CF)

This portion of carbohydrates composed of cellulose, hemicellulose and lignin, even though the latter is not a true carbohydrate, it is included as it is almost always associated with cellulose. The component (CF) serves as the structural and protective parts of plants. It is high in forages and low in grains.

After removal of the fat and water, the feed sample is boiled for 30 minutes, with weak $H_2SO_4$ (1.25%) and then for another 30 minutes with weak NaOH (1.25%). This removes the proteins, soluble sugars and starchs leaving lignin, cellulose and other complex carbohydrates along with the mineral matter. The loss on ignition of the remaining material is defined as crude fiber. This procedure is based on the supposition that carbohydrates which are readily dissolved also will be readily digested by all classes of livestock, and that those which are not soluble under such conditions are not readily digested. Unfortunately it is not so as the treatment dissolves much of the lignin, a non-digestible component. Hence crude fiber is only an approximation of the indigestible material in feedstuffs which is a rough indicator of energy value. Also, the C.F. value is needed for the computation of Total Digestible Nutrient (TDN) of feedstuffs.

Essentially, animal kingdom are uncapable of degrading cellulose or hemicellulose. However, the microscopic life which are habitats of first three sections of the ruminant's stomach and of the caecum and colon of other species, secrete appropriate enzymes capable of hydrolysing the chemical bonds holding the cellulose or hemicellulose molecules together with lignin. Large intestines of many animals including human beings also contain similar microbes thus aid in CF digestion to some extent. In all cases, the end products are volatile fatty acids and gases which are absorbed from the site of production.

Table .64

Digestibility of CF by Various Species

| *Species* | *Where digested* | *% Digested* |
|---|---|---|
| Ruminants | Rumen, Colon | 50–90 |
| Horse | Caecum, Colon | 34–40 |
| Pig | Caecum, Colon | 3–25 |
| Rabbit | Caecum | 16–18 |
| Guinea pig | Caecum | 43–40 |
| Dog | Caecum | 10–30 |
| Human | Small and large intestine | 25–35 |
| Poultry | Caeca | 20–30 |

**Factors affecting Utilisation of C.F.**

1. *Age of the animal*

In general, young animals are less able to digest cellulose than adults.

2. *Nutritional habits of the animal*

It is easy to demonstrate increasing digestibility of CF with an increasing length of time that fiber has been a part of the diet.

3. *Nutrient make up of the diet*

Microflora of the digestive tract requires other nutrients for their utilisation of CF and thereby for their growth. If diets are poor in proteins, vitamins & minerals utilisation of CF will be affected.

4. *Species of animals*

Ruminants are classed by their power of CF. They have sufficient rooms to accomodate huge number of microbes in comparison to single stomached animals who can digest CF through microbial enzymes present in either caecum or in large intestines.

5. *Age of feeds rich in CF*

Digestibility of forage gradually declines as it becomes more matured. This property is due to the heavy deposition of lignin in the CF portion which renders the feedstuff less digestible.

6. *Preparation of Feedstuffs*

Feeds rich in crude fiber when treated with alkali are converted into more degradable form wich are then easily digested by the enzymes of microbes. The property is due to ease at which rigid bonds of lignocelluloses are broken down such as in straw.

## Nitrogen-free Extract (NFE)

The relatively soluble carbohydrates are classified as the nitrogen-free extract (NFE) and include the mono-and disaccharides plus the starches and perhaps a part of the hemicelluloses, based on their relative solubility and digestibility and some cellulose and pentosans along with a limited amount of lignin.

There is no practical method for exact determination of the NFE portion of feedstuffs. Rather, it is determined mathematically by subtracting all other from 100 :

$$\text{NFE }\% = 100 - \left( \begin{array}{c} \text{Moisture }\% + \text{Crude protein }\% + \text{Ether extract }\% \\ + \text{Crude fiber }\% + \text{Ash }\% \end{array} \right)$$

For feeding purposes this calculation has proved satisfactory, although it is not too accurate.

## LIGNIN

Plants have evolved substances that impart resistance to biological degradation. One class comprises the phenylpropanoid substances which include lignin, flavones, coumarines, tannins and isoflavones. Lignin which has the highest molecular weight of the class, limits the availability of cell wall carbohydrates to digesting microorganisms and adds rigidity to cell wall structure. Feed chemists have lumped the various phenyl-propanoid compounds as "*Crude lignin*", which are all indigestible as true lignin.

### Composition of Lignin

The term lignin is not a single substance but a group of substances having very close chemical components and physical characteristics. In general, true lignin is a polymer of one or more of the three aromatic compounds namely: (1) *p*-coumaryl alcohol, (2) coniferyl alcohol, (3) sinapyl alcohol which renders it three dimensional physical stature.

During biosynthesis of lignin, the conversion of mixtures of *p*-coumaryl, coniferyl and synapyl alcohol undergo extremely complex affair. It does not involve a simple chain reaction through the aliphatic double bond but instead a repeated random condensation of smaller units at various points in the molecule, through processes initiated by enzymatic phenol oxidation takes place.

All lignins are not identical in chemical structure. Based on the monomeric units these may be *grouped into three classes*. The alcohol ratio influences not only the methoxyl content of the lignin but also its structure.

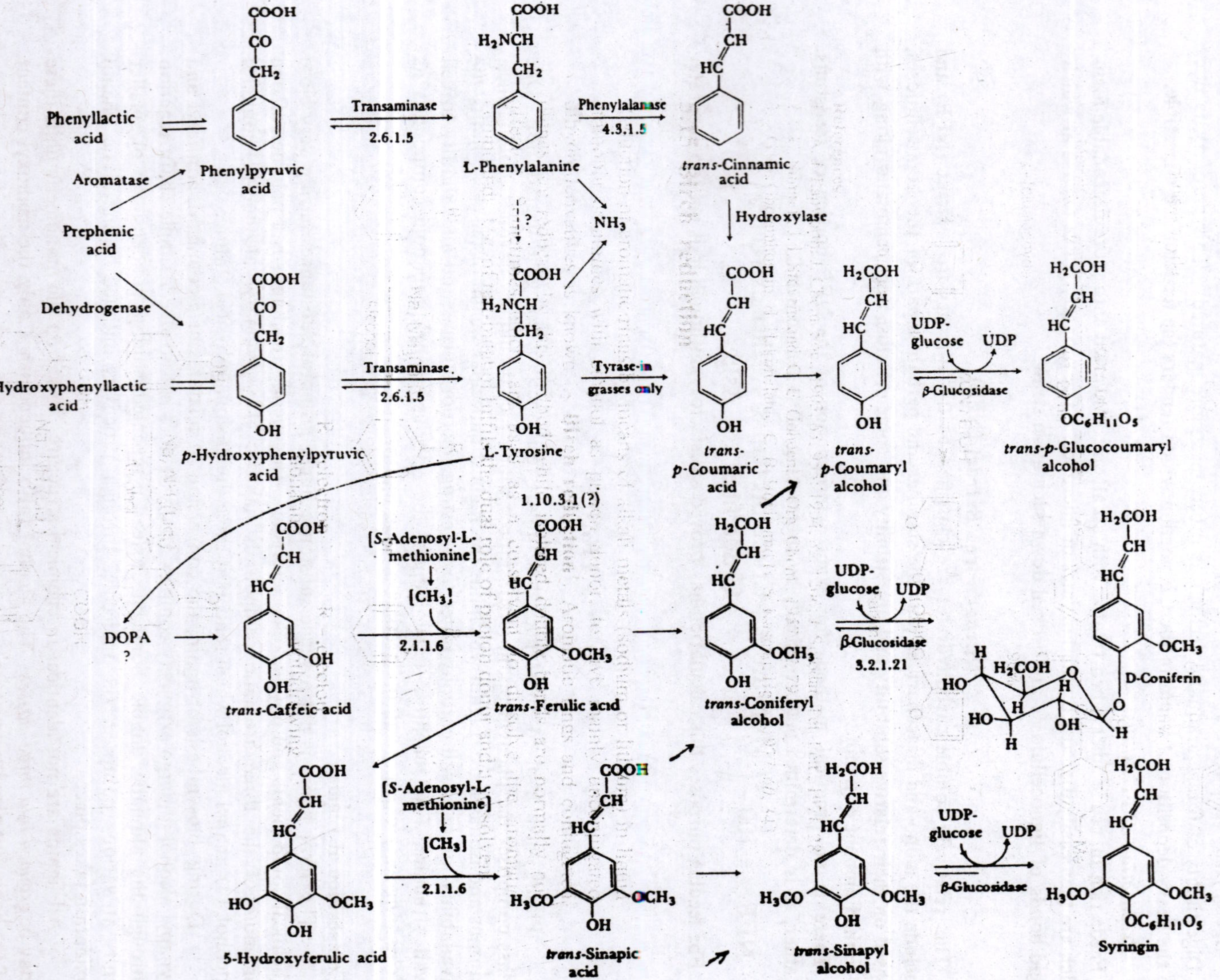


**Fig. 17**. Metabolic pathway leading from prephenic acid to the monomeric precursors of lignin, *p*-coumaryl, coniferyl and sinapyl alcohols.

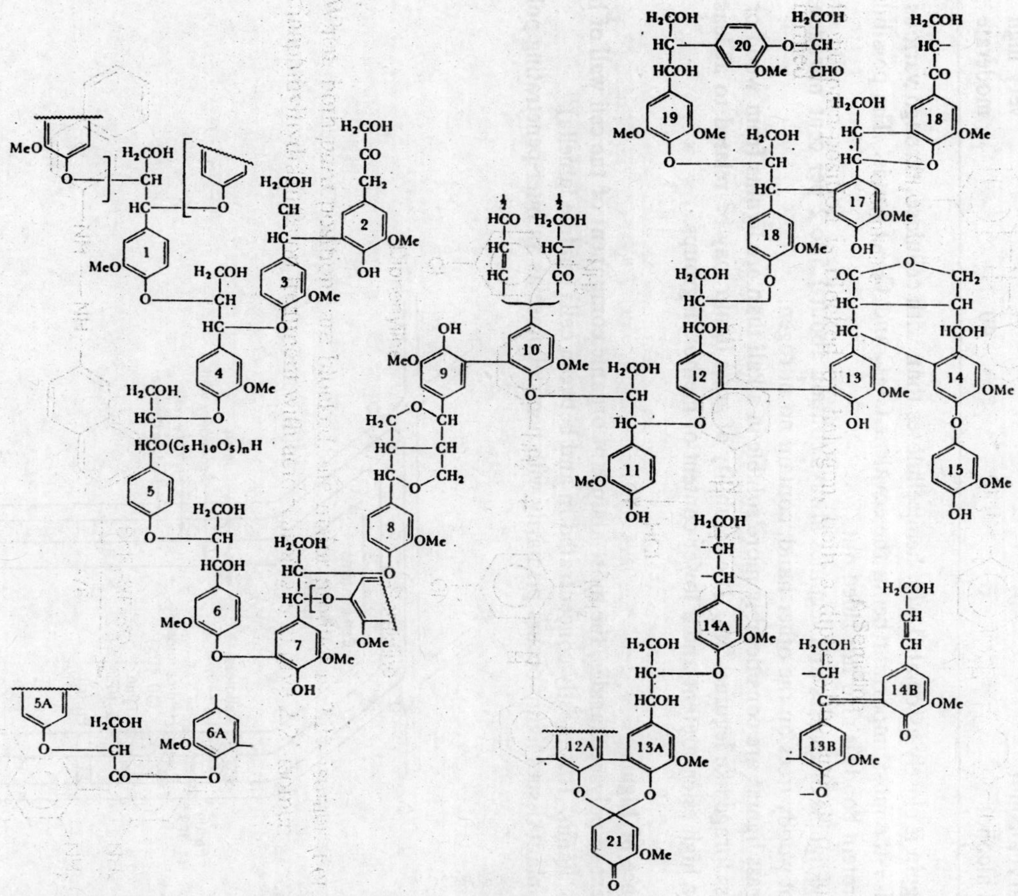

**Fig. 18.** A schematic formula reflecting most of the structural features and the approximate composition of a softwood lignocellulose fragment.

| Units (%) | Softwood lignin (~15-16% methoxyl content) | Hardwood lignin (~21-22% methoxyl content) | Grass herbage lignin (variable methoxyl %) |
|---|---|---|---|
| Coniferyl alcohol | 80 | 56 | moderate |
| *p*-coumaryl alcohol | 14 | 4 | very high |
| Synapyl alcohol | 6 | 40 | moderate |

Lignin is closely associated with hemicelluloses than with celluloses through various types of bonds—the most important being the covalent C—C and C—O bonds. The possibility of lignin-protein bonds is also not ruled out.

The lignins of grasses and legumes always contain about 1.5 to 2 per cent nitrogen. The lignins of woody trees on the other hand, contain no nitrogen.

Grass lignins are considerably more soluble in alkali than are lignins from wood or from non-grass forage like legumes etc. The solubility of grass lignin may be related to at least two factors: a high ester content and a lower content of methoxyl groups.

**Occurrence of Lignin**

Next to polysaccharides, the most abundant organic component of the cell wall of higher plants is lignin. It is mostly concentrated in and between cells (middle lamella).

In plant tissues lignin occurs primarily with hemicellulose as an inter-penetrating polymer

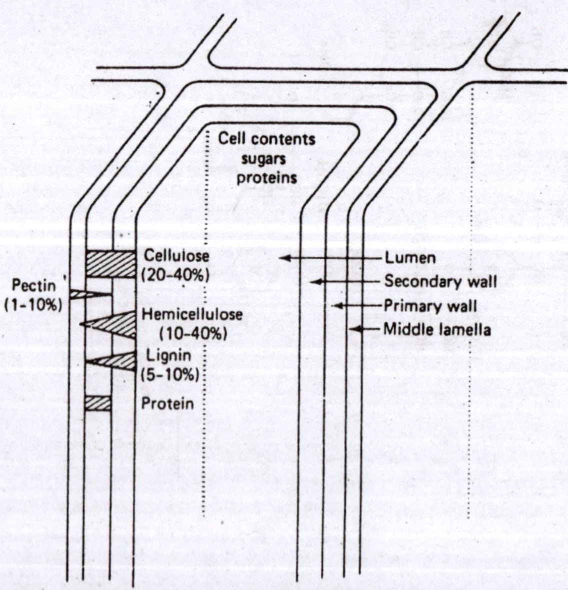


**Fig. 19** Schematic representation of the structure of a forage plant cell showing the component layers. The relative amounts of each of the carbohydrate fractions in the respective layers are depicted by the shaded areas, e.g., hemicellulose largely in the secondary wall; pectin largely in the middle lamella. The figures in parentheses are amounts often found in forage dry matter.

network which surrounds cellulose fibrils in the cell wall. Lignin is found in the woody parts of plants such as cobs, hulls and the fibrous portion of roots, stems and leaves. Hardwood contain the most lignin of any plant. Its content increases steadily as the growing plant matures and the chemical linkage specially with hemicellulose markedly reduces the digesti-

**Table 65**

**Composition of some lignocellulosic materials (% dry weight)**

| | Cellulose | Hemicellulose | Lignin |
|---|---|---|---|
| Coniferous wood | 40-50 | 20-30 | 25-35 |
| Deciduous wood | 40-50 | 30-40 | 15-20 |
| Cotton | 94 | 2 | 0 |
| Bagasse | 40 | 30 | 20 |
| Nut shells | 26-30 | 25-30 | 30-40 |
| Maize cobs | 45 | 35 | 15 |
| Maize stalks | 35 | 25 | 35 |
| Wheat straw | 30 | 50 | 15 |
| Paper | 85-99 | 0 | 0-15 |
| Newsprint | 50 | 20 | 30 |
| Sorted refuse | 60 | 20 | 20 |
| Rice straw | 31 | 40 | 10 |
| Maize straw | 32 | 38 | 13 |
| Berseem | 15 | 34 | 8 |
| Lucerne | 46 | 10 | 7 |

Source: Punj, M.L., Kochar, A.S. and Bhatia, I.S. 1971. *Indian J. Anim. Sci.*, 31: 536.

**Contribution of lignin in plant properties**

| Function of lignin | Plant property |
|---|---|
| Energy storage system. | Photosynthesis. |
| Permanent bonding agent between cells, resulting in composite structure of wood. | Resistance to mechanical stresses such as compression and blending. |
| Impediment to penetrate of destructive enzymes, inhibitor to enzymic degradation of other plant components. | Resistance to biochemical stresses such as microbial attack, infection and wounding. |
| Antioxidant, UV light stabiliser, flame retardant. | Resistance to chemical stresses such as atmospheric degradation, UV light radiation. |
| Water proofing agent*. | Resistance to physical chemical stresses, response to humidity, water balance and transport, nutrient transport. |

Source: Punj, M.L. and Jakhmola, R.C.—Proceedings of 5th Animal Nutrition Research Workers' Conference, 1986.

* Lignin a biological plastic, decreases water permeation across cell walls in the conducting xylem tissues, thus preventing water leakage from cell walls.

bility. In grass forage bonds predominate as ester bonds, while in legume forage bonds are mostly ether, neither of which are attacked by mammalian or microbial enzymes elaborated by anaerobic organisms. Aerobic organisms and fungi can break the linkage, resulting in the rotting of forages and wood that we observe in nature.

**How lignin depresses digestibility of carbohydrates of roughages?**

As a plant matures, its crude fibre content situated in the cell wall also increases. The increased materials are cellulose, hemicellulose, pectin and lignin. The oldest theory is that of physical incrustation and entrapment of nutrients by lignin. Thus as the plant accumulates lignin, the accessibility of carbohydrates mostly of hemicelluloses and celluloses to the rumen microorganisms decreases.

An alternative mechanism has been suggested as due to covalent bonds between hemicelluloses and lignins which are very strong. Thus lignin is tightly bound to plant polysaccharides at various points. These bonds prevent swelling of plant fibre and thereby resist microbial fermentation.

## Degradation of Lignin

Since lignin is inhibiting the digestibility of the structural carbohydrates of roughages in animals markedly, it is necessary to remove it or to at least break the barrier between the microbial enzymes and the substrate. Various methods of degradation so far attempted are summarised as follows:

### A. Physical treatments

**1. Grinding and ball milling**

Plant materials when subjected to reduction of their particle size by mechanical ball milling etc. probably split C—O and C—C bonds of lignin components thereby facilitate better enzyme action on cellulose and hemicellulose portions.

**2. Steam treatment**

It has been reported that the steam treatment of sugarcane bagasse (7 kg/cm$^2$ for 30 minutes) improved the digestibility and voluntary feed intake by about 55-60 per cent. Further high pressure than recommended may degrade carbohydrates to phenolic compounds and furfurol, which are usually toxic to microorganisms. The method is not suitable under small scale farming conditions since it requires costly pressure tight reactor and steam.

**3. Irradiation**

Irradiation by X-ray or gamma rays of 500 KGY on lignocellulose components leads to effective hydrolysis of the material. The method involves high cost and technology.

### B. Chemical methods

**1. Dilute alkali (NaOH)**

Sodium hydroxide has been used for delignification with success. It swells the fibre, cleavage the alkali labile lignin-carbohydrate bonds and may dissolve out some lignin without destroying (changing the structure) it. But the present cost of this compound prohibits its use due to economic considerations.

**2. Ammonia**

Use of urea as ammonia source is also used in place of NaOH delignification. About 4-8 per cent urea is dissolved in water and added evenly to the straw. The urea is turned into $NH_3$ by urease. After about three weeks, the reaction process is completed, and the straw which is now about 10-20 per cent more digestible is fed to animals. One of the major criticisms is the 40-60 per cent loss of ammonia gas and the consequent high cost of treatment.

**3. Sodium hypochlorite**

By treating sodium hypochlorite and acetic acid on roughages, the lignin is completely oxidised and the oxidation products are washed out leaving holo-celluloses (cellulose and hemi-cellulose) completely free from lignin. The recovery of holo-celluloses in straw was found to be about 75 per cent of initial material. In 36 hours of incubation, the holo-cellulose prepared from wheat straw was almost completely digested but the method involves significant expenditure.

The oxidation products of lignin are *p*-coumeric, ferulic and synapic acids, out of which *p*-coumeric acid has been found to be toxic to certain rumen microbes. Therefore, oxidation products of lignin and residual chemicals must be removed before feeding the treated materials to animals.

## C. Bio-degradation of lignin

Lignin destruction is possible by the use of lignin-destroying fungi or bacteria. All known lignin digesting organisms are aerobic. Effective fermentation (lignin destruction) may require energy input to keep the culture supplied with oxygen. Biological degradation of lignin requires a considerable time—weeks to months. Some control over the culture to avoid microbial destruction of the released carbohydrates would seem necessary, while some lignin-destroying organisms may depend on freed carbohydrate (in case of roughages, this may be holocellulose) for growth.

Lignin destruction proceeds by conversion of aromatic groups (ring structure compounds) to vicinal quinones followed by cleavage of aliphatic (straight chain) dicarboxylic acids ultimately converted into $CO_2$ and $H_2O$. This process can proceed anaerobically in the case of simple phenols, but appears to be restricted in condensed polyphenols (lignin).

It has now been indicated that the enzyme *ligninase* contains a heme-porphyrin which is oxidised by $H_2O_2$ to become a powerful oxidising agent, capable of drawing electrons out of the phenolic rings in lignin thereby breaking apart the polymer. The optimum pH for this reaction is suggested to be around 3.0.

The future of delignification of cellulosic wastes depends heavily upon economics. Most processes are expensive relative to energy and labour. In consideration of the probable future rise in energy cost, long term improvement may lie in the area of plant genetic rather than with chemical treatments.

**Microbes involved in bio-degradation of lignin**

There are three types of fungi apart from some yeasts and bacteria living on dead wood, which actually degrade one or more wood components, that is soft rot fungi, brown rot fungi and white rot fungi.

Many fungi of the white rot type are known to metabolise lignin, cellulose and other fibrous components. Firstly, the greatest challenge is to select white rot fungi species, by screening and careful selection, which selectively degrade only lignin and not cellulose. Secondly, we need to select those strains which can be grown in unsterilised conditions. And thirdly, care should be taken to choose those strains which do not produce toxins. The Indo-Netherlands research project at present running in four centres of this country might solve some of our above problems.

Once solved, the present shortage of 38 per cent dry fodder of the country will be minimised by increasing digestibility per cent of the available roughages.

## OTHER METHODS FOR PARTITIONING CARBOHYDRATES

**Since 1960 efforts to find alternative schemes of greater precision to evaluate forages have shown promise. Dr. P.J. Van Soest in 1965 developed a method which makes use of the concept that the dry matter of plant origin consists of two principal parts: *Cell wall* and *Cell contents.***

**Table 66**

**Division of Forage Organic Matter by System of Analysis Using Detergents (Van Soest, 1966)**

| *Fraction* | *Components* | *Nutritional available* | |
|---|---|---|---|
| | | *Ruminant* | *Non-ruminant* |
| Cell contents | Lipids | Virtually complete | Highly available |
| (*soluble in neutral detergent*) | Sugars, organic acids, and water soluble matters | ,, | ,, |
| | Starch | ,, | ,, |
| | Non-protein nitrogen | ,, | ,, |
| | Soluble protein | ,, | ,, |
| | Pectin | ,, | ,, |
| Cell wall | | | |
| (Fibre insoluble in neutral detergent) | | | |
| (1) *Soluble in acid detergent* | Hemicellulose | Partial | Very low |
| (2) *Insoluble in acid detergent* | Cellulose | ,, | ,, |
| (acid detergent fibre) | Lignin | Indigestible | Indigetible |
| | Lignified nitrogen compounds | ,, | ,, |
| | Heat damaged protein | ,, | ,, |
| | Silica | ,, | ,, |

Plant cell contents consist of sugars, starch, soluble carbohydrates, pectin, non-protein nitrogen, protein, lipids and miscellaneous other water-soluble materials, including minerals and several vitamins. True digestibility is almost complete, averaging 98 per cent.

The cell walls of feeds of plant origin are not uniformly nutritious, in the sense that their principal components consist of cellulose, hemicellulose, silica, lignin, etc., singly or in such combinations as nitrogen-hemicellulose or lignocellulose differ widely in nutrition availability depending on the kind and maturity of the plant as well as on the age and species of the animal fed. Nitrogen-hemicellulose are not at all digestible. Chemical procedure to estimate various organic components are given below after Van Soest method.

Van Soest and Moore at U.S.D.A. have found high correlation of the *in vivo* digestibility of the cell contents, of the cell wall, and of the lignin with the *in vitro* data. Their formula for predicting the *in vivo* apparent digestibility of cattle feed (as dry matter) is:

$$0.98 \text{ NDS} + \text{W} (147.3 - 78.9 \log \text{lignin}) + 12.9 \text{ per cent}$$

in which 12.9 per cent is the constant percentage of the weight of the feed due to metabolic dry matter. NDS and lignin are expressed as percentages of a unit weight of feed. If the constants of this equation are, in fact, constants for feeds in general, it means that we will have a valid, entirely in *in vitro* method of describing the nutritionally available energy of feedstuffs.

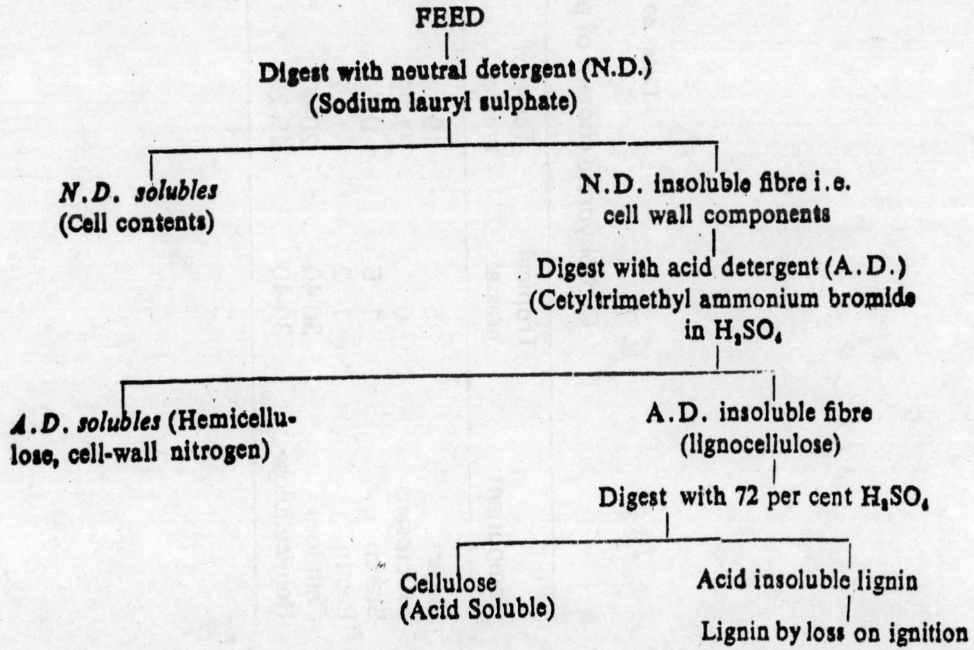

**Table 67**

Carbohydrate content of plant tissues, % of DM.

| Component | Tropical grasses | Temp. grasses | Cereal seeds | Alfalfa | Green vegetables |
|---|---|---|---|---|---|
| Sugars | 5 | 10 | negl. | 5-15 | 20 |
| Fructosans | 0 | 1-25 | 0 | 0 | -- |
| Starch | 1- 5 | 0 | 80 | 1- 7 | low |
| Pectin | 1- 2 | 1- 2 | negl. | 5-10 | 10-20 |
| Cellulose | 30-40 | 20-40 | 2- 5 | 20-35 | 20 |
| Hemicellulose | 30-40 | 15-25 | 7-15 | 8-10 | low |

## LIPIDS

Lipids include all substances extractable from biological materials with the usual fat solvents (ether, chloroform, benzene, carbon tetrachloride, acetone, etc.) and are important constituents of plant and animal tissue. These are important energy storage compounds of animal kingdom and structural compounds. The modern discoveries established the concept of the dynamic state of lipid metabolism. Fatty acids from the depots are being constantly mobilised and transported. A portion of absorbed fatty acids also degraded in the same way while others are combined with glycerol and transported back to the depots. All of these reactions are so balanced that mixtures of fatty acids in the depots, blood and organs tend to remain at equilibrium condition. In the proximate analysis of foods lipids are included in the ether extract portion which actually contains glycerides of fatty acids, free fatty acids, cholesterol, lecithin, alkalies, volatile oils, etc. The ether extract will differ in composition among different foods particularly in sterol content and also wax. Since this has no energy value it will affect the energy value of the entire ether extract. The useful energy of dietary ether extract is its gross energy minus that found in subsequent faecal excretion. However, when faeces are extracted with ether, soaps that may have been formed in the intestinal tract from free fatty acids and calcium will not be removed. This incomplete recovery of the faecel fat gives erroneously high value, for the digestibility of the ration fat, particularly in practical diets containing relatively high calcium content.

## CLASSIFICATION OF LIPIDS

Unlike polysaccharides and proteins, lipids are not polymers—they lack a repeating monometric unit. Lipids have been classified in several different ways. The present classification is on the basis of whether they are *saponifiable* or *nonsaponifiable.* (Saponification is the alkaline hydrolysis of lipids, particulaly of glyceride, that yields sodium or potassium salts of fatty acids-soap).

The saponifiable lipids are further subdivided according to their hydrolysis products.

## SAPONIFIABLE LIPIDS

### Fats and Oils

Like Carbohydrates, the fats contain the elements carbon, hydrogen and oxygen but they are relatively much richer in carbon and hydrogen as shown below.

| | Carbon | Hydrogen | Oxygen |
|---|---|---|---|
| Fat | 77 | 12 | 11 |
| Starch | 44 | 6 | 50 |

Because of this large proportion of hydrogen in addition to carbon and the fact that much more atmospheric oxygen instead of internal oxygen must be used to oxidise them, fats

Table 68

| A. *Saponifiable Lipids* | *Hydrolysis products* |
|---|---|
| 1. Fats and Oils | Fatty acids and glycerol |
| 2. Waxes | Fatty acids and long chain alcohols. |
| 3. Phospholipids. | |
| (i) Phosphoglycerides | Fatty acids, glycerol, phosphoric acid, and a polar alcohol group. |
| (ii) Sphingolipids | Fatty acids, sphingosine, phosphoric acid, and a polar alcohol group. |
| 4. Glycolipids | Fatty acids, sphingosine or glycerol and one or more monosaccharides |
| **B.** *Non-Saponifiable Lipids* | |
| 1. Steroids | |
| 2. Prostaglandins | |
| 3. Fat soluble vitamins | |
| 4. Terpenes | |

produce much more heat than carbohydrates or protein. The burning of 1 gram of hydrogen produces 34.5 kcal while one gram of carbon gives only 8 kcal.

Fats and Oils are the most abundant lipids found in nature. Both types of compounds are

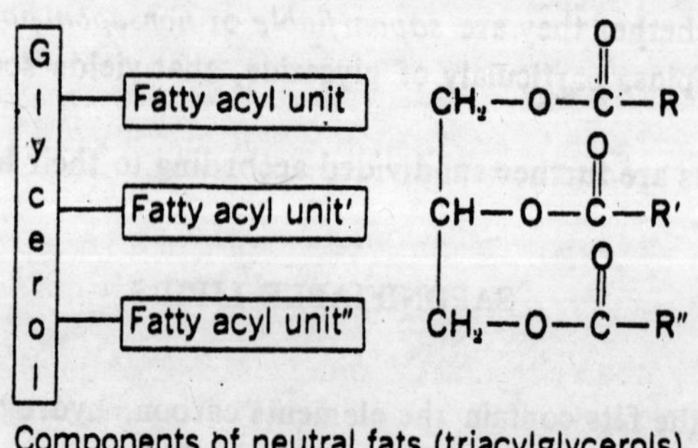


Components of neutral fats (triacylglycerols)

called *"Triacylglycerols"* because they are *esters* compound of *three fatty acids* joined to *glycerol,* a trihydroxy alcohol. Formerly these compounds were called triglycerides.

Further classification of triacylglycerols is made on the basis of their physical states at room temperature. It is customary to call a lipid a *fat* if it is a solid at 25°C, and an *oil*, if it is a liquid at the same temperature. These differences in melting points reflect differences in the degree of unsaturation of the constituent fatty acids. Furthermore, lipids obtained from animal sources are usually solids, whereas oils are generally of plant origin. Therefore, we commonly speak of *animal fats* and *vegetable oils.*

Acylglycerols are esters of one, two, or three fatty acids with the trihydroxy alcohol,

$$\begin{array}{c} H \\ | \\ C_{17}H_{35}-\overset{\overset{O}{\|}}{C}-O-C-H \\ | \\ C_{17}H_{35}-\overset{\overset{O}{\|}}{C}-O-C-H \\ | \\ C_{17}H_{35}-\overset{\overset{O}{\|}}{C}-O-C-H \\ | \\ H \end{array} \qquad \begin{array}{c} H \\ | \\ C_{11}H_{23}-\overset{\overset{O}{\|}}{C}-O-C-H \\ | \\ C_{15}H_{31}-\overset{\overset{O}{\|}}{C}-O-C-H \\ | \\ C_{17}H_{33}-\overset{\overset{O}{\|}}{C}-O-C-H \\ | \\ H \end{array} \qquad \begin{array}{c} H \\ | \\ C_{17}H_{31}-\overset{\overset{O}{\|}}{C}-O-C-H \\ | \\ C_{17}H_{31}-\overset{\overset{O}{\|}}{C}-O-C-H \\ | \\ C_{17}H_{31}-\overset{\overset{O}{\|}}{C}-O-C-H \\ | \\ H \end{array}$$

Glyceryl stearate (Tristearin) (a simple triacylglycerol) mp 71°C

Glyceryl lauropalmitooleate (a mixed triacylglycerol)

Glyceryl linoleate (Trilinolein) (a simple triacylglycerol) mp 9°C

glycerol. As mentioned earlier, these are designated as simple or mixed acylglycerols depending upon the number of different fatty acids present in the molecule. Tristearin, for example, indicates a simple triacylglyceride containing only stearic acid in the molecule, whereas 1-oleo-2-stearo-3 palmitin is a triacylglycerol containing oleic, stearic and palmitic acids.

Triacylglycerols are a form of stored energy in animal tissues (adipose cells) and are commonly referred to as neutral fat.

**The fatty acids**

The main constituents of all lipids are fatty acids. Fatty acids consists of an alkyl chain with a terminal carboxyl group, and the simplest configuration is a completely saturated straight chain. The basic formula is $CH_3—(CH_2)_n—COOH$. They consist of chains of carbon atoms with (4 to 30) with a methyl group at one end and a carboxyl group at the other end. Short chain fatty acids contain 4 to 6 carbon atoms, medium chain fatty acids contain 8 to 12 carbon atoms, and long chain fatty acids contain more than 12 carbon atoms.

Fatty acids of animal origin are usually quite simple in structure, that is, their fatty acids are straight chained and may contain up to 6 double bonds, nearly always with a *cis* configuration. Bacterial fatty acids may be staturated, monoenoic (one double bond), branched chain or may contain a cyclopropane ring (lactobacillic acid). Plant fatty acids are variable, may contain acetylenic bonds, epoxy, hydroxy and keto groups.

**Saturated fatty acids**

There are fatty acids in which after methyl carbon each of the carbon atoms in the chain has two hydrogen atoms attached $CH_3—CH_2—CH_2—C$. Examples of the acids in this series are shown in Table.

**Table 69**

**Saturated fatty acids.**

| | | |
|---|---|---|
| Acetic | $CH_3COOH$ | Major end product of carbohydrate fermentation by rumen organisms |
| Propionic | $C_2H_5COOH$ | An end product of carbohydrate fermentation by rumen organisms |
| Butyric | $C_3H_7COOH$ | In certain fats in small amounts (especially butter). An end product of carbohydrate fermentation by rumen organisms. |
| Caproic | $C_5H_{11}COOH$ | |
| Caprylic (octanoic) | $C_7H_{15}COOH$ | In small amounts in many fats (including butter), especially those of plant origin |
| Decanoic (capric) | $C_9H_{19}COOH$ | |
| Lauric | $C_{11}H_{23}COOH$ | Spermaceti, cinnamon, palm kernel, coconut oils, laurels |
| Myristic | $C_{13}H_{27}COOH$ | Nutmeg, palm kernel, coconut oils, myrtles |
| Palmitic | $C_{15}H_{31}COOH$ | Common in all animal and plant fats |
| Stearic | $C_{17}H_{35}COOH$ | |
| Arachidic | $C_{19}H_{39}COOH$ | Peanut (arachis) oil |
| Behenic | $C_{21}H_{43}COOH$ | Seeds |
| Lignoceric | $C_{23}H_{47}COOH$ | Cerebrosides, peanut oil |

As the chain length increases these have progressively become less soluble in water, and those with chain lengths of 10 or more are solids at room temperature.

**Unsaturated fatty acids**

An unsaturated fatty acid is one in which a hydrogen atom is missing from each of two adjoining carbon atom—thus necessitating a double bond between the two carbon atoms: $—CH=CH—$. Monounsaturated fatty acid has one double bond; oleic acid is widely distributed in food and body fats. A polyunsaturated fatty acid (PUFA) contains two or more double bonds; linoleic, linolenic and arachidonic acids are nutritionally important examples of this group. Naturally occurring unsaturated fatty acids are almost all of the *cis* configuration, whereas those produced during β-oxidation have the *trans* structure. Examples of unsaturated fatty acids are given in Table.

| Monoenoic fatty acids | | MP°C |
|---|---|---|
| Oleic acid | $CH_3(CH_2)_7CH\overset{cis}{=}CH(CH_2)_7COOH$ | 13 |
| Vaccenic acid | $CH_3(CH_2)_5CH\overset{cis}{=}CH(CH_2)_9COOH$ | 44 |
| **Dienoic fatty acid** | | |
| Linoleic acid | $CH_3(CH_2)_4(CH\overset{cis}{=}CHCH_2)_2(CH_2)_6COOH$ | −5 |
| **Trienoic fatty acids** | | |
| α-Linolenic acid | $CH_3CH_2(CH\overset{cis}{=}CHCH_2)_3(CH_2)_6COOH$ | −10 |
| γ-Linolenic acid | $CH_3(CH_2)_4(CH\overset{cis}{=}CHCH_2)_3(CH_2)_3COOH$ | — |
| **Tetraenoic fatty acid** | | |
| Arachidonic acid | $CH_3(CH_2)_4(CH\overset{cis}{=}CHCH_2)_4(CH_2)_2COOH$ | −50 |
| **Unusual fatty acids** | | |
| α-Elaeostearic acid | $CH_3(CH_2)_3CH\overset{trans}{=}CHCH\overset{trans}{=}CHCH\overset{cis}{=}CH(CH_2)_7COOH$ (conjugated) | 48 |
| Tariric acid | $CH_3(CH_2)_{10}C{\equiv}C(CH_2)_4COOH$ | 51 |
| Isanic acid | $CH_2{=}CH(CH_2)_4C{\equiv}C{-}C{\equiv}C(CH_2)_7COOH$ | 39 |
| Lactobacillic acid | $CH_3(CH_2)_5\overset{CH_2}{CH{-}CH}(CH_2)_9COOH$ | 28 |
| Vernolic acid | $CH_3(CH_2)_4\underset{O}{CH\overset{cis}{-}CH}CH_2CH{=}CH(CH_2)_7COOH$ | — |
| Prostaglandin ($PGE_2$) | 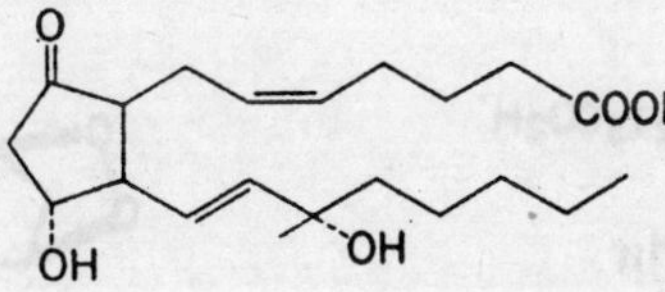 | — |



## Nomenclature

Polyunsaturated fatty acids in the above table have been arranged on the basis of the degree of unsaturation such as (A) Monounsaturated (Monoenoic); (B) Dienoic; (C) Trienoic; (D) Tetraenoic and others. Since fatty acids are straight-chain, aliphatic monocarboxylic acids, the position of a double bond is designated by its distance from the carboxyl end of the molecule. However, in discussing the biological chemistry of fatty acids it is convenient to identify the position of a double bond by its distance from the methyl end of the molecule. The methyl carbon is designated the *n*-carbon irrespective of the length of the chain. Thus linoleic acid is *n*-6. As it has in total 18 carbon and two double bonds, it is designated as 18 : 2. Linoleic and arachidonic acid belong to the same class of fatty acid because in both of them the first double bond from the methyl end is between the 6th and 7th carbons.

### 1. Prostaglandins (Eicosanoids = 20 carbon)

These are hormone like substances, derived from arachidonic acid originally isolated from semen found in the prostrate gland and referred to as prostaglandins. The compounds are

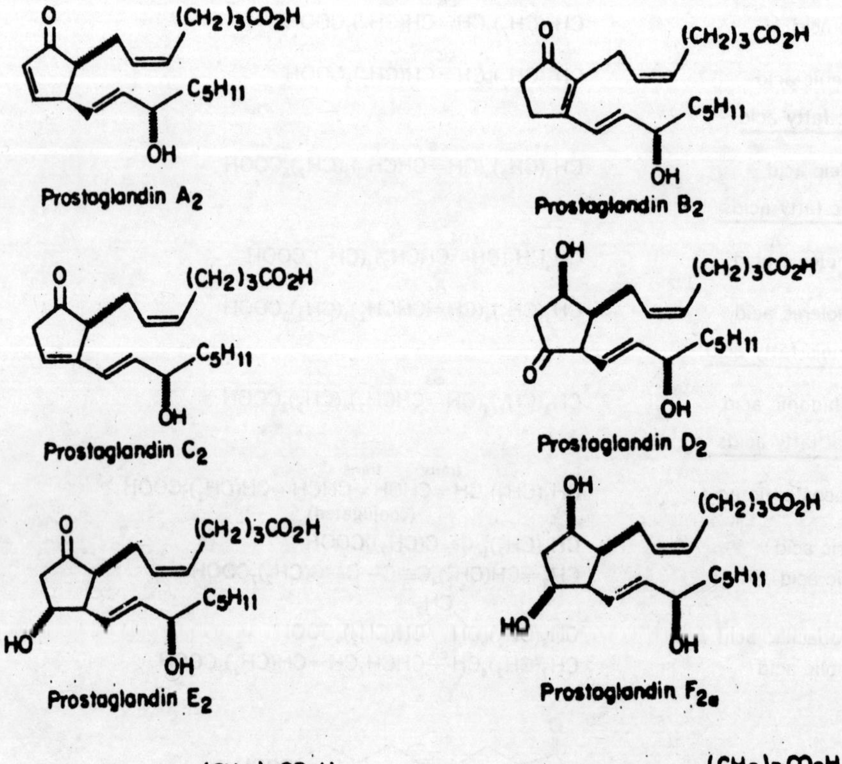

$(CH_2)_3CO_2H$ / $C_5H_{11}$ / OH

Prostaglandin $A_2$

$(CH_2)_3CO_2H$ / $C_5H_{11}$ / OH

Prostaglandin $B_2$

$(CH_2)_3CO_2H$ / $C_5H_{11}$ / OH

Prostaglandin $C_2$

$(CH_2)_3CO_2H$ / $C_5H_{11}$ / OH

Prostaglandin $D_2$

$(CH_2)_3CO_2H$ / $C_5H_{11}$ / HO / OH

Prostaglandin $E_2$

$(CH_2)_3CO_2H$ / $C_5H_{11}$ / HO / OH

Prostaglandin $F_{2\alpha}$

$(CH_2)_3CO_2H$ / $C_5H_{11}$ / OOH

Prostaglandin $G_2$

$(CH_2)_3CO_2H$ / $C_5H_{11}$ / OH

Prostaglandin $H_2$

$(CH_2)_3CO_2H$ / $C_5H_{11}$ / OH / OH

Prostaglandin $I_2$

**Fig. 20 . The nine classes of naturally occurring prostaglandins isolated to date.**

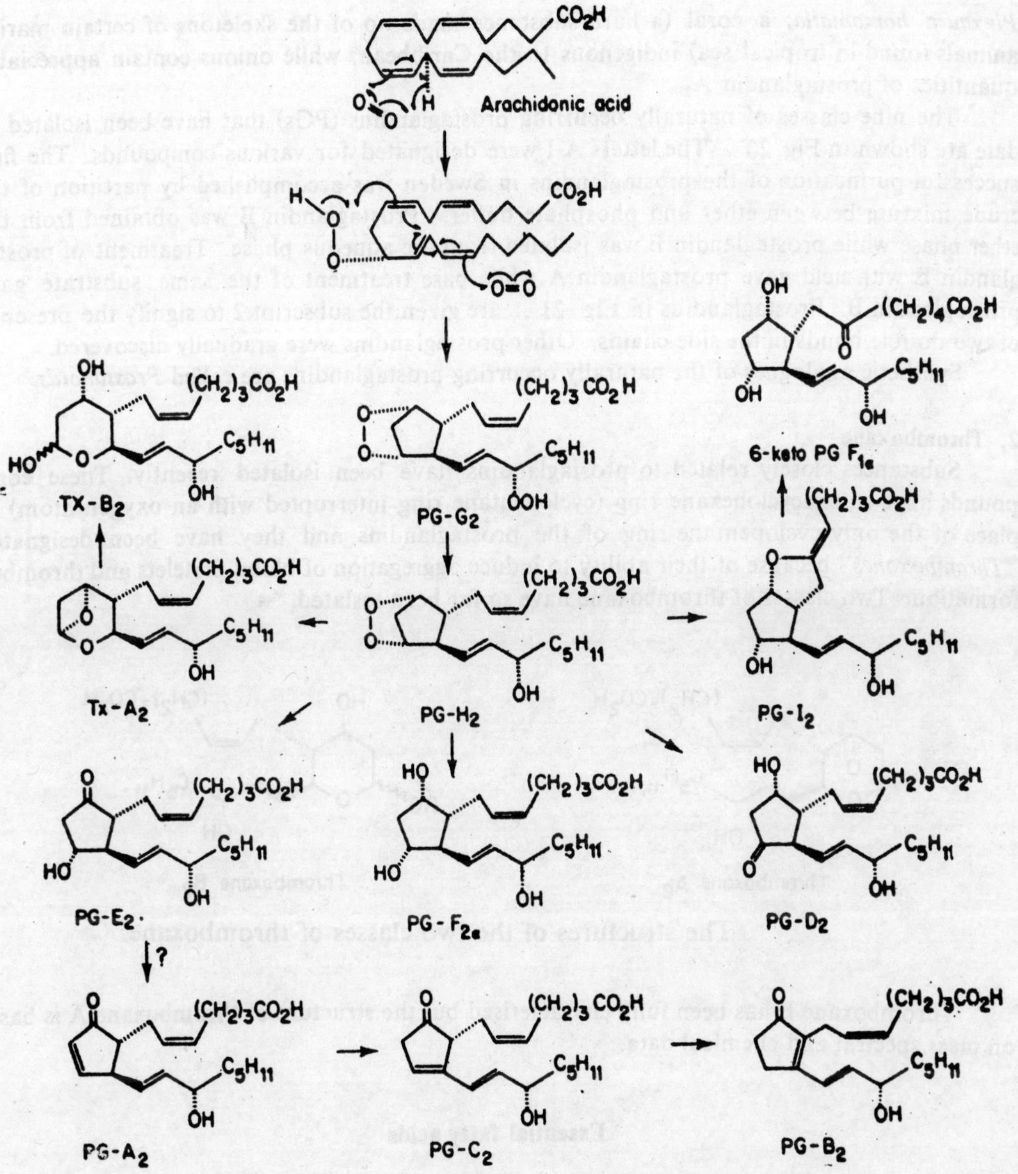

**Fig. 21 . The major pathways of prostaglandin biosynthesis.**

widely distributed in mammalian tissues and have important physiologic and pharmacologic activities. They are synthesized in vivo by cyclization of the centre of the carbon chain of 20-C (ecasanoic) arachidonic acid to form a cyclopentane ring.

The richest sources (300μ g/g) of prostaglandins are the seminal fluids of man and sheep. Lower concentrations (1μ g/g) are detectable in tissues from *inter alia* the uterus, lung, brain, eye, pancreas and kidney. . Prostaglandin $A_2$ 15-acetate has been obtained from the gorgonian

*Plexaura homomalla,* a coral (a hard substance made up of the skeletons of certain marine animals found in tropical sea) indigenous to the Caribbean, while onions contain appreciable quantities of prostaglandin $A_1$.

The nine classes of naturally occurring prostaglandins (PGs) that have been isolated to date are shown in Fig. 20 . The letters A-I were designated for various compounds. The first successful purification of the prostaglandins in Sweden was accomplished by partition of the crude mixture between ether and phosphate buffer. Prostaglandin E was obtained from the ether phase while prostaglandin F was isolated from the aqueous phase. Treatment of prostaglandin E with acid gave prostaglandin A while base treatment of the same substrate gave prostaglandin B. Prostaglandins in Fig 21 . are given the subscript 2 to signify the presence of two double bonds in the side chains. Other prostaglandins were gradually discovered.

Synthetic analogues of the naturally occurring prostaglandins are called *Prostanoids.*

**2. Thromboxane**

Substances closely related to prostaglandins have been isolated recently. These compounds have an oxacyclohexane ring (cyclopentane ring interrupted with an oxygen atom) in place of the only cyclopentane ring of the prostaglandins and they have been designated "*Thromboxanes*" because of their ability to induce aggregation of blood platelets and thrombus formation. Two classes of thromboxane have so far been ioslated.

$(CH_2)_3CO_2H$ $C_5H_{11}$ OH

Thromboxane $A_2$

HO $(CH_2)_3CO_2H$ HO $C_5H_{11}$ OH

Thromboxane $B_2$

**The structures of the two classes of thromboxane.**

**Thromboxane B has been fully characterised but the structure of thromboxane A is based on mass spectral and chemical data.**

## Essential fatty acids

Linoleic acid, the 18 carbon acid with two double bonds, is an essential fatty acid; that is, it cannot be synthesized in the body and must be present in the diet.

In the body linoleic acid is rapidly converted to arachidonic acid, the physiologically functioning polyunsaturated fatty acid.

Linolenic acid, another of the polyunsaturated fatty acids, promotes normal growth in animals but it does not cure the dermatitis that occurs from fatty acid deficiency. It is therefore, not an essential fatty acid and is not a substitute for linoleic acid.

About 50 years ago essential fatty acids (EFAs) were established. At that time linoleic acid and arachidonic acid were considered to be the only two EFAs. By definition, it is strictly only linoleic which is the EFA since animals have the enzymatic capacity to synthesise arachidonic and the intermediary fatty acids -γ- lenolenic acid and dihomo -γ- linolenic acid.

$$\overset{}{CH_3\cdot(CH_2)_4\cdot}\overset{12}{CH{=}CH}\cdot CH_2\cdot\overset{9}{CH{=}CH}\cdot(CH_2)_7\cdot COOH \quad \text{Linoleic acid}$$

↓

$$CH_3\cdot(CH_2)_4\cdot\overset{12}{CH{=}CH}\cdot CH_2\cdot\overset{9}{CH{=}CH}\cdot CH_2\cdot\overset{6}{CH{=}CH}\cdot(CH_2)_4\cdot COOH \quad \gamma\text{-Linolenic acid}$$

↓

$$CH_3\cdot(CH_2)_4\cdot\overset{14}{CH{=}CH}\cdot CH_2\cdot\overset{11}{CH{=}CH}\cdot CH_2\cdot\overset{8}{CH{=}CH}\cdot(CH_2)_6\cdot COOH \quad \text{Homo-}\gamma\text{-linolenic acid}$$

↓

$$CH_3\cdot(CH_2)_4\cdot\overset{14}{CH{=}CH}\cdot CH_2\cdot\overset{11}{CH{=}CH}\cdot CH_2\cdot\overset{8}{CH{=}CH}\cdot CH_2\cdot\overset{5}{CH{=}CH}\cdot(CH_2)_3\cdot COOH$$

Arachidonic acid

Unsaturated fatty acids can be grouped into families depending upon the number of carbon atoms *from the terminal methyl group to the first double bond*, the n-number, e.g.,

$$\overset{1}{CH_3}.\ \overset{2}{CH_2}.\ \overset{3}{CH_2}.\ \overset{4}{CH_2}.\ \overset{5}{CH_2}.\ \overset{6}{CH}{=}CH.\ CH_2.\ CH{=}CH\ (CH_2)_7\ COOH$$

linoleic n-6

$$CH_3.\ (CH_2)_7\ \overset{9}{CH}{=}CH.\ (CH_2)_7\ COOH$$

oleic n-9

$$\overset{1}{CH_3}.\ \overset{2}{CH_2}.\ \overset{3}{CH}{=}CH.\ CH_2.\ CH{=}CH.\ CH_2.\ CH{=}CH.\ (CH_2)_7\ COOH$$

Linolenic n-3

Members of the families with greatest nutritional and metabolic significance are shown in following Table.

Table 70

MEMBERS OF POLYENOIC FATTY ACID FAMILIES

| | | | |
|---|---|---|---|
| Linoleic acid (n-6 series) | 9,12–18:2<br>6,9,12–18:3<br>8,11,14–20:3<br>5,8,11,14–20:4<br>7,10,13,16–22:4<br>4,7,10,13,16–22:5 | Linolenic acid (n-3 series) | 9,12,15–18:3<br>6,9,12,15–18:4<br>8,11,14,17–20:4<br>5,8,11,14,17–20:5<br>7,10,13,16,19–22:5<br>4,7,10,13,16,19–22:6 |
| Oleic acid (n-9 series) | 9–18:1<br>6,9–18:2<br>8,11–20:2<br>5,8,11–20:3 | Palmitic acid (n-7 series) | 9–16:1<br>11–18:1<br>8,11–18:2 |

Animals can synthesise *de novo* fatty acids of the palmitoleate (n-7) and Oleate (n-9) families but the families based on linoleate (n-6) and linolenate (n-3) can be synthesised only if the basic fatty acids are provided in the diet. Interestingly enough, members of all families are modified by the same enzymes (Fig. 22 – 23 ). The formation of the long chain polyunsaturated fatty acids (PUFA) is regulated by competitive inhibition of the enzymes and the conversions within each family depend upon the concentrations of the substances and the products. Thus the presence of an excess of lenolenic acid (n-3) can suppress synthesis of the higher members of the linoleic acid family and vice versa.

In the above Table 70 . note that n-6 family (the linoleic acid family) having 9, 12-18 : 2 shows the position of double bond from methyl end of the molecule are on carbon 9 and 12. Total carbon is 18, and there are in total 2 double bonds.

**Relative activities of EFA**

When compaiing the EFA activity of different fatty acids, water intake capacity of the animal is considered a quantifiable criteria. This changes markedly with changes in skin permeability and water loss induced by EFA deficiency. The relative EFA potencies of a range of fatty acids are shown in Table . . 71 . Those with the highest potency belong to the linoleic acid (n-6 family), with greatest activity being shown by arachidonic acid (5, 8, 11, 14-20 : 4) of n-6 family.

**Table 71**

RELATIVE EFA POTENCIES OF FATTY ACIDS

| *Fatty acid* | *Position of terminal double bond* | *Relative potency* |
|---|---|---|
| 5,8,11,14-20:4 | n-6 | 139 |
| 6,9,12-18:3 | n-6 | 115 |
| 8,11,14-20:3 | n-6 | 102 |
| 9,12-18:2 | n-6 | 100 |
| 11,14-20:2 | n-6 | 46 |
| 3,6,9,12-18:4 | n-6 | 34 |
| 4,7,10,13-19:4 | n-6 | 20 |
| 10,13-19:2 | n-6 | 9 |
| 5,8,11,14-19:4 | n-5 | 49 |
| 5,8,11,14-21:4 | n-7 | 62 |
| 9,12,15-18:3 | n-3 | 9 |
| 7,10,13-19:3 | n-6 | 6 |
| 8,11,14-18:3 | n-4 | 0 |
| 5,8,11-20:3 | n-9 | 0 |
| 8,11,14-22:3 | n-8 | 0 |

From Holman, 1978

The mechanism of conversion of arachidonic acid from lenolenic acid is shown below.

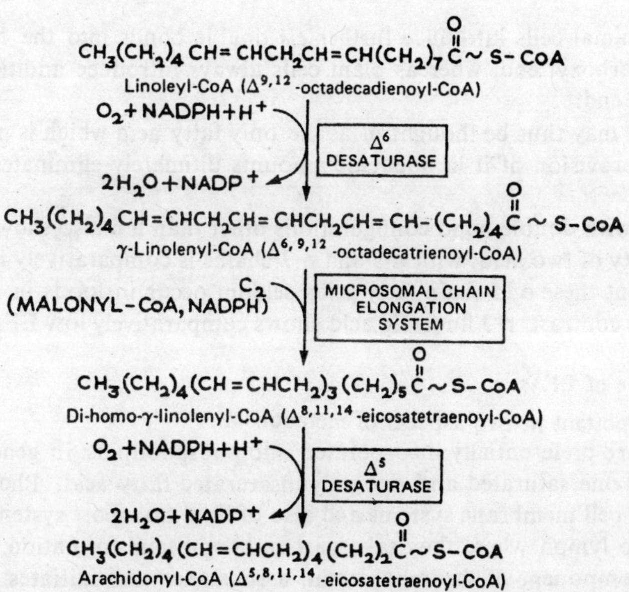


**Fig. 22** Conversion of linoleate to arachidonate.

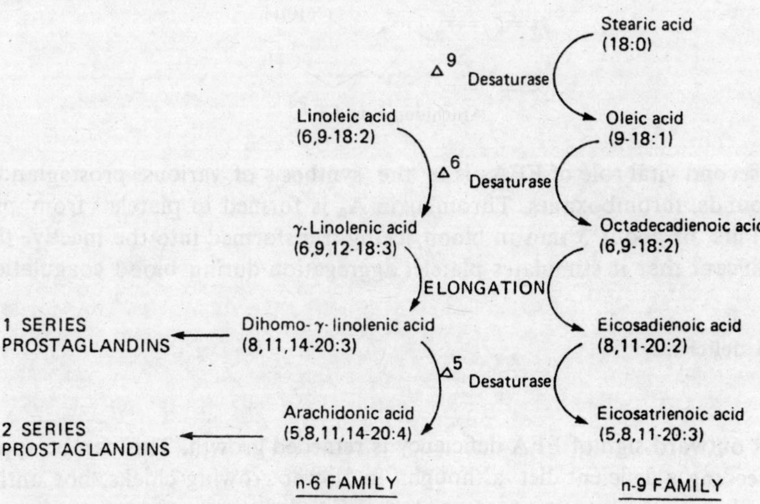


**Fig. 23** Outline of the stepwise parallel metabolism of linoleic acid and stearic acid via common enzymes. The conversion of dihomo-γ-linolenic and arachidonic acids to their respective series of prostaglandins occurs via the intermediate endoperoxides. The other families of fatty acids not shown are the n-3 derived from α-linolenic acid and the n-7 derived from palmitic acid

Note that animal cells introduce further *cis* double bonds into the hydrocarbon chain only toward the carboxyl end, whereas plant cells always introduce additional double bonds toward the methyl end.

Linoleic acid may thus be thought of as the only fatty acid which is perfectly an essential fatty acid, since provision of it in adequate amounts ultimately eliminates all symptoms of EFA deficiency.

Fatty acids with double bond configurations other than n-6 also show some EFA activity (Table 71). Activity of two acids with n-5 and n-7 chains is comparatively high by the criterion of water intake, but these odd-chain fatty acids seldom occur in foods in nutritionally significant amounts. In contrast, n-3 linolenic acid shows comparatively low EFA activity.

**Biochemical role of EFAs**

EFAs are important in two aspects of metabolism.

1. PUFAs are preferentially incorporated into phospholipids: in general a phospholipid molecule contains one saturated and one polyunsaturated fatty acid. Phospholipids are vital constituents of all cell membrane systems and also of lipid transport system through the intestinal wall into the lymph where they take part in lipoprotein formation. One phospholipid (a cephalin) is a component of thromboplastin, a substance that initiates blood clotting, and another (a sphingomyelin) acts as an insulator around nerve fibers.

The structure of arachidonic acid as shown below indicates about its hooked structure. This may be favourable for its binding with cell membranes.

The low melting points of PUFAs may also contribute to fluidity of membranes.

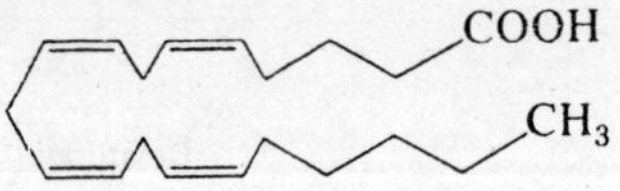

COOH

$CH_3$

Arachidonic acid

2. The second vital role of EFAs is in the synthesis of various prostaglandins and the related compounds, thromboxanes. Thromboxin $A_2$ is formed in platelets from prostaglandin $G_2$, has a half life of about 3 min in blood, being transformed into the inactive thromboxane $B_2$. It is significant that it stimulates platelet aggregation during blood coagulation.

**Effect of EFA deficiency**

*In poultry*

The first outward sign of EFA deficiency is retarded growth. This can be apparent within one week of feeding a deficient diet although, in slower-growing chicks, not until 6 weeks of age. Male chicks seem to be more susceptible to EFA deficiency.

As the deficiency intensifies, the deterioration of membrane structures leads to increased capillary fragility and dermal problems. The skin has a rough, flaky appearance and its increased permeability leads to enhance water loss and consequently greater water consumption. The birds also have a decreased resistance to disease, a poorer efficiency of feed utilisation and faulty feathering. The impairment of lipid transport leads to the formation of fatty livers and, in males, testis size is depressed and the development of secondary sex characteristics is delayed.

Signs of deficiency are much slower to appear if birds are first fed a diet containing EFA. The birds then build up reserves which must be depleted before a deficiency can develop. It has been noted that the time taken for signs to occur in growing broilers fed a deficient diet was proportional to the period during which an adequate diet was fed initially.

Because of their large EFA reserves, adult birds rarely show signs of abnormality if fed a deficient diet. However, if they are reared on a deficient diet or their reserves become depleted, adverse effects occur. Hens suffer from reductions in rate of egg production and egg size while fertility and hatchability of eggs are depressed. Chicks hatching from deficient eggs are small and weak and show the characteristic abnormalities in fatty acid composition.

They also have impaired viability and growth potential, even when fed adequate diets.

**EFA requirements in birds and pigs**

It appears that the EFA requirements of immature and mature poultry are broadly uniform and that under most circumstances a dietary linoleic acid content of 0.9% is adequate. For pig a level of 2-5% of the dietary energy in the diet must come from linoleic acid.

**Table 72**

Fatty Acid Components of Some Common Fats and Oils

| | Component Acids (%)[a] | | | | | | | |
|---|---|---|---|---|---|---|---|---|
| | *Lauric* ($C_{12}$) | *Myristic* ($C_{14}$) | *Palmitic* ($C_{16}$) | *Stearic* ($C_{18}$) | *Oleic* ($C_{18}$) | *Linoleic* ($C_{18}$) | *Linolenic* ($C_{18}$) | *Iodine Number* |
| *Fats* | | | | | | | | |
| Butter | 1-4 | 8-13 | 25-32 | 8-13 | 22-29 | 2-4 | | 26-42 |
| Tallow (beef) | | 2-3 | 24-32 | 20-25 | 37-43 | 2-3 | | 30-48 |
| Lard | | 1-2 | 25-30 | 12-16 | 40-50 | 3-8 | | 46-70 |
| *Edible Oils* | | | | | | | | |
| Coconut oil | 44-50 | 13-18 | 7-10 | 1-4 | 5-8 | 1-3 | | 8-11[b] |
| Olive oil | 0-1 | 0-2 | 7-20 | 2-3 | 53-86 | 4-22 | | 79-90 |
| Peanut oil | | 0-1 | 6-11 | 3-6 | 40-65 | 17-38 | | 84-100 |
| Cottonseed oil | | 0-3 | 17-23 | 1-3 | 23-44 | 34-55 | | 97-112 |
| Corn oil | | 1-2 | 8-12 | 2-5 | 29-49 | 34-56 | | 103-128 |
| Soybean oil | | 0-1 | 6-10 | 2-5 | 20-30 | 50-60 | 2-10 | 120-141 |
| Safflower oil | | | 6-7 | 2-3 | 12-14 | 75-80 | 0-2 | 140-150 |
| *Nonedible oil* | | | | | | | | |
| Linseed oil | | 0-1 | 5-9 | 4-7 | 9-29 | 8-29 | 45-67 | 175-202 |

[a]Totals less than 100% indicate the presence of lower or higher acids in small amounts.

[b]Coconut oil is a highly saturated oil, hence the very low iodine number. It contains an unusually high percentage (53-70%) of the low-melting $C_8$, $C_{10}$, and $C_{12}$ saturated fatty acids. Coconut oil is a liquid in the warmer, tropical climates, but at room temperature in the temperate zone, it is a solid.

**EFA in ruminants**

1) The digesta in ruminants upon entering the small intestine is augmented by the addition of the various digestive secretions associated with doudenum. Levels of linoleic acid in both unesterified and esterified components which generally varies between 0.3 to 0.5% of the energy available at the time of leaving the abomasum while entering the duodenum are therefore increased significantly particularly due to addition of the biliary phosphatidylcholine. However, stearic acid remains the same principal fatty acid in the digesta with linoleic acid accounting for not more than 7% of the total.

**Vegetable fats vs animal fats**

Animal fats differ from vegetable fats in that they contain a greater variety of fatty acids. In addition to the usual saturated $C_{16}$ and $C_{18}$ acids, animal fats have both saturated and unsaturated fatty acids of the $C_{20}$, $C_{22}$ and $C_{24}$ varieties.

Vegetable fats, however, contain a greater proportion of linoleic acid, which is present only in small amounts in animal fats.

**Waxes**

A wax is an ester of a long chain alcohol (usually monohydroxy and a fatty acid. The acids and alcohols normally found in waxes have chains of the order of 12—34 carbon atoms in length. They are not easily hydrolysed as the tracylglycerols and therefore are useful as protecting coatings.

Plant waxes are found on the surfaces of leaves, stems, flowers, and fruits and serve to

$$R-O-\overset{\displaystyle O}{\overset{\|}{C}}-R'$$

Alcohol unit — Fatty acyl unit

Components of waxes

protect the plant from dehydration and from invasion by harmful micro-organisms. (You can polish an apple to a high luster because of the waxes present in its skin).

Animal waxes also serve as protective coatings. They are found on the surface of feathers skin and hair and help to keep these surfaces pliable and water repellant.

**Phospholipids :**

Phospholipids have the useful property of attracting both water soluble and fat soluble substances. In combination with protein, they are constituents of cell membranes and membranes of subcellular particles where they serve as a liaison between fat soluble and water soluble materials that must penetrate the membrane and interact once they have gained entry. In this structural role, phospholipids are not generally available as an energy source. Even a starved animal will retain the phospholipid necessary to maintain the integrity of tissue cells. It is thought that phospholipids take part in fat metabolism by promoting the transp ortation of lipids in the blood stream as lipoprotein complexes.

Phospholipids differ chiefly in the specific compound attached to the phosphate group of the phosphatidic acid core. The fatty acids present in the molecule are usually saturated in the $\alpha$-position (palmitic or stearic) and unsaturated in the $\beta$-position (oleic or linolenic).

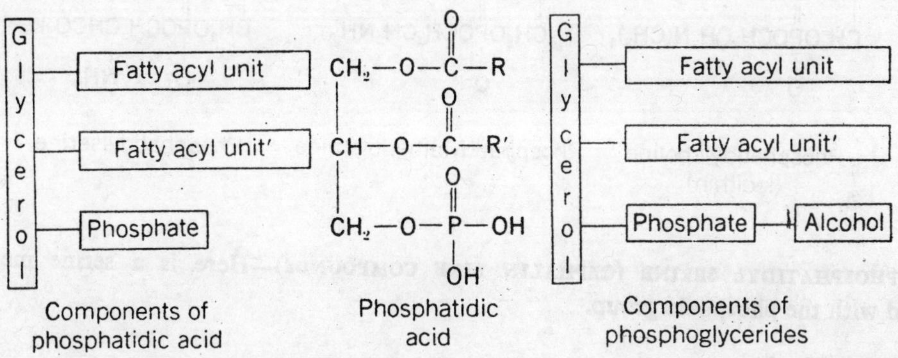

Components of phosphatidic acid | Phosphatidic acid | Components of phosphoglycerides

The main function of phospholipids and other lipids (like CHOL) is the formation of structural membranes within the body to prevent the absorption of water-soluble substances and water evaporation from the skin (11). And, they aid in the transport of fatty acids through the intestinal wall into the *lymph*. One phospholipid (a cephalin) is a component of thromboplastin, a substance that initiates blood clotting, and another (a sphingomyelin) acts as an insulator around nerve fibers.

**Phosphatidic Acid**

**Phosphatidic acids are compounds consisting of glycerol, two fatty acids, and a phosphate group and, as the structure suggests, they easily give rise to triacylglycerols or to phospholipids. Because they are active intermediates in the biosynthesis of other lipid compounds, the phosphatidic acids do not accumulate in tissues in significant amounts.**

**There are 3 common phospholipids found in animal body which are :**

**(a)** PHOSPHATIDYL CHOLINE (LECITHIN)—A choline melecule is attached with the phosphate **group of phosphatidic acid.**

**(b) PHOSPHATIDYL ETHANOLAMINE (CEPHALIN)—In place of choline if an ethanolamine molecule is attached with the phosphate group of phosphatidic acid, then it becomes phosphatidyl ethanolamine or commonly known as cephalin.**

$$\begin{array}{l} CH_2OCOR \\ | \\ CHOCOR \\ | \\ CH_2OPO(O)(O)OCH_2CH_2N(CH_3)_3 \end{array}$$

Phosphatidylcholine (lecithin)

$$\begin{array}{l} CH_2OCOR \\ | \\ CHOCOR' \\ | \\ CH_2OPO(O)(O^-)OCH_2CH_2\overset{+}{N}H_3 \end{array}$$

Phosphatidylethanolamine

$$\begin{array}{l} CH_2OCOR \\ | \\ CHOCOR' \\ | \\ CH_2OPO(O)(O^-)OCH_2CH(NH_3^+)CO_2H \end{array}$$

Phosphatidylserine

**(c) PHOSPHATIDYL SERINE (CEPHALIN LIKE COMPOUNDS)—Here is a serine molecule is attached with the phosphate group.**

**Sphingosine Lipids :**

**Sphingolipids, or sphingomyelins, are derivatives of the basic compound sphingosine also known as 4-Sphingenine.**

**In sphingolipids the amino group of the sphingosine is attached to a fatty acid and the terminal alcoholic group to phosphocholine.**

Sphingosine: OH; Fatty acylamido unit; Phosphate-Alcohol OR Glycoside

Components of sphingolipids

$$\begin{array}{l} CH_3 \\ | \\ (CH_2)_{12} \\ | \\ CH \\ \| \\ HC \\ | \\ CHOH \\ | \\ CHNHCOR \\ | \\ CH_2OPO(O)(O^-)OCH_2CH_2\overset{+}{N}(CH_3)_3 \end{array}$$

Sphingomyelin

$$\begin{array}{l} CH_3 \\ | \\ (CH_2)_{12} \\ | \\ CH \\ \| \\ HC \\ | \\ CHOH \\ | \\ CHNHCOR \\ | \\ CH_2O\text{–(galactose: OH, OH, OH, HO)} \end{array}$$

Cerebrosides

**Sphingomyelins occur in large amounts in brain and in the myelin sheath of nerve tissue and derive their name from the structure.**

### Glycolipids (Cerebrosides)

Glycolipids, as their name implies, are sugar containing lipids. The simplest glycolipid is *Cerebroside,* in which there is only one sugar residue, either glucose or galactose. More complex glycolipids, such as *gangliosides,* contain as many as seven sugar residues. In animal

$$CH_3-(CH_2)_{12}-CH=CH-\underset{OH}{CH}-\underset{NH-\underset{O}{C}-R}{CH}-CH_2O-\text{galactose}$$

*The structure of galactocerebroside (galactolipid).*

cells, glycolipids, like sphingomyelin are derived from sphingosine. The sugar molecule(s) is attached with the primary hydroxyl group of sphingosine instead of phosphoryl choline as in sphingomyelin. The compound is abundant in the myelin sheath of nerves and in brain tissue.

## NONSAPONIFIABLE LIPIDS

### Steroids

The steroids constitute a large group of cyclic compounds that have a common basic structural unit of a phenanthrene nucleus linked to a cyclopentane ring. They include a number of biologically important compounds as the sterols, the bile acids, the adrenal hormones and sex hormones. They are often found in association with fat. They may be separated from fat after the fat is saponified, since they occur in the "unsaponifiable residue". All of the steroids have a similar nucleus resembling phenanthrene (rings A, B and C) to which a cyclopentane ring (D) is attached. However, the rings are not uniformly unsaturated, so the parent (completely saturated) substance is better designated as cyclopentaneperhydrophenanthrene. The positions of the steroid nucleus are numbered as is shown.

Perhydrocyclopentanophenanthrene

The individual compounds belonging to the steroid group differ in the number and positions of their double bonds and in the nature of the side chain at carbon atom 17. Methyl groups are frequently attached at positions 10 and 14 (constituting Carbon atoms 19 and 18). If the compound has one or more hydroxyl groups and no carbonyl or carboxyl groups, it is *sterol,* and the name terminates in -ol. If it has one or more carbonyl or carboxy-groups, it is a *steroid.*

**Cholesterol**

Cholesterol, the principal sterol of vertebrates is a wax-like substance found in all body cells, is extremely essential to normal body functions as animals can not live without it.

**Distribution**

Cholesterol does not occur in plants. Being a major sterol the compound is present virtually in all cell surfaces and intracellular membranes. It is specially abundant in the myelinated structure of the brain and central nervous system. In contrast to the situation in plasma, most of the cholesterol in cellular membranes occurs in the free, unesterified form. Its name is derived from the source ( Greek, *chole,* bile ; *stereos,* solid ) as it can be isolated from gallstone as a white crystalline solid.

**Function**

Cholesterol furnishes the nucleus for the synthesis of 7-dehydrocholesterol, a precursor to vitamin D. It is also the immediate precursor of the bile acids that are synthesised in the liver, it is the precursor of adrenocortico hormones as well as of male ( testosterone ) and female sex hormones estrogens ( estradiol ).

**Synthesis**

Although the de novo biosynthesis of cholesterol occurs in virtually all cells, this capacity is greatest in certain tissues, particularly the liver, intestine, adrenal cortex, and reproductive tissues, including ovaries, testes and placenta. Ruminants are exception in that the intestinal mucosa and possibly adipose tissue are the major sites of biosynthesis.

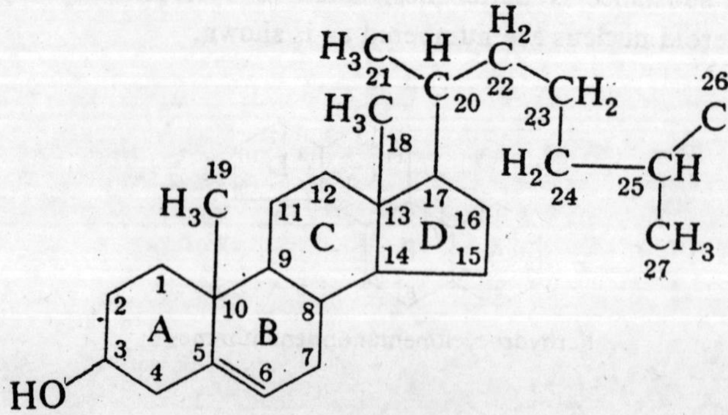

Cholesterol

The compound is synthesised entirely from acetyl coenzyme A by condensation reactions of isoprene units. The major steps of reactions are as follows :

1) Acetyl-CoA is converted to mevalonic acid by condensation.
2) Mevalonic acid is transformed to squalene.
3) Squalene is converted into lanosterol and then to cholesterol.

In the first step two molecules of acetyl CoA condense to form acetoacetyl CoA. A third molecule of acetyl CoA reacts with acetoacetyl CoA and forms a branched chain compound 3-hydroxy-3-methylglutaryl CoA ( HMG-CoA ) by HMG-CoA reductase enzyme.

## Regulation of synthesis

Free cholesterol at higher concentration through receptors of the cell membranes slows down the biosynthesis of the new cholesterol molecules by inhibiting the enzyme HMG-CoA reductase. Fasting also inhibits the production of cholesterol whereas saturated fats at high level tend to accelerate the production at cellular level.

**The regulation of serum cholesterol level, however, is dependent not only upon the rate of synthesis but also upon the rate of degradation and excretion of cholesterol in liver. Some cholesterol is excreted in the bile as such, and may be reabsorbed from the intestine and rest will pass through faeces.**

## Transportation

Actually, only about 30% of the total circulating cholesterol occurs free as such ; approximately 70% of the cholesterol in plasma lipoproteins exists in the form of cholesterol esters where some long chain fatty acids, usually linoleic acid, is attached. The presence of ester bond by long chain fatty acid enhances the hydrophobicity of cholesterol. The concentration of the compound varies considerably and is increased during periods of stress, physical activity and over eating. In apparently normal human adults values ranges from 150-250 mg/100 ml serum, although a level above 200 mg/100 ml serum is now considered undesirable. This value is almost twice the normal concentration of blood glucose. For transportation in blood, esterified cholesterol is complexed with water soluble proteins ( lipoproteins ). Lipoproteins generally are classified according to their density and origin. There are four broad categories : chylomicrons ( density of less than 1·006 g/ml and made in the intestine ), very low-density lipoproteins ( VLDLs ), density of less than 1·006 and made mainly in the liver, low-density lipoproteins ( LDLs ), density between 1.006-1.063, and high density lipoproteins ( HDLs ), density varies 1·063-1·21.

Low density lipoproteins are the chief carriers of cholesterol.

## Absorption

It is slowly absorbed from the intestinal tract and enters the body via the lymphatic system. The proportion of absorption of dietary cholesterol is always poor.

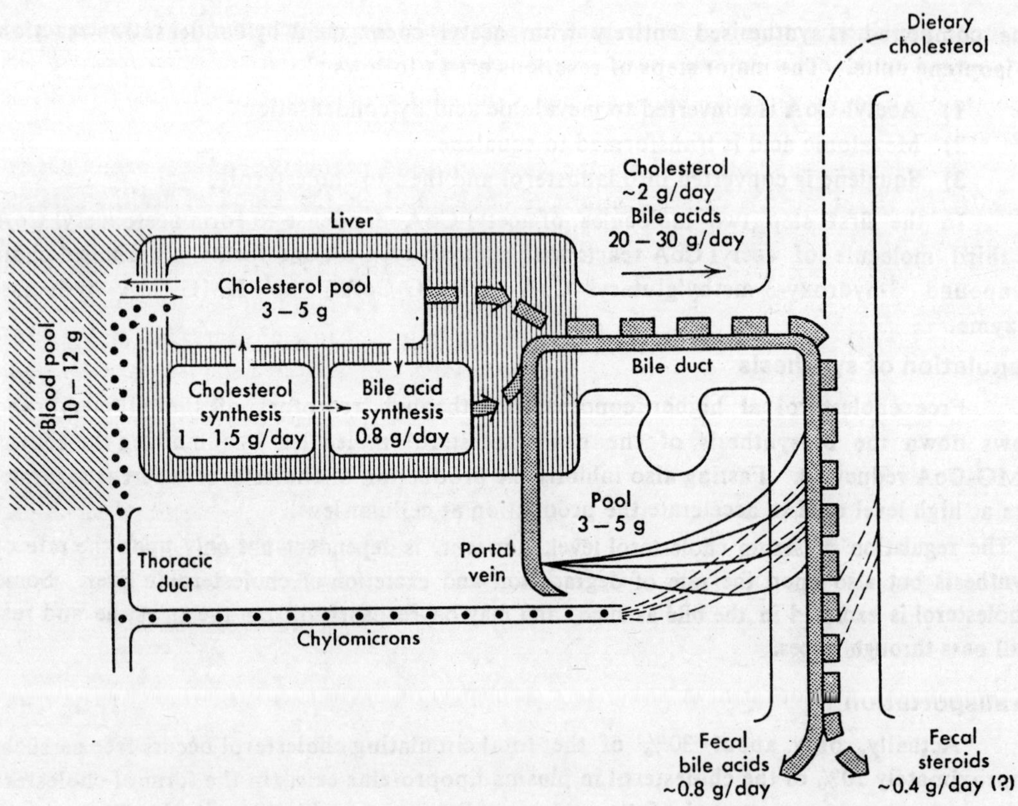


**Fig. 24** Cholesterol and bile acid absorption, secretion, and excretion.

## Sources in feed

Only animal food furnish cholesterol. Liver, whole egg ( contains 250 mg of cholesterol ), kidney, brain, fish are rich sources. Much smaller concentration are found in whole milk, cream, butter, cheese and meat. Ruminant feed contain traces of cholesterol.

## Relationship with Heart diseases

Cholesterol has received much publicity because of the correlation between the cholesterol level in the blood and certain types of heart diseases like atherosclerosis, coronary heart diseases and stroke. The disorder underlying both heart attack and stroke is atherosclerosis, characterised by the building up of deposits ( plaques ) on the inner surfaces of the arteries. If a blood clot forms in such a constricted artery leading to the heart or brain and causes a complete stoppage of blood flow. a heart attack or stroke occurs almost instantly. In atherosclerotic plaques, the lipid in highest concentration is cholesterol. Present in lower concentration are two other types of lipids—phospholipids and triacylglycerols.

The lipid hypothesis carries the assumption that the intake of dietary cholesterol in the form of food products of animal origin would be responsible for elevated blood cholesterol. This question has been extensively studied in different subgroups of the population. The opinion of the American Council on Science and Health ( 1980 ) is given below :

"The intake of cholesterol in the form of food products of animal origin has an insignificant effect on the concentration of cholesterol in the blood of healthy persons representative of the population in general."

It is fact that dietary saturated fat is more implicated in atherosclerosis rather than dietary cholesterol. Thus it must be realised from recent findings that dietary cholesterol is not the sole cause rather a number of factors enter into the cause of heart disease, many of which are more important than cholesterol ; among them, stress, heredity, hypertension, diabetes mellitus, smoking, lack of exercise and obesity.

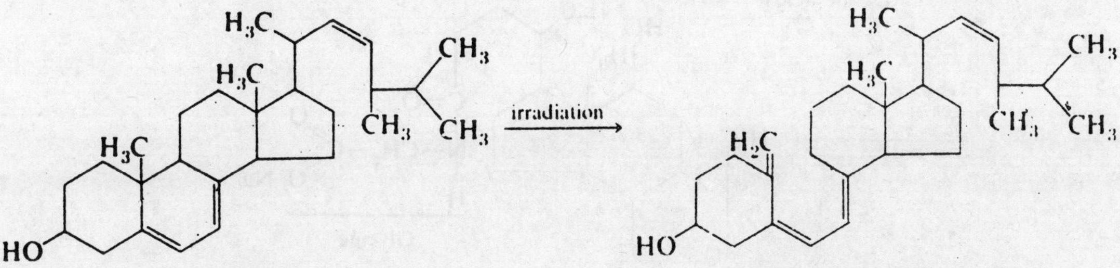

$H_3C$ $CH_3$ $H_3C$ $CH_3$ $CH_3$ $H_3C$ HO — irradiation → $H_3C$ $CH_3$ $H_3C$ $CH_3$ $CH_3$ $H_2C$ HO

Ergosterol  Vitamin $D_2$ (ergocalciferol)

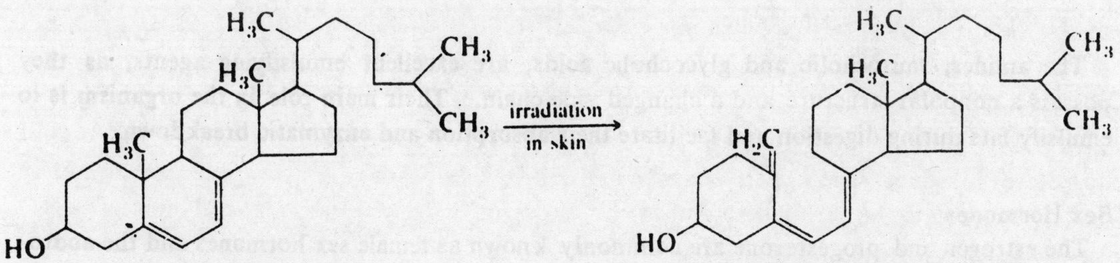

$H_3C$ $CH_3$ $H_3C$ $CH_3$ $H_3C$ HO — irradiation in skin → $H_3C$ $CH_3$ $H_3C$ $CH_3$ $H_2C$ HO

7-Dehydrocholesterol  Vitamin $D_3$ (cholecalciferol)

**Ergosterol**

Ergosterol occurs in ergot and yeast. It is important as a precursor of vitamin $D_2$. When ergosterol is irradiated with ultraviolet ligh⁺, it changes into vitamin $D_2$.

**Bile acids**

Human liver contains 3 different bile acids—cholic, deoxycholic and chemodeoxycholic. The last one is microbial in origin and is absorbed from intestinal contents. The bile acids have a

**five carbon side chain at carbon 17 terminating in a carboxyl group which is bound by an amide linkage to amino acids glycine and taurine**

Cholic acid
(a bile acid)

**Taurocholic acid**

Glycine

Sodium glycocholate
(a bile salt)

**The amides, taurocholic and glycccholic acids, are excellent emulsifying agents, as they possess a nonpolar structure and a changed side chain. Their main role in the organism is to emulsify fats during digestion and facilitate their absorption and enzymatic breakdown.**

**Sex Hormones**

**The estrogen and progesterone are commonly known as female sex hormones and the androgens as male sex hormones. Of the estrogens, estradiol is produced in the ovaries and estrone and estriol formed as a result of enzymatic transformations of estradiol. Progesterone, which is also produced in the ovaries, is related more closely to the androgens in structure.**

Estrone

Testosterone

Progesterone

Androsterone

**Testosterone is produced in the testes and biochemically transformed to androsterone, which is the product found in urine.**

## Prostaglandins

**There are a group of biologically active lipids that are derived from a 20-Carbon unsaturated fatty acid containing a five membered ring. Prostaglandins were first found in the prostate gland but are now known to occur in most, if not all, mammalian tissues. At present, 16 prostaglandins have been discovered ; they are found in extremely minute amounts in a**

PGE$_1$ PGE$_2$ PGA$_1$

PGA$_2$ PGF$_{1\alpha}$ PGF$_{2\alpha}$

PGB$_1$ PGB$_2$

**Structure of some naturally occuring Prostaglandins**

| | $F_{2\alpha}$ | | $E_2$ |
|---|---|---|---|
| **opposing effect** | vasoconstriction<br>raised blood pressure<br>bronchoconstriction | | vasodilation<br>reduced blood pressure<br>bronchodilation |
| **effect restricted to F2α** | luteolytic activity | | |
| **common effects** | | spasmogenic activity on smooth muscles of gastrointestinal tract | |
| **predominant effect of E2** | | | spasmogenic activity on uterus (increased frequency of contraction |

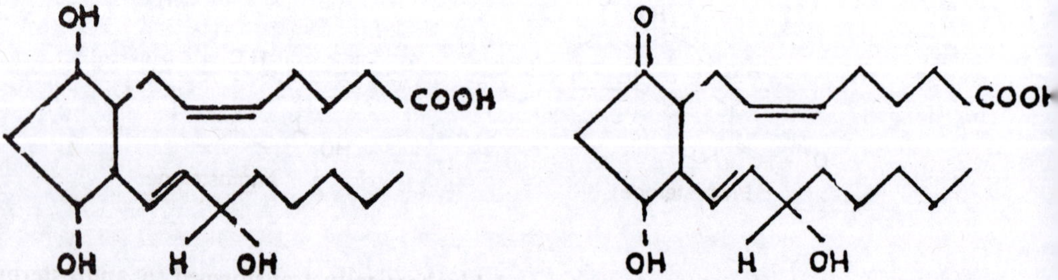

Activity spectrum of PGE2 and PGF2α: a comparision

variety of body tissue and biological fluids, including the menstrual fluid of women.

They are synthesised in the cell membranes from 20-carbon polyunsaturated fatty acids, the arachidonic acids containing 4, carbon-carbon double bonds. During their transformation into various prostaglandins they are cyclized and take up oxygen.

Prostaglandins have been classified into three major classes, the A, E, and F series. They are distinguished on the basis of the functional groups about the cyclopentane ring : the E type is a β-hydroxy ketone, the F series are 1, 3-diols, and those in the A series are L, β-unsaturated ketones. The subscript numerals 1, 2 or 3, refer to the number of double bonds in the six chains.

The prostaglandins have a very short half-life, soon after release they are rapidly taken up by cells and inactivated.

Physiological effects of the Prostaglandins.

1. *Inflammation*

Prostaglandins appear to be responsible for bringing about inflammation. Inflammatory reactions most often involve the joints (rheumatoid arthritis), skin (psoriasis), and eyes. Inflammation of these sites is frequently treated with corticosteroids that inhibit prostaglandin synthesis. Prostaglandins $E_1$ and $E_2$ on administration induce the signs of inflammation that include redness and heat (due to arteriolar vasodilation) and swelling and edema results from increased capillary permeability.

2. *Pain and Fever*

It has been observed that pyrogen activates the prostaglandin biosynthetic pathway, resulting in the release of $E_2$ in the region of the hypothalamus where body temperature is regulated. Aspirin, which is an antipyritic drug, acts by inhibiting cyclo-oxygenase, the enzyme required for the synthesis of prostaglandin.

3. *Reproduction*

The prostaglandins have been used extensively as drugs in the reproductive area. $F_2$ and $E_2$ have been used to induce parturition and for the termination of unwanted pregnancy. There is also evidence that E series of prostaglandins may play some role in infertility in males.

4. *Gastric Secretion & Peptic Ulcer*

Syntnetic prostaglandins have proven to be very effective in inhibiting gastric acid secretion in patients with peptic ulcers. The inhibitory effect of E series appears to be due to inhibition of cyclic AMP formation in gastric mucosal cells. Prostaglandin also accelerates the healing of gastric ulcers.

5. *Regulation of Blood Pressure*

The vasodilator prostaglandins, E, A and $I_2$, lower systemic arterial pressure, thereby increasing local blood flow and decreasing peripheral resistance. There is hope the compounds may eventually prove useful in the treatment of hypertension.

6. *Platelet Aggregation and Thrombosis*

Certain prostaglandins, especially $I_2$, inhibit platelet aggregation, whereas $E_2$ and $A_2$ promote this clotting process.

## FUNCTIONS OF LIPIDS

1. Fats are the most concentrated forms of stored energy in animal kingdom as plants store most of their energy in the form of carbohydrates primarily as starch. It furnish more than twice (2.5 times) as many calories, gram for gram, as do carbohydrates and proteins.
2. Lipids provide insulation for the vital organs, protecting them from mechanical shock and maintaining optimum body temperature.
3. Lipids like phospholipids which contain both polar and non polar groups are an integral component of cell membrane structure. For example, nearly half the mass of the erethrocyte membrane is comprised of various phospholipids and as such are associated with transportation across cellular membrane.
4. Polyunsaturated fatty acids, particularly arachidonic acid, are the precursors of the highly active prostaglandins.
5. Cholesterol—the special lipid is the intermediate precursor of various steriod hormones and of bile, which facilitate the absorption of fat soluble vitamins, particularly vitamin D, from the intestine.
6. The deficiency symptoms which are produced in animals due to lack of intake of essential

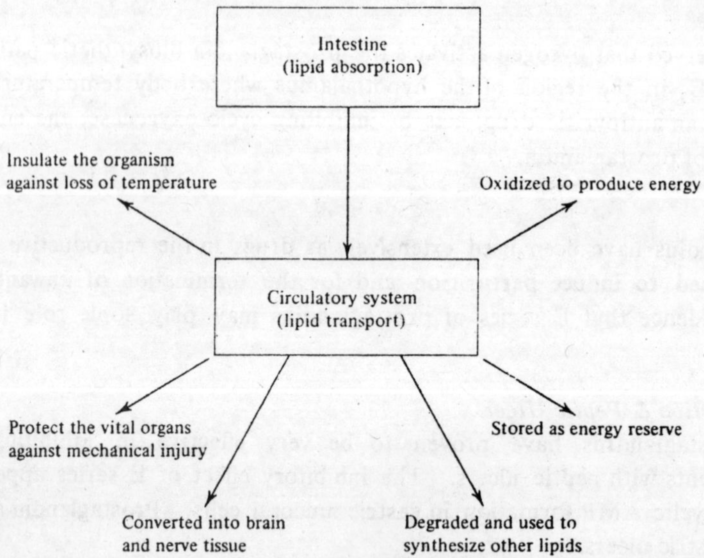


**Fig. 25** Metabolic fate of lipids.

**fatty acids are overcome by feeding such unsaturated fatty acids.**

7. **It improves palatability of feeds for all classes of animals. Even in the case of poultry, where taste is not a measurable factor, additional fat tends to reduce dustiness of feed and to overcome problems associated with acceptibility of feed particles that are too fine.**
8. **It delays the sensation of hunger as it requires a longer period of time to pass through the stomach than carbohydrates and protein.**
9. **It lubricates feed processing equipment.**

**However, the following problems are inherent in the incorporation of fats in feeds :**

1. Animal fats can become rancid
2. **Fats at higher percentage may get deposited around vital organs.**

## PLANT LIPIDS

**The leaves of higher plants contain up to 7 per cent of their dry weight as lipids, some of which are present as surface lipids, the others as components of leaf cells.**

The surface lipids are:

1. Mostly of wax, a term referred to the esters of long-chain alcohols with fatty acids which form a major fraction of the surface lipid mixture.

2. Long-chain (C 29) hydrocarbons, free fatty acids, alcohols, ketones and cutin in some plant epidermal cells of the thick outer part known as cuticle.

The major leaf lipids are those associated with leaf cells at their cellular membranes. The lipids of plasma membranes, mitochondria and endoplasmic reticulum are predominantly

$CH_3(CH_2)_7CH{=}CH(CH_2)_7CH_2.O.CO.CH_2(CH_2)_7CH{=}CH(CH_2)_7CH_3$

**Wax esters**

*Structural*

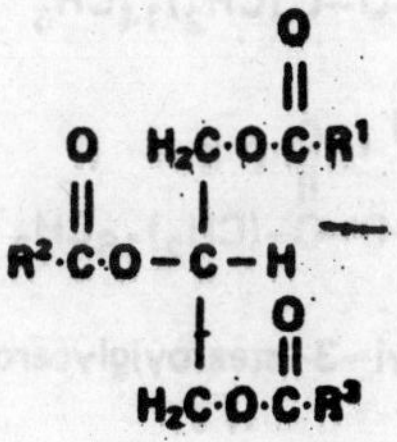

**Triacylglycerols**

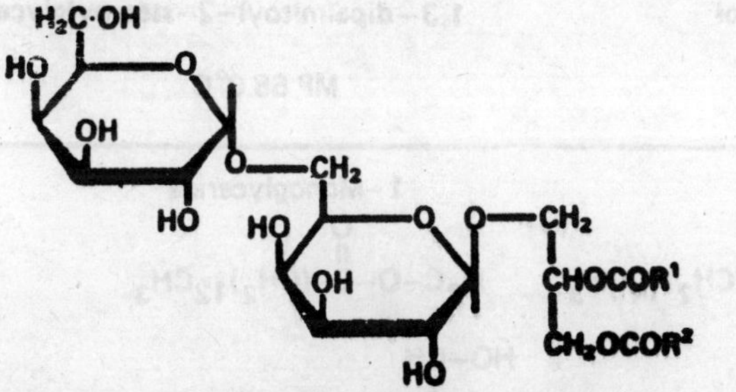

x = choline, ethanolamine, serine, inositol, glycerol

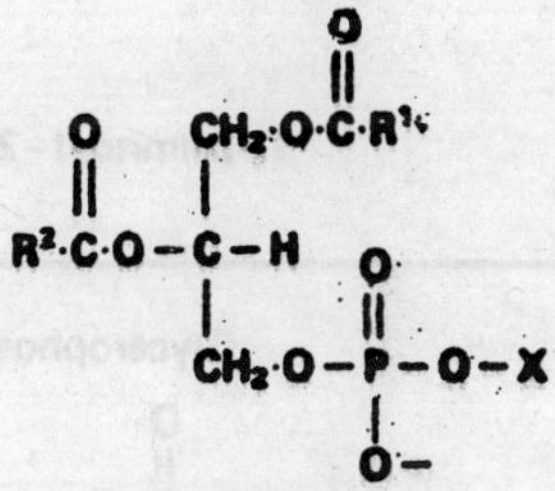

**Phosphatidyl-x**

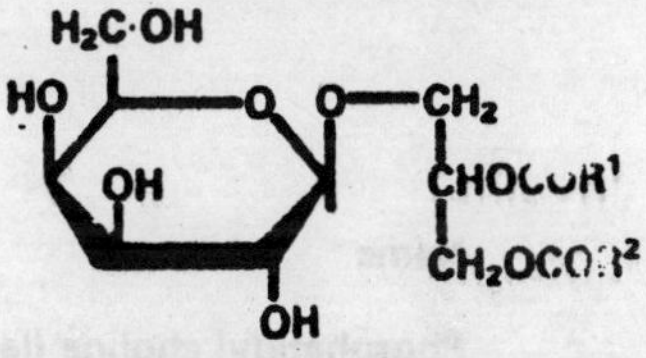

**1,2-diacyl-[α-D-galactopyranosyl-(1′ → 6′)-β-D-galactopyranosyl(1′ → 3)]-sn-glycerol**

(Digalactosyl diacylglycerol)

**1,2-diacyl-[β-D-galactopyranosyl(1′ → 3)]-sn-glycerol**

(Monogalactosyl diacylglycerol)

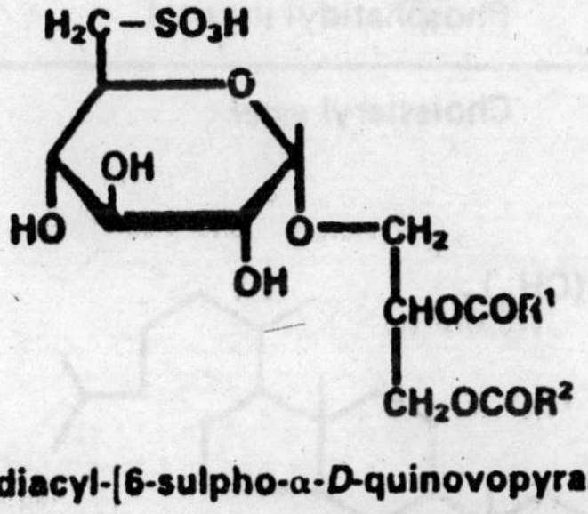

**D-quinovose is 6-deoxy-D-glucose. Note the carbon-sulphur bond.**

**1,2-diacyl-[6-sulpho-α-D-quinovopyranosyl-(1′ → 3)]-sn-glycerol**

(Plant sulpholipid (sulphoquinovosyl-diacylglycerol))

**Fig. 26** Structures of some important plant lipids

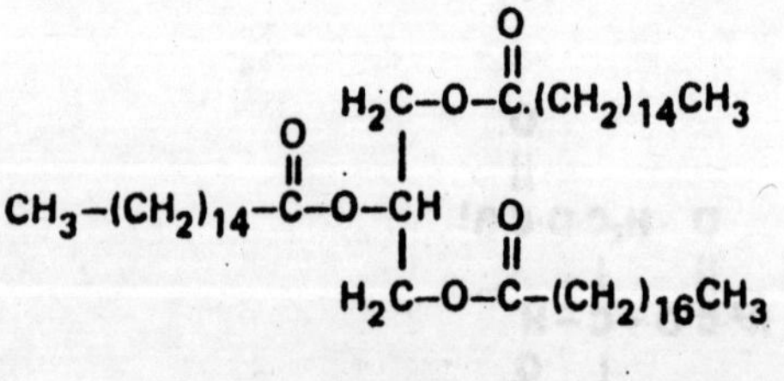

## Triglycerides

$$CH_3-(CH_2)_{14}-\overset{O}{\overset{\|}{C}}-O-CH(CH_2-O-\overset{O}{\overset{\|}{C}}(CH_2)_{14}CH_3)(CH_2-O-\overset{O}{\overset{\|}{C}}-(CH_2)_{16}CH_3)$$

1,2–dipalmitoyl–3–stearoylglycerol

MP 62.5°C

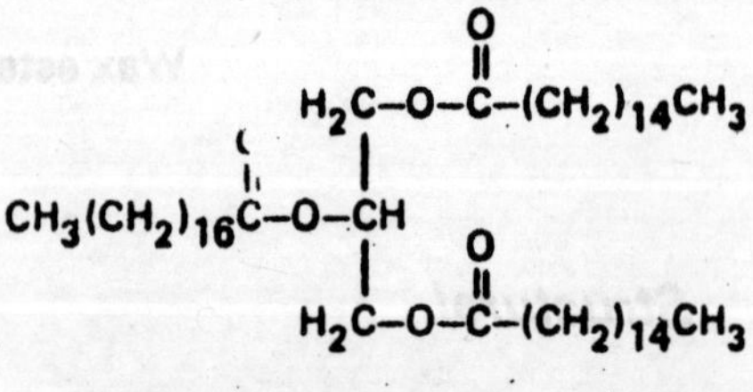

$$CH_3(CH_2)_{16}\overset{O}{\overset{\|}{C}}-O-CH(CH_2-O-\overset{O}{\overset{\|}{C}}-(CH_2)_{14}CH_3)(CH_2-O-\overset{O}{\overset{\|}{C}}-(CH_2)_{14}CH_3)$$

1,3–dipalmitoyl–2–stearoylglycerol

MP 68.0°C

---

### 1,2–Diglyceride

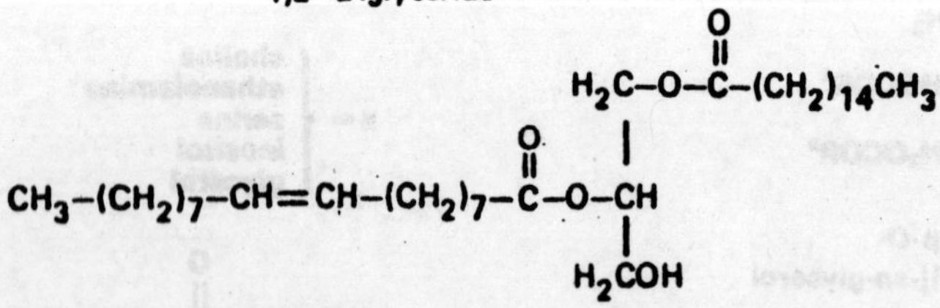

$$CH_3-(CH_2)_7-CH=CH-(CH_2)_7-\overset{O}{\overset{\|}{C}}-O-CH(H_2C-O-\overset{O}{\overset{\|}{C}}-(CH_2)_{14}CH_3)(H_2COH)$$

1–palmitoyl–2–oleylglycerol

### 1–Monoglyceride

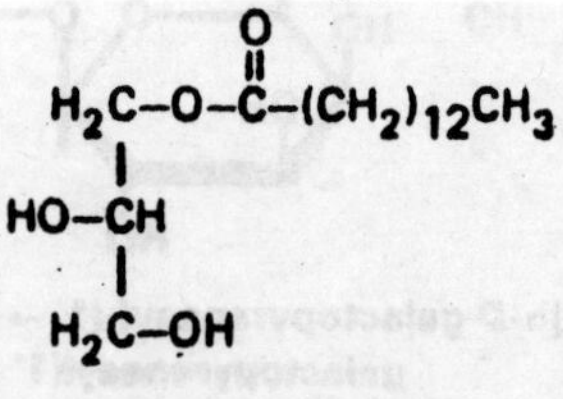

$$H_2C-O-\overset{O}{\overset{\|}{C}}-(CH_2)_{12}CH_3,\quad HO-CH,\quad H_2C-OH$$

1–myristoylglycerol

---

### Glycerophospholipids

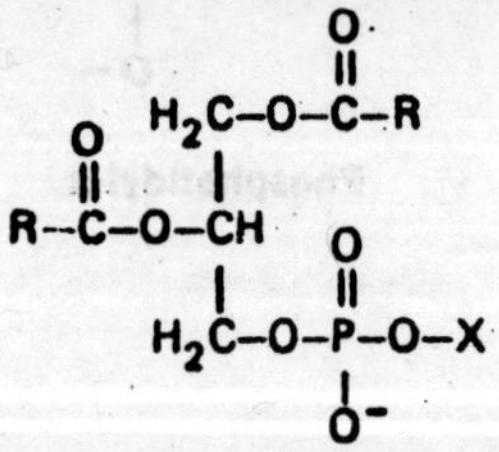

$$R-\overset{O}{\overset{\|}{C}}-O-CH(H_2C-O-\overset{O}{\overset{\|}{C}}-R)(H_2C-O-\overset{O}{\overset{\|}{P}}(O^-)-O-X)$$

| X | Name |
|---|---|
| Choline | Phosphatidyl choline (lecithin) |
| Ethanolamine | Phosphatidyl ethanolamine |
| Serine | Phosphatidyl serine |
| Myo-inositol | Phosphatidyl inositol |

---

### Sphingomyelin

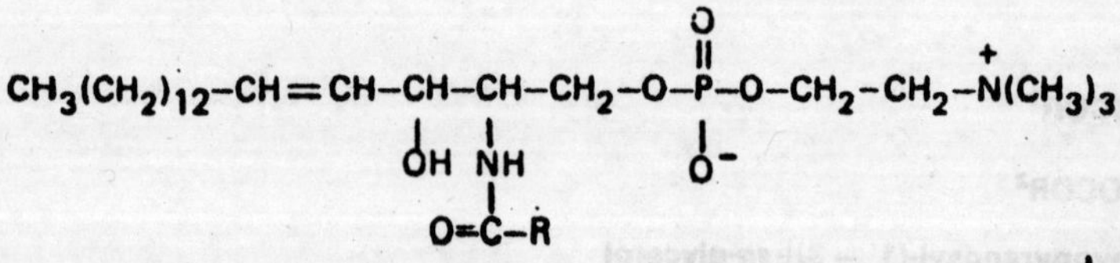

$$CH_3(CH_2)_{12}-CH=CH-CH(OH)-CH(NH-\overset{}{C}(=O)-R)-CH_2-O-\overset{O}{\overset{\|}{P}}(O^-)-O-CH_2-CH_2-\overset{+}{N}(CH_3)_3$$

### Cholesteryl ester

$$R-\overset{O}{\overset{\|}{C}}-O-\text{(cholesterol ring)}$$

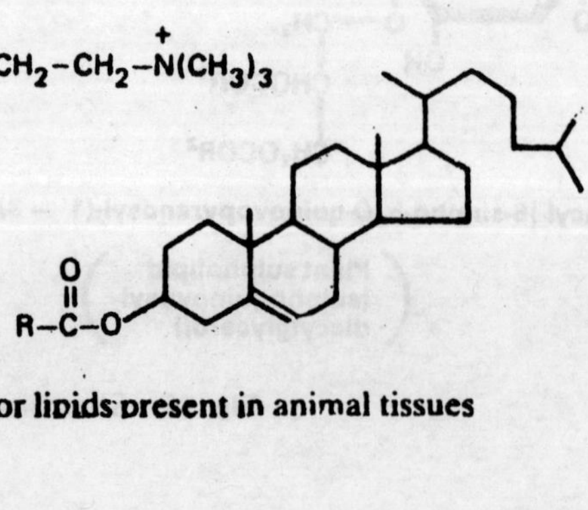

Fig. 27 Structure of major lipids present in animal tissues

**Table 73**

SOME COMMERCIALLY IMPORTANT OIL SEED CROPS

| *Seed* | *Oil content* (%) | *Major fatty acid(s)* | *World total of oil production*[c] ('000 metric tons) 1976 | 1982/3 | *Chief producing areas* | *Major uses* |
|---|---|---|---|---|---|---|
| Soya bean (*Glycine hispida*) | 13–20 | 9,12-18:2 | 10250 | 14700 | USA, Brazil, China | Margarine, cooking oil, salad oil, ice cream, paints, soap |
| Groundnut (peanut) (*Arachis hypogaea*) | 45 | 9,12-18:2 | 3160 | 2900 | India, China, Africa, USA | Margarine, cooking oil, salad oil, ice cream |
| Coconut (*Cocos nucifera*) | 63 | 12:0 | 3130 | 3200 | Philippines, Indonesia | Margarine, cooking oil, soap, lubricants |
| Sunflower (*Helianthus annuus*) | 40 | 9,12-18:2 | 2809 | 5800 | USSR, Argentina | Margarine, cooking oil, salad oil, soaps, paints |
| Oil palm: Palm oil | 50[a] | 16:0, 9-18:1 | 2660 | 5000 | W. Africa, Malaysia, | Margarine, shortenings, biscuit |
| Palm kernel oil (*Elaeis guineensis*) | 50[b] | 12:0 | 527 | 900 | Indonesia | fats, frying fat, biscuit and confectionery fats, ice cream, soap |
| Rape (*Brassica napus*) | 35–40 | 13-22:1 9-18:1 in zero erucic varieties | 2520 | 4600 | India, China, Canada, Poland, France, Sweden | Margarine, cooking oils, salad oils, lubricants |
| Cotton (*Gossypium hirsutum*) | 15–23 | 9,12-18:2, 9-18:1 | 2500 | 3300 | USSR, China, USA | Margarine, cooking oils, salad oils |
| Olive (*Olea sativa*) | 15 | 9-18:1 | 1370 | 2000 | Italy, Spain, Greece | Salad oils, preserving oils, soaps |
| Linseed (*Linum usitatissimum*) | 30–40 | 9,12,15-18:3 | 630 | 760 | Canada, USA, Argentina | Paints, varnishes and other industrial uses |
| Sesame (*Sesame indicum*) | 50 | 9-18:1, 9,12-18:2 | 610 | 660 | India, China, Mexico | Table oils |
| Castor (*Ricinus communis*) | 45 | OH-18:1 | 280 | 370 | Brazil, India | Paints, lubricants, plastics |
| Tung (*Aleurites fordii*) | | 9,11t,13t-18:3 | 115 | 100 | Argentina | Paints, varnishes |

[a]: % of mesocarp
[b]: % of kernel
[c]: 1982/3 are forecast figures

*phospholipids* which are not fundamentally different from those located in animal membranes: phosphatidyl choline, phosphatidyl ethanolamine, phosphatidyl serine, phosphatidyl inositol and phosphatidyl glycerol.

Phosphatidyl glycerol is the major phospholipid of the chloroplast membranes but quantitatively more important are the glycolipids:

Mono- and digalactosyl diacylglycerols make up about 40-50 per cent of the membrane lipid.

Chlorophylls make up about 20 per cent.

Sulphoquinovosyl diacylglycerol accounts for 5 per cent of chloroplast membrane lipids (not found in animal membranes).

The fatty acid composition of plant membrane lipids is very simple — five fatty acids generally account for over 90 per cent of the total:

(a) Palmitic, (b) hexadecenoic, (c) oleic, (d) linoleic, and (e) alpha-linolenic.

The surface lipids on the other hand contain a wider spectrum of fatty acids with chain lengths from C 10 to C 30 while the cutins contain a high proportion of C 18 hydroxy acids.

Plants store the excess lipids in seed cotyledons, embryo and to some extent in the mesocarp predominantly in the form of structural lipids (phospholipids and glycolipids).

## PROTEINS

In 1838 a Dutch chemist, G.J. Mulder described certain organic material which is "unquestionably the most important of all known substances in the organic kingdom. Without it no life appears possible on our planet." He also used the term *protein* (Greek, *proteios*, first) to describe these vital compounds.

It is now apparent that the name was well chosen. Proteins are the major structural components of animal tissue, just as cellulose provides for the structure of the plants. Proteins are components of skin, hair, wool, eggs, feathers, nails, horns, hoofs, muscles, tendons, connecting, tissue, and supporting tissue such as cartilage. In addition, proteins are involved in communication (nerves), defense (antibodies), metabolic regulation (hormones biochemical catalysis (enzymes), and oxygen transport (haemoglobin). They are utilised in the building of new tissue and in the maintenance of tissue that is already developed. Whereas the carbohydrates and lipids are used primarily as energy sources, the primary function of the protein is body building and maintenance. Lipids and carbohydrates are stored by the body as energy reserves, but proteins are not stored to any appreciable extent. It is possible for animals to survive for a short period of time on a diet consisting of protein, vitamins, and minerals; an animal could not survive over the same period of time on protein-free diet containing lipids, carbohydrates, vitamins and minerals.

Proteins are giant polymeric molecules (composed of various amino acids) that vary greatly in physical properties, size, shape, solubility and biological functions. Although there are more than 200 naturally occurring amino acids, only about 20 are commonly found in most protein and up to 10 are required in the diet of animals because tissue synthesis is not adequate to meet metabolic needs.

In human organism, there may be 100,000 different kinds of proteins. In one estimate it has been noted that in about 1.5 million species of living organisms. there are about $10^{10}$ to $10^{12}$ different kinds of protein molecules. The dry weight of a typical animal cell is composed of about 50 per cent protein of which 90 per cent are the enzymes upon which fundamental cellular function depends. There may be up to 1000 different enzymes in a single cell.

In addition to carbon, hydrogen, and oxygen, all proteins contain nitrogen, and many contain sulphur, phosphorus, and, traces of other elements. The elementary composition of most proteins is remarkably constant at about 51% carbon, 7% hydrogen, 23% oxygen, 16% nitrogen, 1-3% sulphur, and less than 1% phosphorus.

### Amino acids—building blocks of protein

As each flower constitutes a garland, as each brick constitutes an unit of any big wall, similarly each amino acid constitutes an unit of protein. There are about 300 amino acids occur in nature, only 20 of these occur in proteins of all forms of life—plant, animal or microbial.

With only a couple of exceptions, all amino acids contain both an acidic carboxyl (—COOH) and a basic amino (—$NH_2$) group attached to the alpha carbon which is asymmetric (now the term is known as *Chiral* carbon that is bonded to four different groups).

**Properties of amino acids**

**A.** ***Physical properties***

They are colourless, crystalline substances generally soluble in water, slightly soluble in alcohol and insoluble in ether.

On account of the presence of both acidic and basic groups which are readily ionizable, the amino acids, behave as *amphoteric electrolytes* and give both anions and cations in solution (Zwitterion).

$$R-CH(^{+}NH_3)-COOH \underset{OH^-}{\overset{H^+}{\rightleftharpoons}} R-CH(^{+}NH_3)-COO^- \underset{H^+}{\overset{OH^-}{\rightleftharpoons}} R-CH(NH_2)-COO^-$$

Cationic form at pHs below isoelectric pH, Net charge = + 1; Zwitterion form at isoelectric pH, Net charge = 0; Anionic form at pHs above isoelectric pH, Net charge = − 1

Acid-base behavior of neutral amino acids.

The pH at which an amino acid exists in solution as a Zwitterion is called the isoelectric pH that is, the pH at which the amino acid is electrically neutral and has no tendency to migrate towards either electrode. Each amino acid has its own characteristic isoelectric pH. The isoelectric pH of the neutral amino acids ranges from 4.8 to 6.3, that of the acidic amino acids ranges from 2.8-3.2, and the isoelectric pH of the basic amino acids occurs between 7.6 and 10.8.

**B.** ***Chemical properties***

***Due to —COOH group***

(i) They can form esters with alcohols and salts with bases.

(ii) With ammonia, they form the corresponding amides. The amides of aspartic and glutamic acids—*asparagine* and *glutamine*—are of importance in the transport of ammonia in the body.

(iii) Hydrazine ($NH_2NH_2$) will cleave all peptide bonds and convert all the amino acids to the corresponding hydrazides.

***Due to —$NH_2$ group***

(i) They can form salts with acids.

(ii) The amino group can be methylated.

(iii) Nitrous acid will react with amino group to liberate nitrogen and form the hydroxy acid.

(iv) Two amino acids interact by the amino group of one of them combining with the carboxylic group of the other through what is known as the peptide bond.

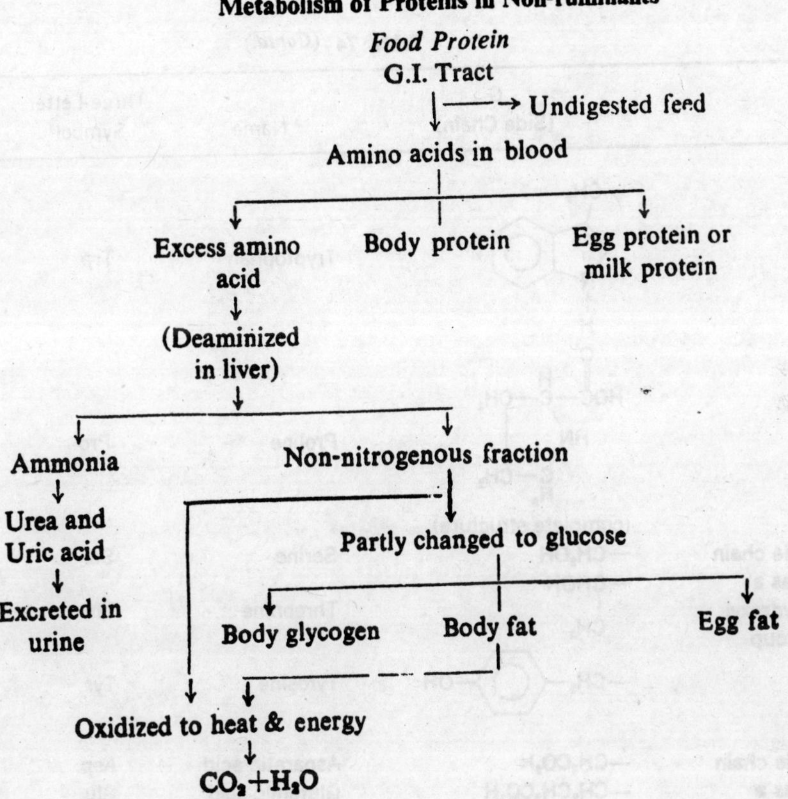


**Table 74**

**Common Amino Acids** $\overset{+}{N}H_3-CH(G)-C(=O)-O^-$

| | G (Side Chain) | Name | Three-Letter Symbol[a] | pI |
|---|---|---|---|---|
| Side chain is nonpolar | $-H$ | Glycine | Gly | 5.97 |
| | $-CH_3$ | Alanine | Ala | 6.00 |
| | $-CH(CH_3)_2$ | Valine | Val | 5.96 |
| | $-CH_2CH(CH_3)_2$ | Leucine | Leu | 5.98 |
| | $-CH(CH_3)CH_2CH_3$ | Isoleucine | Ile | 6.02 |
| | $-CH_2-C_6H_5$ | Phenylalanine | Phe | 5.48 |

**Table 74** *(Contd.)*

| | G (Side Chain) | Name | Three-Letter Symbol[a] | pH |
|---|---|---|---|---|
| | $-CH_2$ (indole ring, N—H) | Tryptophan | Trp | 5.89 |
| | $HOC(=O)-CH-CH_2$; $HN$; $C(H_2)-CH_2$ (complete structure) | Proline | Pro | 6.30 |
| Side chain has a hydroxyl group | $-CH_2OH$ | Serine | Ser | 5.68 |
| | $-CH(OH)CH_3$ | Threonine | Thr | 5.64 |
| | $-CH_2-C_6H_4-OH$ | Tyrosine | Tyr | 5.66 |
| Side chain has a carboxyl group (or an amide) | $-CH_2CO_2H$ | Asparatic acid | Asp | 2.77 |
| | $-CH_2CH_2CO_2H$ | Glutamic acid | Glu | 3.22 |
| | $-CH_2CONH_2$ | Asparagine | Asn | 5.41 |
| | $-CH_2CH_2CONH_2$ | Glutamine | Gln | 5.65 |
| Side chain has a basic amino group | $-CH_2CH_2CH_2CH_2NH_2$ | Lysine | Lys | 9.74 |
| | $-CH_2CH_2CH_2NH-C(=NH)-NH_2$ | Arginine | Arg | 10.76 |
| | $-CH_2-C=CH-N=CH-NH$ (HC—N, CH, N—H ring) | Histidine | His | 7.59 |
| Side chain contains sulfur | $-CH_2S-H$ | Cysteine | Cys | 5.07 |
| | $-CH_2CH_2SCH_3$ | Methionine | Met | 5.74 |

[a] These three-letter symbols are recommended by the Joint Commission on Biochemical Nomenclature of IUPAC IUB.

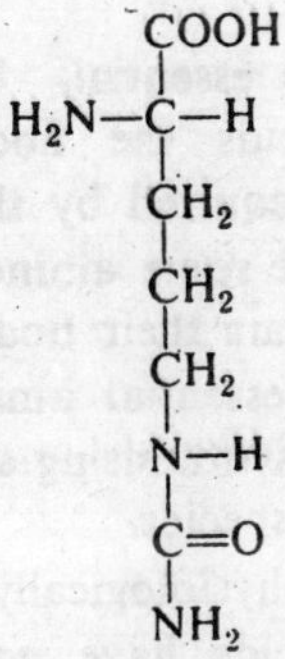

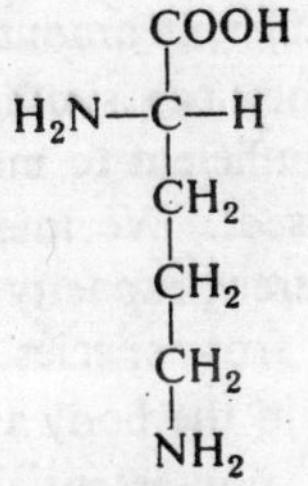

Citrulline

Ornithine

(intermediates in the urea cycle)

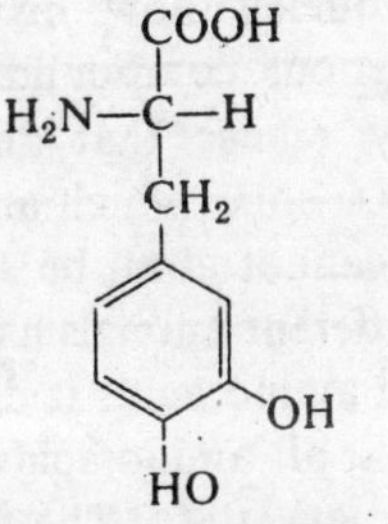

Dihydroxyphenylalanine (DOPA) (intermediate in the formation of adrenaline)

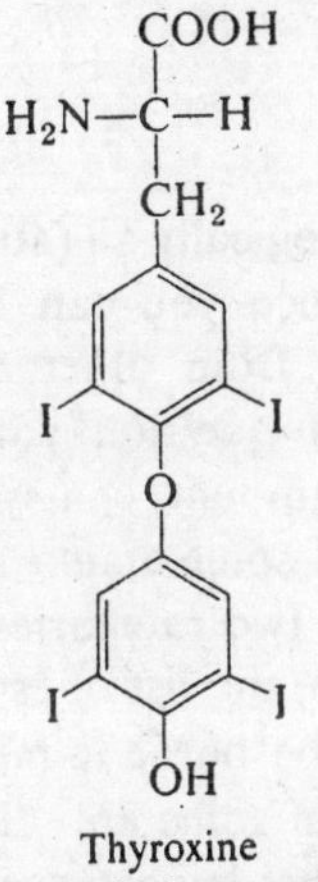

Thyroxine (thyroid hormone)

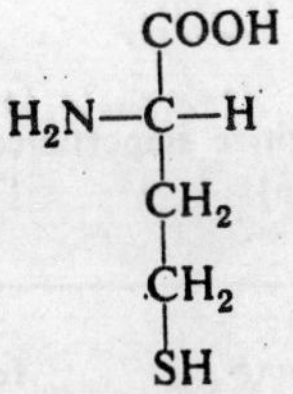

Homocysteine (intermediate in the synthesis of methionine)

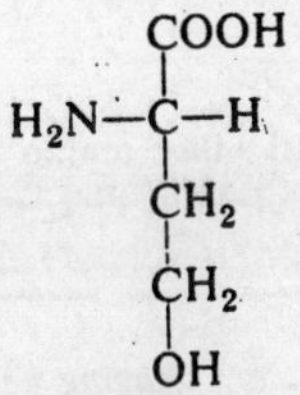

Homoserine (intermediate in the synthesis of threonine)

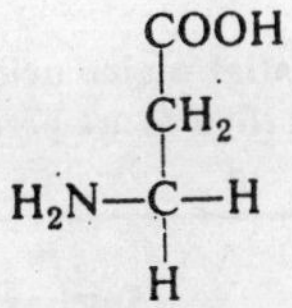

$\beta$-Alanine (component of coenzyme A)

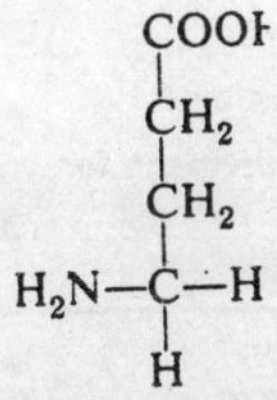

$\gamma$-Aminobutyric acid (involved in the transmission of nerve impulses)

**Some biologically important nonprotein amino acids.**

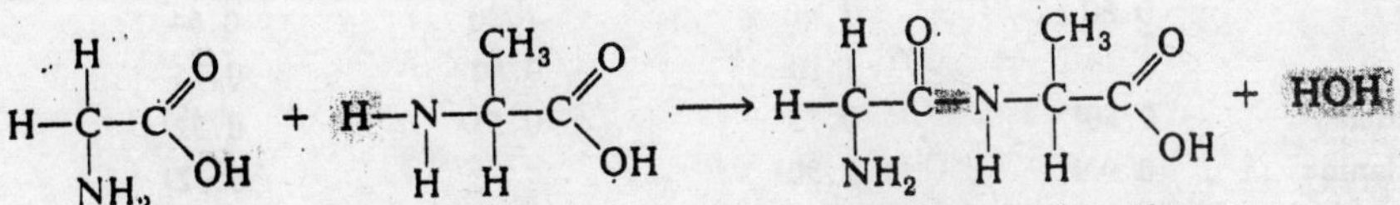

Glycine + Alanine ⟶ Glycylalanine (Gly—Ala) + HOH

One peptide bond

(a)

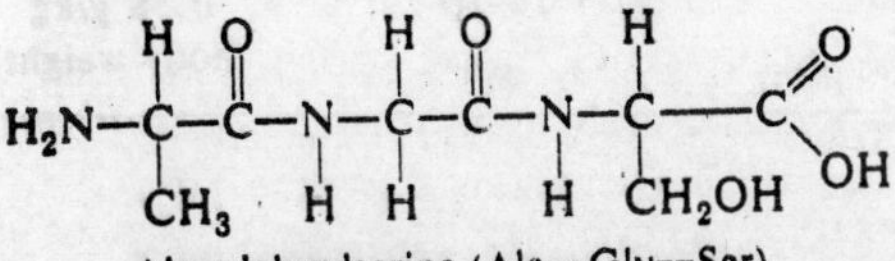

Alanylglycylserine (Ala—Gly—Ser)

Two peptide bonds

(b)

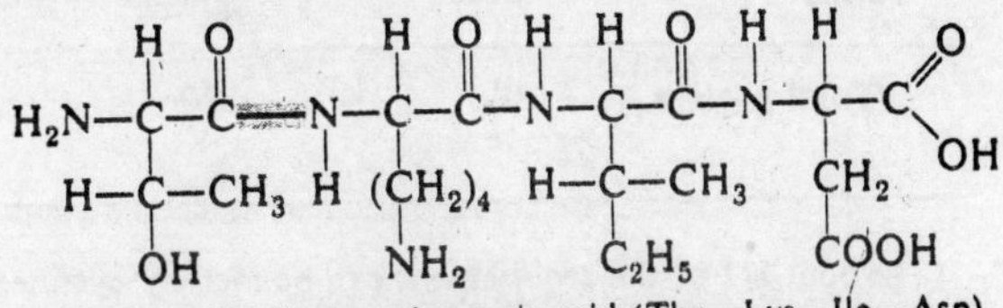

Threonyllysylisoleucylaspartic acid (Thr—Lys—Ile—Asp)

Three peptide bonds

(c)

**(a) Formation of a dipeptide. (b) A tripeptide. (c) A tetrapeptide.**

## ESSENTIAL AMINO ACIDS

**Physiologically all (about 20) amino acids found in animal tissues are essential. Under this circumstance you can ask yourself how many of these amino acids the body cannot synthesise from other nitrogenous compounds in sufficient amount required by the animal.** From this question you may realise that animal body can synthesise some amino acids in sufficient amount, can synthesise some which are not sufficient to maintain their body requirements and some amino acids cannot at all be synthesised. We infer "essential amino acids" of the last two categories. Different animals have different capacity of synthesising amino acid types So, the list of essential amino acids is different from species to species.

It is to be borne in mind that all amino acids found in the body are physiologically essential; out of them some are dietary essential. The dietary non-essential acids have got no less physiological importance. One research philosopher mentioned, "Some are so essential that the body ensures an adequate supply by synthesis.'' However, if the diet does not supply adequate quantity of the "non-essential" ones, they will have to be synthesised from other non-

**Table 75**

**Requirement for each essential amino acid when all other amino acids of nutritive importance are provided (figures are percentages of total diet, except for man)**

| *Amino acid* | *Young rat* | *Starting chicken* | *Laying hen* | *Growing pig* | *Adult man* |
|---|---|---|---|---|---|
| Arginine | 0.20 | 1.20 | 0.80 | 0.22 | — |
| Glycine | — | 1.00 | ? | — | — |
| Histidine | 0.30 | 0.40 | ? | 0.22 | — |
| Isoleucine | 0.50 | 0.75 | 0.50 | 0.53 | 0.70 g/day |
| Leucine | 0.80 | 1.40 | 1.20 | 0.64 | 0.98 |
| Lysine | 0.90 | 1.10 | 0.50 | 0.75 | 0.84 |
| Methionine | 0.60[1] | 0.75[1] | 0.53[1] | 0.52[1] | 0.91[2] |
| Phenylalanine | 0.90[3] | 1.30[3] | ? | 0.52[4] | 0.98[5] |
| Threonine | 0.50 | 0.70 | 0.40 | 0.45 | 0.49 |
| Tryptophan | 0.15 | 0.20 | 0.15 | 0.13 | 0.24 |
| Valine | 0.70 | 0.85 | ? | 0.48 | 0.70 |
| Total protein | 20 | 20 | 15 | 16–18 | 0.55 g/kg body weight |

[1]About 1/2 of the requirement can be met by cystine

[2]About 3/4 of the requirement can be met by cystine

[3]About 1/3 to 1/2 of the requirement can be met by tyrosine

[4]About 1/3 of the requirement can be met by tyrosine

[5]About 3/4 of the requirement can be met by tyrosine.

protein nitrogenous substances or it will come from the essential amino acids that are present. Thus, provision in the diet for adequate quantities of either non-protein nitrogen or of non-essential amino acids must be made to meet the needs of non-essential amino acids. For essential amino acids there is no other alternative except to supply these acids through diet.

The number and types of amino acids which are essential for a particular species are not exactly the same for other species. The requirement varies depending on the age and species of animal, as shown in Table 75.

For ruminants the situation is quite different. The micro-organisms which are common inhabitants in the rumen can utilise any kind of nitrogenous substance present in the animal ration, and converts them into different essential and non-essential amino acids which are deposited as microbial protein and later on utilised by animal body. Thus the problem of essential amino acids arises only in non-ruminants like man, pig, horse, poultry, etc., but not for sheep, goat or cattle except during their very young age when their rumen is not developed to carry this function.

### Classification of Amino Acids

About two dozen amino acids have so far been definitely established as occurring in proteins, and most proteins contain a large proportion of these amino acids while others may be rich in one or other type of amino acids as in silk protein which is specially rich in glycine, about 40 per cent

Amino acids have been classified in various ways. One system classifies them as aliphatic, aromatic and heterocyclic amino acids, depending upon the presence of chain and ring structure. Another system classifies them according to the number of amino and carboxyl groups present in the molecule as monoamino monocarboxylic acids, monoamino dicarboxylic acids, etc. Again they are classified according to reaction in solution as neutral, acidic and basic amino acids. From the nutrition point of view these acids are further classified as essential or non-essential type based on whether the body can or cannot synthesise the particular type of acid as per requirement. Lastly, the amino acids are also classified into three groups according to their catabolic fates as (*i*) *Glucogenic*, (*ii*) *Ketogenic*, and (*iii*) *Glucogenic and/or Ketogenic* based on the major end products formed from degradation of carbon skeletons of various amino acids.

The general class, subclass, nature, molecular weight and abbreviations of all common 20 amino acids are thus listed in Table 76 in a classified manner.

### Glucogenic and Ketogenic Amino Acids

After absorption of amino acids mostly from the jejunum portion of the small intestine these are largely utilised as such for the synthesis of various protein and other non-protein nitrogenous compounds. A significant portion of absorbed amino acids, after shaking off of their amino ($NH_2$) group either by deamination or by transamination, are also utilised as a carbon skeleton for the synthesis of other non-nitrogenous compounds as glucose (the process is known as *Gluconeogenesis*) or some other ketones. The physiological conditions which encourage the acids to follow such glycogenic and/or ketogenic pathway are either fasting or at diabetes mellitus condition or at situations when the animals are on low levels of dietary carbohydrates.

If amino acids are fed one at a time to a starving phlorizinised dog it has been observed that some give rise to glucose in the urine, while others give rise to acetoacetic acid. A few give rise to neither. In such an animal about 60 gms of glucose are formed and excreted in the urine for each 100 gms of protein metabolised; this means, 60 per cent of protein is potentially glucogenic. Thus it has been proved that amino acids differ in yielding products from the degradation of their carbon skeleton and accordingly amino acids are classified into three groups.

1. GLUCOGENIC OR ANTIKETOGENIC AMINO ACIDS. Amino acids belonging to this group, just after deamination, initially form keto acids and immediately change into glucose which may be stored temporarily as glycogen in the liver. The term *Glucogenic* is often used to designate those acids which give rise to TCA cycle intermediates or pyruvate and therefore are on the general pathway to carbohydrate synthesis.

**Table 76**

**Classification of twenty amino acids according to tne structure, molecular weights and nature of the side chain**

| *General class* | *Subclass* | *Nature* | *M. Wt.* | *Amino acid* | *Abbreviation* |
|---|---|---|---|---|---|
| Basic | | G | 174 | Arginine | Arg |
| | | G | 154 | Histidine | His |
| | | GK | 146 | Lysine | Lys |
| Acidic | | G | 133 | Aspartic acid | Asp |
| | | G | 147 | Glutamic acid | Glu |
| Neutral | Aliphatic Straight chain | G | 89 | Alanine | Ala |
| | | G | 75 | Glycine | Gly |
| | Branched chain | GK | 131 | Isoleucine | Ilu |
| | | K | 131 | Leucine | Leu |
| | | G | 117 | Valine | Val |
| | Hydroxy | G | 105 | Serine | Ser |
| | | GK | 119 | Threonine | Thr |
| | Sulfur-containing | G | 121 | Cysteine | Cys |
| | | — | 240 | Cystine | Cysscy |
| | | G | 149 | Methionine | Met |
| | Aromatic | GK | 165 | Phenylalanine | Phe |
| | | GK | 204 | Tryptophan | Try |
| | | GK | 181 | Tyrosine | Tyr |
| | Imino | G | 131 | Hydroxyproline | Hypro |
| | | G | 115 | Proline | Pro |

G = Glucogenic
K = Ketogenic

2. KETOGENIC AMINO ACIDS. *Ketogenic* refers to those amino acids which give rise to acetyl CoA and consequently the potential fatty acid producers. During starvation, diabetes mellitus or other defects in carbohydrate metabolism acetyl CoA accumulate and will be converted into one of the three ketone compounds—aceto acetic acid, acetone and β-hydroxybutyric acid.

Under ordinary conditions ketogenic amino acids after deamination will yield keto acids which during the subsequent oxidation (through the stage of acetoacetic acid) to carbon dioxide and water will yield energy. Although leucine is the only truly ketogenic amino acid, several other amino acids such as tryptophan, lysine, tyrosine, etc., are also catabolised to form some acetyl CoA or acetoacetic acid.

3. GLUCOGENIC AND/OR KETOGENIC. Amino acids of this group can give rise to both glucose and ketone bodies. They include isoleucine, lysine, phenylalanine, tyrosine, threonine and tryptophan.

## Classes of Proteins

### Classification

### According to Solubility

When proteins are classified according to their solubilities, two major families are the fibrous and globular proteins. Fibrous proteins that are insoluble in water include the following.

1. ***Collagens***—in bone, teeth, tendons, skin, and soft connective tissue. When such connective tissue is boiled with water, its collagen changes to gelatin, a much more soluble form. The change of this collagen to gelatin when meat is cooked is an important preliminary step to later digestion.
2. ***Elastins***—in many places where collagen also occurs, but particularly in ligaments, the walls of blood vessels, and the necks of grazing animals. Elastin has little hydroxyproline, no hydroxylysine, and is rich in hydrophobic side chains. Cross-links between elastin strands are important to its recovery after stretching. Elastin is not changed to gelatin by hot water.
3. ***Keratins***—in hair, wool, animal hooves, nails, and porcupine quills. The keratins are exceptionally rich in disulfide links.
4. ***Myosins***—proteins in contractile muscle.
5. ***Fibrin***—the protein of a blood clot, formed from a more soluble form, fibrinogen, when clotting must occur.

Globular proteins that are soluble in water or water containing certain salts include the following.

1. ***Albumins***—in egg white; in circulation in the blood where they perform various duties—buffers, carriers of lipids, carbohydrates, metal ions, and other small things that otherwise would not be soluble in blood. Albumins are soluble (or easily dispersed colloidally) in pure water.
2. ***Globulins***—include the gamma (γ)-globulins, part of the body's defense against infectious diseases. Globulins need the presence of dissolved salts to dissolve.

## Classification According to Composition

The nature of the prosthetic group in conjugated proteins provides another way of classifying proteins.

1. *Glycoproteins*—proteins with sugar units attached; γ-globulin is an example. The sugar unit is a complex system.
2. *Hemoproteins*—proteins with heme units. Hemoglobin, myoglobin and an enzyme for using oxygen, cytochrome *c*.
3. *Lipoproteins*—proteins carrying lipid molecules.
4. *Metalloproteins*—proteins incorporating a metallic ion; several enzymes have this feature.
5. *Nucleoproteins*—proteins bound to nucleic acids, such as ribosomes and some viruses.
6. *Phosphoproteins*—proteins with an ester between the side chain of a serine residue and a phosphate unit. Milk casein is an example.

## Classification According to Biological Function

Perhaps no other classification quite so clearly dramatizes the enormous importance of proteins.

1. *Enzymes*—All known enzymes are proteins, simple or conjugated.
2. *Contractile proteins*—In muscle both the stationary filaments, myosin, and the moving filaments, actin, are examples.
3. *Hormones*—Growth hormone, insulin and many other hormones are proteins.
4. *Storage proteins*—These store nutrients needed by the organism or used by another species feeding on it. Examples are the seed proteins in grains, casein in milk, ovalbumin in egg white and ferritin, the protein that stores iron for us in the spleen.
5. *Transport proteins*—These carry things from one place in the body to another. Examples are hemoglobin and myoglobin that carry oxygen, serum albumin that carries fatty acids in the blood, ceruloplasmin that carries copper ions, and a globulin that carries iron ions in blood.
6. *Structural proteins*—Proteins that hold structure together. Examples are collagen, elastin, keratin, and proteins in cell membranes.
7. *Protective proteins*—These participate in the body's defensive mechanisms. Examples are antibodies, fibrinogen, and thrombin (both important in the formation of a blood clot), and complement (a material that sometimes participates with antibodies in handling foreign proteins or antigens).
8. *Toxins*—Proteins that are poisons. Examples are snake venom, diphtheria toxin, and the toxic element in bacterial food poisoning, clostridium botulinum toxin.

### Denaturation

A wide variety of reagents and conditions do not hydrolyze peptide bonds but still destroy the biological nature and activity of a protein. When this has happened, the protein is denatured. After denaturation coagulation usually happens. Several of the more common chemicals or conditions that denature a protein are listed in Table 12.2.

**Table 77**

**Chemicals and Conditions That Cause Protein Denaturation**

| Denaturing Agent | How the Agent May Operate |
|---|---|
| Heat | Disrupts hydrogen bonds by making molecules vibrate too violently. Produces coagulation as in the frying of an egg |
| Solutions of urea $(NH_2{-}\overset{\overset{O}{\|}}{C}{-}NH_2)$ | Disrupt hydrogen bonds. Since it is amidelike, urea can form hydrogen bonds of its own |
| Ultraviolet radiation | Appears to operate the same way that heat operates (e.g., sunburning) |
| Organic solvents (e.g., ethyl alcohol, acetone, isopropyl alcohol) | May interfere with hydrogen bonds in protein, since alcohol molecules are themselves capable of hydrogen bonding. Quickly denatures the proteins of bacteria, thus killing them (e.g., disinfectant action of ethyl alcohol, 70% solution) |
| Strong acids or bases | Can disrupt hydrogen bonds. Prolonged action of aqueous acids or bases leads to actual hydrolysis of proteins |
| Detergent | May affect hydrogen bonds |
| Salts of heavy metals (e.g., salts of the ions $Hg^{2+}$, $Ag^{+}$, $Pb^{2+}$) | Ions combine with SH groups. These ions usually precipitate proteins |
| Violent whipping or shaking | May form surface films of denatured proteins from protein solutions (e.g., beating egg white into meringue) |

## FUNCTIONS SERVED BY AMINO ACIDS

**1. SYNTHESIS OF CELL PROTOPLASM.** Proteins being essential constituents of all living cells, amino acids are necessary to build them up.

**2. FOR THE REPAIR OF WEAR AND TEAR.** Tissue proteins break down during metabolism. These damaged parts are repaired with the help of amino acids.

**3. PROTEIN STORAGE.** In mature animals, where nitrogen equilibrium is established, proteins cannot be stored, but can be stored in calves, pregnant animals, etc.

**4. SYNTHESIS OF BILE ACIDS.** The two bile acids, Taurocholic acid and Glycocholic acid, are derived from the amino acids Taurina and Glycine, respectively.

5. SYNTHESIS OF HORMONES. Thyroxine and Adrenaline are derivatives of tyrosine or phenyl-alanine. Insulin is also a protein in nature. Hence intact amino acids are required for synthesis.

6. SYNTHESIS OF ENZYMES. Most of the enzymes are protein in nature. So amino acids are required to build them up.

7. SYNTHESIS OF MILK PROTEINS AND ANTIBODIES. In lactating animals, synthesis of milk proteins are carried out with the help of amino acids from the blood stream. Antibodies in colostrum are globulin in nature.

8. SYNTHESIS OF MELANIN. Melanin, which is the pigment of the skin, choroid, hair, etc., is derived from the amino acid tyrosine or phenyl-alanine.

9. FORMATION OF RHODOPSIN. Rhodopsin, also known as visual purple, is made up of vitamin A and another protein component. Necessary amino acids are required for its synthesis.

10. SUPPLY OF ENERGY. Amino acids break down and liberate energy. One gram of protein is equivalent to 4.3 calories.

11. Absence of protein in proper quantities profoundly affects the digestion of cellulose portion of carbohydrates.

Feeding of excessive amount of protein is just as undesirable as giving too little of it, because the excess amount of proteins cannot be stored in the animal body. They are broken down and the nitrogenous portion is excreted through the kidneys. Excessive feeding of feed rich in proteins causes heating and production of evil smelling faeces and gases and taxation on kidney function.

## NON-PROTEIN NITROGENOUS COMPOUNDS

A considerable variety of nitrogenous compounds which are not classed as proteins occur in plants and animals. In plant analysis these compounds have been frequently classed together as non-protein nitrogenous compounds to distinguish them from "true proteins" determined in routine chemical analysis. In general above 50 per cent of the total non-protein is the free amino acid, followed by the amides. Among others, amines, purines, pyrimidines, nitrates, and alkaloids are noteworthy. In addition many members of the vitamin B complex and some types of lipids contain nitrogen in their structure.

Formerly, the protein requirements were stated in terms of digestible true protein, and as a rule, no allowances were made for the nutrient value of the non-protein portion of the nitrogenous matter. It was later generally accepted that the "amide" had half the nutrient value of true protein and when calculating rations the sum of the digestible true protein and crude protein was halved and the result was called "Protein Equivalent". This was used in place of true protein. However, recent researches have shown that the non-protein nitrogenous compounds play in ruminant system almost an identical role as the true protein. As mentioned earlier, the amides and the amino acids are the only ones which occur to any considerable extent, and they are present in large amounts in only a few of the common feeds. In fast growing plants such substances are abundant and may make up as much as one-third of the total nitrogen. The developing seed is high in non-protein nitrogen at the start but low at maturity. Commonly fed concentrate grain mixture and mature hays contain relatively little non-protein nitrogen.

In addition to the non-protein nitrogen compounds which occur in feed as in free state, there

Table 78

**Non-protein nitrogenous constituents formed from amino acids in animals**

| *Biological compound* | *Amino acid precursor* | *Physiological function* |
|---|---|---|
| Purines and pyrimidines | Glycine and aspartic acid | Constituents of nucleotides and nucleic acids |
| Creatine | Glycine and arginine | Energy storage as creatine phosphate in muscle |
| Glycocholic and taurocholic acids | Glycine and cysteine | Bile acids, aid in fat digestion and absorption |
| Thyroxine, epinephrine and norepinephrine | Tyrosine | Hormones |
| Ethanolamine and choline | Serine | Constituents of phospholipids |
| Histamine | Histidine | A vasodepressor |
| Serotonin | Tryptophan | Transmission of nerve impulses |
| Porphyrins | Glycine | Constituent of hemoglobin |
| Niacin | Tryptophan | Vitamin |
| Melanin | Tyrosine | Pigment of hair, skin, and eyes |

**are a number of other non-protein nitrogenous constituents which are formed either as intermediary or end products of various amino acid metabolism. Some of such non-protein nitrogenous compounds that originate from amino acids are listed with their physiological functions in Table 78.**

## CRUDE PROTEIN (CP)

The protein part of feeding stuff as determined in the routine analysis is really made up of two component parts; one is the true protein occuring in larger proportions, the other is constituted of non-protein nitrogenous compounds. The term crude protein includes both the types as a whole.

The estimation of crude protein in the feeding stuff is determiend by the standard Kjeldhal procedure which gives the estimation of the feed coming from the protein and non-protein nitrogenous compounds. The percentage of nitrogen ($N_2$) is then expressed in terms of crude protein (CP), calculated as mentioned in next page.

$$\text{Percent CP} = \text{Percent } N_2 \times 6.25$$

**The factor 6.25 is used on the assumption that proteins contain 16 per cent nitrogen. (100/16=6.25).**

**So, when we express the total nitrogen content in terms of CP, we make two assumptions: (1) all food protein contain 16 per cent nitrogen, (2) all the nitrogen of the food is present as true protein. Both of these assumptions are unsound. Different food proteins have different**

Table 79

*Factors for converting nitrogen to CP

| Food protein | Per cent $N_2$ | Conversion factor |
|---|---|---|
| Cotton seed | 18.87 | 5.30 |
| Soybean | 17.51 | 5.71 |
| Maize | 16.00 | 6.25 |
| Wheat | 17.15 | 5.83 |
| Egg and Meat | 16.00 | 6.25 |
| Milk | 15.68 | 6.38 |

*From D.B. Jones; 1931. U.S.D.A. Circular 183.

nitrogen contents and therefore different factors should be used in the conversion of nitrogen to protein for individual foods.

The second assumption that the whole of the food nitrogen is present as protein is also false, since many simple nitrogenous compounds such as amides, amino acids, glycosides, alkaloids, ammonium salts may be present in the food.

From practical point of view, as all ruminants can utilise nitrogen from protein and non-protein equally and hence the two assumptions that are made to calculate CP will not affect the ruminants. In the diet of pigs and poultry, cereals and oilseed meals predominate, and in these there is little non-protein nitrogen. Hence in practice there is little to be gained from attempting to distinguish between the two types of nitrogen.

### True Proteins

True proteins are sometimes determined to know the actual nitrogen substances present as only protein. This is done by boiling the feeding stuff with suspension of copper hydroxide in glycerol (Stutzer's reagent) followed by filtration. All the true protein remains on the filter paper and can be determined in the usual manner, while the non-protein nitrogen compounds pass through into the filtrate.

## DEGRADABLE AND UNDEGRADABLE PROTEIN

The protein intake of a ruminant becomes available for maintenance and production in two ways. In the first place it is broken down (degraded) by the microbes in the rumen and used in their own protein synthesis. Later in the digestion process the microbes are themselves digested and the protein they contain becomes available to the animal for their own protein synthesis. On the other hand, some protein is resistant to microbial breakdown (undegraded) and passes unchanged into the small intestine where it is digested and absorbed in the usual way.

At a low level of productivity a cow can meet her protein needs from the microbial protein, i.e., provided by digesting the bacteria and protozoa. In these circumstances, therefore, the diet only needs to contain a supply of degradable protein. High-yielding cows, however, cannot meet all their protein needs from that supplied by the microbes as in general the digestibility of bacterial protein is lower, 0.74 and thus the Net Protein utilisation (NPU) is about 0.59.

**Table 80**

**Soluble and degradable protein in various feedstuffs.**

| Ingredient | Crude protein | % of Crude protein: Soluble | ADF bound | Insoluble available |
|---|---|---|---|---|
| High solubility feeds | | | | |
| Corn sol. + germ meal & bran | 29.4 | 63 | 2.8 | 35 |
| Corn gluten feed | 22.2 | 55 | 2.6 | 43 |
| Rye middlings | 18.3 | 48 | 2.0 | 50 |
| Wheat middlings | 18.4 | 37 | 2.3 | 61 |
| Wheat flour | 15.2 | 40 | .2 | 64 |
| Intermediate solubility feeds | | | | |
| Oats | 12.9 | 31 | 4.8 | 64 |
| Corn gluten feed w/corn germ | 23.8 | 32 | 3.3 | 65 |
| Cotton waste product | 22.3 | 24 | 1.6 | 74 |
| Hominy | 11.0 | 24 | 2.8 | 73 |
| Soybean meal | 52.3 | 24 | 1.8 | 75 |
| Soybean mill feed | 15.2 | 22 | 14-20 | 57-63 |
| Distillers DG w/sol. | 29.1 | 19 | 15.3 | 65 |
| Low solubility feeds | | | | |
| Cottonseed meal | 44.3 | 12 | 3.1 | 85 |
| Corn | 9.6 | 15 | 5.0 | 80 |
| Brewer's dried grains | 28.9 | 6 | 13.2 | 81 |
| Distillers DG | 26.7 | 6 | 18.8 | 76 |
| Corn gluten meal | 66.2 | 4 | 10.6 | 85 |
| Beet pulp | 8.5 | 3 | 10.9 | 86 |
| Forages and silages | | | | |
| Alfalfa hay | 15-25 | 30 | 10 | 60 |
| Alfalfa dehy | 17-25 | 25-30 | 10-30 | 40-75 |
| Alfalfa silage[2] | 17-25 | 30-60 | 15-40 | 0-50 |
| Corn silage[2] | 9 | 30-40 | 10-30 | 30-60 |

[1] Degree of degradability of insoluble available fraction: 1—very resistant, 5—very degradable.

[2] Higher moisture silages tend to have greater soluble NPN while low DM silages may have greater heat damage.

About 20% of bacterial nitrogen comprise nucleic acid. This fraction ot the crude protein is essentially wasted as these are degraded to form urea in the post-ruminal section of the gastro-intestinal tract. There is thus a great demand of undegradable protein in the diet of high yielders. This is also true for young ruminants where the rumen has not developed at all.

The protein in silage and barley is highly degradable (85%), and, therefore, supplies only a small amount of undegradable protein. On the other hand some high protein concentrates, e.g. soybean meal. fish meal etc., contain a higher proportion of undegradable protein, and these feeds should be used as protein supplements in the concentrate mixes of high yielding cows. In U. K. some feed manufacturers use this knowledge as a sales feature for their compound feeds and high protein supplements.

The feeding standards for dairy cows and the protein content of feeds may in the future, be given in these terms. For further information on degradable protein one may refer "Evaluation of Protein Quality for Ruminants" written in this book.

## Methods to Increase Utilisation of Crude Protein in Ruminants.

In plants, the protein is largely concentrated in the actively growing portions, especially the leaves and seeds. In animals, proteins are much more widely distributed than in plants.

Crude protein refers to all nitrogenous compounds (true protein + non-protein $N_2$) in a feed. It is determined by finding the $N_2$ content and multiplying the result by 6.25. The nitrogen comes from true protein as well as from non-protein nitrogen fraction. In fresh herbage as much as 30% of the $N_2$ may be in NPN form. Seeds such as maize grain or soybean seed also contain NPN which may be as high as 30—40% at the immature stage while levels reach as low as of 4-5% at maturity. Thus the amount and chemical nature of nitrogenous compounds in the diet may be extremely variable.

The amount of protein, its digestibility and the balance of essential amino acids are important factors that must be considered in balancing rations. In general, animal proteins are superior to plant proteins for monogastric animals due to the presence of all essential amino acids in proper ratio. Fortunately, the amino acid content of proteins varies from various plant and animal sources. Thus, the deficiencies of one protein source may be improved by combining it with another. It is for this reason that a combination of protein feeds in a ration is usually recommended when the person formulating the ration does not have access to specific amino acid values of the feeds to be used.

### Amino Acid Availability in Non-ruminants.

Amino acid availability is critical in the nutrition of non-ruminants since they do not have the ability to systhesise certain essential amino acids. Therefore, non-ruminant nutritionists not only calculate total protein intake by a non-ruminant but also the proportion of each amino acids present in that. In recent years requirement of all essential amino acids in nonruminant species are calculated instead of total protein requirements. A deficiency, and sometimes an excess, of a particular amino acid can severely affect production though total protein levels appear to be adequate.

**Amino Acid Availability in Ruminants**

Since the great bulk of dietary protein fed to ruminants is subject to microbial attack in the rumen, methods of protecting a portion of protein from ruminal degradation are matter of current investigations. It has been estimated that 20 percent of the nitrogen found in the crude protein fraction of the ruminal microorganisms is actually nitrogen from nucleic acids. This fraction of crude protein is essentially wasted as the nucleic acids are, for the most part degraded to form urea in the postruminal section of the gastrointestinal tract. Moreover, the true protein fraction from ruminal microorganisms is not as digestible as the dietary protein in many cases.

It has been observed that when amino acids and high quality proteins such as casein have been infused in the abomasum by-passing ruminal degradation, it always lead in improved $N_2$ retention, more rapid wool growth, greater milk production, and so forth. Qualitatively, ruminants have the same essential amino acid requirments as non-ruminants on a tissue level. Therefore, if certain essential amino acids are deficient in microbial protein, maximum performance cannot be achieved.

Many factors influence the rate of protein degradation such as (1) secretion of urea into the rumen via saliva and of ammonia through the rumen epithelia, (2) absorption of ammonia and other nitrogenous compounds by rumen epithelia, (3) recycling of bacterial and protozoal proteins in the rumen, (4) protein solubility and (5) flow rate through the rumen. The last two factors are most important.

Dietary proteins are degraded in proportion to their solubility in the ruminal fluid, For this reason, it may not be advantagious to feed ruminants high protein feeds which are highly soluble. Zein, a protein present in maize, is extremely insoluble, thus 40-60% is escaping ruminal breakdown. On the other hand, casein is highly soluble and is almost totally degradable in the rumen.

Various methods of protecting protein from ruminal degradation are described below :

1. *Heat treatment*

When protein feeds are heated, free amino groups within and between forms cross linkages which not only reduces the solubility but also reduce the surface of the protein for enzymatic attack.

2. *Treatment of proteins with tannins*

Tannins form hydrogen bonds with proteins, thereby protects protein from enzymatic degradation. As the treated protein travels down the digestive tract, the acidity of the fluids is altered and the tannin-protein complex dissociates.

3. *Treatment with formaldehyde*

The aldehyde reacts with free amino groups and N-terminal groups to form Schiff bases and cross-linkages between protein chains thus reduces the solubility of the protein and protects it from enzymatic degradation. Once the treated protein enters into a highly acid medium in the abomasum, the reaction is reversed and the protein is degraded.

4. *Encapsulation of amino acids*

The theory of encapsulating specific amino acids appears to be an easy, efficient means of ruminal bypass but yet the technique has not proven to be entirely successful.

5. *Use of amino acid analogues*

**Only one analogue, methionine hydroxy analogue (MHA) produced variable but promising result. The compound is less soluble in ruminal fluids than methionine and thereby much of it escapes degradation in the rumen.**

## MINERALS

Animal body contains about 3 percent minerals, which are constant constituents of animal tissues. These may be defined as those elements which remain mostly as ash when plant and animal tissues are burned. In animal body there are about 30-40 mineral elements which occur largely in the various parts of their body. Calcium and phosphorus account for three-fourths of the mineral elements in the body (49 percent calcium, 27 percent, phosphorus and 24 percent other elements). A predominant part of the mineral material in the animal body is located in the skeletal tissue (bones and teeth). In the four human bodies analysed in the laboratories of H.H. Mitchell of U.S.A., an average of 98.3 percent calcium, 87.0 percent of the phosphorus and 86.0 percent of the total mineral matter (ash) was found in the skeleton. Out of 30-40 mineral elements which are found in animal body, a large number of these are not essential for body processes. Their presence in a tissue may be purely adventitious, due to their ingestion with the food, their inbibition in water, or their inhalation with air during respiration. In fact the essentiality of any mineral element is known from its metabolic role in the animal body from the criteria as mentioned below:

1. it is present in all healthy tissues of all animals;
2. its concentration from one animal to the next is fairly constant;
3. its withdrawal from the body induces reproducibly the same structural and physiological abnormalities regardless of the species studied.
4. its addition either prevents or reverse these abnormalities.

**Table 81**

**APPROXIMATE CONTENT OF ASH IN ANIMALS**

| *Species* | *Ash content* (per cent of live weight)* |
|---|---|
| Cattle | 2.8/3.5 |
| Sheep | 2.9/3.4 |
| Swine | 3.2/2.8 |
| Dog | 2.1/3.6 |
| Rabbit | 2.6/5.6 |
| Rat | 1.5/5.6 |
| Mouse | 1.7/5.6 |
| Chicken | 1.9/4.2 |

* The figure to the left of the oblique indicates ash content at birth: the figure to the right of the oblique indicates ash content in mature animals.

(5) the abnormalities induced by deficiency are always accompanied by pertinent, specific biochemical changes; and
(6) these biochemical changes can be prevented or cured when the deficiencies are prevented or cured.

Elements which do not meet these exacting requirements occur more or less constantly in highly variable concentrations in living tissues. They include aluminium, antimony, mercury, cadmium, vanadium, silicon, rubidium, silver, gold, lead, bismuth, titanium and others.

Table 82

PERCENTAGE CONTENTS OF ASH IN ANIMAL ORGANS AND TISSUES

| *Organ or tissue* | *In crude substance* | *In dry substance* |
|---|---|---|
| Bones | 33–35 | 58–61* |
| Hide | 0.8–0.9 | 2.4–2.8 |
| Liver | 1.3–1.4 | 4.4–4.8 |
| Kidneys | 1.1–1.3 | 5.6–6.5 |
| Muscles | 0.9–1.1 | 4.0–4.8 |
| Blood | 0.7–0.8 | 3.7–4.2 |

* In dry defatted substance.

Table 83

APPROXIMATE PERCENTAGE CONTENTS OF MINERAL ELEMENTS IN BODY ASH OF ADULT ANIMALS

| *Element* | *Content (%)* |
|---|---|
| Calcium | 28.5 |
| Phosphorus | 16.6 |
| Potassium | 4.8* |
| Sulphur | 3.6 |
| Chlorine | 3.5 |
| Sodium | 3.7 |
| Magnesium | 1.1 |
| Iron | 0.15 |

* Varies in different animal species.

In general, *purified diet experiment* is conducted to know initially about the essentiality of any element. In such experiments, the animals are fed with ration made up of all pure ingredients such as for protein—purified uncontaminated casein, for carbohydrate—purified uncontaminated starch, for oils or fats—purified stripped lard or purified oil of maize or any other vegetable oil in stripped condition by which oil is made free of any other factor as oil soluble vitamins or any other compounds. For minerals and vitamins, individual purified items are added except that particular one about which we are interested to know the essentiality. Thus due to absence

**of that item in the ration, the experimental animal will develop some deficiency symptoms within a reasonable period of feeding purified diet. If the missing element is really an essential one, upon addition of it in ration where it was missing, the deficiency symptoms will be cured.**

**Twenty-one such elements have uptil now been proved to be essential and there is some**

**Table 8.4**

**The essential mineral elements and their approximate concentration in animal body.**

| *Macro-elements* | | | | *Trace of micro-elements* | *ppm mg/kg* | *Possibly essential mineral elements* |
|---|---|---|---|---|---|---|
| *Principal cations* | *%* | *Principal anions* | *%* | | | |
| Calcium | 1.5 | Phosphorus | 1.0 | Manganese | 0.2-0.5 | Arsenic |
| Magnesium | 0.04 | Chlorine | 0.11 | Iron | 20.80 | Barium |
| Sodium | 0.16 | Sulfur | 0.15 | Copper | 1.5 | Bromine |
| Potassium | 0.3 | | | Iodine | 0.3–0.6 | Cadmium |
| | | | | Zinc | 10-50 | Strontium |
| | | | | Fluorine | 2.5 | |
| | | | | Vanadium | 50-500 ppb | |
| | | | | Cobalt | 0.02-0.04 | |
| | | | | Molybdenum | 1-4 | |
| | | | | Selenium | 1-2 | |
| | | | | Chromium | 0.08 | |
| | | | | Tin | 1.5–2.0 | |
| | | | | Nickel | ? | |
| | | | | Silicon | ? | |

**evidence that six other elements may also be essential. Table 84 gives an idea of the amount of such essential mineral elements present in the animal body.**

**Many of the essential or non-essential elements may be toxic if their amounts are higher than usual level which cause disorder in normal metabolic disturbances. Selenium is an example of an essential mineral which is toxic at quite low levels in the diet while fluorine is another example of a mineral believed to be essential which in excess amounts produces toxicity. When any specific mineral is present at too high a level it may cause a metabolic deficiency of another mineral element by inhibiting the absorption of the latter; such is the case where a high level of molybdenum causes a conditioned copper deficiency. This fact is sufficient enough to emphasise that an imbalance of mineral elements—as distinct from a single deficiency—is equally effective to cause mineral deficiency. Supplementation of any diet with minerals should be done with proper care. In modern age the use of radioactive isotopes has advanced our knowledge of**

mineral nutrition and it is hoped that in the near future we may know much more through this type of experiment.

Over 80 per cent of the total mineral matter is found in the skeleton, giving strength and rigidity to the bones and teeth; the remaining mineral elements occur in the tissues and in the blood where they are frequently in organic combination and play an essential part in many of the body functions.

## The Principal Functions of Minerals

The 1·5 essential elements serve the body in many different ways. As constituents of the bones and teeth, they give rigidity and strength to the skeletal structures. They are also constituents of the organic compounds, such as protein and lipids, which make up the muscles, hair, hoofs and horns, blood and other soft cells of the body. They are important in maintenance of homeostasis in the internal fluids; maintenance of cell membrane equilibrium and thereby exert characteristic effects on the irritability of muscle and nerves. They also activate enzyme systems; involve in direct or indirect effects on the functions of endocrine glands; effect on the symbiotic microflora of the GI tract. Lastly the quality and quantity of all animal products like milk, wool, eggs and meat are affected by the presence or absence of minerals in the body.

### 1. The structural function of minerals

(i) Bone and teeth: Normal adult bone may be considered to have the following approximate composition.

*Composition of fresh bone*

| | | | | |
|---|---|---|---|---|
| **Water** | **45 per cent** | | **Calcium** | **36 per cent** |
| **Ash** | **25 „** | ⟶ | **Phosphorus** | **17 „** |
| **Protein** | **20 „** | | **Magnesium** | **0.8 „** |
| **Fat** | **10 „** | | **Others** | **46.2 „** |
| | | | | **100 „** |

The organic matrix of bone in which the mineral salts mainly of calcium, phosphorus and carbonate, with small amounts of magnesium, sodium, strontium, lead, citrate, fluoride, hydroxide and sulphate are deposited consists of a mixture of collagen, mucopolysaccharides and protein carbohydrate complexes.

(ii) Minerals are also necessary for the formation of hair, hoofs and horn.

(iii) A small amount is present in all soft tissues, which quantitavely may be small but are vital for life processing.

(iv) Blood cells contain a small amount of minerals for the normal functioning of blood cells. Haemoglobin of R.B.C. contains $Fe^{++}$ without which blood will not be able to carry $O_2$ or $CO_2$.

**2. Minerals and homeostasis**

Homeostasis is the constancy of the chemical composition and physico-chemical properties of the internal medium of the organism. These include body temperature, osmotic pressure of fluids, hydrogen ion concentration, and concentration and ratio of biologically active ions. Minerals present as soluble salt in the cell medium, interstitial fluid, blood and lymph, participate directly or indirectly in maintaining the above parameters at a constant level.

(i) *Maintenance of ionic equilibrium*: Salts, when dissolved in liquids, are fully or partly dissociated into electrically charged ions--cations and anions. Cations are formed by metals ($Na^+$, $K^+$, $Ca^{2+}$, $Mg^{2+}$, etc.), while anions are formed by acid residues ($Cl^-$, $HCO_3^-$, $SO_4^{2-}$, $HPO_4^{2-}$, $H_2PO_4^{2-}$). The ammonium ion ($NH_4^+$) is also a cation, while organic acids and proteins are anions.

Under normal conditions all liquids in the organism are electrically neutral, since the sum of the positive ions (cations) is equivalent to the sum of the negative ions (anions).

The ions in the body fluids together with the other components, produce a certain level of osmotic pressure, maintain the equilibrium of cell membranes, affect the condition of tissue colloids (by maintaining them in the requisite state of dispersion), help regulate the acid-base equilibrium and, in addition, fulfil other functions specific to each individual ion.

(ii) *Maintenance of osmotic pressure*: The osmotic pressure within the organism is an important physiological factor which promotes the migration of water and of soluble substances in the tissues. The dissolved salts produce a certain osmotic pressure in the body fluids. Ionised salts, which dissociate into ions in solution, increases the osmotic pressure to a greater extent than do non-electrolytes (urea, glucose) in equal molar concentrations. The reason for this is the fact that osmotic pressure is determined by the overall number of non-dissociated molecules, colloidal particles and ions.

(iii) *Maintenance of acid base equilibrium*: Blood and intercellular fluid have a weakly basic reaction (pH 7.3-7.4), while the pH in the intracellular fluid is slightly higher that is 7.0-7.2 owing to the intense metabolism of the cells.

The body's buffer systems namely, blood protein as potassium salt of oxyhaemoglobin ($KHbO_2$), phosphate as sodium phosphate ($Na_2HPO_4$) which dissociates with the formation of two sodium ions ($Na^+$) and a secondary phosphate ion ($HPO_4^{2-}$), and the third system is of sodium bicarbonate ($NaHCO_3$), which dissociates into sodium and bicarbonate ions are all involved in maintaining acid-base equilibrium of the body.

$$NaHCO_3 \rightarrow Na^+ + HCO_3^-$$

$$HCO_3^- + H^+ \rightleftharpoons H_2CO_3 \text{ (unstable) decomposes into } CO_2 + H_2O$$

**3. Minerals and the function of cell membranes**

Membranes have a complex chemical structure and participate in major physiological function; generation and transmission of nerve stimuli; intercellular signalling; perception of light, odours and tastes; energy conversion in the cell, changes in enzyme activities; etc. In the form of complex organic compounds, and mainly in the form of ions, minerals are directly related to the structure and functions of membranes.

**4. Minerals and enzyme systems**

Enzymes are the most effective and the most specific of all known catalysts. Catalysis of the enzyme system often requires the presence of not only the enzymes and the substrate, but also of non-protein substances—the cofactors. Both organic compounds like vitamins which act as coenzymes and metallic ions may act as cofactors.

All enzymes which require the presence of metals to achieve their maximum activity may be classed in two groups; (i) metalloenzymes of metallocoenzymes, and (ii) metal activated enzymes.

(i) *Metalloenzymes*: In metalloenzymes the metal is an integral part of the molecule and cannot be removed by dialysis. Enzymes of this type usually contain transition metals (Cu, Fe, Zn), which form highly stable coordination complexes in their active centres.

**Table 85**

SOME METALLOENZYMES IN ANIMALS

| *Enzyme* | *Metal* | *Stoichiometry* | *Source* |
|---|---|---|---|
| Monoamine oxidase | Cu | 1 Cu | Plasma } cattle |
| Uricase | Cu | 1 Cu | Liver } cattle |
| Cytochrome oxidase | Cu | 1 Cu/geminal | Heart } cattle |
| NADH-dehydrogenase | Fe | 4 Fe | Pig heart |
| Succinate dehydrogenase | Fe | 4 Fe | Pig heart |
| Aldehyde oxidase | Fe, Mo | 8 Fe, 2 Mo | Pig heart |
| Pyruvate carboxylase | Mn | 4 Mn | Chick livers |
| Xanthine oxidase | Mo | 1.5 Mo, 8 Fe | Cow milk |
| Carbonic anhydrase | Zn | 1 Zn | Erythrocytes } cattle |
| Carboxypeptidase A | Zn | 1 Zn | Pancreas } cattle |
| Carboxypeptidase B | Zn | 1 Zn | Pig pancreas |
| Alcohol dehydrogenase | Zn | 4 Zn | Horse liver |
| Leucine aminopeptidase | Zn | 4–6 Zn | Pig kidney |
| Glutathione peroxidase | Se | 4 Se | Cattle erythrocytes |

(ii) *Metal activated enzymes*: The metal here is not usually firmly bound to the enzyme, may be almost fully extracted by dialysis at pH 7.0.

The following 15 cations may serve as activators of one or several enzymes: $Na^+$, $K^+$, $Rb^+$, $Cs^+$, $Mg^{2+}$, $Ca^{2+}$, $Zn^{2+}$, $Cd^{2+}$, $Cr^{2+}$, $Cu^{2+}$, $Mn^{2+}$, $Co^{2+}$, $Ni^{2+}$, $Al^{2+}$, $Fe^{2+}$.

### 5. Minerals and hormones

A minimum of hormones are important as because they maintain the ionic equilibria of some metals in various body fluids such as (i) aldosterone for sodium, (ii) parathyroid and, (iii) thyrocalcitonin for calcium.

Minerals are also found to be the structural components of some hormones. The disulphide bridges (-s-s), which interlink the amino acid chains and stabilise the protein structure, are contained in the molecules of several hormones such as insulin, prolactin, oxytocin, vasopressin etc. Hormones of the thyroid gland are found to contain iodine.

### 6. Minerals and symbiotic bacteria

A number of minerals are definitely essential for microorganisms, which produce the metabolites required by the animals. An example of such an element is cobalt, whose salts really serve as food for the microflora. The main function of cobalt is to supply the needs of certain groups of bacteria producing vitamin $B_{12}$ or its analogues (Cobamines, Cobalamins) required by the animals. This process takes place in the forestomachs (rumen, reticulum and omasum) of the ruminants, in the large intestine of monogastric animals and in the cecum of rabbits and hens.

Bacteria are capable of reducing feed sulphates to sulphides, and incorporate the latter into sulphur containing amino acids and proteins. Thus rumen amino acids are synthesised from carbohydrates, ammonia and inorganic sulphur.

**7. Minerals and milk**

Cow's milk contains 5.8 per cent ash or mineral matter on a dry basis. Deficiency of minerals in the diet will ultimately cause poor production.

## ORGANIC CHELATES

The word "chelate' is derived from the Greek word "Chele" meaning "claw" which is a good descriptive term for the manner in which polyvalent cations are held by the metal binding agents. Prior to union with the metal these organic substances are termed as "ligands". Ligand + mineral = chelate element.

Recently, animal nutritionists have come to realize that organic chelates of mineral elements which are cyclic compounds may be the most important factors controlling absorption of a number of mineral elements. A particular element in chelated form may be released in ionic form at the intestinal wall or might be readily absorbed as the intact chelate. Chelates may be of naturally occurring substances such as chlorophyll, cytochromes, haemoglobin, vitamin $B_{12}$, some amino acids, etc., or may be of synthetic substances like ethylenediaminetetracetic acid (EDTA).

Chelates show exceptionally high stability. The bonds between the ligand and the metal ions are of "coordinate" type and occur because of peculiarities in the electron shell of the transition metals. Sometimes the chelates are so stable that the metal ion is released with great difficulty resulting in difficulties in availability by the animal or plant tissues.

In biological systems there are three types of chelates:

**Type I. Chelates that Aid in Transport and to Store Metal Ions**

Chelates of this group behave as a carrier for proper absorption, transportation in the circulatory system and passing across cell membranes to deposit the metal ion at the site where needed.

(a) Among amino acids, cysteine and histidine are particularly effective metal binding agents and may be of primary importance in the transport and storage of mineral elements throughout the animal body.

(b) Ethylenediaminetetracetic acid (EDTA) and other similar synthetic ligands also may improve the availability of zinc and other minerals.

**Type II. Chelates Essential in Metabolism**

Many chelates of animal body are holding metal ions in such a cyclic fashion which are absolutely necessary to be in that form to perform metabolic function. Vitamin $B_{12}$, cytochrome

1. Oxalic acid $+ Ca^{++} \longrightarrow$ Insoluble Calcium Oxalate

*Oxalic acid* *Insoluble Calcium Oxalate*

2. EDTA $+ 2Zn^{++} \longrightarrow$ Zn chelate

$N-CH_2-CH_2-N$

EDTA
*(Ethylenediaminetetra acetate)*

**Chelates as example number 1 interfere with absorption while Chelates like number 2, serve to transport and to store metal ions.**

**enzymes and haemoglobin are some of the examples of this type. Haemoglobin molecule without its content of ferrous form of iron will be of no use in transporting oxygen.**

**Type III. Chelates Which Interfere with Utilisation of Essential Cations**

**There are some chelates found in the body which might have accidentally formed and are of no use to the subject. Rather, those chelates may be detrimental for the proper utilisation of the element. Phytic-acid-Zn chelate or oxalic acid calcium chelate are examples of this type.**

## Interaction of Minerals with Each Other and with Other Nutrients

Minerals may interact both with each other and with other nutrient and non-nutritive factors. This interaction, which may be *synergistic* (elements which mutually enhance their absorption in the digestive tract and jointly fulfil some metabolic function at the tissue or cell level) or *antagonistic* (elements which inhibit the absorption of each other in the digestive tract and produce effects on any biochemical function in the organism), takes place in the feed itself, in the digestive tract and during tissue and cell metabolism.

From the practical point of view knowledge of these mechanisms makes it possible to prevent undesirable forms of such interactions and the appearance of secondary mineral insufficiency in animals.

### Mutual interactions between minerals

Owing to their liability and their tendency to form bonds, minerals are much more liable to interact than are other nutrient substances.

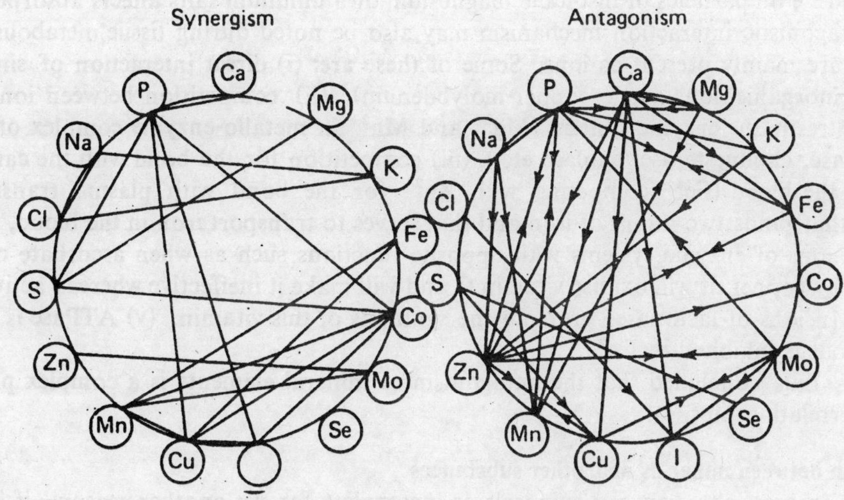


Metabolic interactions of essential elements

### Synergism

The synergism of minerals in the gastrointestinal tract and at the tissue and cell metabolism renders the following interactions possible:

(i) *At the gastrointestinal tract*: (a) due to direct interaction between elements (Ca with P, Na with Cl, Zn with Mo), the level of absorption enhances provided the elements are at proper ration; (b) due to indirect interaction by stimulating the growth and activity of the microflora in the forestomachs and in the intestine by some specific mineral such as cobalt causes intensification of microbial biosynthetic processes.

(ii) *At the time and cell metabolism level*: (a) direct interaction between elements in structural processes such as Ca and P in the formation of bone hydroxyapatite, joint participation of Fe and Cu in the formation of haemoglobin, interaction of Mn with Zn in the conformation of RNA molecules in the liver; (b) simultaneous participation of elements in the active centre of some enzymes such as Fe and Mo in xanthine and aldehyde oxidases, Cu and Fe in cytochrome oxidase are noteworthy examples of synergistic interaction which jointly fulfil metabolic function at the tissue or cell level.

**Antagonism**

As distinct from synergism, which is most often mutual, antagonism may be one- or two-sided. Thus, P and Mg; Zn and Cu inhibit the absorption of each other in the intestine, whereas K inhibits the absorption of Zn and Mn, but not the other way round. Inhibition of absorption of some elements by others in the digestive tract may proceed by the following mechanisms: (i) excess presence of Mg in the diet may form complex magnesium phosphate affect the absorption of both the elements, similarly reaction between Cu and sulphate makes another complex compound, formation of the triple Ca—P—Zn salt in the presence of high Ca in the diet is another example which renders absorption; (ii) some elements when in excess may get adsorbed on the surface of colloidal particles such as fixation of Mn and Fe on particles of insoluble magnesium or aluminium salts affects absorption.

Antagonistic interaction mechanism may also be noted during tissue metabolism where minerals are mainly present as ions. Some of these are: (i) direct interaction of simple and complex inorganic ions (e.g., copper-molybdenum), (ii) competition between ions for the active centres in the enzyme systems ($Mg^{2+}$ and $Mn^{2+}$ in metallo-enzyme complex of alkaline phosphatase, cholinesterase, enolase etc.), (iii) competition for the bond with the carrier substance in the blood ($Fe^{2+}$ competing with $Zn^{2+}$ for the bond with plasma transferrin—a globulin that binds two atoms of iron and that serves to transport iron in the blood, (iv) activation by ions of enzyme systems with opposite functions such as when ascorbate oxidase is activated by copper, it will oxidise vitamin C and will make it ineffective whereas activation by Zn and Mn ions of lactonases promote the synthesis of this vitamin. (v) ATPase is activated by $Mg^{2+}$ but is inhibited by $Ca^{2+}$.

It is thus concluded that the antagonism of mineral elements is a complex process of biotic interrelationships.

**Interaction between minerals and other substances**

The interactions between minerals is incomplete for yet another reason—it ignores a number of other factors which influence the utilisation or metabolism of minerals.

Thus vitamin D affects the absorption of calcium, phosphorus, magnesium, zinc and other elements. Fat affects the absorption of magnesium and calcium. The protein level and the type of protein fed determine the degree of utilisation of phosphorus, magnesium, zinc, copper and other elements in the feed of ruminants, pigs and birds. The opposite relationship is also possible; thus excess molybdenum stimulates the elimination of urea nitrogen from the organism, reduces the biosynthesis of muscle protein, and impairs the flavour of the meat.

In the digestive tract, minerals may form new bonds with organic compounds. Of special interest are internally complexed compounds—chelates—which may stimulate or may inhibit the absorption of minerals.

The ligands (organic substances on which metal ion binds to form chelates) in such compounds may be amino acids (especially glycine, cystine, cysteine and histidine), polypeptides proteins, prophyrins, organic acids (amino-acetic, oxalic, citric, malic, formic and, in particular, phytic acid). Natural feeds with strong chelating properties include dry malt residues and molasses.

It is known that soya, cotton seed, sunflower seed and sesame seed cakes contain insoluble phytates, whose phosphorus and microelements, in particular zinc, are difficult to assimilate. Up to 60 per cent of the phosphorus in soybeans is in the form of phytates. Non-

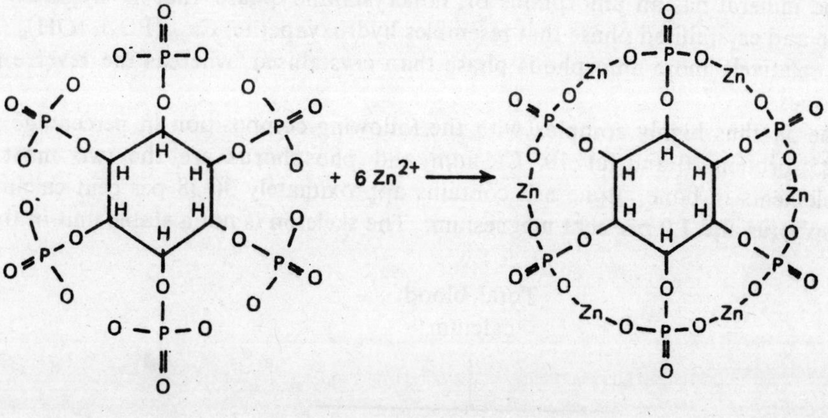

$$+ 6\,Zn^{2+} \longrightarrow$$

Formation of insoluble zinc phytate

ruminants find it difficult to utilise phosphorus and zinc from insoluble zinc phytate although ruminants can easily digest with the aid of the microflora of the forestomachs.

Microelement absorption can be facilitated only by thermal treatment of the feed and also by addition of strong chelating agents such as EDTA, citric or acetic acids. It may be noted that chelates are essential for transport and storing of metal ions, essential for normal metabolism and of course some are undesirable because they interfere with absorption and utilisation of essential cations.

## CALCIUM

Calcium is one of the elements occurring abundantly in nature. It is found as calcium carbonate (chalk, limestone, marble), calcium sulphate (gypsum), calcium theoride (fluorite), dolomite $CaCO_3$, $MgCo_3$ and fluoroapatite $Ca_5\,(PO_4)_3$. Eleven calcium isotopes, including six stable isotopes are known.

Calcium rich vegetable feeds include leguminous grasses and sunflowers, cereal grasses and maize are relatively poor in calcium. The vegetative parts of plants contain more calcium than their reproductive parts. The amount in plants varies with the pH of the soil, the extent of liming, and the concentration of magnesium in the soil, which is antagonistic to calcium. It would appear that the optimum level of calcium in green plants is 40-60 mg per kg dry matter, and any excess content impairs the mineral metabolism of animals.

**Content in body and variations**

The amount of calcium in adult animal body is 1.2-1.5 per cent, calculated in terms of fresh tissue, 3.5-4.0 per cent in dry tissue, and 25-30 per cent calculated in terms of the total body ash. The calcium and the ash levels of the body increase with age; variations in content may also be due to the state of nutrition and species. Nearly 99 per cent of the total body calcium is found in skeletons (bone) and teeth, where the concentration of calcium is fairly constant (36-38 per cent).

Bone mineral has an amorphous or noncrystalline phase that is hydrated tricalcium phosphate and crystallised phase that resembles hydroxyapetite, $Ca_{10} (PO_4)_6 (OH)_2$. The young bone has relatively more amorphous phase than crystallised, whereas the reverse is true for mature bones.

Bone is thus highly complex with the following composition in percentage: Water 45; mineral 25; protein 20 and fat 10. Calcium and phosphorus are the two most abundant mineral elements in bone. Bone ash contains approximately 36-38 per cent calcium, 17 per cent phosphorus and 1.0 per cent magnesium. The skeleton is not a stable unit in the chemical

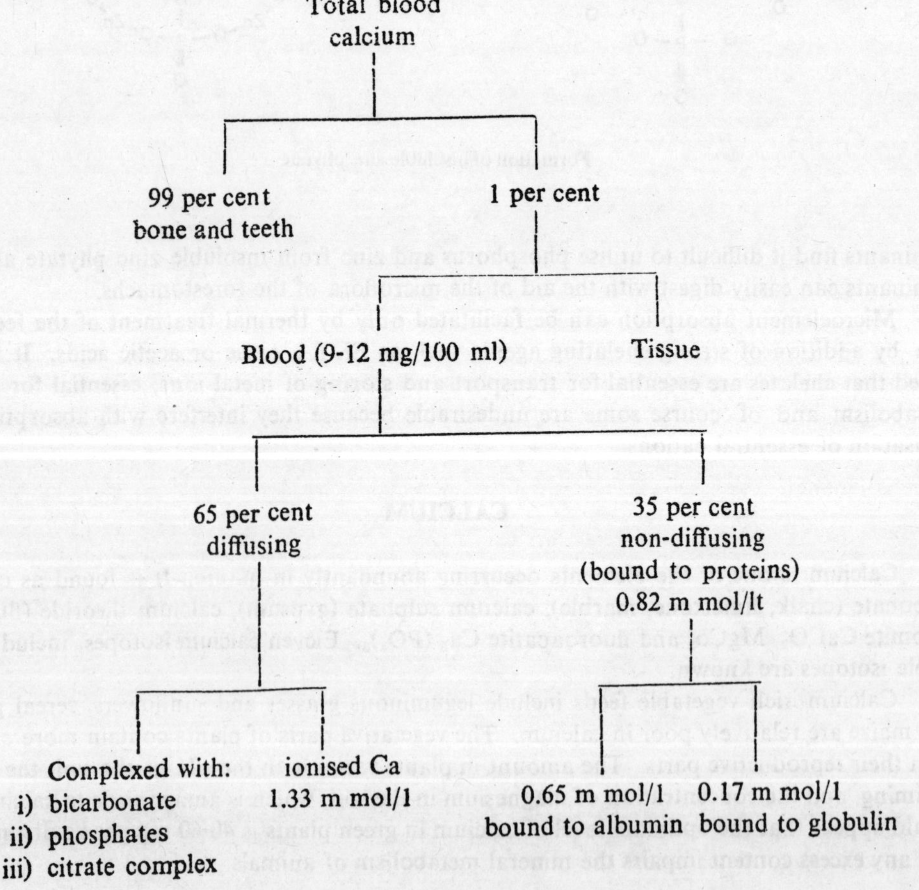

sense; exchange of calcium and phosphorus between bones and soft tissue is always a continuous process.

The 1 per cent of body calcium which occurs outside the bones is widely distributed throughout the organs and tissues including blood for performing vital body functions. Calcium is required for normal blood clotting as it must be present for the formation of thrombin from prothrombin, for muscle contraction, myocardial function, normal neuromuscular excitability, activation of several enzymes and secretion of several hormones and hormone releasing factors.

**Table 86**

**Ranges of Ca in soft tissues of animals**
**(mg/100 g fresh tissue)**

| Tissue | Ca content | Tissue | Ca content |
|---|---|---|---|
| Muscle | 5-14 | Spleen | 9-15 |
| Skin | 6-20 | Lungs | 10-25 |
| Kidneys | 6-20 | Liver | 10-30 |
| Brain | 8-22 | Intestine | 13-15 |
| Heart | 8-25 | Cartilage | 50-95 |

The calcium in the blood plasma of mammals is usually from 9 to 12 mg/100 ml, although that of laying hens may be between 30 and 40 mg/100 ml. Calcium concentration in erythrocytes is negligible (0.14-0.22 mg/g in the liquid phase), but may be higher in membranous structures.

Calcium is present in blood serum as two main fractions—one capable of diffusing through ultrafilters (65 per cent of the total blood calcium) and the other incapable portion (35 per cent). Among the diffusing type bulk portion is ionic $Ca^{2+}$, while about 15 per cent is complexed with bicarbonates, phosphates and citrates.

**Absorption**

Calcium is absorbed into the organism with vegetable feeds and mineral additives. In plants it is bound to proteins and to organic acid anions, while in the additives it appears as carbonate or phosphate. Whatever the actual chemical form it takes, the bulk of the calcium compounds introduced (except for oxalates) is converted by the gastric juice to calcium chloride which is almost completely dissociated into ions. It is believed that the transfer of $Ca^{2+}$ ions across the membranes of the intestinal epithelium involves a special calcium binding protein produced by the influence of vitamin D in the mucous cell. The amount of calcium absorbed largely depends on the activity of the agents which reduce the content of ionised calcium in the intestines. If anions (negatively charged ions) which bind or precipitate calcium (oxalates, phytates, phosphates and possibly sulphates) are present in excess, they may interfere with the absorption of calcium in the intestine. The absorption of both Ca and P is thus favoured by factors which operate to hold them in solution.

The optimum Ca : P ratio for the absorption of both elements in the intestine should not vary other than 1.3 : 1 to 1.5 : 1, which is optimum for efficient absorption. With a marked excess of either in the diets, the faecal excretion of both increases. One function of vitamin D is also to promote calcium and phosphorus absorption as is detailed later through the formation of the calcium binding protein.

Dietary Ca is absorbed largely from the duodenum and in the upper section of the large intestine (jejunum) of most animals. Absorption occurs both by active (energy dependent) and passive (diffusion) transport. Depending on the age of the animals and on other factors, absorption varies between 10 and 50 per cent and is relatively independent of the nitrogen content of the diet.

It has been noted that there is always some endogenous loss of calcium through faeces, irrespective of feeding a very low or optimum amount of calcium in the diet. Thus true absorption of calcium from the feed can only be established by deducting the endogenous losses (largely arising from secretions of the intestinal mucosa) of this element. Depending on the species of animal these endogenous losses vary between 18 and 50 mg per kg of live weight per day.

Once calcium is absorbed in the intestine, it moves through the portal vein into the liver, where its complex compounds are broken down and the calcium forms new compounds, possibly with proteins.

**Excretion**

Under normal conditions both calcium contained in the feed which remains unabsorbed, and calcium of endogenous origin are eliminated from the body through the gastrointestinal tract. Unlike the monovalent ions ($K^+$, $Na^+$) which can almost entirely be absorbed in the intestine, and then eliminated without impairing the homeostatic mechanism of their regulation by the kidneys, calcium which is filtered through the kidney is almost 99 per cent reabsorbed, so that its excretion with the urine is very limited. In principle the above applied to most laboratory and farm animals, with some variation due to age and species. In the case of pigs, rabbits and laying hens excretion of calcium with urine is more intensive than other species. The concentration of calcium in the urine of calves is high (up to 100 mg per cent), because during the first two weeks in the life of ruminants calcium is mainly excreted through the kidneys and not through the intestinal mucosa. Under usual conditions cows excrete between 0.1 and 1 g/day through urine.

**Table 87**

AVERAGE CALCIUM EXCHANGE INDICES IN ANIMALS[71]

| *Calcium* (mg per day) | *Calves* | *Sheep* | *Goats* | *Pigs* |
|---|---|---|---|---|
| Live weight (kg) | 50 | 43 | 72 | 35 |
| Utilized | 5800 | 3000 | 9400 | 11000 |
| Metabolized in body (mg) | 33000 | 20000 | 3200 | 14900 |
| Absorbed | 5300 | 800 | 1100 | 4700 |
| Endogenous faecal | 500 | 500 | 800 | 1450 |
| Eliminated with faeces | 1120 | 2700 | 9100 | 7800 |
| Eliminated with urine | 10 | 50 | 80 | 110 |
| Deposited in skeleton | 15000 | 5000 | 2300 | 13300 |
| Extracted from skeleton | 10300 | 4750 | 2250 | 10200 |

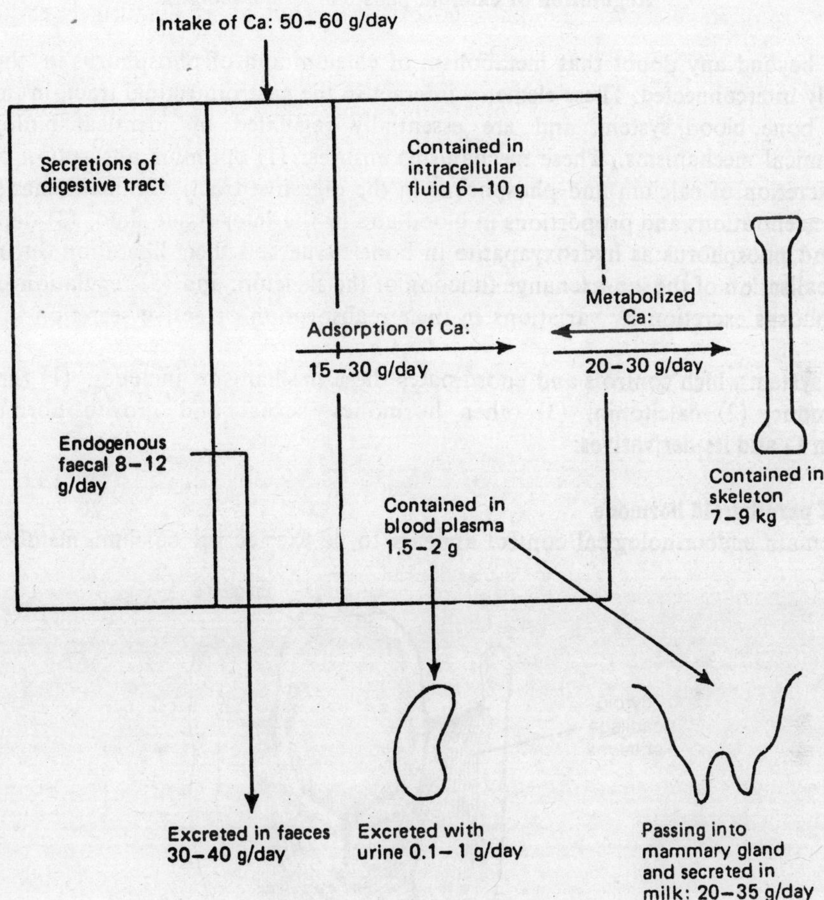


Calcium metabolism in a lactating cow[71]

**Table 88**

**Distribution of faecal and urinary Ca excretion in humans, cattle and rats**

| Species | | Age | Ca intake | Faecal Ca | Urine Ca |
|---|---|---|---|---|---|
| | | | ← | g/day | → |
| Man | | | | | |
| | Male | 11-16 yr. | 1.8 | 1.01 | 0.127 |
| | | 23 | 1.4 | 1.23 | 0.072 |
| | Female | 14-16 | 0.88 | 0.66 | 0.194 |
| | | 55-63 | 0.71 | 0.59 | 0.169 |
| Cattle | | Young adult | 29.00 | 27.00 | 0.500 |
| Rats | | 12 week | 0.044 | 0.02 | 0.0009 |

Source: Bronner, F. 1964. In Mineral Metab., Vol. 2, Part A. Academic Press, New York.

## Regulation of calcium-phosphorus metabolism

It is beyond any doubt that metabolism of calcium and of phosphorus in the body is very closely interconnected. These elements interact in the gastrointestinal tract, in intercellular fluids, in bone blood system, and are essentially regulated by identical biological and physiochemical mechanisms. These mechanisms ensures: (1) optimum absorption and endogenous excretion of calcium and phosphorus in the digestive tract; (2) maintenance of their normal concentrations and proportions in blood and in the inter-tissue fluid; (3) deposition of calcium and phosphorus as hydroxyapatite in bone tissue and their liberation during resorption; (4) realisation of the ion-exchange function of the skeleton; and (5) regulation of calcium and phosphorus excretion by variations in their reabsorption or active secretion in the renal ducts.

The system which controls and coordinates these mechanisms includes: (1) the parathyroid hormone; (2) calcitonin; (3) other hormones—sexual and growth hormones; and (4) vitamin D and its derivatives.

### 1. Role of parathyroid hormone

The main endocrinological control appears to be exerted on calcium metabolism with

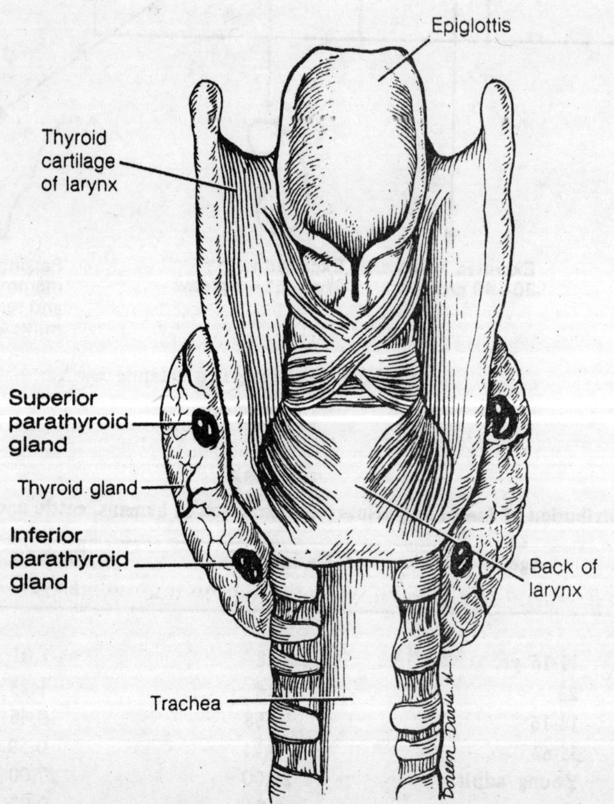


**Fig. 28** The parathyroid glands.

only secondary effects on phosphorus. In fact animals seem to tolerate wide variations in concentration of inorganic phosphorus in the blood without immediate harm whereas calcium is under close control.

The parathyroid hormone secreted by the parathyroid glands is a protein or a polypeptide, with a molecular weight of 9,500, which contains 84 amino acids regulates calcium metabolism and maintains a constant level of blood calcium at 9-12 mg per 100 ml in most species. In young hens, calcium levels in blood may be three to four times higher during egg production.

The plasma calcium occurs in two forms. One capable of diffusing through ultrafilters (65 per cent of the total blood Ca) is in ionised form either free or complexed with bicarbonate, phosphate and citrates, the other fraction is bound with protein including albumins and globulins.

The level of blood calcium is not readily influenced by the dietary intake though there are species differences in this respect. Out of various physiological factors which tend to maintain a constant level of blood calcium in ionised form despite high intakes or marked body losses, the most important is parathyroid hormone. The hormone (1) raises by increasing the mobilisation of calcium from the bones. It is believed that the mechanism is connected with citrate ion which functions as solvent at an environment of temporary low pH, thus facilitating increase osteoclastic (large special cells that erode bone) activity. (2) The second way in which parathyroid hormone acts is by decreasing urinary excretion of calcium but increasing urinary phosphate and lastly (3) the hormone stimulates the reabsorption of calcium in intestine together with vitamin D.

## 2. Role of calcitonin hormone

The hormone also known as thyrocalcitonin is produced in special parafollicular or thyroid C cells of the thyroid gland (in birds and fish it is formed in special organs—ultimobronchial bodies). The hormone is a polypeptide with a molecular weight of 3,500-4,500, consisting of 32 amino acid residues.

The hormone counteracts the effect of parathyroid hormone in that it decreases calcium concentration by cutting down the resorption rate of mineral from the bones. It now seems clear that parathyroid hormone and calcitonin both act in concert to maintain blood calcium at a constant concentration. Parathyroid hormone is secreted in response to hypocalcaemia and cause calcium levels to rise, this action being relatively slow lasts for several hours. In contrast calcitonin lowers the blood calcium and is secreted fast, reaching a peak in the matter of minutes after the hormone is secreted.

## 3. Other hormones affecting Ca-P metabolism

### a) *Sexual hormones*

It is believed that sexual hormones, especially oestrogens, enhance the content of calcium and phosphorus in the body particularly with the production of calcium reserves in the skeleton and their consumption during lactation in cows.

### b) *Growth hormone*

The somatotropic (STH) hormone directly affects one of the bone growth mechanisms by stimulating protein synthesis in the cartilage and bone cells either by inclusion of a large number of amino acids or by regulation of polysaccharide synthesis.

**4. Vitamin D and calcium-phosphorus metabolism**

Vitamin D is the collective name for a family of compounds with antirachitic effects. The most important of these compounds are ergocalciferol (vitamin $D_2$) and cholecalciferol (vitamin $D_3$).

Since the reserves of vitamin D in the tissues are low and are very labile, a regular, uniform intake of vitamin D must be ensured. The concentration of vitamin D in the blood plasms of animals of various species is 1.5-3 micro gram per 100 ml, and in rare cases it touches 5-6 micro gram.

The functional metabolism of vitamin D to activate the target organs of intestine, bone and kidney. Vitamin D must acquire two hydroxyl groups to be active.

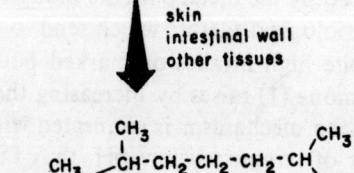

The mechanisms of the principal activity of vitamin D are as follows:

1. Vitamin D or vitamin D derivatives intensify the diffusion of calcium ions across the intestinal wall, by counteracting the factors which reduce the concentration of $Ca^{+2}$ or by increasing the permeability of the membrane of the intestinal epithelium.

2. Vitamin D is essential for the formation or initiation of the special calcium transport system in the intestinal wall.

For the above two functions, vitamin D or cholecalciferol has to be hydroxylated in two stages : (1) in the C-25 position by the liver, (2) in the C-1 position by the kidney which is done under the influence of parathyroid hormone.

If the animal is tending to hypocalcaemia, parathyroid hormone will be secreted which in turn stimulates the synthesis of 1,25-$(OH)_2$ cholecalciferol in the kidney which is the most active metabolite of vitamin D. It stimulates the synthesis of the so-called calcium binding proteins in the cytoplasmic fraction of the epithelial cells.

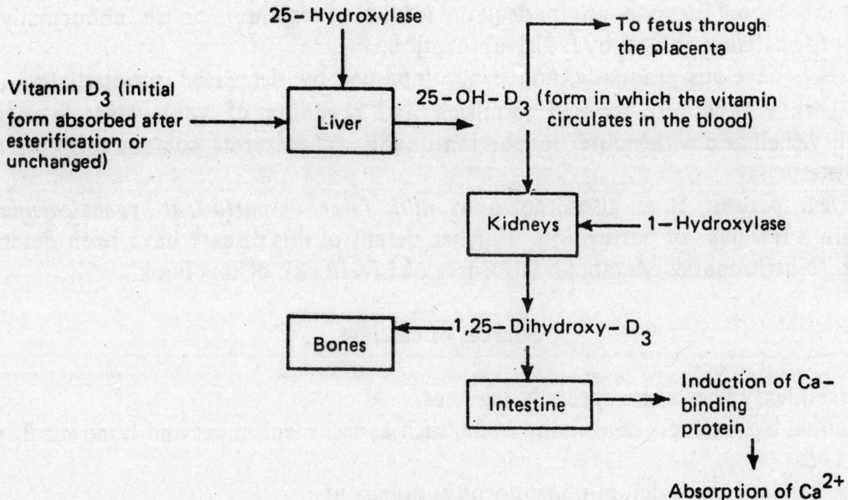


Scheme for vitamin D metabolism

**Effects of calcium deficiency or excess**

If the diet fed to farm animals is deficient in calcium or contains calcium in excess, some of the characteristic clinical symptoms and biochemical changes are manifested.

*Rickets*: The disease occurs only in growing animals due to subnormal calcification caused by a lack of adequate calcium and/or phosphorus in the diet, a decrease in the ability to absorb these inorganic elements, or a suboptimal intake of vitamin D. The primary trouble in rickets lies in the composition of the blood or the fluid bathing the bone, which is characterised by a low level of calcium and/or phosphorus. Characteristic symptoms include stunted growth, impaired or unnatural appetite, distorted spine, ribs (arching back in calves), bowed legs in human.

*Osteomalacia*: The condition in which the mineral content of the bone is depleted without making up for the losses found in adult animals, thus exhibits a continued mineral balance. Such a condition may be the result of a suboptimal intake of calcium and phosphorus, a faulty absorption of these elements, an overactive parathyroid, or the special demands for mineral elements created during pregnancy or lactation.

In osteomalacia the bones are gradually weakened. Such bones break easily, and fractures are common in farm animals as well as in humans suffering from the disease. The posterior paralysis of pregnant sows is frequently the result of fracture of a vertebra and a consequent pinching of the spinal cord.

*Osteoporosis*: A reduction of total bone mass due to resorption of both mineral and organic components. The bone becomes porous and thin over the better part of a life time. This disorder may result from: (1) a dietary deficiency of calcium and/or protein, (2) a lowered calcium absorption, (3) a hormonal disturbance.

It is believed that the rate of bone formation in osteoporosis is normal but the bone resorption takes place at an increased rate from an attempt to maintain the normal level of calcium in the blood, despite an inadequate intake of calcium or an abnormally large requirement for calcium caused by faulty absorption.

The disease develops gradually, and is accompanied by decreased productivity, impairment of digestive function, arrested moulting and shedding of wool. Hens lay eggs with poorer quality shell and with poorer incubation quality. The excreta contain a higher content of phosphorus.

*Parturient paresis*: It is also known as *milk fever* or *parturient hypocalcaemia* which occurs within a few days of parturition. Further details of this disease have been described in the chapter "Nutritional & Metabolic Disorders of Livestock" of this book.

## Sources of calcium

1. Green leafy vegetables specially legumes.
2. Animal by-products containing bone, such as fish meal, meat and bone meal, poultry by-products etc.
3. The calcium and calcium-phosphorus supplements:

| | |
|---|---|
| Oyster shell flour | 37.95 per cent |
| Ground limestone | 35.85 per cent |
| Defluorinated phosphate | 33.00 per cent |
| Steamed bone meal | 30.92 per cent |

## PHOSPHORUS (P at. wt. 31)

Phosphorus is found in every cell of the body, but most of it (about 80 per cent of the total) is combined with calcium in the bones and teeth. About 10 per cent is in combination with proteins, lipids and carbohydrates, and in other compounds in blood and muscle. The remaining 10 per cent is widely distributed in various chemical compounds. The amount of phosphorus present in blood serum is usually within the range of 4-12 mg per 100 ml.

**Functions**

1. Constituents of bone and teeth.
2. A constituent of the high energy compound ATP and thus is necessary for energy transductions essential for all cellular activity.
3. The oxidation of carbohydrate leading to the formation of ATP also requires phosphorus since phosphorylation is an obligatory step in the metabolism of any type of monosaccharides.
4. Phospholipids are constituents of all cellular membranes and are active determinants of cellular premeability.
5. DNA and RNA, the genetically significant compounds responsible for cell reproduction and therefore for growth and for all type of protein synthesis these phosphorylated compounds are absolutely necessary.

**Symptoms of Phosphorus Deficiency**

1. Since phosphorus is required for bone formation, a deficiency can cause rickets or osteomalacia.
2. 'Pica' or depraved appetite has been noted in cattle when there is a deficiency of phosphorus in their diet; the affected animals have abnormal appetite and chew wood, bones, rags and other foreign materials. Although Pica can be developed by other causes—a blood serum analysis of phosphorus may be run to know the exact cause of Pica, i.e., whether Pica is due to phosphorus deficiency or due to other reasons.
3. In chronic phosphorus deficiency animals may have stiff joints and muscular weakness.
4. Low dietary intakes of phosphorus have also been associated with low fertility and low-milk yield in cows and with stunted growth in young animals.

Phosphorus deficiency is usually more common in cattle than in sheep or goat as the latter group tend to have more selective grazing habits and choose the growing parts of plants which happen to be richer in phosphorus.

**Absorption**

*In vitro* studies indicate an active transport (molecules move from a low concentration to area of high concentration and this process requires extra metabolic energy). Excess of magnesium, iron, aluminium, by forming insoluble phosphates, made phosphorus unavailable. Remember, when there is either excess of calcium or excess phosphorus the larger amount interferes with the absorption of the smaller one.

Much of the phosphorus present in cereal grains is in the forms of phytates, which are salt of phytic acid, a phosphoric acid derivative. Insoluble calcium and magnesium phytates occur in cereals and other plant products. In ruminants like sheep and cattle there is no problem to hydrolyze insoluble phytates as rumen microbes produce phytase, an enzyme which changes the insoluble form into soluble form and thus renders the phosphorus available. In pigs some of the phytate phosphorus is made available in the stomach by the action of plant phytase enzymes present in the food. Chicks can utilise only 10 per cent as effectively as disodium phosphate.

**Metabolism**

The metabolism of phosphorus is in large part related to that of calcium, as heretofore. The Ca : P ratio in the diet affects the absorption and excretion of these elements. If either elements is given in excess, excretion of the other is increased. The Ca : P ratio considered most suitable for farm animals other than poultry is generally within the range 1 : 1 to 2 : 1. The proportion of calcium for laying hens is much larger, since they require great amount of this element for egg shell production.

Parathyroid hormone, when it becomes more, increases the serum calcium and lowers the serum phosphorus and vice versa.

Out of the total 4-12 mg of phosphorus per 100 ml of blood 43 per cent are present as free $HPO_4^{--}$; 20 per cent as $NaHPO_4^{-}$; like calcium, magnesium, etc.

**Source**

Grains, grain by-products, concentrates like oil cakes, brans, sterilized bone meal, milk products are the major sources of phosphorus.

## POTASSIUM ($K^+$ at. wt. 39)

Potassium is the chief cation of the intra-cellular fluid and plays a very important part along with sodium, chloride and bicarbonate ions, in the osmotic regulation of the body fluids. Nerve and muscle cells ase specially rich in potassium.

**Functions**

1. Maintenance of acid-base equilibrium
2. Maintenance of osmotic pressure
3. Nerve transmission
4. Heart beat relaxation
5. Activates certain enzymes
6. Potassium ion is necessary for carbohydrate and protein metabolism but the mechanism by which it acts is not clear
7. It also aids in the uptake of certain amino acids by the cell.

**Deficiency Symptoms**

Overall muscle weakness characterized by:

1. Weak extremities
2. Poor intestinal tone with poor intestinal distension
3. Cardiac weakness
4. Weakness of the respiratory muscle.

The potassium content of plants is generally very high. The amount present in grass dry matter, for example, being frequently above 2.5 per cent; so that it is normally ingested by animals in larger amounts than any other element. Consequently it is extremely unlikely that potassium deficiency could occur in farm animals under natural conditions. Fortunately dietary excess of potassium is normally rapidly excreted from the body, chiefly in the urine. High intake interferes with the absorption and metabolism of magnesium in the animal.

## SODIUM ($Na^+$ at. wt. 23)

The value of salt has been recognized for centuries. The common expression "worth his salt" and even the word "salary" all derive from the high value placed upon salt throughout history.. Unlike potassium, sodium is present in the extracellular fluid. The sodium concentration within the cells is relatively low, the element being replaced largely by potassium and magnesium. Only one-third of the total body sodium is present in the skeleton, rest all in body fluids.

**Functions**

1. Maintains body fluid pH
2. Regulates body fluid volume
3. Takes active part in nerve functions (transmission) and muscle contraction
4. Functions in the permeability and carrier of the cells

**Deficiency Symptoms**

1. Growth failure and reduces the utilisation of digested protein and energy
2. Dehydration—decreases plasma and body fluid volume
3. Vascular disturbances—decrease cardiac output, decrease arterial pressure and increase hematocrit
4. Corneal keratinization
5. Nervous disorder
6. In hens egg production is adversely affected as well as growth. Experiments carried out on rats fed on low sodium diets resulted in reproductive disturbances
7. Salt (NaCl) deficiency is maintained by an intense craving for salt, a lack of appetite, a generally haggard appearance, lustreless eyes and a rough haircoat. In milking cows there is a rapid loss of weight and a decline in milk production. In high producing cows collapse may be sudden and death may rapidly ensue.

Sodium metabolism is regulated primarily by aldosterone, a hormone of the adrenal cortex which promotes the reabsorption of sodium from the kidney tubules. In the absence of this hormone, sodium excretion is increased and symptoms of deficiency ensue.

**Sources**

All animal products, especially meat meals and foods of marine origin are richer sources; vegetable origin have comparatively low sodium contents. The commonest source is common salt.

## SULPHUR (S at. wt. 32)

Sulphur is present in all cells of the body, primarily in the cell proteins containing amino acids, cystine, cysteine and methionine. The hormone insulin, the two vitamins biotin and thiamine also contain sulphur. In addition to these other organic compounds such as heparin, glutathione, conzyme-A, lipoic acid, taurocholic acid also contain sulphur. Wool is rich in cystine and contains about 4 per cent sulphur. Keratin, the protein of hair, hoofs, etc., is rich in sulphur containing amino acids. Small amounts of inorganic sulphates, with sodium and potassium are present in blood and other tissues.

**Sources and Metabolism**

The main (if not the only) sources of sulphur for the body are the two sulphur containing amino acids as mentioned above. Elemental sulphur or sulphate is not known to be utilised. Organic sulphur is mainly oxidised to sulphate and excreted as inorganic sulphate. The metabolic importance of some sulphur-containing compounds reside in the easy interconvertibility of disulphide and sulphydryl groups in oxidation reduction reactions.

Deficiency of this element in the body is not usually considered, since the intake is mainly in the form of protein and a deficiency of sulphur would indicate a protein deficiency. However, in ruminant diets in which urea is used as a partial nitrogen replacement for protein nitrogen, sulphur may be limiting for the synthesis of cysteine, cystine and methionine. There is evidence that sodium sulphate can be used by the micro-organisms more efficiently than elemental sulphur.

## MAGNESIUM ($Mg^{++}$ at. wt. 24)

About 70 per cent of the total magnesium is found in the skeleton, the remainder being distributed in the soft tissues and fluids. The normal magnesium content of blood serum in cattle is within the range of 1.7 to 4 mg magnesium per 100 ml blood serum, but the levels below 1.7 frequently occur without clinical symptoms of disease.

**Functions**

1. An essential component of bone.
2. Magnesium ion activates enzymes like phosphatases and the phosphorylation reaction involving ATP. Among the later groups are glucokinase, phosphoglucokinase, creatine transphosphorylase, arginine transphosphorylase, etc.
3. Controls the irritability of neuromuscular system.

**Symptoms of Deficiency**

Symptoms due to a simple deficiency of magnesium in the diet have been reported for a number of animals. In rats fed on purified diets the symptoms include tetany which is exhibited by (a) redness of exposed skin surface, (b) hyperirritability, (c) cardiac arhythmia, (d) marked vasodilation.

In adult ruminants a condition known as *hypomagneseamic tetany* associated with low blood levels of magnesium has been recognised since the early thirties. The condition is known as *Grass tetany or Grass staggers* characterized by (a) convulsions, (b) hyperirritability, (c) twitching of the facial muscles, (d) staggering gait and ultimately tetany. Tetany is usually preceded by a fall in blood serum magnesium to amount 0.5 mg per 100 ml.

Symptoms can be reversed by injecting magnesium sulphate at an early time. but in practice this is sometimes difficult.

The exact cause of grass tetany is yet unknown, although a dietary deficiency may be a factor.

Some research workers consider that the condition may be caused by a cation-anion imbalance in the diet. Others suggest that soils which are heavily fertilized with $(NH_4)_2SO_4$ and when cattles are pastured on such soils develop the disease as ammonium interferes with absorption of magnesium. Still others suggest that excessive ruminal ammonia production may be the cause.

Experimental magnesium deficiency has been produced in dogs, rabbits, guinea pigs and chicks. In most cases the deficiency diseases are similar to those of rats and cattle. Magnesium deficient chicks grow slowly for about one week, then growth stops and they become lethargic.

**Source**

Green fodders, pericarp of cereal grains, bran, cotton seed cake and linseed cake are good sources of magnesium. When hypomagneseamic tetany is likely to occur it is generally considered that about 50 gm of magnesium oxide should be given to cows per day as a prophylactic measure.

## TRACE ELEMENTS

### IRON (Fe at. wt. 56)

About 65 per cent of the total body iron is present in the form of haemoglobin (which contains about 0.34 per cent of the element). Myoglobin accounts for another 4 per cent, 1 per cent in the form of various heme enzymes that control intracellular oxidation, 0.1 per cent in the form of transferrin in the blood plasma, 15 per cent stored in the form of ferritin or hemosiderin and 10–15 per cent probably in other forms. Broadly, iron is utilized in the body for (a) transport of oxygen to the tissues, (b) for maintenance of oxidative enzyme system within the tissue cells and (c) it is also concerned in melanin formation. Without all these important functions life would cease within a few seconds.

**Absorption from Gastrointestinal Tract**

Iron is present in most of the animal feed as in ferric iron ($Fe^{+++}$). It is reduced in the acid medium of the stomach to ferrous form ($Fe^{++}$), the form necessary for absorption. The metal is absorbed almost entirely in the upper part of the small intestine, mainly in the duodenum. By an active process it is absorbed probably as a complex with amino acids and is then carried to the mucosal cells of the intestine where it combines with a protein, *apoferritin*, to form *ferritin*.

Absorption is related to the requirements of the animal body. It is greatly increased if the body stores are reduced or the rate of formation of red blood cells are increased. In such cases, the iron portion of ferritin is more utilised and thus the mucosal cell becomes rich in apoferritin, which are further utilised to bind more and more of digested iron. When all the available apoferritin has become bound to iron form as ferritin, any additional iron that arrive at the binding site is rejected, returned back to the lumen of the gut and passes away for excretion. This means that the reserve ferritin present in mucosal cells correlates with body's need for iron. Thus, the two most important factors which control iron absorption are:

1. The state of iron stores in the body.
2. The state of the activity of the bone marrow.

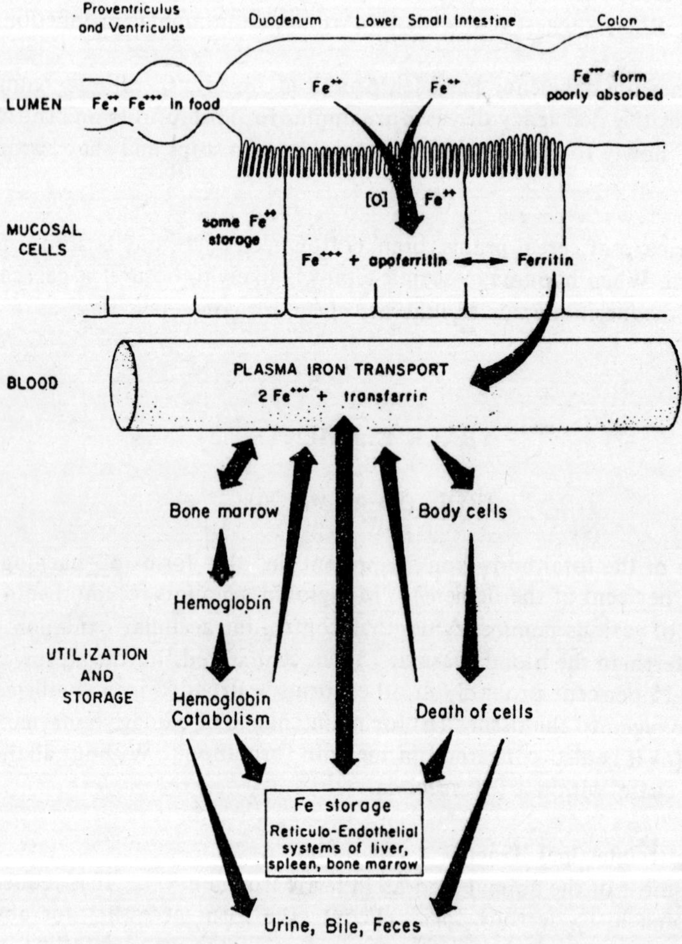


**Fig. 29** Iron Metabolism in Chicken

**Transport and Storage of Iron**

Mucosal ferritin delivers ferrous iron to the portal blood circulation. **Here the iron is again converted back to the ferric state by oxidation. As ferric iron it combines with a plasma $\beta_1$ globulin (carrier protein) to form a ferric-protein complex known as *Transferrin*. It serves a complex function since it must both *accept* iron that is being absorbed from the intestinal tract or from the degenerated red blood cells and *deliver* it to the bone marrow for haemoglobin synthesis, to reticuloendothelial cells for storage, to the placenta for foetal needs and to all other cells for the synthesis of iron containing enzymes.**

When the total quantity of iron in the body is more than the apoferritin storage pool can accommodate, some of it is stored in an extremely insoluble form called *hemosiderin.*

The body does not excrete iron. All the iron present in the plasma is bound to protein and this does not appear in the urine. An insignificant iron loss occurs in the desquamation of cells from the skin and from the epithelium of urinary and respiratory tracts. In human being the more important is the iron loss in the menstrual blood.

**Table 89**

BIOLOGICAL FUNCTIONS OF IRON COMPOUNDS[79]

| *Compounds* | *Main sources* | *Function* | *Mol. wt* | Fe *content* (g atom/mol) |
|---|---|---|---|---|
| Heme-containing compounds: | | | | |
| haemoglobin | Erythrocytes | Oxygen transport | 67000 | 4 |
| myoglobin | Skeletal muscles | Oxygen transport | 16500 | 1 |
| Heme-containing enzymes: | | | | |
| cytochrome oxidase (EC 1.9.3.1) | Heart muscle | Electron transfer | 290000 | 3 |
| cytochrome C | Heart muscle | Electron transfer | 12400 | 1 |
| catalase (EC 1.11.1.6) | Horse erythrocytes | Peroxide decomposition | 250000 | 4 |
| peroxidase (EC 1.11.1.7) | Horse radish | Peroxide decomposition | 40000 | 1 |
| Compounds which do not contain heme: | | | | |
| succinate dehydrogenase (EC 1.3.99.1) | Heart | Electron transfer | 200000 | 4 |
| reduced NAD dehydrogenase (EC 1.6.99.3) | Heart | Electron transfer | 550000 | 16–18 |
| xanthine oxidase | Milk | Electron transfer | 290000 | 8 |
| ferritin | Liver | Iron reserves | 450000 | 3000 |
| transferrin | Blood plasma | Transport of iron | 90000 | 2 |
| conalbumin | Egg white | Transport of iron | 87000 | 2 |

**Deficiency Symptoms**

A deficiency may result from inadequate intake (e.g., a high cereal diet, low in animal protein) or inadequate absorption, (e.g., gastrointestinal disturbances such as diarrhoea or intestinal disease) as well as from excessive loss of blood. Deficiency symptoms may be narrated as below:

1. Since more than half the iron present in the body occurs as haemoglobin, a dietary deficiency of iron would clearly be expected to effect the formation of this compound. The

red blood cells contain haemoglobin and in any interruption of haemoglobin formation will result in anemia. In pigs and chickens there is a development of microcytic (small red cell) and hypochromic anemia while in calves the anemia is of microcytic normochromic type.

2. Skin colour may be redden.
3. Decrease growth rate.

**Sources of Iron**

Green leafy materials, most leguminous plants and seed coats are excellent sources. Bone meal, glandular meal, liver and meat meal are other good sources.

## ZINC (Zn at. wt. 65)

Zinc has been found in every tissue in the animal body. The element tends to accumulate in the bones rather than the liver, which is the main storage organ of many of the other trace elements. Most of the zinc in blood is present in the erythrocyte. The element is poorly absorbed from the intestine, virtually all zinc in food being excreted in the faeces, and only small amount in the urine. The amount excreted in urine is not influenced significantly by the intake or by the concentration in the blood plasma, suggesting that the zinc contained in the urine is derived from metabolic processes in the kidney. Traces are present in bile and somewhat more in pancreatic juice and milk.

**Table 90**

ZINC METALLOENZYMES[79]

| *Enzymes* | *Designation* (EC) | *Cofactors of enzymes* | *Mol. wt.* | *g-atom Zn/mol* | *Source* |
|---|---|---|---|---|---|
| *Peptidases and esterases* | | | | | |
| Carboxypeptidase A | 3.4.2.1 | None | 34300 | 1 | Pancreas of cattle |
| Carboxypeptidase B | 3.4.2.2 | None | 34300 | 1 | Pancreas of pigs |
| Carbonic-anhydrase | 4.2.1.1 | None | 30000 | 1 | Erythrocytes of cattle |
| Alkaline phosphatase | 3.1.3.1 | None | 89000 | 4* | *Escherichia coli* |
| Neutral protease | | None | 44700 | 1–2 | *Bacillus subtilis* |
| Renal dipeptidase | | None | 47200 | 1 | Kidneys of pigs |
| *Dehydrogenases* | | | | | |
| Alcohol dehydrogenase | 1.1.1.1 | NAD | 150000 | 4 | Yeasts |
| Glutamate dehydrogenase | 1.4.1.2 | NAD | 1000000 | 2–6 | Liver of cattle |
| Maleic acid dehydrogenase | 1.1.1.3.7 | NAD | 40000 | 1 | Heart of cattle |
| D-lactate-cytochrome reductase | 1.1.2.4 | NAD | 50000 | 4–6 | Yeast |

* Two g-atoms are required for the catalytic activity of the enzyme; and the other two to maintain the quaternary structure of its molecule.

**Biochemical Functions**

Zinc is an integral part of the enzyme *carbonic anhydrase*, which is present in especially high concentration in the red blood cells. This enzyme is responsible for rapid combination of carbon dioxide with water in the red blood cells of the peripheral capillary blood and for rapid release of carbon dioxide from the pulmonary capillary blood into the alveoli of the lungs.

Zinc is also a component of *lactic dehydrogenase* and, therefore is important for the inter-conversions of pyruvic acid and lactic acid. Also, zinc is a component part of some *peptidases* and therefore is important for digestion of proteins in the gastrointestinal tract. High concentrations have been found in the skin, hair and wool of animals.

**Deficiency Symptoms**

1. Retarded growth
2. Disorders of the bones
3. Skin diseases
4. Disorders of the feathers and hair coat
5. Reduced efficiency of feed utilisation
6. Delayed sexual maturity, sterility and loss of fertility
7. Severe zinc deficiency also causes loss of appetite in swine, poultry and cattle
8. Parakeratosis (a skin disease characterized by sore and itchiness), a naturally occurring disease of pigs, cattle, has been shown to be due to zinc deficiency.
9. Leg abnormality in poultry is a common feature of zinc deficiency. The defect is characterised by stiff and unsteady gait, shortening and thickening of the leg bones, apparent failure of cartilage cell development in the epiphyseal plate region of the long bone.

**Sources**

The element is fairly well distributed. Wheat standard middlings, safflower seed oil meal, molasses, fish meal with solubles are rich sources. Yeast is another very good source.

## COPPER (Cu at. wt. 64)

Although Boutigny demonstrated the presence of copper in animals in 1833, its importance in nutrition was not recognised until Hart et al. (1928) of the University of Wisconsin showed that addition of both copper and iron is necessary for haemoglobin formation in rats suffering from anemia produced by feeding a milk diet. The role of copper appears to be that of a catalyst since it is not a part of the haemoglobin molecule. Soon after demonstration of the essential role of copper in haematopoiesis, several enzymes with oxidase functions were shown to contain copper. Among these are *tyrosinase*, *ascorbic acid oxidase* as well as uricase, which contains 550 micro gram of copper per gram of enzyme protein.

In the blood, copper is distributed approximately equal between erythrocytes and plasma, except in late pregnancy, when the concentration rises in the plasma. It is present in erythrocyte in the form of *erythrocuprein*. About 96 per cent of the plasma copper is firmly bound to an $\alpha$-2 globulin as *ceruloplasmin*, the form in which copper is transported in the body. *Cerebrocuprein* is another form of copper protein isolated from human brain by Porter and

Folch (1957). It differs from erythrocuprein in that the copper of cerebrocuprein reacts directly with diethyl dithiocarbamate.

Interest in copper nutrition was markedly increased when in the 1930's certain diseases of sheep and cattle in various parts of the world were shown to be due to copper deficiency. The first that copper deficiency is responsible for a disease known as "*salt sick*" in cattle came from Florida (U.S.A.). In 1933 a report from Holland showed that copper deficiency was responsible for the disease of sheep and cattle characterised by diarrhoea, loss of appetite and anemia, called "*Lechsucht*". Bennetts and Chapman (1937) in Australia showed that a disease of lambs called "*enzootic ataxia*" was due to a copper deficiency and could be prevented by feeding copper to the ewes during pregnancy. These studies led to an extensive mapping of the copper deficient areas in most parts of the world. In all copper deficient areas the situation was markedly similar, as follows: (*a*) Sheep and cattle failed to thrive unless supplied with extra copper, either directly or indirectly; (*b*) blood and liver of the copper deficient animals contained copper levels which were greatly below normal, and (*c*) the forages and the soils contained low levels of copper.

### Copper Content of the Body

A normal adult human contains approximately 100-150 mg of copper, or 1.5-2.0 ppm. Similar concentrations of copper occur in the bodies of the adult animal species. The body of the new born calf apparently is much richer in copper than that of any of the other species. By far the largest concentration of copper is in the liver. The liver copper level reflects the dietary intake; with high copper levels it may be increased manifold.

**Table 91**

COPPER-CONTAINING ANIMAL PROTEINS WITHOUT CATALYTIC PROPERTIES

| *Protein* | *Source* | *Molecular wt.* | *Copper content* (%) | *Copper content* (g-atom/mol) |
|---|---|---|---|---|
| Ceruloplasmin | Blood plasma | 160000 | 0.32 | 8 |
| Hemocuprin | Erythrocytes in cattle | 35000 | 0.34 | 2 |
| Erythrocuprin | Erythocytes in man | 33000 | 0.32-0.36 | 2 |
| Hepatocuprin | Liver of mammals | - | 0.34 | - |
| Cerebrocuprin | Brain of cattle | 30000 | 0.29 | 2 |
| Mitochondrocuprin | Liver of newborn calves | - | 3-5 | - |

### Deficiency Diseases

1. *Spontaneous fracture of bone*. Bone defects in grazing cattle and sheep on copper deficient pastures are characterized by spontaneous fracture and a condition very similar to rickets in young calves and osteoporosis in older animals.

2. *Demyelination of the central nervous system*. Severe ataxias have occurred in lambs and calves in various parts of the world and is known as *Sway back* or *Swing back* or *Gingin rickets* or

*Enzootic neonatal ataxia.* The last name has been widely accepted throughout the world. Two types of neonatal ataxia are now recognised in lambs: (1) a common acute form occurs in new born lambs and (2) a delayed type often occurs in which clinical symptoms are not observed for several weeks or sometimes months after birth. In both diseases the symptoms are characterised by spastic paralysis, incoordination of the hind legs, a stiff and staggering gait and an exaggerated swaying of the hind quarters. Some lambs are completely paralyzed or ataxic at birth and die immediately.

3. *Pigmentation and structure of hair and wool.* A syndrome consisting of achromotrichia, alopecia and dermatitis is the most sensitive index of copper deficiency in the rabbit occurring even before a pronounced anemia. In sheep, copper deficiency produces a lack of black wooled sheep, and characteristic loss of "*crimp*" from the fibers of all wool. This has been found in Merino sheep, which normally have a crimpy wool, grow relatively straight when allowed to graze on copper-deficient fields. Copper content of the wool is decreased but more interesting is an increase in sulphydryl groups and a decrease in disulphide linkages, which likely accounts for change in protein structure and change from crimpy to straight wool.

4. *Fibrosis of the myocardium.* A disease condition in cattle in Australia known locally as "*falling disease*", characterised by sudden death, usually without any preliminary signs. The anemia associated with 'falling disease' is of the macrocytic hypochromic type. The disease appears to be interrelated with complicating factors since it disappears spontaneously in each summer in spite of continued very low copper intake.

5. "*Scouring*" (*diarrhoea*) *in cattle.* Severe diarrhoea has been observed in many parts of the world. In Holland it was called "*scouring disease*", and in New Zealand, "*peat scours*". Scouring is known to be accentuated in areas containing excess molybdenum and low amounts of copper. In high molybdenum areas it has been believed to be due to molybdenum toxicosis and is referred to as "*teart*".

6. *Aortic rupture.* Recently in the University of Missouri (U.S.A.), it has been found that copper deficiency in chicks produces dissecting aneurysm of the aorta and various bone deformities, all in all resembling lathyrism.

7. *Decreased reporductive capacity and milk production.* Many experimental reports are accumulating to show the above effect on copper deficiency states.

**Source**

Under normal conditions the diet of farm animals is likely to contain adequate amounts. Copper level of the soil is an index of the copper content of the corps. Liver and glandular meal contains about 90 ppm. Among other good sources, cron distillers dried solubles, dried whey, peanut meal, cotton seed meal and fish meal are noteworthy.

## MANGANESE (Mn at. wt. 55)

Kemmerer, Elvehjem and Hart (1931) were probably the first to demonstrate manganese to be an essential element in nutrition. A diet composed exclusively of milk cause poor growth and poor reproduction in mice which were corrected by supplementing the diet with manganese. It was soon found that manganese is also required by the rat and that high mortality, testicular degeneration and poor lactation accompany manganese deficiency. Interest in manganese nutrition was greatly stimulated by the discovery of Wilgus, Norris Heuser (1936) that a deficiency of this element was responsible for a crippling disease of chickens known as "*perosis*" or "*slipped tendon*".

The highest concentration of manganese is in bone followed by pituitary gland, pineal gland, lactating mammary gland, liver, gastrointestinal tissue, kidney and pancreas. Blood contains about 12-18 micro gram, about 2/3rd of which is in the blood cells. An interesting observation has been that lactating gland of the rabbit contains about ten times as much manganese as the non-lactating tissue, significance not known.

**Absorption of Manganese**

Absorption and final excretion of manganese appears to depend upon formation of natural chelates, (the word 'chelate' is taken from the Greek word *chele* meaning "claw") which is a fairly good descriptive term for the manner in which polyvalent cations are held by the metal binding agents. A metal chelate is formed as a ring structure produced by attraction between the positive charges of certain polyvalent cations and any two or more sites of high electronegative activity in a chemical compound. The bonds are known as "coordinate" bonds and occur because of peculiarities in the electron shells of the transition metals, specially chelates with bile salts. It is excreted in the faeces primarily via the bile and is probably reabsorbed as bile bound manganese. It appears likely that each manganese atom may recirculate several times before it is finally excreted. Therefore, manganese in the gastrointestinal tract represents a manganese pool which is in more rapid equilibrium with the tissues than it is with the outside environment. Excretion rate is effected by the presence of diet and not by the presence of other metal ions.

**Biochemical Functions**

1. Manganese has been reported to be effective in the *in vitro* activation of the following enzymes: Arginase, cysteine desulphydrase, thiaminase, deoxyribonuclease, enolase, intestinal prolinase and glycyl-L-leucine dipeptidase.

It is also thought to be required for (1) oxidative phosphorylation in mitochondria; (2) fatty acid synthesis (as a manganese chelate of acetoacetyl-S-coenzyme-A); (3) acetate incorporation into cholesterol and mucopolysaccharide synthesis.

2. Manganese metabolism is believed to be involved in amino acid metabolism, not only because of its activation of some of the hydrolysing enzymes (i.e., arginase), but also because it forms chelates with amino acid in which pyridoxal may participate. These complexes of amino acid, pyridoxal and manganese are transported in the body more rapidly than are amino acids alone. This links protein metabolism to manganese turnover.

3. Wakil *et al.* (1957) have demonstrated that manganese is an activator in the synthesis of fatty acids *in vitro*. It has also been found that manganese is involved in mucopolysaccharide synthesis and bone matrix cell maturation in chicks. Lastly it is believed that manganese also has a direct effect upon calcification.

**Deficiency Diseases**

Symptoms of manganese deficiency in mammals (rats, mice, rabbits) are similar but not identical. The nature and severity of symptoms depend upon the previous nutritional history of the experimental animals, specially the carryover of manganese from the mother and the manganese content of the diet prior to being placed on manganese deficient diets. Manganese deficiency in these animals is characterised by reduced growth, slightly reduced mineralisation, defective structure of the bones and decreased reproductive performance in both males and females.

In chicks the most dramatic manganese deficiency syndrome occurs which is termed as "*perosis*" and is characterized by gross enlargement and malformation of the tibiometatarsal joint, twisting and bending of the distal end of the tibia, and the proximal end of the tarsometatarsus, thickening and shortening of the leg bones and slippage of the gastrocnemius or Achilles tendon from its condyles. The disease is markedly aggravated by high intakes of calcium and phosphorus which is due to the absorption of manganese by precipitated calcium phosphate in the intestinal tract. Thus manganese is rendered into unabsorbable form.

**Source**

Whole rice is wonderful, contains about 420 ppm, this quality deteriorates when the rice is made polished (18 ppm). All other cereals contain moderate amounts, except for maize which is low in the element. Most green foods contain adequate amounts.

## IODINE (I at. wt. 127)

As early as 1820, a Swiss physician, J. Francois, Coindet, first recommended iodine as a remedy for goiter—a disease results in a swelling of the thyroid gland. As far as is known the role of iodine in the animal body is related solely to its function as a constituent of thyroxine and other related compounds synthesized by the thyroid gland. Hence, a deficiency of iodine first causes the structural and then physiological abnormalities of thyroid gland and thereby affect entire animal body.

The adult animal body contains less than 0.6 parts per million of iodine, one third of which is concentrated in the thyroid gland, the rest is present in all tissues; next to the thyroids, ovary, muscle and blood tend to have the highest concentration.

**Absorption and Formation of Thyroid Hormone**

The element is absorbed as iodide from any portion of the alimentary tract, most readily perhaps from the small intestine. On reaching the thyroid gland iodide is quickly oxidized to

**Table 92**

IODINE CONTENT IN ORGANS AND TISSUES OF CALVES[75]

| *Tissue* | *Content* (μg% fresh tissue) |
|---|---|
| Whole blood | 6.3–7.8 |
| Blood serum | 6.1–7.4 |
| Hair | 1.7–3.2* |
| Hide | 2.7–4.0* |
| Liver | 8.0–8.1 |
| Kidneys | 7.0–7.2 |
| Lungs | 5.0–5.2 |
| Thyroid gland | 24–38† |

* Depending on the iodine content in the diet.
† mg% fresh tissue.

iodine and bound to the tyrosine molecules of thyroglobulin a glycoprotein. In the thyroglobulin molecule, iodine is present primarily as (*i*) 3-monoiodotyrosine; (*ii*) 3,5-diiodotyrosine; (*iii*) 3,5,3,5-tetraiodothyronine (thyroxine) and (*iv*) 3,5,3-triiodothyronine. On hydrolysis of thyroglobulin, thyroxine and other iodinated compounds are released into the blood stream.

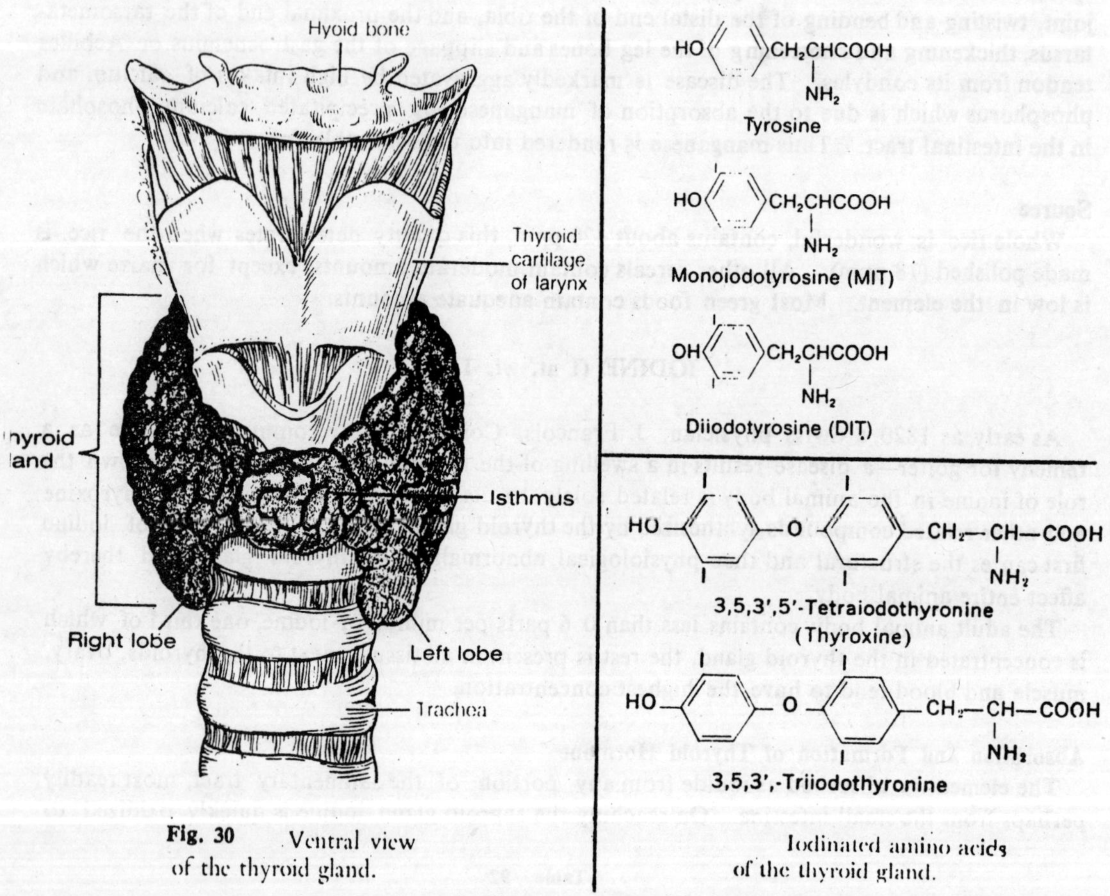


**Fig. 30** Ventral view of the thyroid gland.

Iodinated amino acids of the thyroid gland.

## Metabolic Functions

The functions of thyroxine and thyronine and therefore of iodine are as follows:

1. Exercises control of the rate of energy metabolism or level of oxidation of all cells (calorigenic effect).
2. Influences physical and mental growth and differentiation or maturation of tissues.
3. Affects other endocrine glands, especially the hypophysis and the gonads.
4. Influences neuromuscular functioning.
5. Affects circulatory dynamics.

6. Thyroxine has an effect on the integument and its outgrowths, hair, fur, and feathers.
7. Influences the metabolism of food nutrients, including various minerals and water.

In cold blooded animals thyroid hormone action is manifested mainly by (1) an effect on the differentiation and function of the nervous system, (2) an effect on the skin and its derivatives, and (3) a role in metamorphosis.

**Symptoms of Deficiency**

Iodine deficiency is characterised by endemic goiter, resulting in cretinism and myxedima. Iodine deficiency greatly retards general growth, including a delayed osseous development which results in dwarfism in humans known as "*cretinism*". Severe deprivation of iodine is accompanied by a delay in almost all developmental processes. There is retarded mental development in the young and mental dullness and apathy in both young and old. *Myxedima* is characterized by a dropsy-like swelling (edema), specially of the face and hands, slow pulse rate, dryness and wrinkling of the skin, falling of hair and dulling of mental activity.

**Sources**

Foods of marine origin are very rich in iodine. Among common animal feeds, fish meal, meat and bone meal, molasses are the richest sources. Synthetic iodized salts are more commonly used by the farmers.

## COBALT (Co at. wt. 59)

The first evidence that cobalt is an essential mineral nutrient for ruminants came from a group of Australian investigators, (Lines, 1935; Marston, 1935; Underwood and Filmer, 1935).

A number of disorders of cattle and sheep characterized by an emaciation and listness typical of mal-nutrition have been recognized for many years and have given a variety of local names, some of which are descriptive of the disease and some of which merely reflect the district or area in which the deficiency occurs. Thus the disease was known as *bush sickness* in New Zealand, *coast disease* in South Australia, *wasting disease* in western Australia, *nakuruitis* in Kenya, *pining* in Great Britain etc. The most appropriate scientific designation for all these conditions is *enzootic marusmus.* All these names clearly indicate the occurrence of cobalt deficiency in many areas of the world including Australia, New Zealand, U.S.A., Canada, middle and northern Europe, and many parts of Asia.

Progress in understanding the mode of action of cobalt in the animal organism was slow until after the discovery that the anti-pernicious anemia factor in liver, subsequently designated vitamin $B_{12}$, is a cobalt compound containing almost 4 per cent of the metal. Within three years of that discovery complete remission of all signs of cobalt deficiency in lambs was secured with parenteral injections of vitamin $B_{12}$. Thus it has been proved that cobalt deficiency in ruminants is actually a vitamin $B_{12}$ deficiency brought about by the inability of the rumen micro-organisms, in the lack of dietary cobalt, to synthesize sufficient vitamin $B_{12}$ to meet the need of ruminant tissues for the vitamin. The other function of cobalt in animal nutrition has so far been demonstrated as the activating ion in certain enzyme reactions.

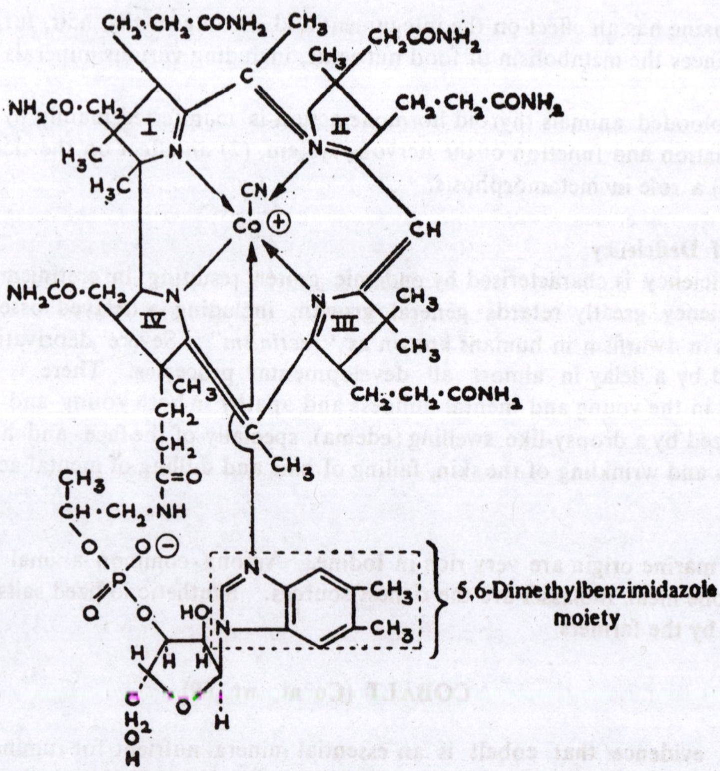

Cobalt as a component of Vitamin $B_{12}$ (Cyanocobalamin)

5,6-Dimethylbenzimidazole moiety

**Deficiency Symptoms in Ruminants**

The syndrome of cobalt deficiency in sheep, goat and cattle is essentially that of starvation. There is a gradual wasting of the animals. With this, there develops the usual straggly, rough wool in sheep, severe anemia with almost complete appetite failure. As the condition becomes more advanced, the animal is dull, listless, and because of the anemia all the exposed skin surface around the eyes and mouth take on a blanched or pale anemic look. The oxygen carrying capacity of the blood is markedly reduced and the blood volume may be severely reduced. There is a total absence of body fat, on the other hand the liver becomes fatty. As the cobalt deficiency state progresses the concentration of cobalt and vitamin $B_{12}$ decline to subnormal levels in the liver and kidneys (which are the main sites of vitamin $B_{12}$ storage). The levels of vitamin $B_{12}$ in the blood serum also decline significantly below those of normal animals.

**Prevention and Control**

Cobalt deficiency in ruminants can be cured or prevented through treatment of the soils or pastures with cobalt-containing fertilizers. It has been found that single dressings of cobalt sulphate at the rate of 4 oz. to 8 oz. per acre raised the cobalt content of pasture from 0.04 to 0.19 and 0.39 ppm respectively.

**The provision of salt licks containing about 0.1 per cent cobalt is a satisfactory procedure.**

**Sources**

**Although all plants and animal materials commonly used in the feeding of farm animals contain cobalt in trace amounts, but in general the legumes are richer sources. This also depends on the amount of cobalt in the soil. Cereal grains are poor in cobalt. Among animal feeds except the livermeal which may contain 0.2 ppm or more, the rest are mostly poor sources of cobalt. The cobalt content of milk and milk products is even lower, although it is possible to increase the cobalt of cow's milk several-fold by heavy supplementation of the cow's diet with cobalt salts. Normal pastures have a cobalt content in the dry matter within the range 0.1 to 0.25 mg/kg.**

**Cobalt Toxicity**

**Cobalt salts are not particularly toxic to animals, and there is wide margin between the levels which may be administered to prevent deficiency conditions. Unlike copper, cobalt is poorly retained by the body tissues and the excess will always be eliminated from the body. The toxic level of cobalt for cattle is 40 to 50 mg. cobalt per 100 lb. body weight daily. Sheep are less susceptible to cobalt toxicosis.**

## MOLYBDENUM (Mo at. wt. 96)

**Although molybdenum has been known for several decades to be toxic when consumed in excessive amounts, knowledge of its nutritional essentiality stemmed from the fact that two enzymes of the animal tissues, (1) xanthine oxidase and (2) liver aldehyde oxidase contain molybdenum as an essential part of the molecule. Xanthine oxidases catalyse the oxidation of many different substrates including purines, aldehydes pterins and reduced diphosphopyridine nucleotide (NADH). The level of these enzymes in the tissues have been shown to be affected by the levels of dietary molybdenum.**

**Table 93**

MOLYBDENUM-CONTAINING ENZYMES

| *Enzyme* | *Designation (EC)* | *Other cofactors* | *Substrate* | *Product* |
|---|---|---|---|---|
| Xanthine oxidase | 1.2.3.1 | FAD, Fe | Xanthine, purines | Uric acid |
| Aldehyde oxidase | 1.2.3.1 | FAD, Fe | RCHO | RCOOH |
| Assimilatory citrate reductase | 1.9.6.1 | FAD, cytochrome B | $NO_3^-$ | $NO_2^-$ |
| Respiratory nitrate reductase | 1.9.6.1 | FAD, cytochrome C | $NO_3^-$ | $O_2^-$ |
| Nitrogenase | | ? | $N_2$ | $NH_3$ |

**A nutritional role of molybdenum has also been demonstrated in young lambs, where addition**

of the element as molybdate to a diet low in molybdenum increased liveweight gains. Similar growth stimulating effect have been observed in chicks and poults. Although in animal body about 1 to 4 ppm of molybdenum has been found but yet the amount required per day in the diets of the animal have not been worked out.

The effects of excess molybdenum in cattle, however, have been known for almost 30 years. A condition in cattle known for a long time in England as *"teartness"* has been identified as a molybdenum poisoning. It occurs when the forage contains 0.002 per cent or more of the element. Recently, potentially toxic levels in soils and forages have also been found in Canada and in New Zealand where the clinical toxicity is known as "peat scours".

The chief symptoms of molybdenum poisoning are extreme diarrhoea and consequent weight losses, and a decreases in production. The diarrhoea due to molybdenum poisoning can be restored by the administration of copper sulphate. The interrelationship between molybdenum and copper is as follows:

In the normal metabolism of both ruminant and monogastric animals, there is an antagonism between molybdenum and copper which is markedly affected by the sulphur content of the diet. It was shown that sheep on a low molybdenum diet (less than 0.1 ppm dry weight) rapidly accumulated copper in their livers resulting in a typical copper toxicity. Conversely, when the diet is high in molybdenum (5 ppm) sheep may develop a clinical copper deficiency. Sulphate administration also results in an increased excretion of molybdenum in the faeces, suggesting a reduction in the rate of molybdenum absorption from the gut.

**Sources**

| | *Molybdenum (ppm)* | | |
|---|---|---|---|
| Cabbage | 1.00 | Peas | 1.40 |
| Liver and glandular meal | 1.80 | Alfalfa meal (dehydrated) | 0.35 |
| Soyabeans, whole | 2.50 | Cereals | trace or nil. |

## CHROMIUM (Cr at. wt. 24)

The amount of chromium in body tissue is maximum at birth, falls quite rapidly during the early years of life and then levels off throughout the rest of life.

Schwarz and Mertz of Maryland in U.S.A. as early as in 1959 have reported that chromium in the trivalent form ($Cr^{+++}$) is needed for the normal glucose utilization. The importance lies in the fact that trivalent chromium acts as a cofactor with insulin at the cellular level, through the formation of a complex with membrane sites, insulin and chromium.

In the metabolism of lipids chromium might have got a significant role since it has been observed that when chromium is added to low chromium diets it reduces the level of serum cholesterol.

Similarly chromium also involves in protein metabolism. Rats fed diets having deficiency in protein and chromium showed an irregularities during incorporation of certain amino acids, such as methionine, serine, etc., into the protein of their hearts.

## FLUORINE (F at. wt. 9)

Fluorine as fluoride is present in various tissues of the body, particularly in bone and teeth. Normal bone contains 0.01 to 0.04 per cent of fluorine as an integral part of the molecule and thus is an essential mineral.

**Physiological Functions**

(1) By combining with calcium phosphate, fluorine hardens tooth enamel and so helps to guard against tooth decay.

(2) It enhances growth in rats: 2.5 ppm of fluoride in the diet produce an optimal rate of growth in this species.

(3) In adults the osteoporosis is retarded by fluorine.

*Absorption and excretion.* About 90 per cent of the dietary fluorine is absorbed from the small intestine although large amounts of dietary calcium, aluminium and fat will depress its uptake. Excess amount of plasma fluorine which could not be deposited in bones and teeth is excreted in the urine, with the result that the level of fluoride in blood plasma is quite constant. At the time of low intake, the plasma level is maintained from the release of fluorine from bones and teeth.

*Deficiency symptoms.* Excess of fluorine are more of a concern than are deficiencies in livestock production because of its presence at moderate concentrations in the forages and in drinking water; also because of its presence at high (3-4 per cent) levels in variety of natural phosphate sources.

The only reported fluorine deficiency have been noted in children in the form of excessive dental caries.

*Supplementation.* No need has ever been felt for supplementing livestock with fluorine since most, if not all, livestock rations seem to contain adequate amount of fluorine. In case of real necessity, addition of 1 ppm to the drinking water should suffice.

*Toxicity.* The element at higher concentration is very much toxic to all classes of livestock. It has been estimated that a level in the diet above 20 mg per kg of the dry matter or from 8 to 9 mg of fluorine per kilo of body weight given to cattle causes a condition described as "Fluorosis". in which the following symptoms have been noted.

1. Teeth become pitted and worn until the pulp cavities are exposed.
2. Drastic reduction in appetite
3. Disturb osseous metabolism
4. Causes fatty degeneration
5. Inhibit certain enzymes concerned with carbohydrate and lipid metabolism (e.g., glucose-6-phosphate dehydrogenase, ATPases, lipase, alkaline phosphatase).

*Note.* Mineral mixture containing rock phosphate might carry more than 0.1 per cent fluorine. Their use should be made after defluorination.

## SELENIUM (Se at. wt. 34)

It has been confirmed in 1935 by the scientists of South Dakota Experiment Station, U.S.A.

that selenium of forages causes toxicity by promoting alkali disease or blind staggers in cattle. Interest in selenium was enhanced greatly by the discovery in 1957 that selenium in traces (0.05 to 0.2 ppm) is an essential nutrient despite its toxicity in larger intakes. Animals grazing on certain soils suffered from retarded growth and reproduction troubles which could be overcome by the feeding of traces of the element. M.L. Scott and associate of Cornell University have confirmed that selenium at a level of approximately 0.15 ppm is required for prevention of dietary liver necrosis in vitamin E deficient rats, exudative diathesis in vitamin E deficient chicks, and also for pancreatic degeneration of chicks.

**Types of Selenium Compounds**

The most common inorganic forms of selenium are selenic acid, selenates and selenites, which are the selenium analogues of sulphuric acid, sulphurous acid, sulphates and sulphites. Plants and micro-organisms have been shown to be able to replace the sulphur in cystine, and methionine with selenium, thereby producing selenocystine and selenomethionine.

In ruminants a large percentage of the ingested selenium appears to be incorporated by the rumen micro-organisms into the selenoanalogues of cystine and methionine. These may be absorbed by the animals and deposited in the tissues in the form of selenoamino acids.

**Absorption, Transport and Excretion of Selenium Compounds.** Inorganic selenite and selenocystine are absorbed for the intestine by passive processes whereas selenomethionine is absorbed by an active transport mechanism.

After absorption the compound gets binded with $\alpha_2$ and $\beta_1$ globulin fractions of the plasma. From this selenium binding protein, selenium is then transferred to erythrocytes (RBC). Uptake by the erythrocytes is influenced by adequate intracellular reduced glutathione.

Selenium intake in excess of that which can be bound by proteins are methylated. In mammals this methylation occurs in two steps: (1) formation of dimethyl selenide; and (2) further conversion of dimethyl selenide to trimethyl selenonium ion which is water soluble and represents the normal excretory product of moderate excess of dietary selenium. At the time of excess intake, the transformation of dimethyl to trimethyl stops at certain stage and then the dimethyl selenide, being a volatile compound is excreted through expired air imparting a garlic odour to the breath.

**Physiological Functions**

1. Acts as non-specific antioxidant,
2. Protects against peroxidation in tissues and membranes,
3. Participates in the biosynthesis of ubiquinone,
4. Participates in hydrogen transport along the respiratory chain.
5. Prevents degeneration and fibrosis of the pancreas in chicks.
6. Selenium influences the absorption and retention of vitamin E and of triglycerides in at least three ways:
   (a) It is required to preserve the integrity of the pancreas, which in turn allows normal fat digestion, normal lipid-bile salt micelle formation, and thus normal vitamin E absorption.
   (b) Since selenium is an integral part of the enzyme, *glutathione peroxidase* (0.34 per cent of selenium), this converts reduced glutathione to oxidized glutathione and at the

same time destroys peroxides by converting them to harmless aocohols.

$$\underset{(A)}{2GSH} + \underset{\text{Peroxide}}{H_3O_2} \longrightarrow GSSG + 2H_2O$$

Thus a portion of reduced glutathione (A) is spent to destroy the toxic compound peroxide. In the same way it also destroys fatty acid hydroperoxides (general structure ROOH) through reactions catalyzed by the glutathione peroxidase as below.

$$2GSH + ROOH \longrightarrow GSSG + ROH + H_2O$$

This prevention of attack by peroxides upon the polyunsaturated fatty acids of the lipid membranes of cells thus greatly reduces the requirement of Vitamin E.

Oxidised glutathione is again regenerated by the activity of the enzyme glutathione reductase

$$GSSG \xrightarrow[NADPH + H^+ \text{——} NADP^+]{\text{(Glutathione reductase)}} 2\ GSH$$

(c) Selenium acids in some unknown way in the retention of vitamin E in the blood plasma.

*Note.* Vitamin E reduces selenium requirement in at least two ways:

(a) By maintaining body selenium in an active form or by preventing its loss from the body.

(b) By preventing a chain reactive auto-oxidation of the lipid membranes thereby inhibiting the production of hydroperoxides. This reduces the amount of selenium containing glutathione peroxidase needed to destroy the peroxides formed in the cells.

**Toxicity**

Selenium poisoning afflicts grazing animals if the forage contains 5 ppm or more of the element, or if the plants consume by the animals are grown on soil containing more than 0.5 ppm of selenium. Within plants grown on seleniferous soil, the highest concentration of selenium is in the leaves; less is found in the stem and still less in the seed.

The mechanisms by which selenium experts its toxic effects in animals appear to be through its competition with sulphur compounds or because of its strong affinity for sulphur in the formation of sulphur-selenium complexes.

The symptoms of selenium poisoning disease *Alkali disease* (blind staggers) which occur in horses cattle and sheep are as follows:

1. Dullness and lack of vitality,
2. Emaciation and roughness of haircoat,
3. Loss of hair,
4. Grating of teeth,
5. Stiffness of the joints and lameness,
7. Paralysis of the swallowing and respiratory mechanism.

*Note*: Certain species of plants contain 10-30 mg/kg of selenium and are potentially dangerous for the grazing animals.

Table 94

THERAPEUTIC EFFECT OF SELENIUM

| *Pathological symptoms* | *Rats* | *Mice* | *Rabbits* | *Minks* | *Piglets* | *Sheep* | *Calves* | *Foals* | *Chicks* | *Turkey poults* |
|---|---|---|---|---|---|---|---|---|---|---|
| Muscular dystrophy | ++ | +++ | +++ | + | +++ | +++ | +++ | +++ | ++ | ++ |
| Myocarditis | + | +++ | + | +++ | + | +++ | +++ | + | ++ | + |
| Liver necrosis | +++ | +++ | +++ | ++ | +++ | + | + | + | ++ | + |
| Kidney necrosis | +++ | +++ | – | +++ | – | – | – | – | – | – |
| Impaired growth | ++ | ++ | – | – | +++ | +++ | +++ | ++ | +++ | ++ |
| Exudative diathesis | = | = | = | = | = | = | = | = | +++ | +++ |
| Atrophy of the pancreas | +++ | +++ | – | – | – | – | – | – | – | – |
| Lung haemorrhages | ++ | + | +++ | – | – | – | – | – | – | – |
| Anaemia | + | + | + | + | + | ++ | ++ | + | +++ | +++ |
| Parodontosis | ++ | ++ | – | – | – | ++ | – | – | – | – |
| Calcification | +++ | – | – | – | – | +++ | +++ | – | – | – |
| Change in blood serum ratio | ++ | +++ | – | – | – | – | – | – | +++ | +++ |

Symbols: +++ high therapeutic effect; ++ moderate prophylactic effect; + selenium compound was not invariably active; – selenium studies were not carried out; = disease is not encountered.

**Sources:** Selenium is widely distributed in the animal body and is found in highest concentration in the kidney cortex, pancreas, pituitary and liver. The amount of selenium in feedstuffs is highly variable, due largely to differences in soil selenium content in the areas where feed is grown. Fish meal contains a good amount of selenium (1.2 to 5 μg/gram).

**Relationship to Vitamin E**

Some of the disorders of animals induced by dietary means are responsive either to selenium or to Vitamin E, indicating that a close relationship exists between the two nutrients. However, certain diseases are apparently caused by a deficiency which responds specifically to one nutrient but not to the other. The role of selenium in hydroperoxide destruction through glutathione peroxidase activity, serves to clarify the interrelationships between vitamin E and cystine as a precursor of glutathione.

If vitamin E prevents fatty acid hydroperoxide formation, and the sulphur containing amino acids (as precursors of glutathione) and selenium are involved in peroxide breakdown, all of these nutrients would obviously lead to a similar biochemical results, i.e., lowering in the tissues of the concentrations of peroxides or products induced by them. Certain tissues or subcellular components that are inherently low in glutathione peroxidase would not be affected by selenium, but would still be protected by Vitamin E, which acts as an antioxidant by a mechanism not involving glutathione peroxidase.

## VITAMINS

When animals are maintained on a chemically defined diet containing only purified proteins, carbohydrates, and fats, and the necessary minerals, it is not possible to sustain life. Additional factors present in natural foods are required, although often only minute amounts are necessary. These "accessory food factors" are called vitamins. A vitamin is now generally accepted to be an organic compound which (*a*) is component of natural food but distinct from carbohydrates, fat, protein, and water; (*b*) is present in normal foods in minute amounts; (*c*) essential for development of normal tissue and for normal health, growth and maintenance; (*d*) when absent from the diet or not properly absorbed or utilized, causes a specific deficiency disease or syndrome; and (*e*) cannot be synthesized by the host and therefore must be obtained either from the diet or from the micro-organisms of the intestinal tract. The latter characteristic distinguishes a vitamin from a hormone; it is possible, however, that a substance may be a vitamin in one species and a hormone for ano her. Ascorbic acid, for example, is a vitamin for man, monkeys, and guinea pigs, but may be called a hormone in all other animals since they are capable of producing it by biosynthesis.

The vitamins have no chemical resemblance to each other, but because of a similar general function in metabolism they are considered together.

Early studies of the vitamins emphasized the more obvious pathologic changes which

**Table 95**

**Some typical differences between fat and water soluble B vitamins**

| *Fat soluble vitamins* | *Water soluble B vitamins* |
|---|---|
| **1. Chemical composition** | |
| The group contains only carbon, hydrogen and oxygen. | Along with carbon, hydrogen and oxygen the group also contains either nitrogen, sulphur or cobalt. |
| **2. Occurrence** | |
| Fat soluble vitamins can occur in plant tissue in the form of a provitamin, which can be converted into vitamin in the animal body. | No provitamins are known for any water soluble B vitamins. |
| Vitamins are not universally distributed rather are completely absent from some tissues. | Water soluble B vitamins are universally distributed in every living tissues. |

Table 95 (*Contd.*)

| *Fat soluble vitamins* | *Water soluble B vitamins* |
|---|---|
| **3. Physiological action** | |
| **The members of this group are required for the regulation of the metabolism of structural units and each member appears to have one or more specific and independent roles.** | **Water soluble B vitamins almost collectively concerned with the transfer of energy in every cell.** |
| **4. Absorption** | |
| **Absorbed from the intestinal tract in the presence of fat and thus related with factors which govern fat absorption.** | **In general, the absorption is a simple process as there is a constant absorption of water from the intestine.** |
| **5. Storage** | |
| **Any of the fat soluble vitamins can be stored wherever fat is deposited. The amount to be stored depends upon the intake.** | **Water soluble B vitamins are not stored in the same way or to the same extent.** |
| **6. Excretion** | |
| **Members of this group are excreted usually through faeces.** | **The water soluble B vitamins may also be present in the faeces (though sometimes only because of bacterial synthesis) but their chief pathway of excretion following metabolic use is through urine.** |

occurred when animals were maintained on vitamin deficient diets. Increased knowledge of the physiologic role of each vitamin has enabled attention to be concentrated on the metabolic defects which occur when these substances are lacking. and we may therefore refer to the biochemical changes as well as to the anatomical lesions which are characteristic of the various vitamin deficiency states.

Before the chemical structures of the vitamins were known it was customary to identify these substances by letters of the alphabet (A, B, C, etc.). This system is gradually being replaced by a nomenclature based on the chemical nature of the compound or a description of its source or function.

The vitamins are generally divided into two major groups: fat soluble and water soluble. The fat soluble vitamins, which are usually found associated with the lipids of natural foods, include vitamins A, D, E, and K. The vitamins of the B complex and vitamin C comprise the water soluble group.

Vitamin C is the only member of the water soluble group that is not a member of the B family and its functions and characteristics are so different from the B vitamins that it requires special discussion. Consequently while making a differential study between fat and water soluble vitamins (Table 96) the consideration of Vitamin C has been excluded.

Table 96

**Summary of the metabolic activities of vitamins**

| *Vitamin* | *Metabolic activity* | *Deficiency symptoms* |
|---|---|---|
| **Lipid Soluble** | | |
| Vitamin A (Retinol, Retinal and Retinoic acid) | 1. Oxidation-reduction activity, visual cycle<br>2. Necessary for normal synthesis of chondrotin sulphate | Cattle and pigs—skin conditions, xerophthalmia.<br>Poultry—retarded growth, high mortality. |
| Vitamin D ($D_2$=ergocalciferol, $D_3$=cholecalciferol) | 1. Absorption of calcium from intestine<br>2. Necessary for calcification of bone matrix | Young animals—rickets; old animals—osteomalacia. |
| Vitamin E (α-tocopherol) | 1. Inhibits autoxidation of unsaturated fatty acids | Most animals fail to reproduce young cattle and lambs—muscle degeneration—chick — cerebra degeneration. |
| Vitamin K (Phylloquinine) | 1. Necessary for the hepatic synthesis of proconvertin | Chicks—delayed clotting time of blood. |
| **Water Soluble** | | |
| Thiamine ($B_1$) | 1. Decarboxylation of pyruvic acid<br>2. Transketolase reaction of hexosemonophosphate shunt | Emaciation, weakness, and nervous disorders (polyneuritis of chicks and Chastek paralysis of foxes) |
| Riboflavin ($B_2$) | 1. Biosynthesis of flavin nucleotide (FAD, FMN)<br>2. Used in oxidation-reduction reactions | Pigs—retarded growth, skin, conditions, eye diseases; chicks—curled toe paralysis. |
| Nicotinamide | 1. Component of pyrimidine nucleotides (DPN and TPN)<br>2. Necessary for biological oxidation-reduction | Pigs—Poor growth, enteritis, dermatitis; dogs—black tongue |
| Vitamin $B_6$ (Pyridoxine, Pyridoxal Pyridoxanine) | 1. Amino acid metabolism<br>2. Active transport across cell membrane | Pigs—anemia and convulsions<br>Chicks—slow growth, convulsions |
| Pantothenic acid | 1. Component of acetylcoenzyme A<br>2. Acyl carrier protein | Pigs—slow growth, skin conditions, "goose step": chicks—slow growth, dermatitis |
| Folic acid | 1. Co-factor in "active methyl" or one carbon metabolism | Rare in farm animals but will cause anemia and poor growth |
| Choline | 1. Necessary for synthesis of lecithin<br>2. Lipid metabolism | Slow growth, fatty livers |

Table 96 (*Contd.*)

| *Vitamin* | *Metabolic activity* | *Deficiency symptoms* |
|---|---|---|
| Biotin | 1. Necessary for the incorporation of $CO_2$ into organic compounds | Dermatitis and weight loss |
| Vitamin $B_{12}$ (Cyanocobalamin) | 1. Glutamic acid metabolism<br>2. Certain alcohols and synthesis of nucleic acids | All animals—slow growth wasting sickness in cattle |
| Vitamin C (Ascorbic acid) | 1. Oxidation-reduction reactions | Farm animals do not require this vitamin, but deficiency in man, monkey and guinea pig produces Scurvy |

## FAT SOLUBLE VITAMINS

### VITAMIN A

Vitamin A was the first of the accessory food factors to be identified as a component of specific foods. In 1913 McCollum and Davis reported that rats failed to grow on diets containing carbohydrates, protein fats, and salts. Addition of eggs promoted growth and established that the missing factor was a fat soluble substance. Finally vitamin A was isolated in large amounts from fish liver oils by Karrer in 1931. It was not until the late 1940's however, that synthetic vitamin A became available on the commercial market.

It may now be noted that 1.0 international unit (IU) of vitamin A is supplied by: 0.30 μg of all-*trans* vitamin A alcohol or 0.344 μg of all-*trans* vitamin A acetate or 0.55 μg of all-*trans* vitamin A palmitate or 3.0 μg of β-carotene in cattle or 1.0 μg of β-carotene in chicken and in swine it is equivalent to 1.8 μg of β-carotene.

**Chemistry.** Vitamin A exists in animal products largely as the alcohol—Retinol, and it is stored in the animal body in combination with fatty acids. Palmitic acid appears to be the preferred fatty acid. During the participation of Vitamin A in metabolic functions, the esterified molecule becomes free.

The alcohol retinol is converted *in vivo* to an aldehyde Retinal, isolated from the retina and is the form in which the vitamin functions in dark adaptation. A synthetic derivative, retinoic acid, possesses some vitamin A activity and is believed to be normal metabolite in the *in vivo* degradation of the vitamin.

The general term vitamin A includes a number of isomeric compounds which have various degrees of vitamin A activity (p. 327–328).The *cis-trans* isomers of retinol result from configurational differences at the double bonds in the side chain as illustrated below. Retinal and retinoic acid also exist in *cis-trans* isomeric forms.

Retinol and Retinal are interconvertible and Retinoic acid is a normal *in vivo* metabolite of retinol and retinal. It appears that retinoic acid cannot be converted to retinal or retinol since the acid will promote growth and maintenance in rats but is ineffective in preventing night blindness or in supporting normal reproduction.

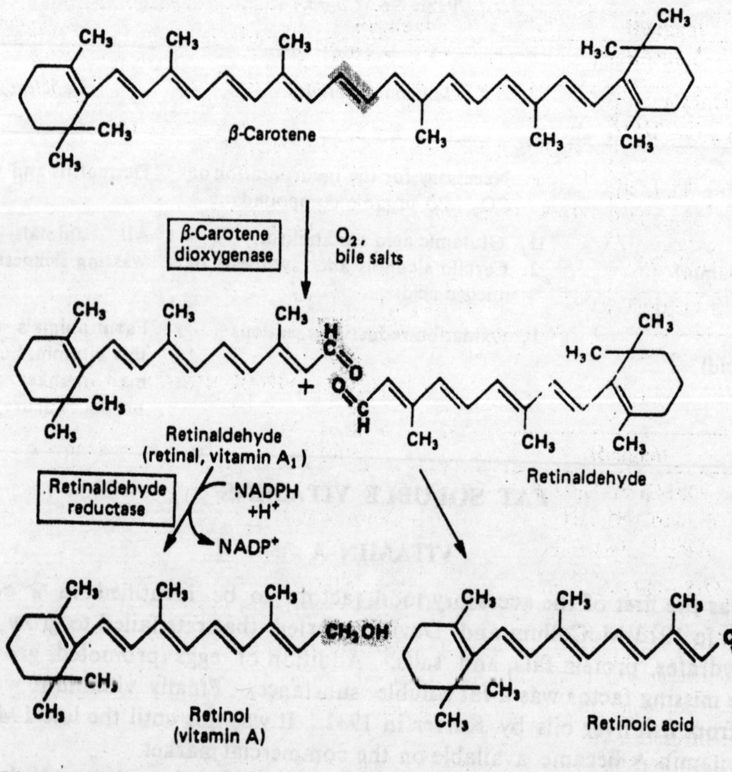

β-Carotene

β-Carotene dioxygenase

$O_2$, bile salts

Retinaldehyde (retinal, vitamin $A_1$)

Retinaldehyde

Retinaldehyde reductase

NADPH $+H^+$

$NADP^+$

$CH_2OH$

Retinol (vitamin A)

Retinoic acid

**Fig. 31** · β-Carotene and its cleavage to retinaldehyde. The reduction of retinaldehyde to retinol and the oxidation of retinaldehyde to retinoic acid are also shown.

**Table 97**

**CONVERSION OF BETA-CAROTENE TO VITAMIN A FOR DIFFERENT SPECIES**[1]

| Species | Conversion of mg of Beta-Carotene to IU of Vitamin A | | IU of Vitamin A Activity (calculated from carotene) |
|---|---|---|---|
| | (mg) | (IU) | (%) |
| Standard (rat) | 1 | 1,667 | 100 |
| Cattle | 1 | 400 | 24.0 |
| Dairy cattle | 1 | 400 | 24.0 |
| Sheep | 1 | 400–500 | 24.0–30.0 |
| Swine | 1 | 500 | 30.0 |
| Horses | | | |
| Growth | 1 | 555 | 33.3 |
| Pregnancy | 1 | 333 | 20.0 |
| Poultry | 1 | 1,667 | 100 |
| Mink | Carotene not utilized | | — |
| Man | 1 | 556 | 33.3 |

[1]Adapted from the *Atlas of Nutritional Data on United States and Canadian Feeds*, NRC-National Academy of Sciences, 1972, p. XVI, Table 6.

Vitamin A molecule contains a β ionine ring with an unsaturated side chain. The molecule is derived by the cleavage of the mid-point of the polyene connecting the β ionine in one side

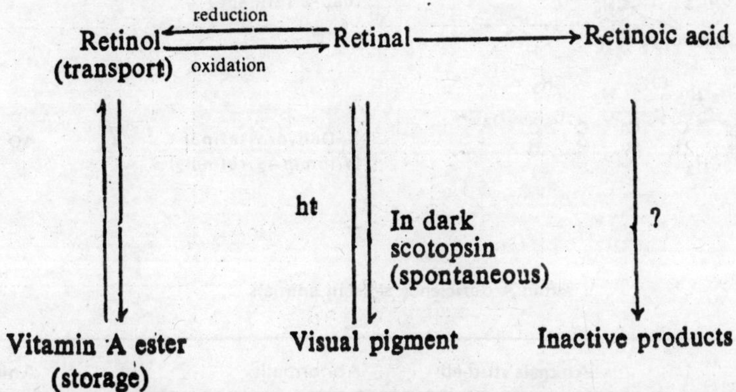


and in other side may be β ionine as in β carotene, or α ionine or some other rings as found in other carotinoids. As it is mentioned earlier, vitamin A in animal body exists largely as the alcohol retinol with the following structural formula:

$$\text{(ring: } CH_3, CH_3 \text{ on C; } H_2C, H_2C, C, C, CH_3\text{)} - C - CH = CH - \overset{CH_3}{C} = CH - CH = CH - \overset{CH_3}{C} = CH_2 - (R)^*$$

*If R is $CH_2OH$, then it is Retinol.
If R is CHO, then it is Retinal,
If R is COOH, then it is Retinoic Acid.

The Vitamin is a pale yellow crystalline solid, insoluble in water but soluble in fat and various fat solvents. It is readily destroyed by oxidation on exposure to air and light. A related compound with the formula $C_{20}H_{27}OH$, found in fish, has biological activity much lower than that of vitamin A and has been designated dehydroretinol or vitamin $A_2$.

Isomeric forms of vitamin A.

| Isomeric form | Relative Biological Activity CHICKS | RATS |
|---|---|---|
| *Trans*-Retinol | 100 | 100 |
| 13-*cis* Retinol | 50 | 75 |

| | | CHICKS | RATS |
|---|---|---|---|
| (structure; steric hindrance) | 11-*cis* Retinal (neo-b-retinene) | ? | 47 |
| (structure) | 3-Dehydro-retinol (vitamin $A_2$, retinol$_2$) | ? | 40 |

Viatmin A deficiency signs in animals.

| Abnormality | Animals studied |
|---|---|
| **General** | |
| Anorexis | Rat, fowl, farm animals |
| Growth failure and weight loss | Rat, fowl, farm animals |
| Xerosis of membranes | Rat fowl |
| Roughened hair or feathers | Rat, birds, farm animals |
| Infections | Rat, birds, farm animals |
| Death | Rat, birds, farm animals |
| **Eyes** | |
| Night blindness | Rat, farm animals |
| Xerophthalmia | Rat, bovine |
| Keratomalacia | Rat |
| Opacity of cornea | Rat, bovine |
| Loss of lens | Rat, bovine |
| Papilloidema | Bovine |
| Constriction of optic nerve | Bovine, dog |
| **Respiratory system** | |
| Metaplasia of nasal passages | Fowl |
| Pneumonia | Rat, bovine |
| Lung abscesses | Rat |
| **GIT** | |
| Metaplasia of forestomach | Rat |
| Enteritis | Rat, farm animals |
| **Urinary system** | |
| Thickened bladder wall | Rat |
| Cystitis | Rat |
| Urolithiasis | Rat |
| Nephrosis | Rat |

| Abnormality | Animals studied |
|---|---|
| **Liver** | |
| Metaplasia of bile | Rat |
| Degeneration of Kupffer cells | Rat |
| **Nervous system** | |
| Incoordination | Rat, bovine, pig |
| Paresis | Rat, pig |
| Nerve degeneration or twisting | Rat, dog, rabbit, bovine, bird, pig |
| Constriction of optic foramina | Bovine, dog |
| Bone formation | |
| Defective modeling | Dog, bovine |
| Restriction of brain cavity | Dog |
| **Reproduction** | |
| Degeneration of testes | Rat |
| Abnormal estrus cycle | Rat, bovine |
| Resorption of fetuses | Rat |
| **Congenital abnormalities** | |
| Anophthalmia | Pig, rat |
| Microophthalmia | Pig, rat |
| Cleft palate | Pig, rat |
| Aortic arch deformation | Rat |
| Kidney deformities | Rat |
| Hydrocephalus | Rabbit, bovine |
| **Miscellaneous** | |
| Increased cerebro-spinal fluid pressure | Bovine, pig |
| Cystic pituitary | Bovine |

## Physiological Role and Deficiency Symptoms

1. VITAMIN A AND VISION. Vitamin A is essential for the formation of rhodopsin (visual purple), needed for vision in dim light. 11-cis-retinol of the blood is converted to an aldehyde 11-cis-retinal by an enzyme alcohol dehydrogenase. This compound spontaneously in dark

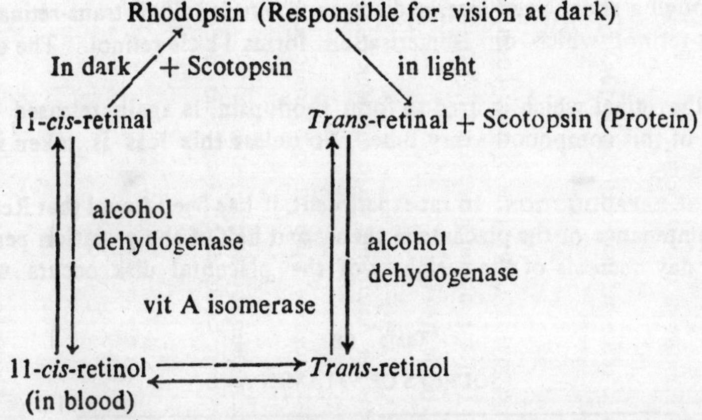


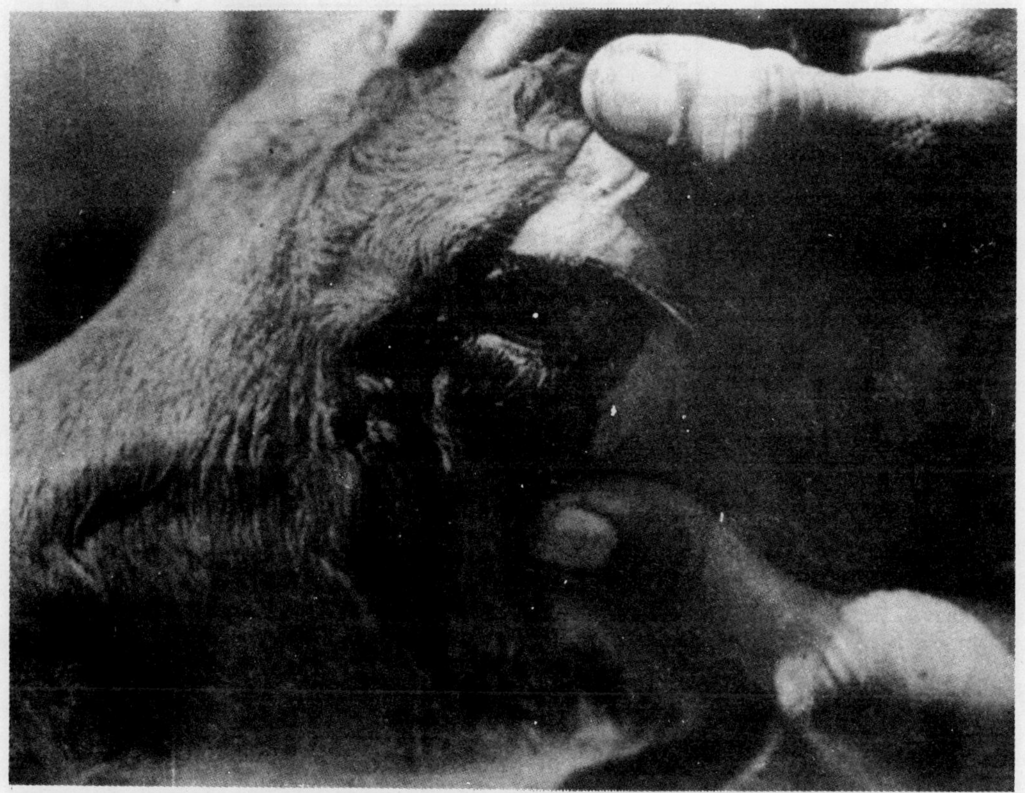

**Fig. 32** Vitamin A deficiency if allowed to continue will lead to xerophthalmia (abnormal dryness of the surface of the conjunctiva).

combines with a protein known as scotopsin and forms Rhodopsin which is responsible for vision in dim light. In bright light condition Rhodopsin changes into (*a*) trans-retinal and (*b*) scotopsin through a short lived intermediate compounds. This trans-retinal again transforms into trans-retinol which on isomerisation forms 11-cis-retinol. The scheme is given in previous page.

Although here the retinal which is used to form rhodopsin is again released as retinal but there is some loss of this compound every time. So unless this loss is taken into care, night blindness is inevitable.

2. VITAMIN A IN REPRODUCTION. In rat experiment, it has been found that Retinol or Retinal is required for maintenance of the placenta in the second half of the gestation period (22 days). At about the 16th day necrosis of the periphery of the placental disk occurs with resorption

Table 98

SOURCES OF VITAMIN A

| Feed Classification | Excellent<br>Greater than 45,360 IU/lb (100,000 IU/kg) | Good<br>4,536–45,360 IU/lb (10,000–100,000 IU/kg) | Fair<br>454–4,536 IU/lb (1,000–10,000 IU/kg) |
|---|---|---|---|
| Fish | Fish-liver oils:<br>Cod<br>Halibut<br>Herring<br>Menhaden<br>Pilchard<br>Salmon<br>Shark<br>Swordfish<br>Tuna<br>Whale | Eel<br>Whitefish | Carp<br>Halibut<br>Herring<br>Oyster<br>Salmon<br>Sardines |
| Meat | Beef liver<br>Calf liver<br>Chicken liver<br>Pig liver<br>Sheep liver | Beef kidney<br>Pig kidney<br>Sheep kidney | |
| Dairy and poultry products | | Butter<br>Cheese<br>Cream<br>Dried milk<br>Egg yolk, raw | Whole milk |
| Forages | Alfalfa meal<br>Most legume hays<br>Most grass hays | Most fresh grass and legumes | |
| Vegetables and grains | Carrots | Corn<br>Hominy<br>Soybeans | Peanuts |
| By-products | | Distillers' grains | |

of the fetus. In male there is failure of spermatogenesis. The damage can be reversed in both sexes by retinol.

3. SYNTHESIS OF MUCOPOLYSACCHARIDES (MPS). Mucus epithelial cells are distributed throughout the body as in respiratory tract, alimentary tract, reproductive tract, etc. Vitamin A is concerned in the synthesis of MPS by doing activation of sulphate molecule which is an important element of MPS. In its absence keratinization of epithelial cells take place which thus affects.

(a) *Respiratory*—due to keratinized tissue, cold and sinus trouble tend to be more severe
(b) *Alimentary tract*—leads of diarrhoea
(c) *Genito-urinary tract*—accounts for the high incidence of kidney and bladder stones through interference with elimination of urine
(d) *Reproductive tract*—directly interferes with normal reproduction.

4. DEVELOPMENT OF BONE. It is concerned with normal development of bone through a control exercised over the activity of osteoclasts and osteoblasts of the epithelial cartilage.

A failure of the spinal and some other bone to develop normally results in turn a pressure on the nerves and in their degeneration. Blindness in calves results from a constriction of optic nerve caused by a narrowing of the bone canal through which it passes. Avitaminosis can result in deafness in dogs, owing to an injury to the auditory nerve.

In practice severe deficiency symptoms are unlikely to occur an adult animals except after prolonged deprivation. Grazing animals generally obtain sufficient amount of provitamin—carotinoids, from pasture grass and normally build up liver reserves.

In poultry on a diet deficient in vitamin A, the mortality rate is usually high. Early symptoms include retarded growth, weakness, ruffled plumage and a staggering gait Yellow maize, dried grass or other green feed, or alternatively cod or other fish liver oils or vitamin A concentrate, can be added to the diet.

5. GROWTH. Because of stimulant for building new cells of epithelial in nature and for bones where it controls the osteoclastic and osteoblastic activity, vitamin A definitely interferes with growth.

**Sources of Vitamin A.** Plant kingdom contains no vitamin A. It is the precursor like different carotinoids which are the potent forms of vit-A present in the plant kingdom.

Synthetic vitamin A can be obtained in pure form.

## VITAMIN D

The disease rachitis, now commonly called rickets, is known to mankind since ancient times. In 1950 Infant rickets was described by Glisson in England. The desease was prevalent especially among the children of the lower classes of people in England (and other sections of the world) for centuries. Infection was early postulated as a cause of the disease. Around London the abundance of fog was held responsible by some to be a contributing factor. In other words, the lack of sunshine due to the fog was a predisposing factor.

In 1918 Mellanby produced the first clear-cut experimental rickets in dogs by feeding only milk. Rickets developed regularly on such diets. In 1919 Huldschinsky demonstrated marked clinical improvement in severely rachitic children by applying ultraviolet rays on their bodies, In 1931 Angus and co-workers isolated crystalline vitamin D upon ultraviolet irradiation of ergosterol. This was named calciferol and is referred to as vitamin $D_2$. Later on vitamin $D_3$ was isolated by irradiation of 7-dehydrocholesterol. It is now established that small amounts of 7-dehydrocholesterol is associated with skin of animals, and thus ultraviolet light, from the sun or from artificial sources, is able to activate and yield vitamin $D_3$ to the body.

**Chemical nature.** Several forms of vitamin D exist; although not all of these are naturally occurring compounds. For nutritional purposes the two most important D vitamins are $D_2$ (ergocalciferol) and $D_3$ (cholecalciferol). Ergocalciferol is produced from ergosterol which occurs in plants, while cholecalciferol is derived from 7-dehydrocholesterol. Ultraviolet light is the main power which converts the pro-vitamins into vitamin D. There is no vitamin $D_1$; the original proposal for such a vitamin was later shown to be an error, since the material was found to be a mixture of calciferol and some impurities. The value of other forms of vitamin D cannot be accurately assessed at present, since small amounts may occur in natural sources and their value, if any, is not established. Vitamin $D_4$ is activated 22-dehydroergosterol. Vitamin $D_5$ is activated 7-dehydrositosterol. The structures of vitamin $D_2$ and $D_3$ are given below: (both differ in side chain only).

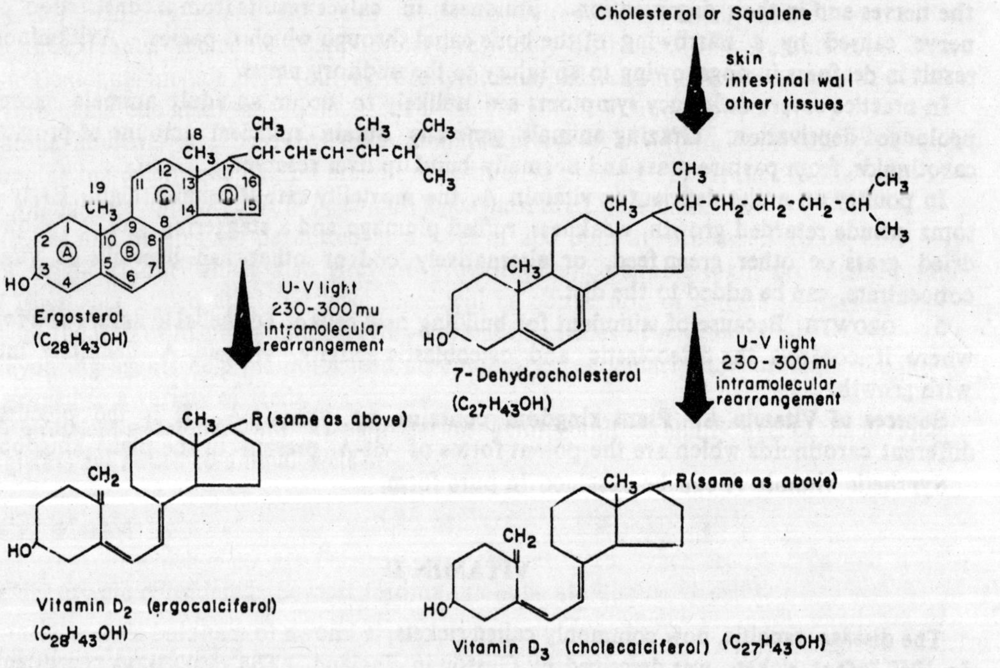

Cholesterol or Squalene

skin
intestinal wall
other tissues

Ergosterol
($C_{28}H_{43}OH$)

U-V light
230-300 mu
intramolecular
rearrangement

7-Dehydrocholesterol
($C_{27}H_{43}OH$)

U-V light
230-300 mu
intramolecular
rearrangement

R (same as above)

Vitamin $D_2$ (ergocalciferol)
($C_{28}H_{43}OH$)

R (same as above)

Vitamin $D_3$ (cholecalciferol) ($C_{27}H_{43}OH$)

**Metabolic Functions**

1. Aids in the absorption of calcium and phosphorus from intestinal tract, which accounts for the antirachitic properties of vitamin D. Whether vitamin D exerts a direct influence on incorporation of calcium into bone has not been resolved.

2. Harrison and Harrison demonstrated a specific function of vitamin D on kidney tubular reabsorption of phosphate. They developed rickets in dogs and then by phosphate clearance studies showed that the administration of large doses of vitamin D definitely increased

phosphate reabsorption. Such action is definitely antirachitic.

3. Addition of vitamin D reduces oxidation of citric acid and a high citrate concentration is found in kidney, bone and blood but not in liver. As citrate has nothing to do with bone growth, the high citrate level which is also accompanied by more citrate excretion has no known physiological role.

4. It has been found that vitamin D increases the activity of the enzyme phytase in the rat intestine. This enzyme hydrolysed food phytic acid (grains primarily), yielding inorganic phosphate. However, the increased enzyme activity does not liberate sufficient inorganic phosphate to account for the antirachitic action of vitamin D.

5. Vitamin D also stimulates release of calcium rather than uptake of calcium by kidney mitochondria.

6. It has been found by, De Luca (1964), that vitamin D stimulates incorporation of phosphorus into phospholipids of intestinal mucosa.

**Deficiency Symptoms**

1. In young animal vitamin D deficiency results in rickets and retarded growth. Rickets includes skeletal deformities characterized by (*i*) enlarged junctions between bone and cartilages, (*ii*) curvatures of the bones and in severe cases, (*iii*) weakening of muscular tissue and particular susceptibility to infection.

2. In older animals vitamin D deficiency causes osteomalacia, where there is reabsorption of bone already laid down.

3. In poultry, a deficiency of vitamin D causes the bones and beak to become soft and rubbery; growth is usually retarded and the legs may become bowed.

Vitamin $D_2$ and $D_3$ have the same potency for cattle, sheep and pigs, but vitamin $D_2$ has about 1/35th of the potency of $D_3$ for poultry. One μg of vitamin $D_3$ is equivalent to 40 international units (IU).

**Sources**

In its active from vitamin D is not well distributed in nature except in some dried roughages. In animal kingdom it is abundant in fish liver on entire body oil. Milk is a very poor source of vitamin D. Fresh green alfalfa forage has zero vitamin D value whereas sun cured hay contain on an average 200 I.U. per 100 gms.

## VITAMIN E

The earliest indication that natural food contain material specifically concerned with reproduction is found in a report by Mattil and Conklin (1920). They indicated that rats fed on a milk diet supplemented with yeast (B vitamin) and iron were unable to bear young. In 1922 Bishop and Evans announced the existance of a factor X in certain foods for normal rat, reproduction. In the year 1936, Evans and his colleagues isolated pure Vitamin E from the unsaponifiable fraction of wheat-germ oil. The active substance was later termed by Evans as "vitamin E", and now at least eight compounds with E activity are known to occur in a variety of plant and animal tissues. These are called "tocopherols". The name tocopherol was derived from the Greek *tokos* (childbirth) and phero (to bear), but the influence of tocopherols is vastly greater than influencing reproduction in rats.

The synthesis of α-tocopherol was accomplished in 1938 by Smith in U.S.A. and Karrer in Switzerland

**Chemistry of Tocopherols**

In reality vitamin E is a group of vitamins. There are about eight naturally occurring tocopherols and toco-trienols with vitamin E activity have so far identified. They differ from

α Tocopherol

β Tocopherol

γ Tocopherol

δ Tocopherol

α Tocotrienol

β Tocotrienol

γ Tocotrienol

δ Tocotrienol

**Chemical structures of naturally occurring tocopherols and toco-trienols**

each other in the number and position of the methyl groups round the ring of the molecule. All have the same physiological properties, although α-tocopherol is the most active and this is the main tocopherol in animal tissue and that is why tocopherol in this form is now synthesised commercially.

Among tocopherols the four compounds so far identified are α-tocopherol (5,7,8-trimethyl tocol), β-tocopherol (5,8-dimethyl tocol) γ-tocopherol (7,8-dimethyl tocol) and δ-tocopherol (8-methyl tocol). Relative to α-tocopherol the biological activities of β-and γ-tocopherols are 40 and 8 per cent respectively

Among toco-trienols, (three double bonds in the side chain) α,β,γ and δ-are noteworthy. The structural formulae are given in previous page. Except α-toco-trienol which has got 20 per cent biological activity of α-tocopherol, other toco-trienols have very little activity. There is no evidence of inter-conversion between the different tocopherols.

Tocopherols are yellow, oily liquid, remarkably stable to heat (even at above 100°C) and acids but not to alkalies. It oxidizes very slowly.

Tocopherols are largely found in wheat germ oil and in other grain oil portion. In animal body the compound is mostly found in body fat. There is some evidence that all α-tocopherol in heart muscle is localised in the mitochondria.

Tocopherols are potent antioxidants and function at least in part in protecting other nutrients, such as vitamin A and polyunsaturated fatty acids from destructive oxidation. It also protects coenzyme Q. Since coenzyme Q is involved in the transfer of electrons, additional studies on this relationship to vitamin E may serve to resolve a current controversy—whether α-tocopherol is an integral part of an enzyme system also.

The degradation of α-tocopherol in the animal body is presented in a diagramatic sketch as below. α-tocopherol is converted to tocopheryl quinone, its biological activity is then

($FeCl_3$)
$+H_2O$ $-2H^+$ $-2e$
Vit. C (in rat)
α-tocopherol
α-tocopheroxide (unstable) hemiacetal of α-tocopherylquinone
not in rat
H Br heat
$AuCl_3$
HCl + Vit.C not in rat
$H^+$ irreversible
$-2H^+$ $-2e$
$Na_2S_2O_4$ or Vit.C
α-tocopherylhydroquinone (unstable)
α-tocopherylquinone (stable)

**Oxidation products of α-tocopherol**

**Table 99**

**Pathology of vitamin E deficiency**

| Condition | Animal | Tissue affected | Prevented by Vitamin E | Prevented by Selenium |
|---|---|---|---|---|
| **I. Reproductive failure** | *Female:* Rat, Hen, Turkey | Vascular system of embryo | Yes | No |
| Embryonic degeneration | Ewe | | No* | Yes** |
| Sterility | *Male:* Rat, Guinea pig, Hamster, Dog, Cock | Male gonads | Yes | No |
| **II. Liver Blood, Capillaries, etc. Brain** | | | | |
| Liver necrosis | Rat, Pig, Mice, Chick | Liver | Yes | Yes |
| Erythrocyte destruction | Rat, Chick, Premature infant | Blood (RBC hemolysis) | Yes | No |
| Blood proteins loss | Chick, Turkey, Pigs | Serum albumin | Yes | Yes |
| Encephalomalacia | Chick | Cerebellum (Purkinje cells) | Yes | No |
| Exudative diathesis | Chick, Turkey, pigs | Capillary walls | Yes | Yes |
| Kindney degeneration | Rat, Monkey Mink | Tubular epithelium | Yes | Yes |
| Steatitis | Mink, Pig, Chick | Depot fat | Yes | Yes |
| **III. Nutritional Myopathies** | | | | |
| Nutritional muscular dystrophy | Rabbit, Guinea pig Duck, Chick, Turkey | Skeletal muscle | Yes | No or only partially |
| Stiff lamb | Lamb, Kid | Skeletal muscle | Yes | Yes |
| White muscle disease | Calf, Sheep, Mouse, Mink | Skeletal and heart muscle | Yes | Yes |
| Myopathy of gizzard | Turkey poult | Gizzard, heart, skeletal muscle | Yes | Yes |
| Cardiac muscle abnormlaites | Cattle, Lambs, Poultry, Rats, Monkey, Rabbits | Heart | Yes | Yes |

*Not in selenium-deficiency diets

**When added to diets containing vitamin E

lost and the reaction is not ordinarily reversible. α-tocopheroxide apparently is reversibly converted to α-tocopherol to a limited extent in the presence of adequate ascorbic acid.

**Biochemical Functions**

1. It is well established that vitamin E acts as an antioxidant in the cellular level. Thus for an example it prevents the oxidation of unsaturated fatty acids, mostly present in all cell wall components.

2. Vitamin E also participates in normal tissue respiration possibly (*i*) aid in some unknown way the function of cytochrome reductase system and (*ii*) to protect the lipid structure of mitochondria from oxidation destruction.

3. Aids the normal phosphorylation of creatine phosphate, ATP—which are all high energy phosphate compounds of the body.

4. It is also involved in the synthesis of ascorbic acid (vitamin C) and ubiquinine (coenzyme) and in the metabolism of nucleic acid (DNA) probably by regulating the incorporation of pyrimidines into the nucleic acid structure and sulphur amino acid.

**Pathology of Vitamin E Deficiency**

Early experiments showed the importance of vitamin E only in rat reproduction, but further studies showed that reproduction is only affected in some species but not in all species. The effect of vitamin E deficiency has been found in various nature in different animals. Some of the vitamin E deficiency has been found cured by adding selenium to the diet. How a mineral can substitute a vitamin deficiency is a mystery. Table 68 is a list of pathology of vitamin E deficiency in different species, it also shows where selenium can replace vitamin E.

**Table 100 SOURCES OF VITAMIN E**

| Feed Classification | Excellent<br>Greater than 136 mg/lb (300 mg/kg) | Fair<br>14–136 mg/lb (30–300 mg/kg) | Poor<br>0–14 mg/lb (0–30 mg/kg) |
|---|---|---|---|
| Fish | | | Most fish meals<br>Fish solubles |
| Dairy and poultry products | Colostrum | | Milk |
| Forages | | Alfalfa<br>Bluegrass<br>Orchardgrass | |
| Vegetables and grains | Rice bran oil<br>Safflower oil<br>Sunflower oil | Coconut oil<br>Corn germ meal<br>Corn gluten meal<br>Corn oil<br>Rice<br>Sesame oil<br>Soybeans<br>Wheat germ | Barley<br>Corn<br>Milo<br>Oats |
| By-products | | Distillers dried grains<br>Distillers dried solubles | |

**Sources**

NOTE: Encephalomalacia—Damage to the brain, edema and hemorrhage cerebellum.
Muscular dystrophy—wasting way of muscle.
Steatitis—Inflammation of addipose tissue.
Exudative diathesis—Blood serum oozed into the tissues.

## VITAMIN K

Vitamin K was identified in 1935 by Dam as a factor present in green leaves which prevented a hemorrhagic syndrome observed in chicks maintained on a low fat diet. The new fat soluble vitamin was designated as vitamin K for the Danish word, *Koagulation.* The purified compound was isolated from alfalfa by Dam and associates in 1939.

It is now well established that vitamin K is an essential metabolite for humans and for all laboratory and farm animals. The dietary vitamin K requirement of animals depends upon many modifying factors. Among these are factors affecting (1) the availability of the vitamin from various foods and foodstuffs; (2) its stability in foods and/or the innate stability of the vitamin K supplement being fed; (3) its gastrointestinal microbial synthesis, including the site of synthesis in the tract; (4) its absorbability which depends upon the level of dietary fat, adequate bile secretion, competition for absorptive and/or transport mechanisms by high levels of other fat-soluble vitamins and freedom from coccidiosis or other intestinal disturbances; (5) its destruction in the gestrointestinal tract, such as possible destruction by action of Coccidia, *Capillaria*, or other parasites; and (6) interference with its metabolic activity, such as by sulphaquinoxaline, dicoumarol, warfarin, etc.

**Chemical Nature**

A number of compounds are known to have vitamin K activity. Naturally occurring compounds come from two sources: (1) Phylloquinone ($K_1$) series occurs in all green leafy mate-

$CH_2-CH=C(CH_3)-CH_2-(CH_2CH_2CH(CH_3)CH_2)_3H$

Vitamin $K_1$ (green leafy vegetables)
Phylloquinone

Vitamin $K_3$ (menadione)

$(CH_2CH=C(CH_3)-CH_2)_6H$

Vitamin $K_2$ (intestinal bacteria)
Menaquinone-4

Dicoumarol

rials, (2) Prenylmenaquinone ($K_2$) series occurs in the intestine by the microbial syinthesis. Among so many synthetic compounds, Menadione ($K_3$) is noteworthy. It is about 3.3 times as active biologically as the naturally occurring vitamins. This property may be due to the fact that menadione is slightly water soluble which aids rapid absorption than the other two natural compounds which are fat soluble. The chemical structure of above three compounds are given in page 389.

**Table 101**

Relative biological activity of several forms of vitamin K.[a]

| | Activity relative to that of natural vitamin $K_1$ (phylloquinone-4) |
|---|---|
| Phylloquinone-1 | 5 |
| Phylloquinone-2 | 10 |
| Phylloquinone-3 | 30 |
| Phylloquinone-4 | 100 |
| Phylloquinone-5 | 80 |
| Phyloquinone-6 | 50 |
| Menaquinone-2 | 15 |
| Menaquinone-3 | 40 |
| Menaquinone-4 | 100 |
| Menaquinone-5 | 120 |
| Menaquinone-6 | 100 |
| Menaquinone-7 | 70 |
| Menadione | 40-150[b] |
| Menadione sodium bisulfate | 50-150[b] |
| Menadione dimethylpyrimidinol bisulfate | 100-160[b] |

[a] From P. Griminger. 1966. Vitamins and Hormones 24:605.
[b] Activity depends on relative stabilities of preparations used and on presence or absence of sulfaquinoxaline in the test diet.

**Biochemical Function**

The site of the metabolic action of vitamin K is in the liver. The main function has been attributed in its participation in the blood clotting mechanism. R.E. Olson (Science, 1964) has proposed that vitamin K is needed for the formation of the specific mRNA which directs the synthesis of prothrombin and several other plasma proteins concerned with blood clotting.

**Role of vitamin K in blood coagulation**

In animal body when blood flows through various blood vessels (arteries and veins) normally it does not clot due to the presence of heparin, a naturally occurring polysaccharide composed of D-glucuronic acid and D-glucoseamine. The compound originates from the white blood corpuscles (Basophil) as secretion and acts by preventing the conversion of *prothrombin* (a proenzyme, proteinous nature found in blood plasma but produced in the liver) to *thrombin* (the active enzyme) required for conversion of plasma *fibrinogen* into threads of *fibrin* of the blood clot.

When any blood vessel is damaged blood will escape. To prevent blood loss cessation of bleeding (*Haemostasis*) must follow. There are 3 phases to haemostasis.

The first phase is constriction of the injured vessel to diminish blood flow distal to the injury. This is thought to be a direct response of the blood vessel mediated through sympathetic nervous system. This is a temporary phenomenon.

The second phase consists of formation of a loose platelet plug, or *white thrombus*, at the site of injury. Collagen, the major macromolecule of all connective tissues (here of blood vessels) become exposed and acts as a binding site for blood platelets which then undergo disurption of their internal structure and release *thromboxane* (a newer compound formed in platelets from prostaglandin $G_2$) and ADP.

The ADP causes the surfaces of nearby platelets to become sticky and, as a result, increasing numbers of platelets adhere to the edge of the cut and form into a growing platelet

**Table 102**

**Factors Involved in Blood Coagulation**

| *Factor number* | *Name* | *Type of factor and origin* |
|---|---|---|
| I | Fibrinogen | A plasma protein produced in the liver |
| II | Prothrombin | A plasma protein produced in the liver |
| III | Tissue thromboplastin | A complex mixture of lipoproteins that contains one or more phospholipid substances that is released from damaged tissues |
| IV | Calcium ions | An ion in the plasma that may be acquired in the diet and from skeletal structures |
| V | Proaccelerin (labile factor, accelerator globulin) | A plasma protein produced in the liver |
| VI | Not utilized | |
| VII | Serum prothrombin conversion accelerator (stable factor, proconvertin) | A plasma protein produced in the liver |
| VIII | Antihemophilic factor (antihemophilic globulin) | A plasma protein produced in the liver |
| IX | Plasma thromboplastin component (Christmas factor) | A plasma protein produced in the liver |
| X | Stuart factor (Stuart–Prower factor) | A plasma protein produced in the liver |
| XI | Plasma thromboplastin | A plasma protein produced in the liver |
| XII | Hageman factor | A plasma protein |
| XIII | Fibrin stabilizing factor | A plasma protein |

*Each factor is a proenzyme*

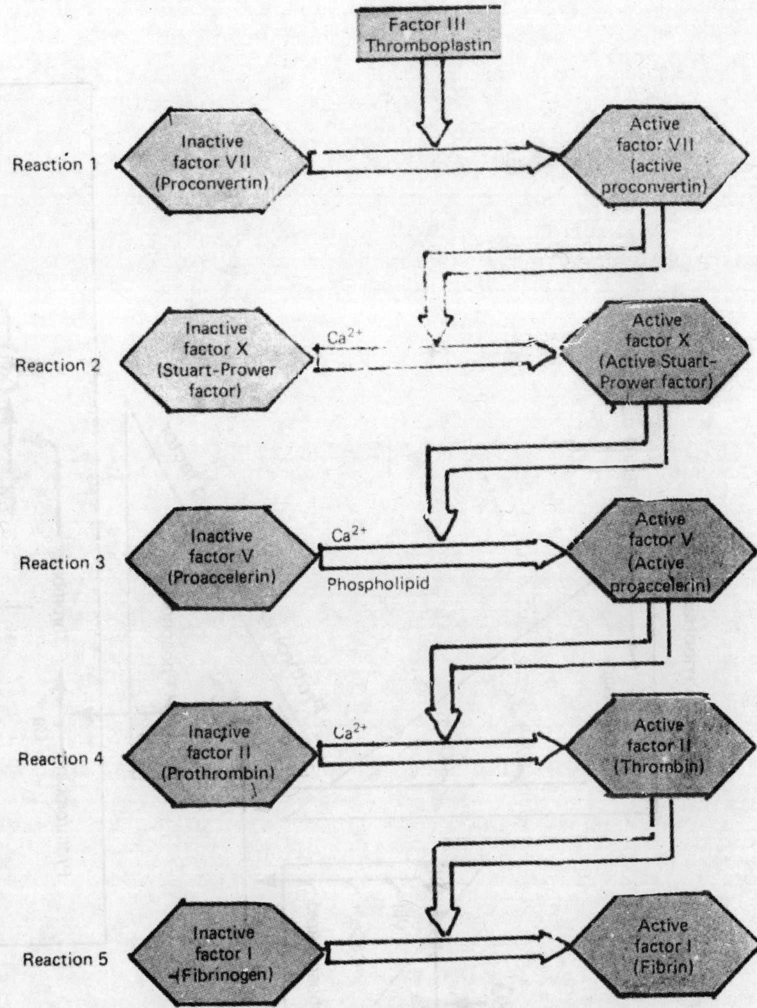


A series of five reactions occur in one of the mechanisms by which blood clots. The first reaction is initiated by thromboplastin, which activates proconvertin. The product of each reaction catalyzes the next reaction. Thus, proconvertin catalyzes reaction 2 and the product of reaction 2 catalyzes reaction 3, etc. In the final reaction, thrombin catalyzes the conversion of fibrinogen to fibrin.

Vitamin K is required for synthesis of clotting factors VII, IX, X. In patients treated with coumarin anticoagulants, which are vitamin K antagonists, an inactive precursor of prothrombin circulates in the plasma, and the related delay in blood clotting is measured by the test known as the prothrombin time

plug or clump. This action may occlude small vessels and slow or stop bleeding, although the plug is generally not strong enough to withstand the pressures of larger vessels, The platelets also release chemicals that may facilitate the first phase (vaso constriction), as well as chemicals that are involved in third phase, i.e., in the process of blood coagulation.

The third phase is the formation of *red thrombus* (blood clot) consists of red cells and

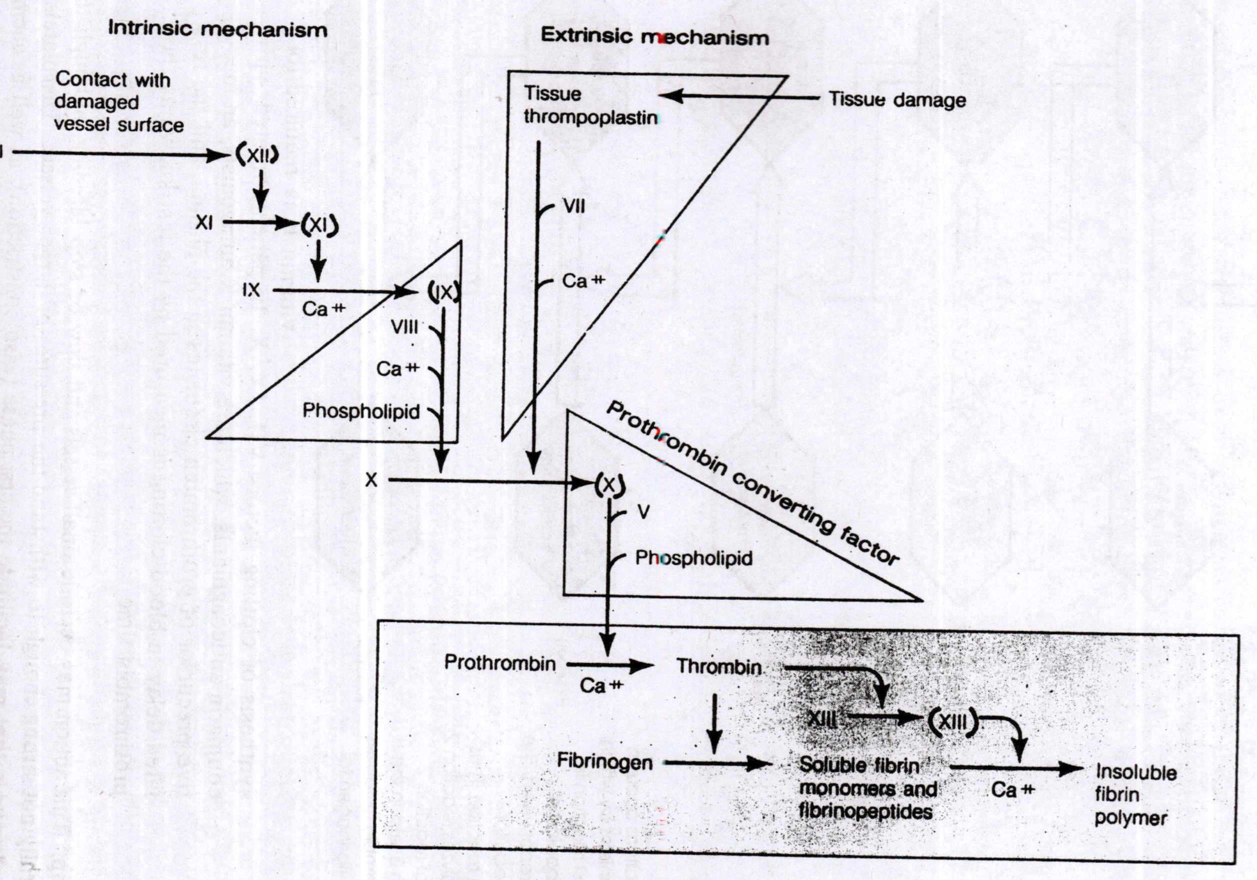


**Fig. 33** The sequence of events that leads to the formation of a fibrin clot. The factors that are indicated in ( ) are activated factors. See the text for a detailed discussion.

fibrin. The red thrombus morphologically resembles the clot formed in a test tube. During this process a pale, yellow fluid called serum exudes from the clot. The process is very complex and involves a number of different factors (proenzymes), many of which are present in blood plasma (Table . 102|.).

Basically, clot formation involves the conversion of a soluble protein called *fibrinogen* (normally present in the plasma but produced in the liver also known as Factor I) into an insoluble polymer called *fibrin.* This conversion requires the enzymatic action of a factor called *thrombin,* which is produced from an inactive plasma protein precursor called *prothrombin.*

Prothrombin converting factor when produced from thromboplastin (thrombokinase) of injured tissues in it is said as *extrinsic pathway* of formation of red thrombus (blood clot). When the same compound is produced from disintegrating blood platelets in an area of restricted blood flow or in response to the injury of the vessel wall without tissue injury by releasing the enzyme thromboplastin (thrombokinase) it is said as *intrinsic pathway* of formation of red thrombus (blood clot).

Both extrinsic and intrinsic pathways ultimately ends up with prothrombin converting factor which then works as a final common pathway—the activation of prothrombin to thrombin and the thrombin-catalyzed conversion of fibrinogen to the fibrin clot.

Vitamin K is involved in at least four steps in clot formation: (1) a plasma thromboplastin component (Factor IX), (2) a tissue thromboplastin component (Factor VII), (3) "Stuart" factor (Factor X), (4) prothrombin (Factor II). The exact mode of action in each reaction is unknown.

A simplified form of blood clotting reactions are as follows:

(1) Platelet factor + Plasma protein accelerators $\xrightarrow{Ca^{++}}$ Thromboplastin

(2) Plasma thromboplastin + Prothrombin + Conversion factor = Thrombin

(3) Fibrinogen $\xrightarrow{+\text{Thrombin}}$ Fibrin + Peptide

(a glycoprotein enzyme) (responsible for clot)

**Apart from this important biochemical function, vitamin K has been found to be involved in electron transport and oxidation phosphorylation.**

**Deficiency Symptoms**

**A. AVIAN SPECIES. Symptoms of vitamin K deficiency occur most frequently in chicks or poults about 2–3 weeks after they are placed on vitamin K-deficient diet. Sulphaquinoxaline in the feed or in the drinking water increases the incidence and severity of the symptoms. Gross deficiency of vitamin K results in such a prolonged blood clotting time that severely deficient chicks may bleed to death from slight bruise or other injury. Borderline deficiencies often cause small haemorrhagic blemishes. Haemorrhages may appear on the breast, legs, wings, in the abdominal cavity and on the surface of the intestines. Chicks show an anemia which in part may be due to loss of blood, or to the development of a hypoplastic bone marrow.**

**B. RUMINANTS.** Although vitamin K is synthesized in the rumen of cattle and other ruminants in adequate amounts under normal conditions but deficiency symptoms occur when spoiled sweet clover forage is fed. Link and associates of the University of Wisconsin (Link 1944) showed that when sweet clover hay undergoes spoilage with certain molds, the coumarin which it contains is converted to dicumarol, an anti-vitamin of K and at the same time a bleeding syndrome develops throughout the animal body. This disease is called *"sweet clover poisoining"* or *"bleeding disease"* and has been shown to be caused by the antivitamin K action of the dicumarol.

**Source**

*Milligram of Vit-$K_1$ per 100 gms. edible portion*

| | | | |
|---|---|---|---|
| Cabbage | 250 | Grass meal | 20 |
| Cauliflower | 275 | Soyabeans | 190 |
| Spinach | 334 | Wheat bran | 80 |

It is present in most green leafy materials, some of which are shown above. Among animals products egg yolk and fish meal and generally good sources. The vitamin is destroyed by light, acid, alkali and different oxidising agents.

## WATER SOLUBLE VITAMINS

## VITAMIN C

Historically the disease scurvy (marked by weakness, anemia, spongy dental gums, and mucocutaneous haemorrhages), become widely recognized when man learned to build ships capable of long sea voyages, and it is probably true that on long-term explorations more deaths were caused by scurvy than any other single factor. Vitamin C deficiency not only was prevalent on long sea voyages because fresh foods were unavailable, but also was epidemic over parts of the world during times of famine and war.

Of the mammals, only man, the monkey, Indian fruit bat, and the guinea pig require the vitamin from dietary source, other species possess the necessary enzymes to synthesize ascorbic acid. Thus farm animals do not require a dietary source of this vitamin.

Ascorbic acid was first isolated by Szent-Gyorgyi (1928) from-orange juice, cabbage juice and adrenal cortex; he named the compound hexuronic acid in recognition of the six carbon atoms in the molecule.

**Chemical Nature and Metabolism**

Vitamin C is chemically known as L-ascorbic acid. Highly soluble in water and slightly soluble in alcohol. Stable in dry crystalline state but oxidised quickly in solution. The acid is a derivative of hexose, it can be classified as carbohydrates. It occurs in two active forms: ascorbic acid (reduced form) and dehydro ascorbic acid (the oxidized form). If the latter is oxidised further to diketogulonic acid, the compound loses its biological activity.

Ascorbic acid $\underset{+2H}{\overset{-2H}{\rightleftharpoons}}$ Dehydroascorbic acid $\longrightarrow$ Diketogulonic acid

L-gulonolactone $\xrightarrow[\text{(enzyme)}]{\text{L-gulonolactone oxidase}}$ 2-keto-L-gulonolactone $\xrightarrow{\text{spontaneously}}$ Vit. C

Species capable of synthesising vitamin C can do it from glucose, via glucuronic acid and gluconic acid lactone.

**The enzyme L-gulonolactone oxidase is deficient in man, monkey, Indian fruit bat and guinea pig and hence vitamin C cannot be synthesised by these mammals. On the other hand farm animals have the ability to synthesise this vitamin in their body as per requirement. Thus we can say that vitamin C is essential for all groups of animals but it is not a dietary essential for any farm animals.**

**The acid is absorbed from the small intestine and excreted through urine. The plasma level of vitamin C is in close relation with that of intake. In body there is no storage but tissues functions at a very high metabolic rate have been observed to have a high ascorbic acid content.**

**Biochemical Functions**

1. **Vitamin C is essential for the collagen (an albuminoid which is the main supportive protein of all connective tissue, predominantly found in the gums) formation.**
2. **It aids for the conversion of folic acid to its active form tetrahydrofolic acid.**
3. **Vitamin C is also involved in the hydroxylation of proline, lysine and aniline—which are important for normal physiology of the animal.**
4. **It aids iron to stay in reduced state, which is very important for the body**
5. **Participates in the synthesis of steroid hormones by the adrenal cortex.**
6. **It involves in the metabolism of lipids as blood cholesterol level appear to fall with the administration of ascorbic acid and rise due to deficiency of vitamin.**
7. **It aids for the conversion of tryptophan to serotonin.**

**Deficiency Symptoms**

Deficiency symptoms for farm animals is unknown. For man, monkey and guinea pigs extensive study has been made. The classical manifestation of severe ascorbic acid deficiency is termed scurvy. The gross lesions observed are those related to degeneration of the collaginous intracellular substance. The disease is characterised by weakness, swollen tendor joints, delayed healing of wounds, spongy haemorrhagic friable gums, loose teeth, and small haemorrhages which may appear anywhere throughout the body, particularly near the bones and joints and under the skin and mucus membrane due to increased fragility of the capillaries.

**Source**

Vitamin C, unlike the vitamin B, is not universally distributed, being absent from eggs and seeds and in general from bacteria, yeasts and protozoa. The outstanding dietary sources of vitamin C are fresh fruits and leafy vegetables. Interestingly enough, for poor man green chilli is a good source. The richest fruit source known is a west Indian cherry called acerola (4.0 mg./gm.). Well-known sources include all citrus fruits and tomatoes. Less regard but good additional sources, include cabbage, sweet potatoes, white potatoes. Other sources are seasonal such as berris, melons, guavas, pineapple etc.

Animal products as a whole are poor sources. Cereal grains have no vitamin C. Raw cow's milk is a fair source; but some is lost is pasteurisation.

## THE VITAMINS OF THE B COMPLEX

The vitamins included under this complex all have the property of being soluble in water and most of them are components of enzyme systems.

Complete agreement has still not been reached concerning which substances should be considered as B vitamins, but those listed here under B complex are generally accepted as members of the B complex. Many writers include choline, inositol and *p*-aminobenzonic acid with the B vitamins.

It is possible that the requirements of different animal species vary. In recent years it has become apparent that the activity of the intestinal flora in synthesizing vitamins of the B group explains species differences. In general we can say that microbial synthesis of the B complex in the digestive tract can supply part of the requirements of all monogastric animals. For ruminants the entire requirements of B vitamins are synthesised by the microbes in their digestive tract. Deficiency symptoms in farm animals do occur only in pigs and poultry.

## THIAMINE (VITAMIN $B_1$)

The disease beriberi had been known for several centuries before its dietary origin was recognized. Beriberi is characterized by extensive damage to the nervous and cardiovascular system and may be accompanied by severe muscle wasting (dry beriberi) or edema (wet beriberi). In the late nineteenth century, Eijkmann, working in a hospital laboratory in Batavia, Dutch East Indies, discovered that a polyneuritis (characterized by a peculiar head retraction obviously of neurological origin) in chickens with symptoms similar to beriberi in humans was produced by feeding an experimental diet of polished rice. It did not occur when brown rice was substituted for polished rice or when rice polishings were added to the polished rice diet.

In 1926. Jansen and Donath. successors of Eijkmann succeeded in crystalizing vitamin B. in pure form. The identification of the structure of the vitamin and its synthesis was accomplished in 1936 by Williams and co-workers in the same laboratory.

**Chemistry of Thiamine.** Thiamine (aneurine, vitamin $B_1$) is a complex nitrogenous base composed of a pyrimidine and a thiazole ring; it is available commercially in hyrdochloride form.

$$\text{Thiamine chloride: pyrimidine ring } (NH_2,\ CH_3) -CH_2-N^+ \text{ thiazole ring } (CH_3,\ C=C-CH_2-CH_2OH,\ C-S,\ H),\ Cl^-$$

*Thiamine Chloride*

Due to the presence of a hydroxyl group at the end of the side chain thiamine easily forms esters with phosphorus of ATP. In the esterified form the molecule becomes active and this active molecule is known as cocarboxylase (thiamine pyrophosphate or TPP). The structure of thiamine pyrophosphate is shown below:

$$\underset{\text{Thiamine}}{R-CH_2-CH_2OH} + ATP \xrightarrow[\text{enz}]{Mg^{++}} \text{pyrimidine}(NH_2,\ CH_3)-CH_2-N^+ \ldots C(CH_3)=C-CH_2CH_2-O-P(=O)(OH)-O-P(=O)(OH)-OH$$

Thiamin pyrophosphate (TPP)
(cocarboxylase)

**Deficiency Diseases.** Deficiency of thiamine in humans (onset of beriberi) occurs first as a numbness of the legs, later with pain in the calf muscle, severe exhaustion, finally emaciation and paralysis. The patient has difficulty in breathing, there is an abnormal enlargement of the right side of the heart and a decrease in the rate of the heart beat. The most characteristic feature of the disease is the so called "*peripheral neuritis*". This is often accompanied by contractions of the feet and severe weakness of the wrists. The brain may be affected. Under these conditions the desease has been termed "*cerebral beriberi*" or "*Wernicke's encephalopathy*".

Symptoms in animals, termed *polyneuritis*, are particularly characterized by unthrifitiness, paralysis convulsions and in birds (pigeons, chicks etc.) there is a characteristic paralysis of the neck muscles which causes the head to be drawn back against the back of the bird so that the break is pointed straight up in a "*star-grazing*" attitude.

Paralysis appears to be due to accumulation in the brain and muscles of lactic acid. This results from the fact that the pyruvate which builds up during cocarboxylase deficiency is quickly converted to lactic acid.

Evidence indicates that the myelin sheath of the nerves and the white matter of the brain are the tissues most seriously affected. The exact cause of the deterioration of this tissue has not yet been shown.

Vitamin $B_1$ is not stored to any great extent in the animal body. Symptoms begin to appear, therefore, within a very short time following consumption of deficient diets. The severity of the symptoms is in direct proportion to the degree of the deficiency.

**Biochemical Function**

Thiamine, in the form of the thiamine diphosphate (thiamine pyrophosphate or TPP) is the coenzyme for the decarboxylation of keto acids such as pyruvic acid. The decarboxylation reaction with pyruvic acid is as follows:

$$CH_3-\overset{\overset{O}{\|}}{C}-COOH \xrightarrow[(TPP)]{\nearrow CO_2} CH_3-\overset{\overset{O}{\|}}{C}-H$$

*Pyruvic acid* *Acetaldehyde*

Table 103

**SOURCES OF THIAMIN**

| Feed Classification | Excellent<br>Greater than 4,536 mcg/lb (10,000 mcg/kg) | Good<br>454–4,536 mcg/lb (1,000–10,000 mcg/kg) | | Fair to Poor<br>45–454 mcg/lb (100–1,000 mcg/kg) | |
|---|---|---|---|---|---|
| Fish | | Meals:<br>Carp<br>Clams<br>Cod<br>Haddock<br>Lobster | <br>Mackerel<br>Oysters<br>Salmon<br>Shad | Meals:<br>Flounder<br>Halibut<br>Herring<br>Pike<br>Sardines<br>Scallops | <br>Shrimp<br>Smelt<br>Sturgeon<br>Trout<br>Tuna<br>Yellow perch |
| Meat | Lean pork | Brain<br>Heart | Kidney<br>Liver | | |
| Dairy and poultry products | | Whole egg | Milk<br>Whey | Cheese | |
| Forages | | Alfalfa | | | |
| Vegetables and grains | Corn germ meal<br>Linseed meal<br>Rice bran<br>Soybean oil meal<br>Wheat germ<br>Wheat middlings | Barley<br>Carrots<br>Copra meal<br>Corn<br>Cottonseed meal<br>Millet | Oats<br>Peanut meal<br>Rice<br>Sesame meal<br>Soybean oil meal<br>Wheat | | |
| By-products | Dried brewers' yeast | Baker's compressed yeast<br>Citrus pulp | Distillers dried solubles<br>Torula yeast | | |

## RIBOFLAVIN (VITAMIN $B_2$)

In the early days of vitamin research it was believed that the antiberiberi factor represented a single vitamin. After thiamine was isolated, however, it became clear that at least two factors were involved, a heat labile fraction which was the true antiberiberi vitamin and a heat stable fraction essential for rat growth. The latter fraction for sometime was thought to be only one substance and was named vitamin $B_2$ in Great Britain and Vitamin G in the United States. Subsequently the heat stable fraction was shown to be not one vitamin but a mixture of several vitamins (later indentified as riboflavin, pyridoxin, nicotinic acid, and pantothenic acid). The orange-yellow colour of riboflavin and its natural fluorescence in solution undoubtedly aided in its discovery since its presence in extracts from foods and other biological materials could be confirmed with the naked eye.

The vitamin was first isolated from egg white and called "*ovoflavin*". Compounds later isolated by other groups from milk and liver were designated "*lactoflavin*" and "*hepatoflavin*" respectively. The name riboflavin was adopted only after the compound was shown to contain ribose in the molecule and has since been changed to riboflavin (IUPAC, 1960).

Riboflavin was synthesized independently by Kuhn *et al.* (1935) at Heidelberg and Karrer *et al.* (1935) at Zurich.

Riboflavin consists of a dimethyl-isoalloxazine nucleus combined with ribose. The vitamin is an orange-yellow crystalline substance, very slightly soluble in water or acid solution. In neutral or acid media it is stable to heat. It is highly soluble in alkaline solution.

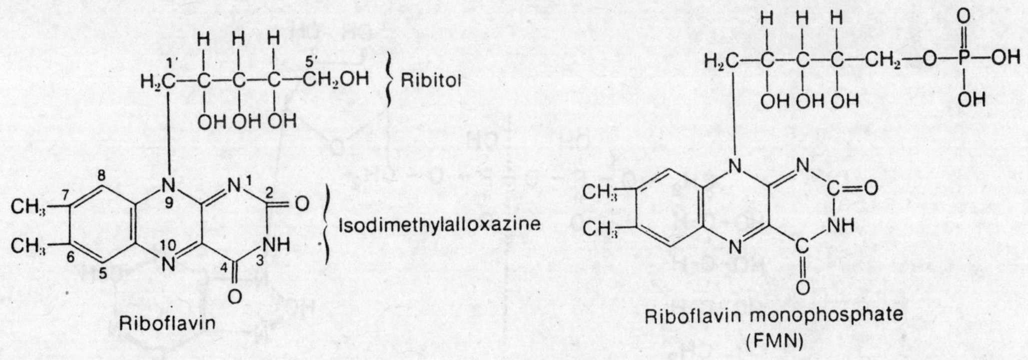

Ribitol

Isodimethylalloxazine

Riboflavin

Riboflavin monophosphate (FMN)

**Deficiency Symptoms**

Riboflavin forms the prosthetic part of over a dozen enzymes in the animal body. Among these are cytochrome reductase, diaphorase, xanthine oxidase, l-and d-amino acid oxidases, histaminase, and others, all of which are vitally associated with oxidation reduction involved in cell respiration. These are essential enzymes for growth and tissue repair in all animals. Many tissues may be affected by riboflavin deficiency. It appears, however, that the two most severely affected tissues are the epithelium and the myelin sheaths of some of the main nerve trunks.

Ariboflavinosis in humans produces a cheilosis (severe dermatitis and fissures at the corners of the mouth), angular somatitis, glossitis and seborrheic dermatitis. The seborrheic dermatitis is usually found in the nasolabial region near the inner and outer canthi of the eyes, behind the ears, and on the posterior surface of the serotum. The eyes are also affected. Ocular manifestations include photophobia, indistinct vision, itching burning and circumcorneal capillary engorgement with invasion of the superficial strata of the eye by small capillaries.

While there are other disease disorders which will also produce each of these symptoms, and therefore, one symptom taken alone is not necessarily suggestive of ariboflavinosis, the occurrence of a number of these symptoms together makes up a syndrome which, with a history of poor dietary intake of foods rich in riboflavin, can be used as a diagnosis of ariboflavinosis. If the symptoms disappear after treatment with riboflavin, the diagnosis is confirmed.

Severe riboflavin deficiency in chicks causes a marked swelling and softening of the sciatic and branchial nerves. The sciatic nerves usually show the most pronounced effects. They may reach a diameter four to five times normal size. The affected nerves show degenerative changes in the myelin sheaths of the main peripheral nerve trunks. These changes cause a continual stimulation of the sciatic nerve which produces a contraction of the toes and development of the typical symptoms of riboflavin deficiency in the chick known as "*curled-toe paralysis*".

## Metabolic Function

Riboflavin in the form of flavin monouncleotides (FMN) and flavin adinine dinucleotide (FAD) acts as the prosthetic group of several enzymes involved in biological oxidation-reduction reactions. These enzymes serve as bridges over which hydrogen atoms can pass berween two other molecules. In its reduction and oxidation riboflavin alternately accepts and releases

FMN

FAD

Flavin mononucleotide (FMN) and flavin adinine dinucleotide (FAD).

two hydrogen atoms. Reactions catalyzed by flavoproteins may be divided into three groups:

1. Reactions in which enzyme removes hydrogen, not from the primary substrate but from an intermediate carrier *e.g.*, from reduced pyridine nucleotide.
2. Reactions in which the enzyme removes hydrogen directly from substrate such as succinic and choline which are transformed to fumaric and betaine aldehyde respectively.
3. Catalyze the reactions of molecular oxygen *e.g.*, xanthine oxidase and oxygen to produce uric acid.

Table 104

SOURCES OF RIBOFLAVIN

| Feed Classification | Excellent<br>Greater than 4.5 mg/lb (10 mg/kg) | Good<br>.45-4.5 mg/lb (1-10 mg/kg) | Fair to Poor<br>.00-.45 mg/lb (.0-1 mg/kg) |
|---|---|---|---|
| Fish, meal | | Anchovy<br>Herring<br>Menhaden<br>Pilchard<br>Whitefish | |
| Meat | Liver | Meat and bone meal | |
| Dairy and poultry products | Buttermilk<br>Dried milk<br>Whey | Casein | |
| Forages | Alfalfa hay | | |
| Vegetables and grains | Peanut meal | Barley<br>Beans<br>Corn<br>Milo<br>Oats<br>Rice bran<br>Soybeans<br>Wheat | Polished rice |
| By-products | Distillers' dried solubles<br>Yeast | Blood meal<br>Cottonseed<br>Distillers' dried grains<br>Feather meal | Bakery products |

## NIACIN AND NIACINAMIDE

The terms niacin and niacinamide have replaced the older terms nicotinic acid and nicotinic acide amide (nicotinamide). The latter names were found to be undesirable because of confusion and the unwanted belief by many that they were physically related to nicotine.

Funk had isolated nicotinic acid from rice polishings as early as 1914, but he did not realize that it was a vitamin. In fact he was searching for an antiberiberi factor but discarded it when it was ineffective against beriberi! However, the discovery of niacinamide as component of coenzyme II (NADP) concerned in hydrogen transport (oxidation-reduction system) by Warburg and Christian (1935) suggested that the substance was of metabolic importance. When Elvehjem et al. (1938) were able to cure black tongue in dogs with niacinamide isolated from liver, niacin was firmly established as the pellagra-preventive factor (from the Italian *pelle agra* means rough skin). Subsequently curing of pellegrous humans with niacin in their ration became a common practice.

*Chemical Nature:* Niacin (or nicotinic acid) is pyridine-3-carboxylic acid. Niacinamide (or nicotinic acid amide) is the acid amide of niacin. Although niacin is frequently termed as vitamin but it has been established that niacin has to be first converted to its amide for vitamin function as niacinamide is the form in which the vitamin is found in its physiologically active combinations. The structure of niacin and niacinamide is as follows:

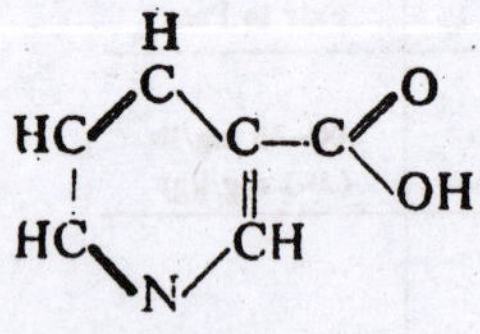

(*Nicotinic acid*) 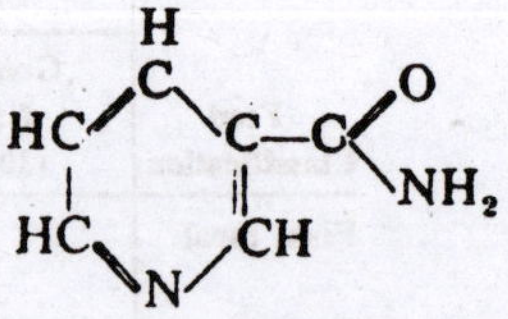 (*Niacinamide*)

**Biochemical Function**

Two well defined coenzymes containing nicotinamide are: (1) Diphosphopyridine nucleotide (DPN), or coenzyme I (Co I), or NAD (nicotinamide adenine dinucleotide); (2) Triphospho-

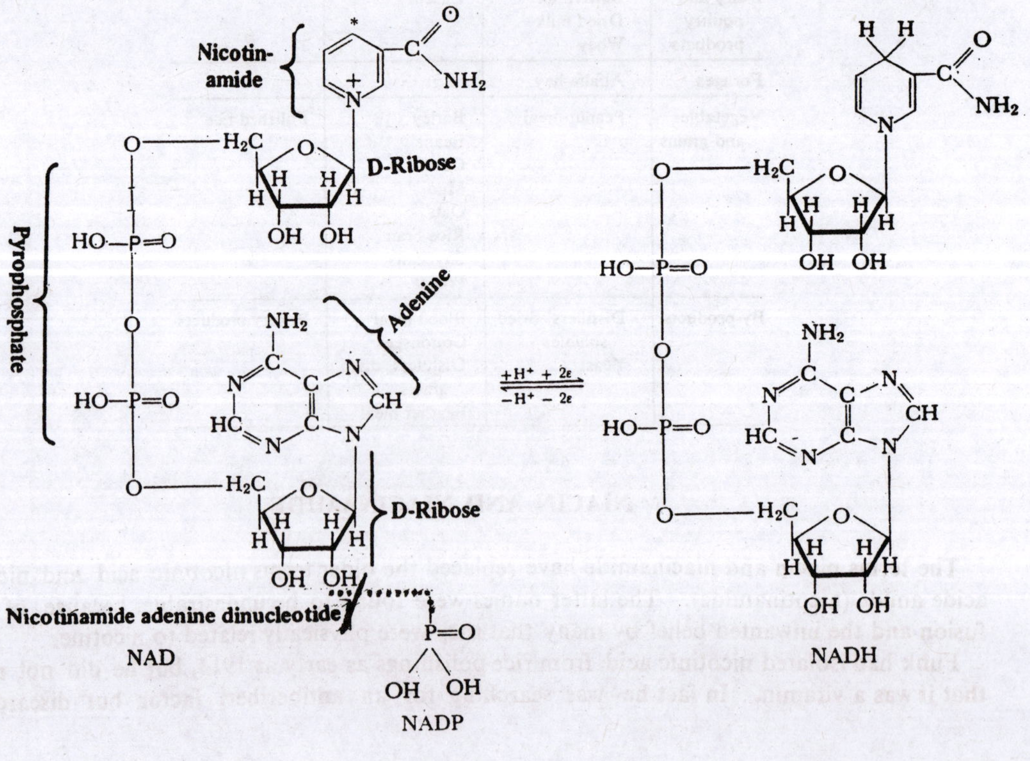

Nicotinamide · D-Ribose · Pyrophosphate · Adenine · D-Ribose

$\underset{-H^+ - 2e}{\overset{+H^+ + 2e}{\rightleftharpoons}}$

Nicotinamide adenine dinucleotide
NAD

NADP

NADH

**Table 105**

**Many of the substances belonging to vitamin B group as are found to act as coenzymes or prosthetic groups of enzymes are summarised below. Details already discussed in the text.**

| *Growth factor or vitamin* | *Structure* | *Related prosthetic group or coenzyme* | *Function* |
|---|---|---|---|
| Thiamine (vitamin $B_1$) | Pyrimidine ring: $CH_3$—C(=N—CH=)—C($N{=}CNH_2$)—$CH_2$—; Thiazole ring: $^+N$(CH—S)—C($CH_3$)=C—$CH_2CH_2OH$ (Pyrimidine ring, Thiazole ring) | Thiamin pyrophosphate | Transfer of some aldehyde groups, e.g., pyruvate dehydrogenase system, transketolase. |
| Lipoic acid, | S—S bridging $CH_2$ and $CH_2$—$CH_2CH_2CH_2CH_2COOH$, ring closed by $CH_2$ | Enzyme-bound lipoic acid | Acceptance of some aldehyde groups and their oxidation to acyl complexes, e.g., pyruvate dehydrogenase compler |
| Pantothenic acid | $HOCH_2$—C($CH_3$)($CH_3$)—CH(OH)CONHCH$_2$CH$_2$COOH | Coenzyme A | Acyl transfer and alteration, e.g., pyruvate dehydrogenase system, fatty acid oxidation. |
| Nicotinic acid (niacin) | Pyridine ring (HC, HC, H–C, CH, N) with CCOOH — Nicotinic acid (niacin); Pyridine ring with CCONH$_2$ — Nicotinamide | NAD, NADP | Transfer of H = $e^-$ + $H^+$ |

| Growth factor or vitamin | Structure | Related prosthetic group of coenzyme | Function |
|---|---|---|---|
| Riboflavin | 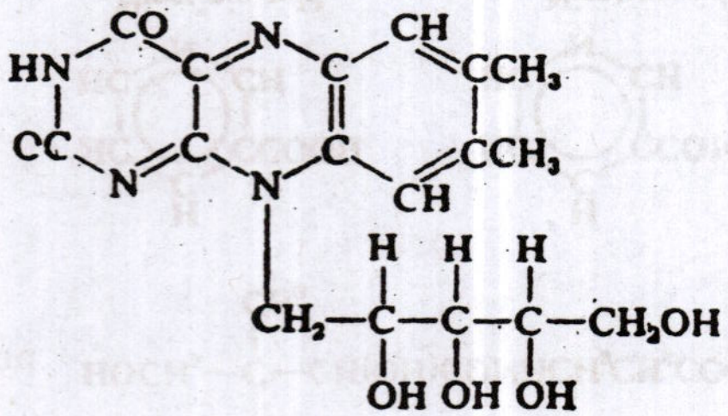 (isoalloxazine ring with ribityl chain: $CH_2-CH(OH)-CH(OH)-CH(OH)-CH_2OH$) | FMN, FAD | Transfer of H ≡ $e^- + H^+$ |
| Pyridoxal and derivatives ($B_6$) | 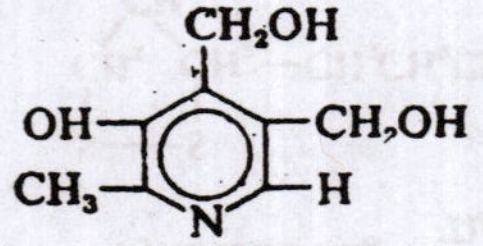 Pyridoxine; 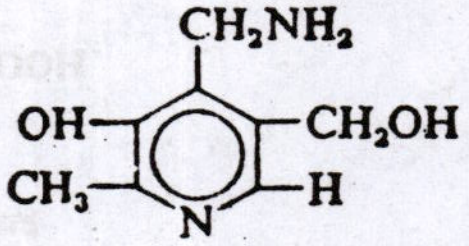 Pyridoxamine | Pyridoxal phosphate | Transfer of amino groups, generally by the formation of Schiff's bases, e.g., aminotransferases, serine hydroxymethyltransferase. |
| Folic acid | 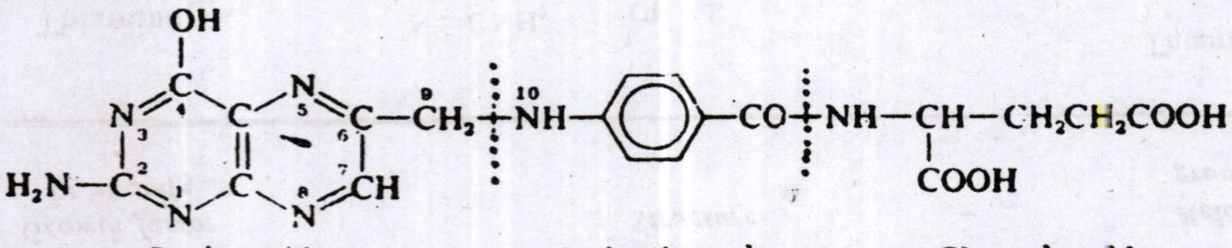 Pterin residue — $CH_2$ — NH — p-Amino-benzoic acid residue — CO — NH — CH(COOH) — $CH_2CH_2COOH$ Glutamic acid residue | Tetrahydrofolic | Transfer and interconversion of $C_1$ units at level of oxidation of formate, formaldehyde and methanol, e.g., in purine synthesis, serine transhydroxymethylase, methionine synthesis. |

| Growth factor or vitamin | Structure | Related prosthetic group of coenzyme | Function |
|---|---|---|---|
| **Cyanocobalamin ($B_{12}$)** | 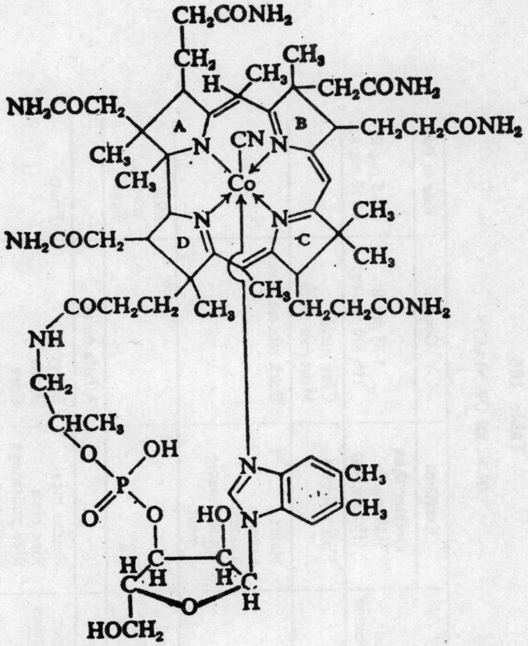 | Cobamide coenzymes | 1. Molecular rearrangements and formation of methyl groups.<br>2. The isomerisation of methylmalonyl CoA to succinyl CoA in fat metabolism requires a vitamin $B_{12}$ coenzyme. This reaction is extremely important in the overall process of gluconeogenesis, especially in ruminants.<br>3. Vitamin $B_{12}$ catalyzes the production of folacin from conjugated folates and aids in the formation of folacin coenzymes.<br>4. It sustains nerve function through its involvement in carbohydrate metabolism (it is known that vitamin $B_{12}$ maintains glutathione in its biologically active reduced state). |
| 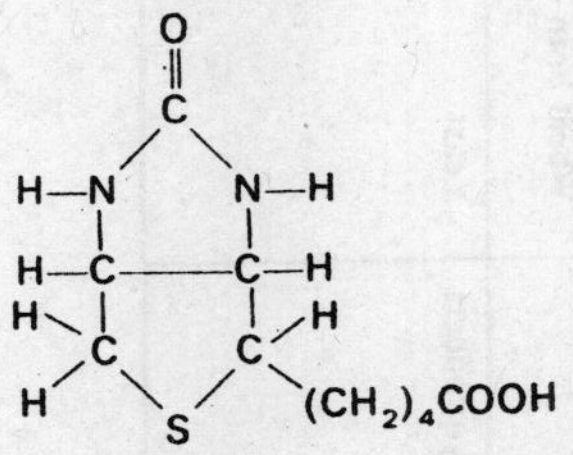 Biotin | Biotin and lipoic acid are both vitamins and coenzymes. They occur mainly in combined forms, covalently bound to proteins through an amide linkage with the ε-amino group of a lysine residue | | In carboxylation reactions, for the biosynthesis of purines, fatty acids, and urea |
| 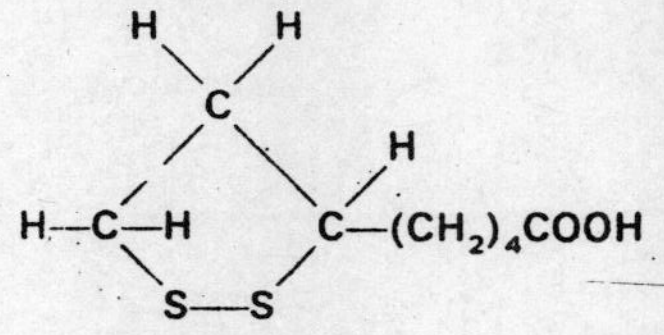 Lipoic acid | | | In generation of acyl groups, acyl group transfer and electron transport |

pyridine nucleotide (TPN), or coenzyme II (Co II), or NADP (nicotinamide adenine denucleotide phosphate).

The primary action of the two coenzymes is to remove hydrogen from substrate as part of dehydrogenase enzymes and transfer hydrogen and/or electrons to the next coenzyme in the chain or to another substrate which then becomes reduced. The enzymes are thus alternately oxidized and reduced.

## Deficiency Symptoms

In chicks, a deficiency produces an enlargement of the tibiotarsal joint, a bowing of the legs, poor feathering and slight dermatitis. A disease characterized by inflammation of the mouth cavity known as "*black tongue*" in fowls is well known. The symptoms of nicotinic acid deficiency in turkeys and ducks while similar are much severe. In swine niacin deficiency is known as "*pig pellagra*" and results in moderate slowing of growth, poor hair and skin condition, occasional vomiting and diarrhoea with foul smelling faeces, particularly involving the large instestine. The large intestine thickens, is very red and appears weak and rotten. Another characteristic symptom is that of high white cell count in the blood.

## Sources

**Table 106**

**SOURCES OF NIACIN**

| Feed Classification | Excellent | Good | Fair to Poor |
|---|---|---|---|
| | Greater than 45 mg/lb (100 mg/kg) | 5-45 mg/lb (10-100 mg/kg) | 0-5 mg/lb (1-10 mg/kg) |
| Fish | Fish solubles | Crab meal<br>Most fish meal | |
| Meat | Heart<br>Liver<br>Kidney<br>White muscle meat | Dark muscle meat | |
| Dairy and poultry products | | | Milk<br>Whey<br>Eggs |
| Forages | | Alfalfa meal | |
| Vegetables and grains | Peanut meal<br>Rice bran<br>Rice polishings<br>Sunflower seed meal<br>Wheat bran | Barley<br>Beans<br>Corn<br>Milo<br>Molasses<br>Oats<br>Rye | Fruits |
| By-products | Yeast | Bakery by-products<br>Brewers' dried grains<br>Distillers' dried grains<br>Meat and bone meal | Feathers |

Niacin requirements are influenced by the protein content of the diet because of the ability of the amino acid tryptophan to supply much of the niacin required by the body which later on is converted to amide. *Sixty mg. of tryptophan are considered to give rise to one mg. of niacin.* Thus if the diet is adequately supplied with protein rich in tryptophan, then the dietary requirement for the niacin should be very low. Moreover, bacterial activity in the intestine contributes niacin which fulfils part of the requirement.

## PYRIDOXINE (VITAMIN $B_6$)

Pyridoxine was first defined by Gyorgy (1934) as "that part of the vitamin B complex responsible for the cure of a specific dermatitis in rats that developed on synthetic rations containing vitamin $B_1$ (thiamin) and vitamin $B_2$ (riboflavin)." The dermatitis of pyridoxine deficiency in rats is a characteristic scaliness around the peripheral parts of the body such as paws and mouth; these areas eventually become denuded as the scales slough off. Hence the vitamin was first indentified as the rat antidermatitis factor. Other names applied to principle included rat acrodynia factor, and *vitamin H*. The term adermin was used by some in European literature.

The vitamin was isolated by Kerestezy (1938) and the synthesis of the vitamin was accomplished by Harris and Folkers in United States. It was not until 1945, however, that the multiple nature of the vitamin was recognized and the other compounds of the complex identified as pyridoxal and pyridoxamine.

### Chemical Nature

Three closely related compounds, pyridoxol, pyridoxal, and pyridoxamine, constitute the group originally known as vitamin $B_6$. Pyridoxine, the previous designation for alcohol form of the vitamin, now is accepted as the group name and is the accepted alternate designation for pyridoxol (IUPAC, 1966). Commercially the vitamin is available in hydrochloride form.

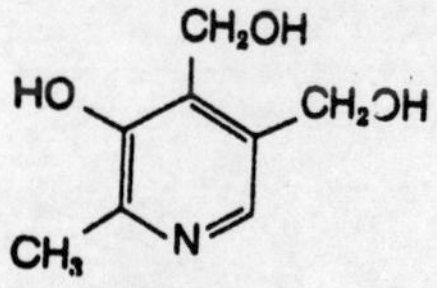

Pyridoxine 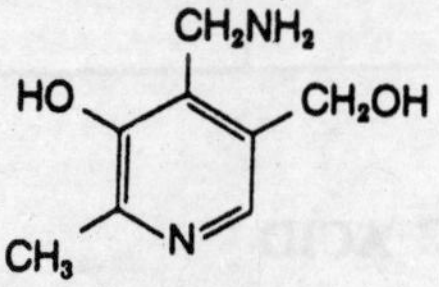 | Pyridoxamine 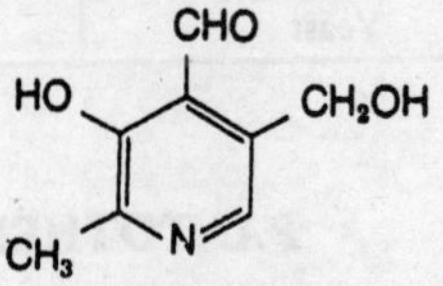 | Pyridoxal 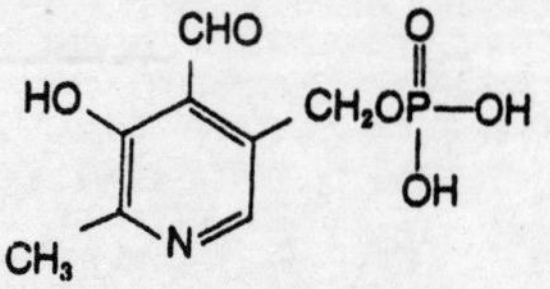 | Pyridoxal phosphate

### Metabolic Function

Of the three related compounds, the actively functioning one appears to be pyridoxal, in the form of the phosphate. Pyridoxal phosphate and other members are essential to amino acid metabolism in several roles: as a coenzyme for decarboxylation, deamination of serine and threonine, transamination, transulfuration, desulfuration of cysteine, the activity of kynureninase, and the transfer of amino acid into cells. Vitamin $B_6$ bound to protein is not easily absorbed, but the vitamin in the free form is absorbed rapidly from the intestine.

### Deficiency Disease

In chicks, a deficiency causes acute convulsion, flatter on the pan, usually starts kicking and generally die. In adult birds with mild deficiency hatchability and egg production are reduced.

A number of symptoms have been reported for pigs which are anorexia, roughness of hair coat, fatty infiltration of the liver, goose step type of gait, convulsions, etc.

In rat characteristic skin lesions appear in the peripheral parts of the body such as paws, nose, ears, tails, etc.

**Table 107**

**SOURCES OF VITAMIN B.**

| Feed Classification | Excellent<br>Greater than 4.5 mg/lb (10 mg/kg) | Good<br>.45-4.5 mg/lb (1-10 mg/kg) | Fair to Poor<br>.05-.45 mg/lb (.1-1 mg/kg) |
|---|---|---|---|
| Fish | | Most fish meals | |
| Meat | Liver<br>Meat and bone meal | | |
| Dairy and poultry products | | Butter<br>Dried milk<br>Eggs<br>Whey | |
| Forages | | Alfalfa meal | |
| Vegetables and grains | Hominy<br>Sesame meal<br>Soybeans, whole<br>Sunflower seed meal<br>Wheat germ | Barley<br>Corn<br>Milo<br>Oats<br>Peanut meal<br>Wheat | Polished rice |
| By-products | Blackstrap molasses<br>Distillers' dried solubles<br>Yeast | Bakery products | Blood meal |

## PANTOTHENIC ACID

Pantothenic acid was isolated and synthesised long before its metabolic role was identified. The vitamin was purified from liver and yeast along with pyridoxine and the two vitamins were separated by adsorption chromatography. Pyridoxine was absorbed on a column of Fuller's earth and subsequently eluted; pantothenic acid was not absorbed and was recovered in the filtrate leaving the column. For this reason, pantothenic acid was designated the *filtrate factor* and pyridoxine, the eluate factor.

At about the same time several groups of investigators were searching for the identification of the vitamin known to be necessary for growth of lactic acid bacteria, prevention of dermatitis in chicks, and prevention of greying of hair in rats. Pantothenic acid was isolated by R.J. Williams and his associates (1938) and synthesised by a group at Merk and Company in 1940. Later tests with the purified vitamin proved it to be the factor required by bacteria, chicks, and rats for preventing the dissimilar deficiency symptoms.

### Chemical Nature

The pantothenic acid molecule is a condensation product of alanine and a hydroxyl and methyl substituted butyric acid, pantoic acid.

```
     OH  CH3  OH  O  H  H  H  O
     |    |    |  ‖  |  |  |  ‖
  H—C — C — C — C—N—C—C—C—OH
     |    |    |        |  |
     H   CH3   H        H  H
  └──────────────┘   └──────────┘
    Pantoic acid       β-alanine
```

*Pantothenic acid*

### Biochemical Functions

Pantothenic acid is the prosthetic group of coenzyme A, an important coenzyme involved in many reversible acetylation reactions in carbohydrate, fat, and amino acid metabolism. The complete enzyme system consists of a specific protein (apoenzyme) combined with the coenzyme moiety. Coenzyme A may act as an acetyl donor or acetyl acceptor. It facilitates condensation

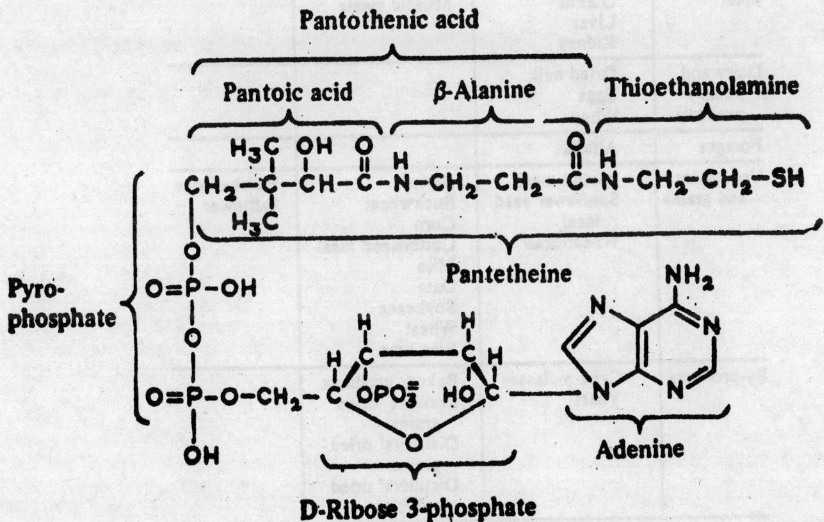


**Structure of coenzyme A**

reactions such as the formation of citrate from oxaloacetate in the Krebs cycle. Coenzyme A also acts as a receiver of acetyl radicals formed in the β-oxidation of fatty acids, and from pyruvate and citrate, and transfer them elsewhere. It conjugates not only with acetyl, but also with acyl groups and with malonyl, the later compound malonyl CoA, being of primary importance in the biosynthesis of fatty acids. . Pantothenic acid, through coenzyme A, is of fundamental importance in the metabolism of all cells.

**Deficiency Symptons**

Affects mainly on three tissues: (1) Nerve—lesions and demyelination. Norris found Riboflavin deficiency causes excessive swelling of nerves but Pantothenic deficiency causes degeneration of sheath, probably both maintain the normal condition of the nerve. (2) Adrenal gland—Acetyl CoA is precursor of cholesterol and thus of steroid hormones of adrenal gland. The anatomic changes of the adrenal gland are accompanied by evidence of functioning inefficiency. (3) Skin—severe dermatitis like biotin deficiency.

In chicks, retarded growth, dermatitis, fatty liver condition, severe edema, subcutaneous haemorrhage are the common symptoms. *"Goose step walk,"* a typical nerve disease is found in case of pigs.

**Table 108**

**SOURCES OF PANTOTHENIC ACID**

| Feed Classification | Excellent<br>Greater than 11 mg/lb (25 mg/kg) | Good<br>2-11 mg/lb (5-25 mg/kg) | Fair to Poor<br>0-2 mg/lb (0-5 mg/kg) |
|---|---|---|---|
| Fish | Fish solubles | Most fish meals | |
| Meat | Glands<br>Liver<br>Kidney | Muscle meats | |
| Dairy and poultry products | Dried milk<br>Eggs<br>Whey | | |
| Forages | Alfalfa | | |
| Vegetables and grains | Peanut meal<br>Sunflower seed meal<br>Wheat bran | Barley<br>Buckwheat<br>Corn<br>Cottonseed meal<br>Milo<br>Oats<br>Soybeans<br>Wheat<br>Rice bran | Polished rice<br>Safflower |
| By-products | Cane molasses<br>Yeast | Bakery products<br>Brewers' dried grains<br>Distillers' dried grains<br>Distillers' dried solubles | |

## FOLIC ACID (FOLACIN)

A deficiency disease found to be folic acid deficiency was first described by Wills (1931) as a "tropical macrocytic anemia" observed in pregnant women patients in Bombay, India, whose diet consisted primarily of white rice and bread. Since the anemia responded to yeast and could be produced in monkeys maintained on similiar monotonous diet it was apparent that the anemia was of nutritional origin.

The development of our present knowledge of folic acid resulted from studies of the nutritional needs of animals, on the one hand, and of bacterial requirements on the other. It is no wonder that this compound has been assigned to a wide variety of designations, since so many test animals and different bacteria have been employed. Also, a variety of symptoms were used as deficiency criteria in animals. Further complications surely resulted from the fact that the vitamin occurs in several chemical forms. A few of the names previously applied to this vitamin include vitamin M (a haematopoietic factor for monkeys), vitamin $B_6$ (chick growth factor), factor R (bacterial growth factor), vitamin $B_{10}$ and vitamin $B_{11}$.

The name folic acid was proposed by Mitchell et al. (1941) for a compound isolated from spinach and shown to be necessary for growth of *Streptococcus faecalis* R. Eventually the structure and synthesis of pteroylglutamic acid were determined by investigators working at Lederle laboratories and Parke Davis Company. A few years later it was clear that all the factors were a form of the vitamin now known as folic acid or pteroylglutamic acid.

**Chemical Nature**

The vitamin consists of a pteridine nucleus, *p*-aminobenzoic acid, and glutamic acid, hence the name pteroylglutamic acid. The portion of the molecule containing pteridine and *p*-aminobenzoic acid is designated pteroic acid. At one time both *p*-aminobenzoic acid and pteroylglutamic acid were considered to be vitamins, but it is now apparent that the species requirement is for one or the other of the two. Pteroylglutamic acid is the vitamin for most mammals, whereas *p*-aminobenzoic acid is essential to certain bacteria that are able to synthesise the larger molecules.

$H_2N$ N N N N OH $CH_2$ H N O H COOH C N C $CH_2CH_2COOH$ H

Pterin Moiety | *p*-Aminobenzoic Group | Glutamic Acid Moiety

Folic Acid (F)

**Biochemical Function**

The active form of the vitamin is tetrahydrofolic acid ($FH_4$), which is formed by reduction of the second ring of the pteridine nucleus with the addition of hydrogen at positions 5, 6, 7 and 8. It is formed from folic acid or dihydrofolic acid ($FH_2$) by action of a reductase and NADH or NADPH serving as carrier. Loss of hydrogen from positions 5 and 6 results in reformation of $FH_2$.

Just as coenzyme A is carrier for acetyl groups, $FH_4$ is carrier for the single carbon groups, may be either formyl (—CHO), formate (H. COOH), or hydroxymethyl (—$CH_2$OH). These are metabolically interconvertible in a reaction catalysed by a NADP—dependent hydroxymethyl dehydrogenase.

in reactions which transfer single carbon units

Tetrahydrofolic acid ($FH_4$)

The one carbon moiety is attached at position 10 or in unstable ring formation at positions 5 and 10 (see following examples).

$N^5$-formyltetrahydrofolic acid ($N^5$-formyl $FH_4$, also folinic acid)

$N^{10}$-formyltetrahydrofolic acid ($N^{10}$-formyl $FH_4$)

The above example appears to be important means for transport of one carbon units. Single carbon units are important in the biosynthesis of purines and pyrimidines and in certain methylation reactions, emphasises the fundamental role of folic acid in growth and reproduction of cells. Because the blood cells are subject to relatively rapid rate of synthesis and destruction, it is not surprising that interference with red blood cell formation would lead to anemia, an early sign of a deficiency of folic acid.

Some specific reactions in which $FH_4$ participates are conversion of glycine to serine, methylation of ethanolamine to choline, methylation of homocysteine to methionine, etc.

### Deficiency Symptoms

The clinical pathology of folic acid deficiency, glossitis, gastrointestinal disturbances, diarrhoea, and reduced erythropoiesis appears to be due to inhibition of mitosis in actively dividing cells such as those of epithelial tissues and bone marrow.

In pigs, macrocytic anemia, lipopenia, megaloblastic arrest, etc., develops. In chicks, poor growth, very poor feathering, depigmentation, anemic appearance and perosis develops.

Table 109

SOURCES OF FOLIC ACID

| Feed Classification | Excellent<br>Greater than 454 mcg/lb (1,000 mcg/kg) | Good<br>136-454 mcg/lb (300-1,000 mcg/kg) | Fair to Poor<br>0-136 mcg/lb (0-300 mcg/kg) |
|---|---|---|---|
| Fish | Herring meal | | Menhaden meal<br>Whitefish meal |
| Meat | Liver | Kidney | |
| Dairy and poultry products | | | Milk<br>Whey |
| Forages | Alfalfa | | |
| Vegetables and grains | Cottonseed meal<br>Linseed meal<br>Soybeans<br>Wheat bran<br>Wheat germ<br>Wheat middlings | Barley<br>Beets<br>Buckwheat<br>Corn<br>Oats<br>Peanut meal<br>Rice<br>Rye<br>Safflower<br>Wheat | Milo |
| By-products | Brewers' dried grains<br>Distillers' dried solubles<br>Yeast | Distillers' dried grains | |

## VITAMIN $B_{12}$

The search for vitamin $B_{12}$ began with the discovery by Minot and Murphy (1926) of the efficacy of liver in the treatment of pernicious anemia. Crystalline $B_{12}$ was isolated independently by two groups, Rickes et al. (1948) in United States and Smith and Parker (1948) in England, and was shown to be active in the treatment of pernicious anemia. It was also well known that chicks required animal protein in their diets in order to maintain adequate growth. The term "*animal protein factor*" (APF) was used to describe this substance which occurs only in foods of animal origin.

### Chemical Nature

Vitamin $B_{12}$ has been isolated in several different biologically active forms. Cyanocobalamin, the principal form of the vitamin contains a cyanide group attached to the central cobalt. The cyanide ion may be replaced by a variety of anions, e.g., hydroxyl (hydroxy cobalamin or $B_{12}$ a) or nitrite nitrocobalamin (or $B_{12}$ c). The biological action of these derivates appears to be similar to that of cobalamin, although hydroxy cobalamin is more active in enzyme systems requiring $B_{12}$ and therefore is used more often than any other forms in experimental studies.

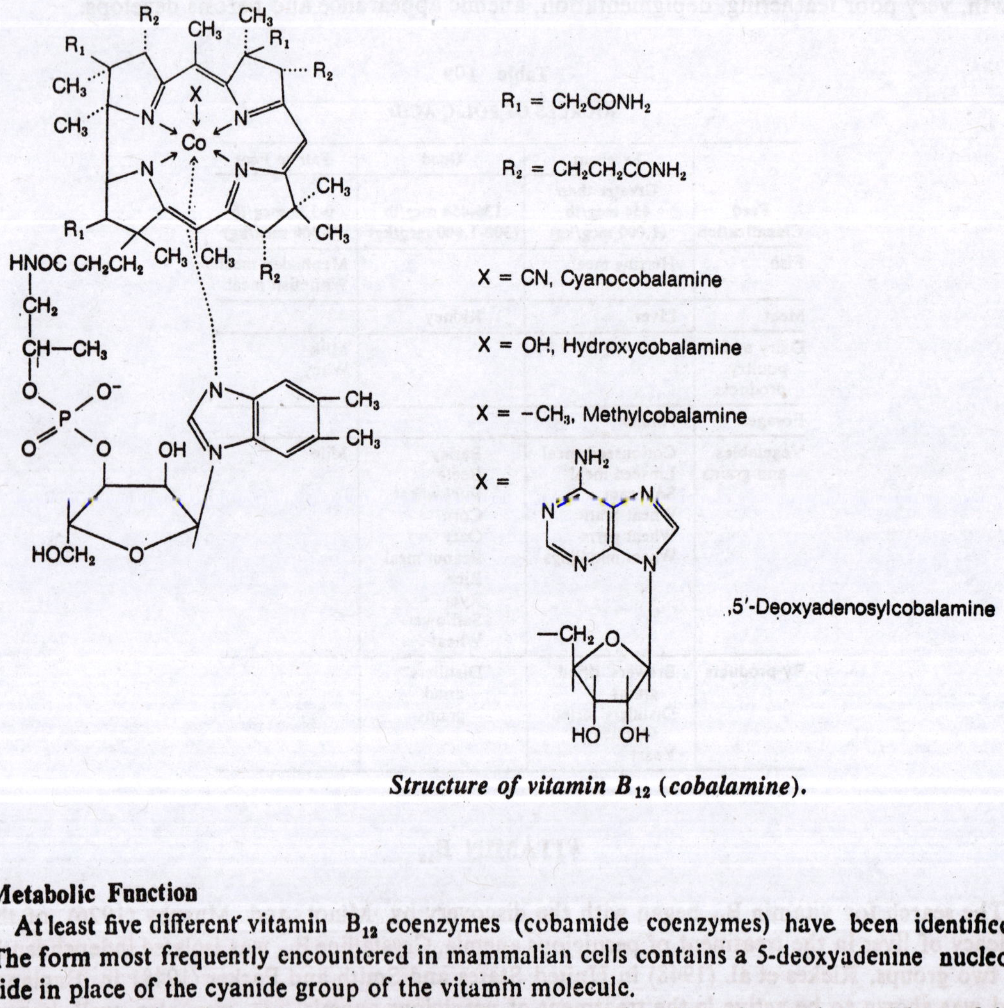

$R_1 = CH_2CONH_2$

$R_2 = CH_2CH_2CONH_2$

X = CN, Cyanocobalamine

X = OH, Hydroxycobalamine

X = $-CH_3$, Methylcobalamine

X = 5'-Deoxyadenosylcobalamine

***Structure of vitamin $B_{12}$ (cobalamine).***

**Metabolic Function**

At least five different vitamin $B_{12}$ coenzymes (cobamide coenzymes) have been identified. The form most frequently encountered in mammalian cells contains a 5-deoxyadenine nucleoside in place of the cyanide group of the vitamin molecule.

The mechanism by which the cobamide coenzyme functions is not clear. Many of its functions appear to be closely linked with $FH_4$ in the metabolism of one carbon groups; it has been suggested that the cobamide coenzyme is required for the interconversion of one carbon units by oxidation reduction reactions. Evidence suggests that the vitamin participates in nucleic acid synthesis, possibly in the conversion of ribose to deoxyribose and in the formation of the methyl group of thiamin. Changes in bone marrow leading to arrested erythrocyte production in pernicious anemia may be related to this function of the vitamin.

Though the mode of actions of folic acid and vitamin $B_{12}$ are referred to similarly in many books, it is believed that they act as coenzymes at different stages in the synthesis of nucleic acids, folic acid and vitamin $B_{12}$ both being required for the formation of deoxyribonucleic acid (DNA) and vitamin $B_{12}$ alone being necessary for the production of ribonucleic acid (RNA). Though folic acid can often substitute for vitamin $B_{12}$ in the maturation of red blood cells it cannot substitute for vitamin $B_{12}$ in maintenance of central nervous system integrity because here the major requirement is for production of RNA rather than DNA.

**Deficiency Symptoms**

In humans, pernicious anemia is the prime symptom. The disease develops either due to lack of vitamin $B_{12}$ in the diet or may be due to lack of a heat labile protein known as "*intrinsic factor*" which is required to "*carry*" vitamin $B_{12}$ across the intestinal mucosa and into the blood stream. The ultimate effect of these two kinds of deficiency results in a lower level of vitamin $B_{12}$ in the body and pernicious anemia crops up.

In chicks and other animals, $B_{12}$ deficiency usually is characterised by poor growth and reproductive failures, with only a slight or no anemia. When pigs are reared indoors on all-plant diets vitamin $B_{12}$ should be included in the diet of pigs.

**Sources**

The origin of vitamin $B_{12}$ in nature is probably the result of microbial synthesis. There is no convincing evidence that the vitamin is produced in the tissues of higher plants or animals. Microbes of the family Actinomycetaceae can synthesise it, although yeast and most fungi apparently do not.

**Table 110**

**SOURCES OF $B_{12}$**

| | Excellent | Good | Fair to Poor |
|---|---|---|---|
| **Feed Classification** | **Greater than 45 mcg/lb (100 mcg/kg)** | **2.3–45 mcg/lb (5–100 mcg/kg)** | **0–2.3 mcg/lb (0–5 mcg/kg)** |
| Fish | Herring meal<br>Liver | | Anchovy meal<br>Menhaden meal<br>White meal |
| Meat | Liver | Meat and bone meal<br>Meat scrap | |
| Dairy and poultry products | | Skimmed milk, dried | Buttermilk, dried<br>Whey, dried |
| Forages | | Alfalfa | |
| Vegetables and grains | | | Corn<br>Soybean meal |
| By-products | Yeast | Distillers' solubles | Distillers' grains<br>Brewers' grains |

## BIOTIN

Biotin was first described as the factor protective against "egg white injury". Rats fed large amounts of raw egg white developed an eczema-like dermatitis, paralysis of the hind legs, and a characteristic alopecia around the eyes, aptly termed *spectacle eye*. Cooked egg white was shown to be non-toxic to rats. This member of the group of B vitamins, has been known by a variety of names including bios factor, vitamin H, and coenzyme R. Duvigneaud and co-workers characterised biotin and published its structure in 1942. Harris and others announced the synthesis of *d*-biotin in 1943. Numerous improvements in synthesis of biotin have been made and at present biotin is readily available to the research worker.

**Chemical Nature**

From the structure it can be said that biotin is a relatively simple monocarboxylic acid. Unlike all other members of the B vitamins, biotin is very slightly soluble in water and alcohol.

In the free state biotin has the structure shown below:

O
‖
C
HN NH
HC—CH
$H_2C$ C—$(CH_2)_4$ COOH
S H

Biotin

**Biochemical Functions**

In biological systems, biotin functions as the coenzyme for carboxylases, enzymes which catalyse carbon dioxide "fixation" or carboxylation. An important example is acetyl-CoA carboxylase, the enzyme which catalyses the reaction of carboxylation in the first step of non-mitochondrial pathway for the synthesis of fatty acids. Biotin also appears to be necessary for synthesis of dicarboxylic acids.

**Deficiency Symptoms**

Experimental biotin deficiency in man, which has been induced by feeding a biotin deficient diet together with large quantities of raw egg white, results in a syndrome characterised by a scaly dermatitis, greyish pallor, extreme lassitude, anorexia, muscle pains, insomnia and a slight anemia.

In chicks biotin deficiency results in dermatitis similar to that occurring in pantothenic acid deficiency. The bottoms of the feet become rough, contain fissures, which show some haemorrhaging. The toes may become necrotic and slough off.

Table 111

SOURCES OF BIOTIN

| Feed Classification | Excellent<br>Greater than .5 mg/lb (1 mg/kg) | Good<br>.05–.5 mg/lb (.1–1 mg/kg) | Fair to Poor<br>0–.05 mg/lb (0–.1 mg/kg) |
|---|---|---|---|
| Fish | | Most fish meals<br>Fish solubles | |
| Meat | | Liver | Muscle meats |
| Dairy and poultry products | | Dried skim milk<br>Eggs<br>Whey | Cheese |
| Forages | | Alfalfa | |
| Vegetables and grains | Safflower | Barley<br>Corn gluten meal<br>Linseed meal<br>Milo<br>Peanuts<br>Rice<br>Soybeans<br>Wheat | Corn<br>Oats |
| By-products | Distillers' dried grains<br>Distillers' dried solubles<br>Molasses<br>Yeast | | Bakery products |

# FEED SUPPLEMENTS, ADDITIVES AND IMPLANTS

## A. FEED SUPPLEMENTS

### What is Supplement ?

*The term, supplement, refers to feedstuffs that are used to improve the value of basal feeds.* They can be used in large quantities, such as protein supplements, or in extremely small quantities, such as trace minerals.

While formulating ration, attention is first given to its dry matter, protein and energy requirements: After this micronutrients such as individual amino acids, minerals, and vitamins are added to correct any deficiency in the ration.

Specific nutrient supplements are now commercially available, thereby permitting the nutritionist to add required amounts of a specific micronutrient or combination of micronutrients in a ration without altering the general makeup of the initial formulation. In general, little or no supplementation of specific amino acid is done in ruminants, although some research with sheep has indicated possible use of methionine hydroxy analogue (MHA) in future. However several amino acids, such as lysine and methionene, warrent careful consideration in feeds for non-ruminants. Mineral and vitamin supplementation is of paramount importance to livestock and poultry. Imbalances, deficiencies or excess of minerals pose major problem. While toxicities of vitamins are rare, deficiencies are, and in this era of highly refined scientific feeding, there can be no excuse for these occurences.

### Mineral Supplements

Almost all feeds contain at least limited amounts of various minerals depending upon the profile of the soil on which they are grown and the genetic variations among its plant species. Apart from such factors, the mineral requirements of animals are highly variable due to age, size, sex, type of production and stage of production.

When using a synthetic compound, the nutritionist often needs to know the percentage of respective elements within the compound. If he knows the chemical formula of the compound, he can establish these percentages quickly. Using calcium carbonate ( $CaCO_3$ ) as an example, the breakdown of the chemical composition is as follows :

**Step 1.** Find out the number of atoms of each element in one molecule. In our example, one molecule of pure $CaCO_3$ breaks down into the following :

*1 atom of Calcium, 1 atom of Carbon, 3 atoms of Oxygen*

**Step 2.** Compute the atomic weight of one molecule of the compound. This is accomplished by multiplying the number of atoms of each element by its atomic weight and adding all of the products. Calcium carbonate yields the following :

| Element | | Number of Atoms | Atomic Weight of the Element | | Product |
|---|---|---|---|---|---|
| Calcium | ... | 1 | 40.00 | | 40.00 |
| Carbon | ... | 1 | 12.00 | | 12.00 |
| Oxygen | ... | 3 | 16.00 | | 48.00 |
| Molecular weight of $CaCO_3$ | | ... | ... | -- | 100.00 |

**Step 3.** Divide the product of each element calculated in step 2 by the total molecular weight of the compound, and multiply by 100 to yield the percentage of each element in the compound.

| | | | |
|---|---|---|---|
| Calcium | $(40 \div 100) \times 100$ | = | 40.00 |
| Carbon | $(12 \div 100) \times 100$ | = | 12.00 |
| Oxygen | $(48 \div 100) \times 100$ | = | 48.00 |
| Total | ... | ... | 100.00% |

It may be noted that supplementation of minerals depend on (1) needs of the particular animal—age, sex, weight and production parameters. (2) types of feed an—all-or high-concentrate ration will require a different mineral supplement than an all-or high-roughage ration.

For mixed feed the following recommendations are applicable to the mineral supplementation.

1. Salt is usually incorporated in the ration at levels of 0.50 to 1.0 per cent.
2. Calcium and phosphorus are added as required to balance the ration.
3. If animals are housed in confinement where they receive little exposure to sunlight, careful attention must be given to provide adequate vitamin D which aids assimilation and utilisation of number of minerals, specially calcium and phosphorus.
4. When the ration is suspected to be deficient in one or more minerals, a trace mineralised salt mixture as available in the market should be provided.

Where animals are primarily on roughage, provide free access to a two compartment mineral box with trace mineralised salt mixture in one side, and in the other side, a mixture of ½ trace mineralised salt mixture and ⅔ dicalcium or steamed bone meal.

Table 112

**Elemental composition of salts used in mineral mixtures**

| *Salt* | *Formula* | *Elements in salt per cent* |
|---|---|---|
| ***Calcium*** | | |
| Calcium carbonate | $CaCO_3$ | 40.05 Ca 59.95 $CO_3$ |
| Dicalcium phosphate, anhydrous | $CaHPO_4$ | 29.46 Ca 22.77 P |
| Dicalcium phosphate, dihydrate | $CaHPO_4.2H_2O$ | 23.29 Ca 18.01 P |
| Tricalcium phosphate | $Ca_3(PO_4)_2$ | 38.76 Ca 19.97 P |
| Calcium sulphate | $CaSO_4$ | 29.43 Ca 70.57 $SO_4$ |
| Bone meal | | 30.00 Ca 15.00 P |
| Oyster shell grit | | 38.00 Ca |
| Ground limestone | | 38.00 Ca |
| ***Chloride*** | | |
| Sodium chloride | NaCl | 60.65 Cl 38.35 Na |
| Potassium chloride | KCl | 47.56 Cl 52.44 K |
| ***Chromium*** | | |
| Chrome alum | $Cr_2K_2(SO_4)_4.24H_2O$ | 10.42 Cr 38.49 $SO_4$ |
| Chromic chloride | $CrCl_3$ | 32.82 Cr 67.18 Cl |
| ***Cobalt*** | | |
| Cobaltous chloride, pentahydrate | $CoCl_2.5H_2O$ | 26.80 Co 32.28 Cl |
| Cobaltous chloride, hexahydrate | $CoCl_2.6H_2O$ | 24.77 Co 29.84 Cl |
| ***Copper*** | | |
| Cupric sulphate | $CuSO_4$ | 39.81 Cu 60.19 $SO_4$ |
| Cupric sulphate, pentahydrate | $CuSO_4.5H_2O$ | 25.46 Cu 38.49 $SO_4$ |
| Cupric chloride | $CuCl_2$ | 47.27 Cu 52.73 Cl |
| ***Fluorine*** | | |
| Potassium fluoride, dihydrate | $KF.2H_2O$ | 20.17 F 41.54 K |
| Sodium fluoride | NaF | |
| ***Iodine*** | | |
| Potassium iodide | KI | 76.45 I 23.55 K |
| Potassium iodate | $KIO_3$ | 59.31 I 18.27 K |
| Calcium iodate | $Ca(IO_3)_2$ | 65.09 I 10.28 Ca |
| Sodium iodide | NaI | 84.68 I 15.32 Na |
| ***Iron*** | | |
| Ferrous sulphate, heptahydrate | $FeSO_4.7H_2O$ | 20.09 Fe 34.59 $SO_4$ |
| Ferrous acetate, tetrahydrate | $Fe(C_2H_3O_2)_2.4H_2O$ | |

Table 112 (*Contd.*)

| *Salt* | *Formula* | *Elements in salt per cent* |
|---|---|---|
| ***Magnesium*** | | |
| Magnesium carbonate | $MgCO_3$ | 28.84 Mg 71.16 $CO_3$ |
| Magnesium sulphate | $MgSO_4$ | 20.19 Mg 79.81 $SO_4$ |
| Magnesium sulphate, heptahydrate | $MgSO_4.7H_2O$ | 9.87 Mg 39.01 $SO_4$ |
| ***Manganese*** | | |
| Manganese dioxide | $MnO_2$ | 63.19 Mn |
| Manganous carbonate | $MnCO_3$ | 47.79 Mn 52.21 $CO_3$ |
| Manganous chloride, tetrahydrate | $MnCl_2.4H_2O$ | 27.76 Mn 35.86 Cl |
| Manganous sulphate | $MnSO_4$ | 36.36 Mn 63.64 $SO_4$ |
| Manganous sulphate hydrate | $MnSO_4.H_2O$ | 32.49 Mn 56.86 $SO_4$ |
| Manganous sulphate tetrahydrate | $MnSO_4.4H_2O$ | 24.63 Mn 43.10 $SO_4$ |
| ***Molybdenum*** | | |
| Sodium molybdate, dihydrate | $Na_2MoO_4.2H_2O$ | 39.66 Mo 19.01 Na |
| Sodium molybdate, pentahydrate | $NaMoO_4.5H_2O$ | 35.15 Mo 8.43 Na |
| ***Nickel*** | | |
| Nickel chloride | $NiCl_2$ | 45.26 Ni 54.74 Cl |
| ***Phosphorus*** | | |
| Orthophosphoric acid | $H_3PO_4$ | 31.61 P |
| Potassium orthophosphate | $K_2HPO_4$ | 17.79 P 44.90 K |
| Potassium dihydrogen orthophosphate | $KH_2PO_4$ | 22.76 P 28.73 K |
| Sodium hydrogen orthophosphate | $Na_2HPO_4$ | 21.82 P 32:40 Na |
| Sodium dihydrogen orthophosphate, hydrate | $NaH_3PO_4.H_2O$ | 22.45 P 16.67 Na |
| Sodium dihydrogen orthophosphate, dihydrate | $NaH_3PO_4.2H_2O$ | 19.86 P 14.74 Na |
| Ammonium phosphate | $(NH_2)_2HPO_4$ | 23.46 P |
| ***Potassium*** | | |
| Potassium chloride | KCl | 52.44 K 47.56 Cl |
| Potassium carbonate | $K_2CO_3$ | 56.58 K 43.42 $CO_3$ |
| Potassium bicarbonate | $KHCO_3$ | 39.05 K, 60.95 HCO |
| Potassium acetate | $KC_2H_3O_2$ | 39.84 K 60.16 Acetate |
| Potassium orthophosphate | $K_3PO_4$ | 55.25 K 14.59 P |
| Potassium sulphate | $K_2SO_4$ | 44.87 K 55.13 $SO_4$ |

Table 112 (*Contd.*)

| | | |
|---|---|---|
| ***Selenium*** | | |
| Sodium selenite | $Na_2SeO_3$ | 45.65 Se 26.60 Na |
| Sodium selenate | $NaSeO_4$ | 41.79 Se 24.34 Na |
| ***Sodium*** | | |
| Sodium chloride | $NaCl$ | 39.35 Na 60.65 Cl |
| Sodium bicarbonate | $NaHCO_3$ | 27.38 Na 72.62 $HCO_3$ |
| Sodium sulphate | $Na_2SO_4$ | 32.39 Na 67.61 $SO_4$ |
| ***Tin*** | | |
| Stannic sulphate | $Sn(SO_4)_2.2H_2O$ | 34.22 Sn 55.36 $SO_4$ |
| ***Vanadium*** | | |
| Sodium orthovanadate | $Na_3VO_4$ | 27.69 V 37.51 Na |
| ***Zinc*** | | |
| Zinc carbonate | $ZnCO_3$ | 52.14 Zn 47.86 $CO_3$ |
| Zinc chloride | $ZnCl_2$ | 47.97 Zn 52.03 Cl |
| Zinc oxide | $ZnO$ | 80.35 Zn |
| Zinc sulphate | $ZnSO_4$ | 40.47 Zn 59.33 $SO_4$ |
| Zinc sulphate hydrate | $ZnSO_4.H_2O$ | 36.42 Zn 53.55 $SO_4$ |

SOURCE: *Poultry Nutrition*, by W. Bolton and R. Blair, Published by Ministry of Agriculture, Fisheries and Food, U.K., 1974, Bulletin No. 174.

**Vitamin Supplements**

Each of the various vitamins perform one or more basic functions in the regulation of various metabolic processes within the body. Vitamin supplements now form an essential part of farm livestock feeding. Animals when feeding under natural conditions, with a free choice from a wide range of feedstuffs, consume, as a rule all the vitamins they require. But under the influence of domestication, and specially of intensive rareing, animals often have no choice in the matter and suffer from vitamin deficiencies either because their artificial diet is too restricted, or because vitamins naturally present have been destroyed during preparation of feed.

For ruminants, only vitamin A needs to be given attention from the standpoint of meeting the dietary needs. Usually all of the vitamin B members are apparently synthesised in the rumen in sufficient quantities to overcome any dietary shortage. Vitamin C is also synthesised within the body tissues in sufficient quantities to meet the animal's need. Where ruminants receive enough exposure to direct sunlight, hardly they will need any supplementation of vitamin D. Most ruminant rations are considered to be more than adequate in vitamin E assuming that required amount of selenium is present to bring about its effective utilisation. Vitamin K is also synthesised in the rumen to meet all the demand. Consequently, it would seem that in most instances ruminants would have no need for vitamin supplementation. However, it has been observed that when ruminants do not find enough of green forages as in summer time, deficiency of carotene and thereby of vitamin A is bound to occur. Similarly during stresses ( vaccination, peak production, antibiotic treatment etc. ) the requirement of almost all vitamins will increase and the ruminants will have to be provided with additional dietary vitamins.

Non-ruminants in general are very much susceptible to vitamin deficiencies as they have no mechanism to synthesise required amounts of vitamins except vitamin C. Under sufficient exposure of sunlight vitamin D requirement may be fulfilled. To-day supplementation of various vitamins to our livestock mav be met from natural as well as from synthetic sources.

## B. FEED ADDITIVES AND IMPLANTS

**What is an Additive ?**

*An additive is a substance that is added to a basic feed, usually in small quantities, for the purpose of fortifying it with certain nutrients, stimulants or medicines other than as a direct source of nutrient.*

In general, the term *"feed additive"* refers to a non-nutritive product that affects utilisation of the feed or productive performance of the animal. Feed additives and implants can be classed according to the mode of action as follows :

**1. Additives that enhance feed intake**

(a) *Antioxidants*

*Antioxidants are compounds that prevent oxidative rancidity of polyunsaturated fats.* Rancidity once develops, may cause destruction of vitamins A, D, and E, and several of the B complex vitamins. Breakdown products of rancidity may react with the epsilon amino groups of lysine and thus affects the protein value of the ration. Ethoxyquin or BHT ( butylated hydroxytoluene) can serve as antioxidants in feed but are unable to prevent peroxidation within the cell.

(b) *Flavouring Agent*

*Flavouring agents are feed additives that are supposed to increase palatability and feed intake.* There is need for flavouring agents that will help to keep up feed intake (1) when highly unpalatable medicants are being mixed, (2) during attacks of diseases, (3) when animals are under stress, and (4) when a less palatable feedstuffs is being fed either as such or being incorporated in the ration.

Ruminants prefer sweet compounds. Additionally cattle and goats respond positively to salts of volatile fatty acids. Horses will often refuse musty feed when there is so little mould that the owner fails to detect it.

**2. Additives that enhance the colour or quality of the marketed product**

Many of the "brain washed" consumers believe that broilers having a deep yellow colour are of top quality. To satisfy them poultryman will often enhance the yellow colour by incorporating xanthophylls into broiler feed. A similar situation exists relative to egg yolk colour. Among various additives, arsanilic acid, sodium arsanilate and roxarsone are added for the purpose.

**3. Additives that facilitate digestion and absorption**

(a) *Grit.* Poultry do not have teeth to grind any hard grain, most grinding takes place in the thick musculated gizzard. The more thoroughly feed is ground, the more surface area is created for digestion and subsequent absorption. Hence, when hard, coarse or fibrous feeds are fed to poultry, grit is sometimes added to supply additional surface for grinding within gizzard. When mash or finely ground feeds are fed, the value of grit become less. Oyster shells, coquina shells and limestone are used as grit.

(b) *Buffers and Neutralisors.* During maximum production stage ruminants are given high doses of concentrate feeds for meeting demands for extra energy and protein requirement of the animal. The condition on the other hand lowers the pH of the rumen. Since many of the rumen microbes cannot tolerate low pH environment, the normally heterogenous, balanced population of microbes become skewed, favouring the acidophilic (acid-loving) bacteria. The condition often leads to *acidosis* and thereby upsets normal digestion.

The addition of feed buffers and neutralisors, such as carbonates, bicarbonates, hydroxides, oxides, salts of VFA, phosphate salts, ammonium chloride and sodium sulphate have been shown to have beneficial effects. Recently the use of baking soda ( $NaHCO_3$ ) has been shown to increase average daily gain by about 10 per cent, feed efficiency by 5 to 10 per cent, and milk production by about 0.5 liter per head per day.

(c) *Chelates.* Chelating agents, such as EDTA, are sometimes used in chick ration for increase zinc absorption. Chelated forms of various trace minerals are now available in market. For further information about chelates, *Chapter 12* may be consulted.

(d) *Probiotic.* The addition of substances which encourage the growth of the desirable microorganisms of gastrointestinal tract are known as probiotics. The addition of molasses, alcohol, ruminal culture all are tried. The value of these substances are still questionable as the immediate environment and type of feed used are probably the most critical factors in establishing a population of microorganisms in ruminants.

**4. Additives that promotes growth and production**

(a) *Antibiotics. These are substances which are produced by living organisms (mould, bacteria or green plants) and which in small concentration have bacteriostatic or bactericidal properties.* They were originally developed for medical and veterinary purposes to control specific pathogenic organisms, but from the work of Stockstad and associates of the American Cyanamid Company (1949), it was discovered that certain antibiotics could increase the rate of growth of young pigs and chicks when included in their diet in small amounts. Soon after this report a wide range of antibiotics have been tested and the following have been shown to have growth promoting properties: penicillin, oxytetracycline (Terramycin), chlortetracycline, bacitracin, streptomycin, tyrothricin, gramicidin, neomycin, erythromycin and flavomycin. Increased weight gain is most evident during the period of rapid growth and then decreases. Differences between control and treated animals are greater when the diet is slightly deficient or marginal in protein, B-vitamins or certain mineral elements.

**Mode of Action of Antibiotics**

1. Antibiotics "spare" protein, amino acids and vitamin on diets containing 1 to 3 per cent less protein, but balance experiments have often failed to show increased nitrogen retention. However, it has been suggested that some antibiotics have a sparing effect on B. vitamins as found in rats and chickens. The materials act by increasing the absorption of these vitamins.
2. Intestinal wall of animals fed antibiotics is thinner than that of untreated animals, which might explain the enhanced absorption of calcium shown for chicks.
3. Reduce or eliminate the activity of pathogens causing "subclinical infection".
4. Reduce the growth of micro-organisms that compete with the host for supplies of nutrients.
5. Antibiotics alter intestinal bacteria so that less urease is produced and thus less ammonia is formed. Ammonia is highly toxic and suppresses growth in non-ruminants.
6. Stimulate the growth of micro-organisms that synthesise known or unidentified nutrients.

**Antibiotics in Pig Feeding**

The good effects of feeding the antibiotic feed supplement is observed with animals given all-vegetable protein diets than those receiving animal protein supplements. The optimum level for most antibiotics in the diet is within the range of 5–15 mg/kg and there is no advantage in exceeding these low levels. Under normal condition of health adding Aureomycin or Terramycin supplement to rations for growing or fattening pigs increases the growth by about 15% reducing the feed intake by 2.5%. A mixture of two or more antibiotics is no more effective than a single effective antibiotic. The greatest increase in the rate of gain from an antibiotic feed supplement occurs during early growth, i.e., the suckling pigs gain more body weight.

**Antibiotics in Poultry Feeding**

Penicillin is more effective than other antibiotics especially to young and growing chicks. It increases the growth rate and this effect is most marked upto 1 month of age. As with pigs, the effect diminishes with age. Growth stimulation has been greatest when the antibiotic penicillin supplement has been added to a ration containing no protein supplements of animal origin or to a ration low in vitamin $B_{12}$. Under hygienic conditions growth increases are small. In "old" (infected) buildings increases of 10–15% in the growth rate of fowls are likely to be obtained with similiar increases in efficiency of feed utilisation. About 5 gm. of procaine penicillin per ton of ration for poultry is needed; but to control diseases, a higher level of 50 gm. or more per ton for feed is used.

Use of a combination of antibiotics has been no more effective than that of a single effective antibiotic. In layers, egg production has not been increased by adding antibiotics to a ration

Table 113

Antibiotics and other antibacterial drugs commonly used as feed additives for improving animal performance.

| | | Approved dose level, | |
|---|---|---|---|
| Name[a] | Approved for use with | g/ton of feed | mg/head/day |
| Arsanilic acid or Na arsanilate | poultry | 40-90 | |
| | swine | 45-90 | |
| Bacitracin* | poultry | 4-50 | |
| | layers | 10-50 | |
| | swine | 10-50 | |
| | beef | | 35 |
| Bacitracin methylene disalicylate* | poultry | 4-50 | |
| | laying chickens | 10-50 | |
| Bacitracin zinc* | poultry | 4-50 | |
| | laying chickens | 10-100 | |
| | swine | 10-100 | |
| | cattle | | 35-70 |
| Bambermycins* | broilers | 1-2 | |
| | swine | 2-4 | |
| Carbadox | swine | 10-50 | |
| Chlortetracycline* (Aureomycin) | poultry | 10-100 | |
| | calves | | 25-70 |
| | feedlot cattle | | 70 |
| | dairy cows | | 70 |
| | lambs | 20-50 | |
| | horses | | 85 |
| | swine | 10-50 | |
| Dichlorvos | swine | 334-500 | |
| Erythromycin* | growing chicks | 4.6-18.5 | |
| | laying chickens | 18.5 | |
| | growing turkeys | 9.25-18.5 | |
| | starter pigs | 10-70 | |
| | growing pigs | 10 | |
| | feedlot cattle | | 37 |
| Furazolidone | poultry | 7.5-10 | |
| | baby pigs | 100 | |
| | sows | 150 | |
| Ipronidazole | turkeys | | 0.00625% |
| Lincomycin* | broilers | 2-4 | |

Table 113 (*Contd.*)

| Name[a] | Approved for use with | Approved dose level, g/ton of feed | mg/head/day |
|---|---|---|---|
| Melengestrol acetate | beef heifers | | 0.25-0.50 |
| Monensin* | cattle | 5-30 | |
| Oleandomycin* | chickens | 1-2 | |
| | turkeys | 1-2 | |
| | swine | 5-11.25 | |
| Oxytetracycline* (Terramycin) | growing chicks and turkeys | 5-7.5 | |
| | laying chickens | 10-15 | |
| | laying turkeys | 10-50 | |
| | swine, 10-30 lb | 25-50 | |
| | 30-200 lb | 7.5-10 | |
| | calf starters & milk replacers | | lb body weight |
| | calves | 25-75 | |
| | feedlot cattle | 75 | |
| | beef cattle | 75 | |
| | dairy cattle | 75 | |
| | sheep | 10-20 | |
| | rabbits | 10 | |
| Penicillin* | chickens, turkeys | 2.4-50 | |
| | swine | 10-50 | |
| Roxarsone | chickens | 22.7-45.4 | |
| | turkeys | 22.7-45.4 | |
| | swine | 22.7-68.1 | |
| Thyroprotein | growing ducks | 100-200 | |
| | dairy cows | | 0.5-1.5 g/100 lb body weight |
| Tylosin* | growing chicks | 4-50 | |
| | laying chickens | 20-50 | |
| | swine | | |
| | starter feeds | 20-100 | |
| | grower feeds | 20-40 | |
| | finisher feeds | 10-20 | |
| | beef cattle | 8-10 | |
| Virginiamycin* | broilers | 5-15 | |
| | swine | 5-10 | |

[a] Many of these drugs are approved for use with others or at higher levels for disease control.

* Antibiotics

which is nutritionally complete. But, if hens are fed on only vegetable product ration, an antibiotic vitamin $B_{12}$ feed supplement may increase both egg production and hatchability.

**Antibiotics in the Diet of Ruminant Animals**

The addition of Aureomycin supplement to calf rations has increased the growth rate of dairy calves specially when there had been much trouble from disease in the herd. It has reduced the incidence of scours and other infectious diseases. Most of the growth improvement occurs before the calves are 8 weeks old. Feeding daily 30 milligrams of Aureomycin or Terramycin per calf is the dose

As far as mature animals are concerned, the results are conflicting. It has been assumed that the inclusion of antibiotics in the diet could be harmful by suppressing the activity of cellulolytic organisms and thus impairing cellulose digestion. In cows neither the milk production nor the fat percentage has been increased. It is similarly of no use in sterile animals and irregular breeders.

Following points should be kept in mind while using antibiotics for animal feeding:

1. Antibiotics should be used only for (a) growing and fattening pigs for slaughter as pork or becon; (b) growing chicks and turkey poults for killing as table poultry.
2. Antibiotics should not be used in the feed of ruminant animals (cattle, sheep and goats), breeding pigs and breeding and laying poultry stock.
3. While adding antibiotics at the recommended level, care should be taken that they are thoroughly and evenly mixed with the feed.
4. For best results, antibiotics should be used with properly balanced feeds. Also, the feeds containing antibiotics should be fed only to the type of stock for which they are intended.
5. Antibiotics are not a substitute for good management and healthy living conditions, or for properly balanced rations.

The use of antibiotic feed supplements or the fortified ration or the medicated feeds is governed by strict State laws in some countries (U.S.A., Canada and U.K.) where they are used for livestock and poultry so that farmers will not run unnecessary risk in using them.

(b) *Arsenicals* In 1949 it was reported that organic arsenicals had growth promoting properties similar to those of antibiotics when added to the diets of chicks. Arsanilic acid. sodium arsanilate are common compounds used.

**5. Additives that alter metabolism**

(a) *Hormones. These are chemicals released by a specific area of the body (ductless glands) and are transported to another region within the animal where they elicit a physiological response.*

Extensive use is being made of synthetic. and purified estrogens, androgens, progestogens, growth hormones and thyroxine or thyroprotein (iodinated casein) to stimulate the growth and fattening of meat-producing animals. There is concern, however, about possible harmful effects of any residues of these materials in the meat or milk for the consumers.

Hormones related to animal growth on the basis of their effect in body can be grouped into two major categories *viz.*, ANABOLIC and CATABOLIC. Somatotropin, thyroxine and androgens are anabolic while estrogen and glucocorticoids belong to catabolic group.

The hormones of the anabolic class by nature exert their effect on both skeleton and protein metabolism. Somatotropin stimulates growth of endochondral bone and epiphysis of long bones while in protein metabolism it aids in nitrogen retention and overall protein synthesis. Thyroxine also stimulates growth of long bones as well as protein synthesis. Testosterone at low dose increases the epiphyseal diameter, promotes muscle growth by augmenting nitrogen retention.

The hormones belonging to catabolic group similarly exert their effect on both skeleton and protein metabolism. Estrogen inhibits skeletal growth although in ruminants it increases nitrogen retention. Glucocorticoids decrease growth of epiphysis and also aid in degrading protein and amino acids and thereby inhibit protein synthesis in extrahepatic tissue.

It is thought that the hormone alters the metabolism so as to increase muscle and bone formation at the expense of fat deposition. Since the energy required to synthesise protein or bone is less than that required to synthesise the same weight of fat, and the amount of water in muscle is greater than in body fat, it follows that a given amount of food will produce a higher live-weight increase due to hormone treatment.

It is an established fact that milk production in the cow will increase following the feeding of thyroprotein or L-thyroxine. The most effective daily dose appears to be about 15 gm per cow in the case of thyroprotein and 100 mg/cow daily for L-thyroxine. The addition of thyroxine or thyroprotein to the diet has increased milk production from 15 to 20 per cent above control animals, if a concomitant increase in energy intake was maintained. If additional feed is not given then the response is muted. A problem which has encountered is that sudden withdrawal of thyroprotein will cause milk production to drop below that of normal control cows, resulting no appreciable increase in the total milk produced in an entire lactation. University of Tennesse investigators found gradual withdrawing of thyroprotein caused milk production to drop only to the expected level or to that of controls. The indications are that feeding thyroprotein for short periods in successive lactation periods does not impair production; feeding the hormone for long periods in successive lactations may have an adverse effect on milk production but adequate proof for this is lacking. Some dairymen have experienced an increase in teat and other injuries and general excitability in thyroprotein fed herd. This is reasonable to expect. The overall seriousness of the problem will vary with a particular situation. During periods of extremely high environmental temperature, , there should be some caution exercised in the artificial induction of a hyperthyroid state.

Some workers have reported increased rates of gain and improved feed efficiency as a result of feeding thyroprotein or thyroxine to growing pigs from the time of weaning to market weight. As in the cow, administration of thyroprotein to lactating cows has been recommended by some investigators, with additional energy intake, lactation would probably be increased.

Studies with fattening lambs have shown that feeding 2-5 mg of stilbesterol daily increased the average daily gain about 20 per cent and reduced the feed per unit of gain. These substances either be given at the rate of 10 mg/day in beef cattle or can be implanted under the skin in the form of pellets in a single dose of 75 gm and 10 mg in sheep. Synthetic oestrogens should never be given to female animals, as otherwise there will be derangement of the breeding behaviour.

The widest application of the use of synthetic estrogenic hormones has undoubtedly been in the field of beef cattle and fat lamb production. The use of synthetic stilbesterol, hexoestrol has attracted more attention in recent years and these are in commercial use as growth promoters in many countries. Optimal amounts of oral dose or implantation of various hormonal compounds as reported by the National Research Council Committee are given in Table 72.

**Table 114**

| | *Products* | *Animal* | *Dosages* | *Method of use* |
|---|---|---|---|---|
| 1. | Diethylstilbesterol | Cattle | 10 mg/day | In feed |
| | | Sheep | 2 mg/day | |
| | (Thyroprotein) | Cattle | 24 to 36 mg | Subcutaneour |
| | | Poultry | 12 to 15 mg | |
| 2. | Diethylstilbesterol plus testosterone | Cattle | 24 mg+120 mg | Subcutaneous |
| 3. | Testosterone propionate+estradiol benzoate | Heifers | 200 mg+20 mg | Subcutaneous |
| 4. | Thiouracil | Swine and Poultry | 0.2% of diet | In feed |
| 5. | Iodinated casein (thyroprotein) | Lactating cows | 15 mg/day | In feed |
| | | Lactating sows | 200 mg/kg diet | In feed |
| | | | 25-50 mg/kg diet | In feed |

SOURCE: *Animal Nutrition*, L. Maynard and J.K. Loosli, 6th edition.

The whole question whether hormones should be used as growth promoters is still debatable, but it seems logical that with any feeding system the economic advantages, however great, should never take precedence over any potential risk to human health. These substances may induce cancer in human beings if taken over a prolonged period through products of the treated animals. The use of such substances in poultry rearing has been prohibited by law in U.S.A.

(b) *Implants. Implants are hormone or hormone like products that are designed to release slowly, but constantly, the active chemicals for absorption into the bloodstream.* These are implanted subcutaneously in the ear. At present three commercial compounds. *viz.*, diethylstilbesterol (DES) synovex ( contain testoterone and estradiol ) and ralgro a trade name for zeranol ( not a hormone but a chemical substance produced by moulds, *Giberella zeae* ) now available in U.S.A.

6. **Additives that affect the health status of livestock**

(a) *Antibloat compounds*

In the market although there are several products claimed as an antibloat compounds but none is 100 per cent effective. One antibiotic oxytetracycline has been found to be highly effective but when used over a period of time, the effectiveness is gradually decreased. Surfactants such as *poloxalene* is used as a preventive for pasture bloat.

Several other products have been shown to be highly effective to prevent bloat are also available in the market.

(b) *Antifungal additives*

Mould inhibitors are added to feed liable to be contaminated with various types of fungi such as *Aspergillus flavus, Penicillium cyclopium* etc. Before adding commercial inhibitors all feedstuff should be dried below 12 cent moisture. Propionic, acetic acid and sodium propionic are added in high moisture grain to inhibit mould growth. Antifungals such as nystathnin and copper sulphate preparations are also in use to concentrate feeds to prevent moulds.

(c) *Anticoccidials*

Various brands of anticoccidials are now available in the country to prevent the growth of coccidia which are protozoa and live inside the cells of the intestinal lining of livestock.

(d) *Antihelmintics* Under some practical feeding conditions anthelmintics have also been used. The compounds act by reducing parasitic infections. Out of many commercial products, DDVP (2,2 dichlorovinyl dimethyl phosphate, has both anthelmintics and separate growth stimulatory effect in cattle.

# 14

# BIOENERGETICS AND ENERGY METABOLISM

## BIOENERGETICS

In this universe, neither energy nor chemical elements can be created or destroyed and the animal system is no exception to this. However, the form of energy and the nature of the chemical compounds present in the animal or ingested in the food are subject to changes through the processes of metabolism in the animal. Nutritional requirement and its efficiency as a growth promoter or as a media for high production in animal system depends upon the nature and the extent of such metabolic transactions.

Bioenergetics or *Biochemical thermodynamics* is the study of the energy changes accompanying biochemical reactions. These reactions, as occurring in every cell are accompanied by an exchange of energy in the system.

### What is Energy?

The term 'Energy' is a combination of two Greek words: *en,* meaning 'in' and *ergon,* meaning 'work'. The Greeks put the two words together to form *energon,* meaning 'active'. Hence energy is that force or power that enables the body to carry on life sustaining activities. Death is the cessation of this activity. Thus energy is the capacity to do work and is derived from mechanics.

### Basic Units of Energy

In contrast to matter which has a mass and a space, energy neither occupies space nor has weight. There is no such thing, for example, as '3 cubic feet' or '4 kg' of energy. *Energy can only be measured by its effects* upon matter. In general greater the effect, the greater the amount of energy. For example, under similar conditions, a stick of dynamite causes more damage to a house (matter) than a firecracker does. The dynamite releases more energy.

The calorie has so long been used as a unit of energy since last two centuries. It is actually a unit of heat since one calorie is the amount of heat required to raise the temperature of one gram of water from 14.5 to 15.5°C at atmospheric pressure. This is also the specific heat of water. In nutritional and physiological studies, the unit of measure is the large calorie or kilocalorie, which is equal to 1000 small calories. Thus a kilocalorie (kcal) is the amount of heat required to raise 1 kg of water to 1°C. 1000 kcal is equal to 1 megacalorie (Mcal) or the Therm. In popular writings, particularly those concerned with human and animal calorie requirements, the term calorie is frequently used erroneously in place of the kilocalorie.

The International Union of Pure and Applied Chemistry (IUPAC) voted to adopt the energy unit as Joule (J) for measuring all forms of energy. The electrical energy required to increase the temperature of water from 14.5°C to 15.5°C has been determined, and average out to 4.1855 joules per 15° calorie. Thus it has been accepted that one small calorie = 4.185 J.

The joule is defined as "the amount of work done by giving a force of 1 newton to displace the point of application of force through a distance of 1 meter. One newton is the force that will give a mass of 1 kg an acceleration of $1 m/sec^2$. By analogy with current practice the units employed would be kilojoule (kJ) and the megajoule (MJ). The advantages of expressing unit of energy as joule is that in the metric system of measurement this unit is suitable for expressing mechanical, chemical or electrical energy as well as in explaining the concept of heat. At present the system has been approved for use in about thirty countries, which has created pressure to replace the calorie with joule as a unit of energy. This pressure has resulted in controversy among nutritional scientists about the pros and cons of discarding the calorie and adopting the joule.

In nutritional work, kilocalories are often rounded off to the nearest 50, which would be approximately to the nearest 200 kilojoules.

Comparisons of physiological fuel values are as follows:

Table 115

| | *Kilocalories/gram* | *Kilojoules/gram* |
|---|---|---|
| Protein | 4 | 17 |
| Fat | 9 | 38 |
| Carbohydrate | 4 | 17 |

**The Kinds and Forms of Energy**

Energy exist in two kinds, *Kinetic* and *Potential*. Potential energy is energy which is stored, or inactive. A stick of dynamite represents a great deal of potential energy. When released, potential energy is capable of causing an effect on matter. However, when it does so it is no longer potential energy. It is kinetic energy, the energy which is in the processes of causing an effect on matter. Kinetic energy can also be measured by determining how much matter it moves in a given period of time, and how far and how fast it moves it.

In addition to the two kinds of energy (potential and kinetic), five more forms are also recognised. These are *chemical, electrical, mechanical, radiant* and *atomic energy*. The last of these atomic energy, has little direct relationship to the normal functioning of living organisms.

CHEMICAL ENERGY. It is the energy possessed by chemical compounds present in every cell. This energy is the most fundamental form of energy in the life processes. Every thought, every nerve impulse, every muscle movement, indeed every activity of any sort shown by living organisms is ultimately traceable to the release of chemical energy. Thus it may be said that animal body is a chemical engine. At rest it transduces the chemical energy present in feed into mechanical work as in the beating of heart and the movements of the diaphragm in respiration.

ELECTRICAL ENERGY. The energy generated in the biological system is due to the movement of electrons. Electrons actually do not flow through the cell in the same manner that they flow along a copper wire. Electrochemical reactions, combinations of electrical and chemical energy, play a large part in the functioning of the brain and the rest of the nervous system.

MECHANICAL ENERGY. The energy directly involved in moving matter. This movement involves the conversion of potential chemical energy into kinetic chemical energy, resulting in the contraction of muscles. Since in many organisms the muscles act upon the bones, which serve as levers, the total movement of such an organism demonstrates kinetic mechanical energy.

RADIANT ENERGY. The energy travels in waves. It includes radio waves, infra-red, ultra-violet rays, X-rays, gamma and cosmic rays. Ultra-violet light present in sunlight or artificially produced radiant energy is necessary for converting sterol molecules into vitamin D. It is only this radiant heat by which all classes of livestocks maintain their heat balance.

### The Transformations of Energy

All forms of energy are interrelated and interconvertible and the process to some extent goes on continuously. Metabolism involves the conversion of chemical energy to other forms of energy for the body's work. This chemical energy is changed to electrical energy as in brain and nerve activity, mechanical energy as in muscle contraction, thermal energy as in regulation of body temperature and to other types of chemical energy as in the synthesis of new compounds. In all these activities of the body, heat is given off.

### Measurement of Energy

The amount of energy locked up by the bonds that hold a molecule of feed stuff together

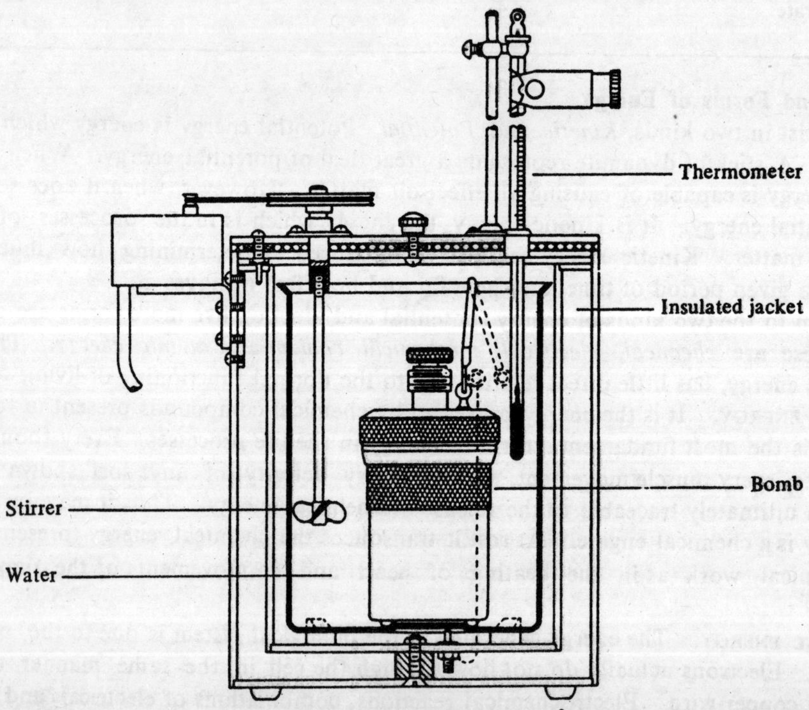


**Fig. 34** Cross section of the oxygen bomb calorimeter. (*Courtesy of the Parr Instrument Company.*)

cannot be determined by direct means. However, the amount of heat energy given off or absorbed when a molecule is formed or decomposed during a chemical reaction is determined by a metal instrument, which is called a *Bomb calorimeter* because its shape resembles that of a bomb. The instrument (Fig. 34) consists of an insulated water jacket containing a known

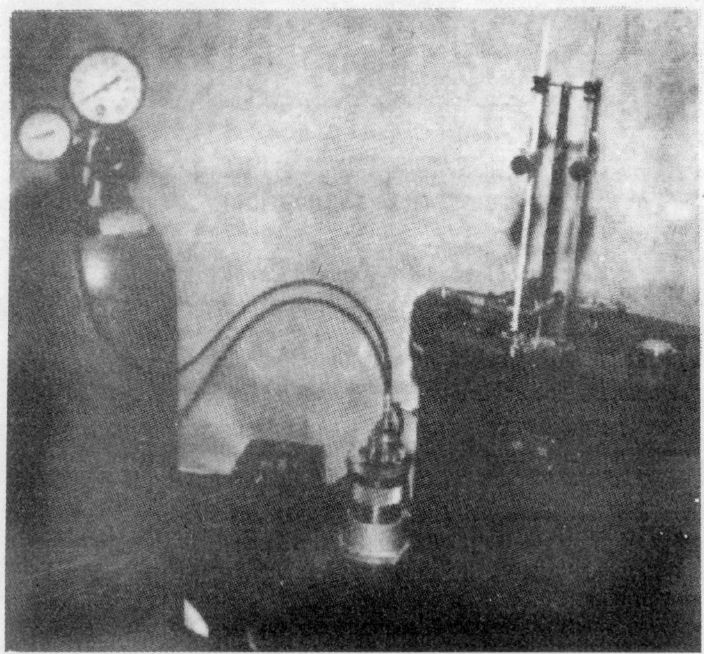

**Fig. 35** A bomb calorimeter. Note bomb being gassed (lower center).

amount of water into which a thermometer, a stirrer to keep the temperature of the water uniform, and a reaction chamber are immersed. The reaction or combustion chamber is known as a bomb. The bomb is a sturdy metal chamber into which the firmly palleted, or otherwise homogeneous substance to be burned, is placed. It is equipped with a valve through which oxygen is introduced to develop a 25 to 30 atmosphere pressure. The combustible substance is ignited in the presence of oxygen pressure by means of magnesium fuse wire sealed within the bomb and connected to an outside switch. As the feed burns, heat produced leads to a rise in temperature of the surrounding water. Thus heat production can be accurately measured from the change in mercury level of the attached thermometer immersed in the water of the jacket. This value, when multiplied by the water equivalent of that instrument, gives the number of calories produced by the burning of the sample.

**Gross Energy (GE)**

This is the total energy of the feed and is mostly determined by bomb calorimeter and sometimes by multiplying the percentage of carbohydrates, proteins and fats with 4.15, 5.65 and 9.40 respectively (Atwater and Bryant, 1899—Gross energy value, kcal/gram). Since none of

**the foodstuffs is completely absorbed; some potential energy, therefore, never enters the body and is excreted in the faeces. Since gross energy includes both digestible and non-digestible components, gross energy has little physiological significance especially in animals that consume large quantities of crude fibre.**

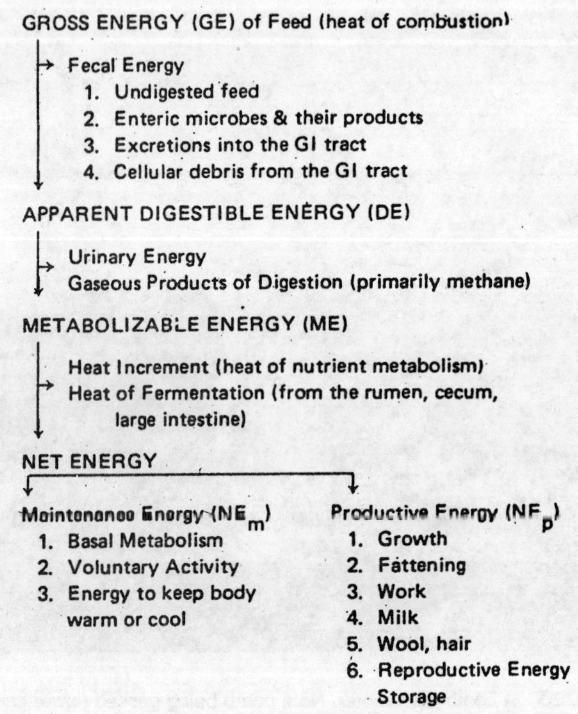

GROSS ENERGY (GE) of Feed (heat of combustion)
Fecal Energy
1. Undigested feed
2. Enteric microbes & their products
3. Excretions into the GI tract
4. Cellular debris from the GI tract
APPARENT DIGESTIBLE ENERGY (DE)
Urinary Energy
Gaseous Products of Digestion (primarily methane)
METABOLIZABLE ENERGY (ME)
Heat Increment (heat of nutrient metabolism)
Heat of Fermentation (from the rumen, cecum, large intestine)
NET ENERGY
Maintenance Energy (NE<sub>m</sub>)
1. Basal Metabolism
2. Voluntary Activity
3. Energy to keep body warm or cool
Productive Energy (NE<sub>p</sub>)
1. Growth
2. Fattening
3. Work
4. Milk
5. Wool, hair
6. Reproductive Energy
Storage


Schematic diagram of energy utilization by animals.

**Digestible Energy (DE)**

The gross energy of a food or other material provides no clue about the amount of energy available for livestock production. The amount of digestible energy is more useful for this purpose. Digestible energy is represented by that portion of feed energy consumed which is not excreted in the faeces. Then the total energy of the feed consumed (GE) is first measured in a bomb calorimeter. The total energy of the faeces is determined in the same way and the difference is called the apparently digestible energy. It can also be calculated from the digested nutrients by the use of the gross caloric factors: Protein 5.65; Carbohydrates 4.15; and Fat 9.45 or from the TDN values as will be described later on in this Chapter.

The method is a direct determination and is one of the most accurate analyses performed in the laboratory. The determination is not as time consuming as the TDN method. It does not account for any loss except that of faecal loss.

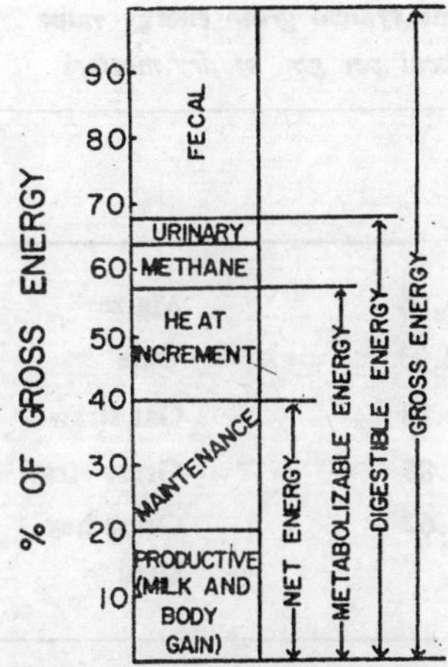


**Fig. 36** Typical proportions of gross energy lost in feces, gaseous products of digestion, urinary energy, heat increment (work of digestion), and that utilized for maintenance and for productive purpose in a lactating dairy cow. Note the various measures of usable energy, digestible energy (DE), metabolizable energy (ME), and net energy (NE). (See also Flatt, 1966; NRC, 1966.)

## Total Digestible Nutrients (TDN)

TDN is not shown in the scheme in Fig. 10-1, but it is a common measure of energy used in ration formulation in the USA for ruminants and swine. TDN is roughly comparable to DE, but is expressed in units of weight or percent. When conversion of TDN to DE is desired, the values used usually are 2,000 Kcal of DE/lb of TDN or 4.4 Kcal/g. TDN is determined by carrying out a digestion trial and summing the digestible protein and carbohydrates (NFE and crude fiber) plus 2.25 times digestible ether extract (crude fat). Fat is multiplied by 2.25 in an attempt to account for its higher caloric value which is about 2.25X that of digestible carbohydrates.

As compared to DE, TDN undervalues protein because protein is not oxidized completely by the body whereas it is in a bomb calorimeter. Multiplication of digestible protein by 1.25 would put TDN on a more comparable basis with DE. The formula for TDN is: TDN = DCP + DNFE + DCF + 2.25(DEE).

Although most nutritionists recognize that TDN or DE tend to overvalue roughages as compared to some version of NE, the popularity of TDN is partially because of the relative ease of obtaining the necessary information and also because of the better understanding of its use by non-professionals. Current NRC publications tend to emphasize other energy values, but it should be pointed out that most of these values for ME or NE were derived from TDN values.

### Metabolisable Energy (ME)

**All of the digestible energy is not available for productive purposes and other energy losses occur. When energy losses in the urine and combustible gases (primarily methane, $CH_4$) are subtracted from the digestible energy, the remaining energy is called the metabolisable energy. Generally the energy losses in the combustible gases and urine account for about 8 and 3 to 5%**

**Table 116**

**Some typical gross energy value**

***(kcal per gm. of dry matter)***

| *Feed constituents* | | *Feed ingredients* | |
|---|---|---|---|
| Glucose | 3.76 | Maize | 4.43 |
| Starch | 4.23 | Oats | 4.68 |
| Cellulose | 4.18 | Oat straw | 4.43 |
| Casein | 5.86 | Grass straw | 4.43 |
| Lactic acid | 3.62 | Grass hay | 4.51 |
| | | Urea | 2.53 |

**Table 117**

**Ranges in loss of dietary gross energy (%)**

| | *Simple stomached animal* | *Non-ruminants herbivores* | *Ruminants* |
|---|---|---|---|
| Faeces | 2–40 | 10–70 | 10–60 |
| Gases (Less than) | 0.5 | 3–7 | 5–12 |
| Urinary | 1–3 | 3–5 | 3–5 |
| Heat increment | 5–30 | 10–35 | 10–40 |
| Net use——→ | 25–50 | 15–50 | 10–35 |

of the gross energy of the feed respectively. Losses are usually greater in ruminants than non-ruminants.

The method significantly represents the useful energy of a feed and is not affected by plane of nutrition nor by the activity of the animal. The urinary and faecal loss are determined by bomb calorimeter while for methane production suitable factors may be employed. The draw-back of this method is that comparison of high and low fibre containing feeds cannot be made by this method.

**Net Energy (NE)**

This is the net remainder of the useful energy after all the losses accounted for faeces, urine, methane and heat increment are subtracted. By this NE represents that part of the feed energy which is actually retained and utilised by the body for its growth or production. As such this is the ideal method of expressing the nutritive energy of a feed. The disadvantages are that

$$NE = GE - \left( \begin{array}{c} \text{fecal} \\ \text{energy} \end{array} + \begin{array}{c} \text{gaseous} \\ \text{product} \\ \text{energy} \end{array} + \begin{array}{c} \text{urinary} \\ \text{energy} \end{array} + \begin{array}{c} \text{heat} \\ \text{increment} \\ \text{energy} \end{array} \right)$$

it is very difficult to have a respiratory chamber or animal calorimeter for the estimation of heat increment. Moreover, it is also a hard job to keep the animals in fast condition required for estimation of heat increment and that heat increment may not be a loss in cold season.

However, a few years ago a relatively simpler slaughter technique was developed at the University of California for determining the net energy requirement for growing and finishing cattle and the net energy value of feeds for this class of cattle. The system includes separate estimates for energy depending on whether it was used for maintenance ($NE_m$) or for body weight gain ($NE_g$). The formula suggested to find out the $NE_m$) is as follows:

$$NE_m = 77 \text{ kcal}/W_k{}^{0.75}$$

Using this formula it has been observed that the average net energy required for maintenance for a beef cattle ranges between 72 to 82 kcal per unit of metabolic size ($W_{kg}{}^{0.75}$).

For determining the net energy for weight gain, Lofgreen and Garrett* observed that the relationship between $NE_g$ and weight gain could be expressed by the following equations:

$$NE_g = (52.72a + 6.84a^2)\ (W_{kg}{}^{0.75}) \text{ for steers}$$

$$NE_g = (56.03a + 12.65a^2)\ (W_{kg}{}^{0.75}) \text{ for heifers}$$

where $NE_g$ is in kilocalories, a is daily weight gain in kilograms, and $W_{kg}$ is the body weight in kilogram.

The $NE_g$ for any feed is determined after feeding it at two levels and estimating the energy deposited as a result of the intake of feed between two levels. Any two levels of feeding above that required for maintenance can be used to determine the $NE_g$ of a ration.

**Heat Increment (HI)**

The increase in heat production after the ingestion of feed has been the subject of much investigation and thought, and a variety of names for the effect have been suggested, for example, specific dynamic action (SDA), specific dynamic effect (SDE), heat increment (HI), calorigenic effect of feed and thermogenic effect of feed.

The cause of heat increment of nutrients is unknown. Several theories have been proposed: (1) the absorbed amino acids excite body cells to a high level of energy metabolism, (2) the energy expense of digestion, absorption, excretion and secretion, (3) energetic inefficiency of the reactions by which absorbed nutrients are metabolised. For example, when glucose is oxidised in the formation of ATP, the efficiency of free energy capture, is only about 44 per cent. The rest amount, i.e., 56 per cent being lost as heat. It seems probable that many or all of these factors contribute to the heat increment. The HI may be expressed in absolute terms (kcal/of feed dry matter) or relative as a proportion of the gross or metabolisable energy.

HI can be reduced somewhat by feeding higher levels of grains. Perhaps this is why we have observed cows on low grain ration eating larger quantities of hay during extreme cold weather (one of nature's provisions for keeping warm).

*Lofgreen, G.P. and W.N., Garrett *Jr.*, *Animal Science*, *27* (1968): 793.

## ENERGY TERMINOLOGY USED IN RATION FORMULATION AND FEEDING STANDARDS

As pointed out in previous discussions on the different categories of energy, GE has no value in itself for evaluation of feedstuffs or animal requirements. DE is often used in the USA, as is TDN, and these require no further explanation at this point. For poultry the NRC recommends the use of ME for chickens and turkeys, and an appreciable amount of information is available on feedstuffs and animal requirements for these species. For swine, DE, TDN or ME values are used in practice.

In Great Britain, the ARC (Agricultural Research Council) has gone along with suggestions of Blaxter and has adopted ME as the preferred base for energy. In the USA, three versions of NE are used in varying degrees for ruminants. These are discussed in succeeding paragraphs.

### Estimated Net Energy [ENE]

Based on some calorimetric work, Moore et al. , developed a formula which allows NE to be estimated from TDN; the resulting value is called ENE. The formula is:

**ENE (as Mcal/100 lb) = 1.39 x %TDN - 34.63**

**or**

**ENE (as Mcal/kg dry matter) = 0.307 x %TDN - 0.764.**

Morrison adopted this formula in the last edition of his book, and it has been used relatively widely as a result. Some dairy nutritionist still favor use of these values, partly because relatively few data are available on NE values of feedstuffs as compared to TDN values.

### Net Energy for Lactation [$NE_\ell$]

Calorimetric experiments have been carried out at the USDA Experiment Station at Beltsville in which the NE requirements for milk production have been studied in high-producing dairy cows, primarily Holsteins, and results have been summarized.

$NE_\ell$ is, in effect, a measure of the total energy requirement of the non-pregnant cow for milk production. The average NE requirement for maintenance was calculated to be 73 Kcal/kg $BW^{0.75}$, which is roughly equivalent to 118 Kcal for ME/$kg^{0.75}$. The amount of NE required for milk production was calculated to be 0.74 Mcal $NE_\ell$/kg of 4% fat-corrected milk. To calculate $NE_\ell$ values from DE or TDN, the authors suggest the equations:

**$NE_\ell$ (as Mcal/kg dry matter)**
**= 0.68 DE (as Mcal/kg DM) - 0.36**
**$NE_\ell$ (as Mcal/kg dry matter) = 0.037 x %TDN - 0.77**

Adjustments can be made in requirements for tissue gain or loss of cows, for excess N intake and for pregnancy. The authors agree that further refinement is needed, but the reader might note that the NRC has adopted this terminology for ther publication on dairy cows.

### Net Energy of Maintenance and Gain [$NE_m$, $NE_g$]

This system, also called the California system (see section on comparative slaughter technique), has come into use and has also been adopted by the NRC for growing beef and dairy cattle. In this scheme the NE for maintenance, $NE_m$, is calculated separately from the $NE_g$, primarily because maintenance is a more efficient process, energetically, than is gain. This causes some complications in formulation of rations. Relatively few feedstuffs have been evaluated with this procedure at this time, although NRC publications give calculated values which were derived with the following formulas. Where DE or TDN are known, ME is first calculated:

$$ME \text{ (as Mcal/kg of feed)} = DE \text{ (as Mcal/kg)} \times 0.82$$

or $ME = 3.615\ TDN$

For NE,

$$\text{Log } F = 2.2577 - 0.2213\ ME$$

(where F = g dry matter/kg $BW^{0.75}$)

$$NE_m = 77/F$$

$$NE_g = 2.54 - 0.0314F$$

or

$$NE_m \text{ (as Mcal/kg dry matter)} = 0.029 \times \%TDN - 0.29$$

$$NE_g \text{ (as Mcal/kg dry matter)} = 0.029 \times \%TDN - 1.01$$

## FORMULAS USED IN CALCULATING DIFFERENT ENERGY VALUES

For the sake of convenience, the various formulas given throughout this chapter for calculating different energy values of feedstuffs are repeated in this section along with some added values for poultry. They are as follows:

$$DE \text{ (as Kcal)} = TDN \text{ (in lb)} \times 2000$$

or

$$DE \text{ (as Kcal)} = TDN \text{ (in g)} \times 4.4$$

ME for swine

$$\underset{\text{(in Kcal/kg)}}{ME} = \frac{DE \text{ (in Kcal/kg)} \times 0.96 - (0.202 \times \text{protein }\%)}{100}$$

ME for poultry

$$\underset{\text{(as Kcal/g)}}{ME} = \text{digestibility (\%)} \times \text{energy equivalents (Kcal/g)}$$

Energy equivalents suggested for pountry are

| | |
|---|---|
| Protein | 3.84 |
| Ether extract | |
| meat and fish meals | 9.49 |
| grains and seeds | 9.33 |
| milk products | 9.21 |
| Carbohydrates (NFE) | |
| grains | 4.2 |
| legume seeds | 4.0 |
| legume leaves & stems | 3.8 |
| milk products | 3.7 |
| Crude fiber | 2.1 |

For ruminants

$$ME \text{ (as Mcal/kg of feed)} = DE \text{ (as Mcal/kg)} \times 0.82$$

$$ENE \text{ (as Mcal/kg dry matter)} = 0.307 \times \%TDN - 0.764$$

$$NE_\ell \text{ (as Mcal/kg dry matter)} = 0.68DE - 0.36$$

$$NE_m \text{ (as Mcal/kg dry matter)} = 0.029 \times \%TDN - 0.29$$

$$NE_g \text{ (as Mcal/kg dry matter)} = 0.029 \times \%TDN - 1.01$$

Note that several formulas are in use for calculating TDN, DE, and so on, based on analytical composition of different feedstuffs.

**Control of Energy in Animal Metabolism**

**The energy in any system may be uncontrolled and destructive, as in an atomic bomb used for warfare; or it may be controlled and constructive, as in an atomic reactor used for research and industry. In the animal body also the energy produced in its many chemical reactions, if "exploded" at once, could be destructive. The mechanism by which energy is retained in the animal system is by *chemical bonding*. The chemical bonds that hold the elements of the compounds together consist of various quantum of energy. So long the compound remains constant, energy is being exerted to maintain the atomic constellation that is characteristic for that molecule. It is in this way that potential energy is stored in the compound. When such compounds are broken into various products, energy is released and it becomes free energy. By nature free energy immediately involves in the bonding of other atoms.**

**Bonds which are involved in exchanging energy are: *Covalent bonds*, *hydrogen bonds* and *phosphate bonds*.**

COVALENT BOND. When two atoms share a pair of electrons, they are joined by a **covalent bond.** Common examples of such bonds are those shared between neighbour carbon atoms in the core of an organic compound ( -C -C -C).

HYDROGEN BOND. This type of bonding takes place between a hydrogen donor group and an acceptor group. Commonly found in peptide linkage. Bonds are weak and can be broken easily. They are less rich in energy than covalent bonds.

HIGH-ENERGY-PHOSPHATE BOND. Phosphate bonds attach the phosphate radical to a compound. Since the phosphate radical is highly labile, more energy is required to bind it and similarly more free energy is released when the phosphate bond is broken. Most of the phosphate bonds are referred to as high energy bonds and are expressed by ~ sign. An example of such high energy compound is adenosine triphosphate (ATP) A—$PO_4$~$PO_4$~$PO_4$.

Examples of low energy phosphate bonds include those formed by the phosphorylation of glucose (glucose-6-phosphate, glucose-1, phosphate) which activates glucose for participation in cell metabolism.

Mechanism of controlling the reaction rate is also an important aspect of energy metabolism as it is this mechanism by which the release of required amount of energy from energy rich compounds is obtained at the time of need at particular cell or tissue. For example some of the chemical reactions that break down proteins if left to themselves (as in sterile decomposition) would span several years. Such reactions must be accelerated or else it might take years to get the necessary energy from a meal. At the same time, they must be regulated so that too fast a reaction will not produce energy in a single explosion. Enzymes, coenzymes and hormones control numerous biological oxidation of the cells.

## The Role of ATP

When fuel molecules are broken down within living organisms, the energy released must be channelled in a useful direction. If it is not captured immediately, the energy is lost for useless work within the cell causing damage to the cells.

None of the energy released is used directly to power chemical reactions. All such energy is stored in small "packages" of energy known as *high energy phosphate bonds.* In this way the energy is available in a common form for all metabolic processes of the cells.

In most living systems, high energy bonds are found in the form of a compound known as adenosine triphosphate (ATP). It is composed of one molecule of adenine and ribose to which are attached three phosphate groups, The last two phosphate groups are jointed to the main body of the molecule by high energy bonds (represented as ~). Upon hydrolysis of the bond which is between the terminal carbon atom and the first phosphate group (which is not a high energy bond) an energy exchange of —1 to —5 kilocalories per mole occurs. When either of the two terminal phosphates are hydrolysed, about —5 to—15 kcal/mole are liberated. These are referred to as high energy bonds. There are also other high energy compounds in nature and a large percentage of those are associated with a terminal phosphate group.

For living organisms there are two advantages to having energy stored in high energy phosphate bonds. First, the energy in such bonds is readily available to the cell for immediate use. The process of extracting the energy from the monophosphate bond is a one-step reaction. Second, and perhaps most important, the amount of energy in a high energy phosphate bond is approximately that amount which is the most useful for producing biochemical reactions. This means that there is less wastage of energy. As a result, biochemical reactions within living

nucleoside group,
ribose — adenine =
adenosine group

Attachment of phosphate or other group is generally at the 5′ position of ribose.

→ adenosine monophosphate group (AMP), adenylic acid or adenyl group

→ adenosine diphosphate group (ADP)

→ adenosine triphosphate (ATP)
High-energy (free energy) is associated with the pyrophosphate linkages of the second and third phosphate groups when they react.

**The ATP molecule is composed of adenine, ribose and three phosphate molecules.**

organisms are quite efficient. They do not release more energy than can be used at any one time.

By virtue of its role in energy transfer mechanisms, ATP is involved in the oxidation and also in synthesis of all proteins, fats and carbohydrates in the body. It provides the energy of muscular contraction so vital to the maintenance of life in the higher forms. ATP is involved in the synthesis of and in many instances is an actual component of several coenzymes involved in tissue respiration. It is also combined with pantothenic acid and cysteamine in the very important coenzyme A (CoA) which acts as an activator of substrates in most intermediary metabolic reactions occurring in living tissues.

**Storage of High-energy Phosphate**

The ATP yield is a rather unstable compound, rapidly utilised in other physiological reactions of the body and is present in small amounts only in tissue. For storage, especially in liver and muscle, any surplus high-energy phosphate is rapidly transferred from ATP to creatine phosphate, the major form of storage in all domestic animals. The terminal pyrophosphate linkage of ATP is hydrolysed and a bond of similar free energy of hydrolysis, a phosphoguanidine linkage, is created by transfer of the phosphate to creatine, forming phosphocreatine.

**Any increase in the concentration of ATP favours the synthesis of phosphocreatine. When ATP concentration falls, phosphocreatine returns the high energy phosphate to yield ATP from ADP.**

**Table 118**

**Some Organophosphates in Metabolism[a]**

| Phosphate | Structure | Free Energy of Hydrolysis[b] | Phosphate Group Transfer Potential[c] |
|---|---|---|---|
| Phosphoenolpyruvate | $CH_2{=}C(CO_2^-)$—O~P(=O)(O⁻)—O⁻ | −14.8 | 14.8 |
| 1,3-Diphosphoglycerate | $^{2-}O_3P$—$OCH_2CH(OH)C(=O)$—O~P(=O)(O⁻)—O⁻ | −11.8 | 11.8 |
| Phosphocreatine | $^-O_2CCH_2$—N($CH_3$)—C(=$^+NH_2$)—NH~P(=O)(O⁻)—O⁻ | −10.3 | 10.3 |
| Acetylphosphate | $CH_3C(=O)$—O~P(=O)(O⁻)—O⁻ | −10.1 | 10.1 |
| Adenosine triphosphate ATP | ⁻O—P(=O)(⁻O)~O—P(=O)(⁻O)~O—P(=O)(⁻O)—O—$CH_2$ (ribose with OH OH, adenine with $NH_2$); bonds ① ② | −7.3 ①<br>−7.3 ② | 7.3<br>7.3 |
| Glucose 1-phosphate | glucose ($CH_2OH$, HO, OH, OH)—O—P(=O)(O⁻)—O⁻ | −5.0 | 5.0 |

**Table 118** (*Contd.*)

| Phosphate | Structure | Free Energy of Hydrolysis[b] | Phosphate Group Transfer Potential[c] |
|---|---|---|---|
| Fructose 6-phosphate | 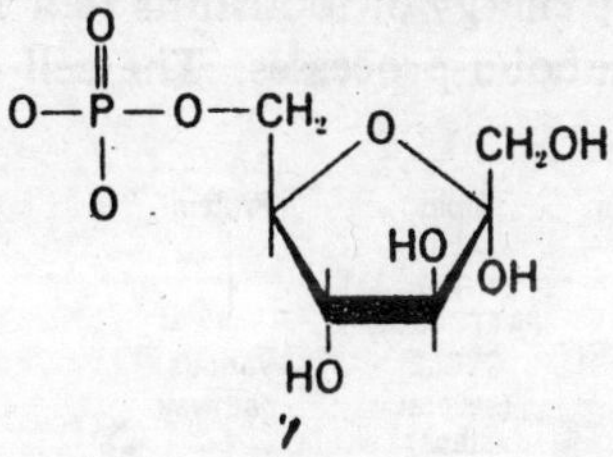 | −3.8 | 3.8 |
| Glucose 6-phosphate | 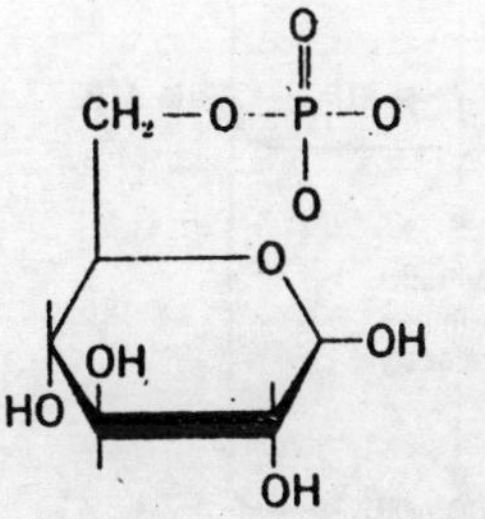 | 3.3 | 3.3 |
| Glycerol 3-phosphate | 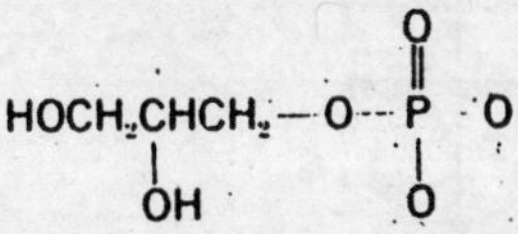 | 2.2 | 2.2 |

[a] Full ionized forms of the structures are shown, but the actual state of ionization varies with the pH of the medium.
[b] In kilocalories per mole.
[c] Simply the free energy of hydrolysis (in kcal/mole) taken as the positive.

**How ATP are formed?**

There are six mechanisms in animal tissues whereby the terminal high energy pyrophosphate bonds of ATP are synthesized. Two occur in the anaerobic glucolysis of glucose via Embenden-Meyerhof pathway as shown below.

(a) 1-3, diphospho-D-glycerate+ADP+inorganic phosphate——————→3 phospho-D-glycerate+ATP

(b) Phospho-enol-pyruvate+ADP+inorganic phosphate————→Pyruvate+ATP

A third mechanism occurs in the oxidative decarboxylation of α-oxo acids to carboxylic acids. The example shown below is that of the oxidative decarboxylation of α-oxoglutarate to succinate.

(c) α-oxoglutarate+oxidized co-enzyme+inorganic phosphate——→Succinate+$CO_2$+ reduced CoA+ATP

The remaining three reactions in which free energy is captured in the terminal pyrophosphate bonds of ATP involve the transfer of pairs of hydrogen atoms from high energy substrates via pyridine nucleotides, flavoproteins, and iron porphyrins to oxygen. The collective process is termed oxidative phosphorylation and takes place in the mitochondria.

**Respiratory chain (electron transport system)**

The oxidation of carbohydrates, fats and proteins via the TCA cycle (Krebs cycle) is the common pathway in the conversion of the energy of foodstuffs to a form that the cell can use at the time of future need in various metabolic processes. The cell extracts the available feed

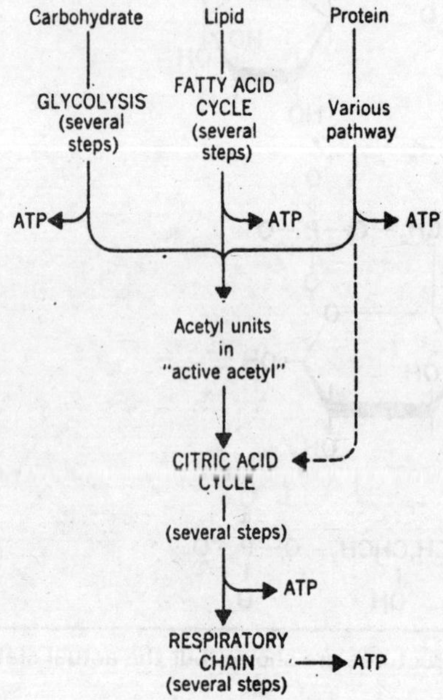


**Fig. 37** The major pathways in biochemical energetics.

energy by a gradual oxidation instead of an abrupt one. An abrupt oxidation would result in a marked liberation of heat. During this gradual oxidation process the substrate is oxidized by a compound that has a slightly higher oxidation potential (a measure of the tendency of a substance to release its electrons when compared to the standard hydrogen electrode) than the initial substrate. This compound is again oxidized by another compound that has a slightly higher oxidation potential. This is continued until a high oxidation potential is reached equivalent to that of oxygen. In this way a small amount of energy is released at each oxidation instead of a sudden release. These oxidation reduction reactions involve the transfer of hydrogen ions and electrons separately. By virtue of such an arrangement of gradual release of energy during oxidative processes, the high energy phosphate transferred to ADP without intervention of oxygen resulting production of ATP.

All the enzymes and cofactors which are necessary for the Krebs cycle and for the conversion of energy are localized in the mitochondria. The mitochondria are small membrane

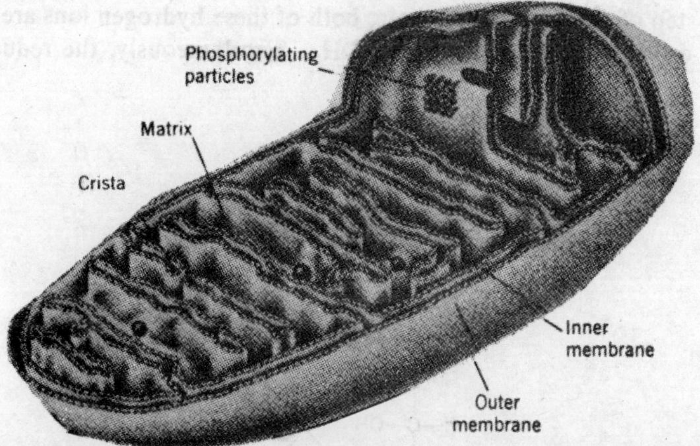


**Fig. 38** . A mitochondrion. Perspective showing the interior of a mitochondrion. Each phosphorylating particle or respiratory assembly contains the respiratory enzymes.

**surrounded granules located throughout the cytoplasm and are often referred to as "power house" of the cell. The enzymes contained within them are fixed in geometrically specific arrays such that they are capable of functioning as extremely efficient assembly lines ( p. 399). The sequence of reactions whereby the reduced forms of coenzymes are reoxidized (ultimately by molecular oxygen) is known as the *respiratory chain* or the *electron transport system.***

**Two hydrogen ions and two electrons (the equivalent of two atoms of hydrogen) are removed from the substrate. The $NAD^+$ molecule accepts both electrons and one hydrogen ion;**

Adenine | Ribose | Pyrophosphate | Ribose | Nicotinamide

Nicotinamide adenine dinucleotide, $NAD^+$

the other hydrogen ion is released into the medium (see page 397).

In the next step of the respiratory chain, both of these hydrogen ions are passed on to the coenzyme FAD, causing its reduction to $FADH_2$. Simultaneously, the reduced form of the

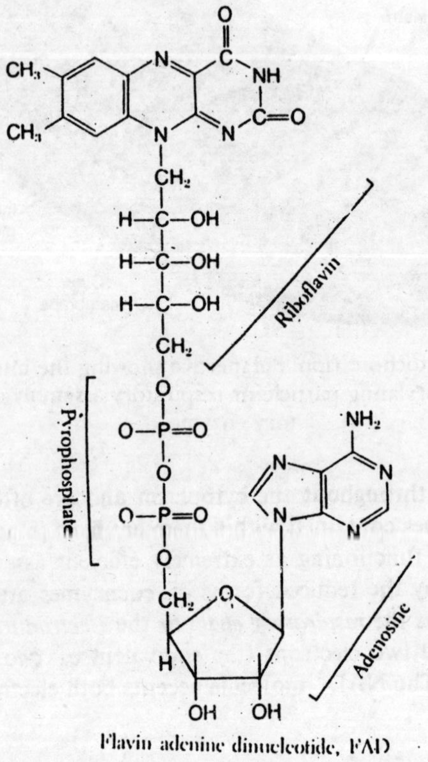

Flavin adenine dinucleotide, FAD

coenzyme NADH is reoxidized, and it is this step that accounts for the regeneration of the $NAD^+$. Again we shall depict only the relevant portion of the FAD molecule.

The coenzyme NAD is the initial electron acceptor in the oxidation of three of the substrates namely isocitrate, α-ketoglutarate and malate. FAD also acts in one case as initial electron acceptor i.e. of succinic acid.

Much controversy has centered about the role of the next electron carrier. Data have been published in support of its participation in the respiratory chain as well as against it. Most workers presently believe that a quinone derivative (tentatively called coenzyme $Q_{10}$) participates in the system between the flavin coenzymes and the cytochromes. It is in this step that the oxidized form of the flavin coenzyme, FAD, is regenerated.

A series of compounds called cytochromes were probably the first entities to be associated with electron transferring reactions. A number of these substances exist, and we have included four of them. However, it seems likely that several more are involved in the respiratory chain. The cytochromes are conjugated protein enzymes. Their coenzymes are iron porphyrins, which resemble here, the normal pigment of haemoglobin. The various cytochromes differ with

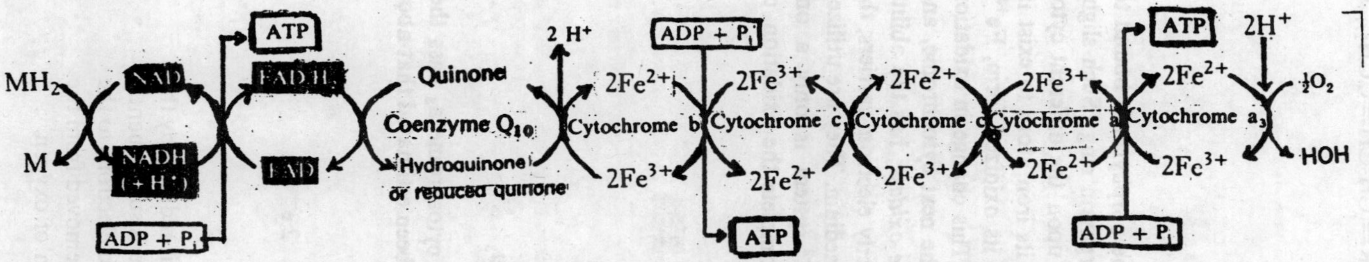

$MH_2$ / M — NAD / NADH (+H⁺) — FADH₂ / FAD — Quinone / Coenzyme $Q_{10}$ / Hydroquinone or reduced quinone — 2 H⁺ — Cytochrome b ($2Fe^{2+}$ / $2Fe^{3+}$) — Cytochrome c₁ ($2Fe^{3+}$ / $2Fe^{2+}$) — Cytochrome c ($2Fe^{2+}$ / $2Fe^{3+}$) — Cytochrome a ($2Fe^{3+}$ / $2Fe^{2+}$) — Cytochrome $a_3$ ($2Fe^{2+}$ / $2Fe^{3+}$) — 2H⁺ + $\frac{1}{2}O_2$ → HOH

ADP + $P_i$ → ATP (three sites)

**The respiratory chain and oxidative phosphorylation.**

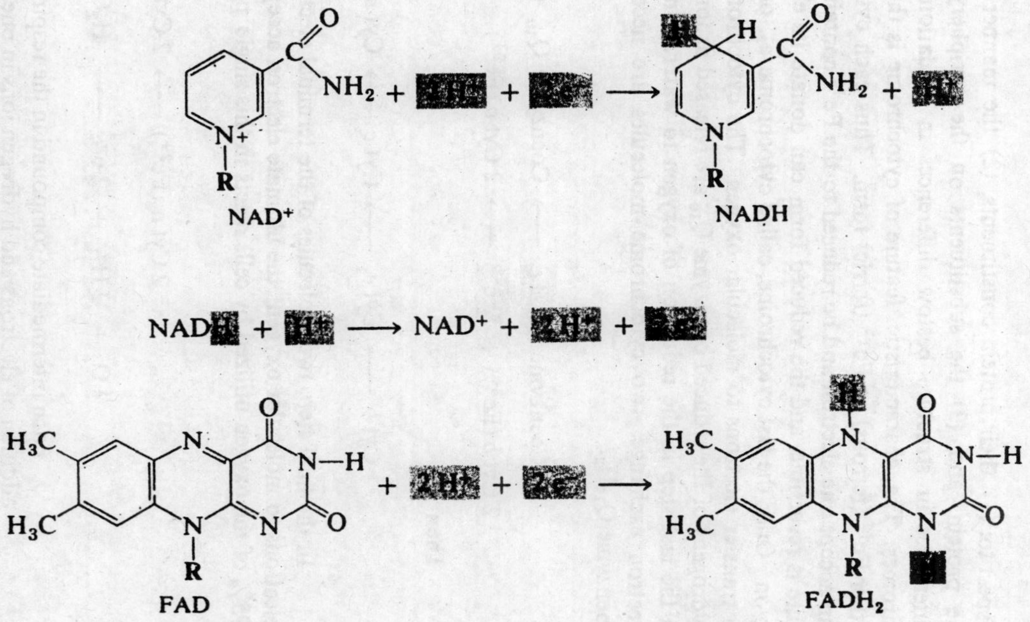

$$NAD^+ + 2H^+ + 2e^- \longrightarrow NADH + H^+$$

NAD⁺ NADH

$$NADH + H^+ \longrightarrow NAD^+ + 2H^+ + 2e^-$$

$$FAD + 2H^+ + 2e^- \longrightarrow FADH_2$$

FAD FADH₂

Quinone ring — Hydroquinone ring

$$\text{CoQ}_{10}\ (\text{oxidized form: quinone ring with } H_3CO, H_3CO, R, CH_3) + 2\ ^{+} + 2e^- \rightleftharpoons \text{Co Q}_{10}H_2\ (\text{reduced form: hydroquinone ring})$$

$$R{=}(CH_2CH{=}\overset{CH_3}{\overset{|}{C}}CH_2)_{10}H$$

$CoQ_{10}$. (oxidized form) Co $Q_{10}H_2$. (reduced form)

respect to: (1) their protein constituents, (2) the manner in which the porphyrin is bound to the protein, and (3) the substituents on the periphery of the porphyrin ring. Such slight differences in structure bestow differences in oxidation potential upon the different cytochromes. The characteristic feature of cytochrome is the ability of its iron atom to exist in either $Fe^{+2}$ (ferrous) or $Fe^{+3}$ (ferric) form. Thus each cytochrome in its oxidized form, $Fe^{+3}$, can accept one electron and be reduced to the $Fe^{+2}$ containing form. This change in oxidation state is reversible, and the reduced form can donate its electron to the next cytochrome, and so on. Only the last cytochrome, called cytochrome $a_3$, or *cytochrome oxidase*, has the ability to transfer electrons to molecular oxygen. The cytochromes are strictly electron carriers; the hydrogens of the reduced coenzyme $Q_{10}$ are released as ions into the medium. They are utilized in the last step in the reduction of oxygen to water. Since $Fe^{+3}/Fe^{+2}$ system is only a one electron exchange, two cytochrome molecules are necessary to complete the oxidation of coenzyme $Q_{10}H_2$.

$$\text{Coenzyme } Q_{10}H_2 \longrightarrow \text{Coenzyme } Q_{10} + 2H^+ + 2e^-$$

$$2\ \text{Cyt}\ b\ (Fe^{3+}) + 2e^- \longrightarrow 2\ \text{Cyt}\ b\ (Fe^{2+})$$

Then

$$\text{Cyt}\ b \longrightarrow \text{Cyt}\ c_1 \longrightarrow \text{Cyt}\ c \longrightarrow \text{Cyt}\ a \longrightarrow \text{Cyt}\ a_3$$

In the final step, two molecules of the terminal electron carrier, cytochrome $a_3$ pass their electrons to molecular oxygen, the ultimate electron acceptor. It has been estimated that about 95% of the oxygen utilized by cells reacts in this single process.

$$2\ \text{Cyt}\ a_3(Fe^{2+}) \longrightarrow 2\ \text{Cyt}\ a_3(Fe^{3+}) + 2e^-$$

$$\tfrac{1}{2}O_2 + 2H^+ + 2e^- \longrightarrow H_2O$$

Each intermediate compound in the respiratory chain is reduced by the addition of electrons and hydrogen ions in one reaction and is subsequently restored to its original form when it delivers the protons and electrons to the next compound. Thus each pair of hydrogen atoms that is removed from the substrates of the Krebs cycle ultimately reduces one atom of oxygen.

**Oxidative phosphorylation**

The process whereby ATP is synthesized as a result of the operation of the respiratory chain is referred to as *Oxidative phosphorylation.* The details of the mechanism which links the formation of ATP to the operation of the respiratory chain are largely unknown. It is known, however, that the energy required for the production of ATP results from the passage of a pair of electrons from one carrier to the next. The electron transport system can be thought to function as a biochemical battery; that is, energy is obtained from oxidation-reduction reactions. The sites on the respiratory chain at which the oxidative phosphorylations are believed to occur are shown in page. 399.

It has been calculated from the difference of oxidation potential that for the oxidation of 1 mole of NADH by molecular $O_2$ to form $H_2O$ there is a total production of 52,000 cal through the cytochrome electron transport system which also leads to the formation of 3 high energy phosphate bonds (3 ATP).

$$NADH+\frac{1}{2}O_2+H^++3ADP+3P_i \longrightarrow NAD^++O_2H+3ATP$$

Taking the average free energy of hydrolysis ($\Delta F$) of each ATP as 7,300, the total energy that will be available from three ATP will be only 7,300×3 calories. Thus the percentage of energy conserved by the respiratory chain

$$=\left(\frac{\text{energy conserved}}{\text{energy available}}\right)(100\%)=\frac{(3)7{,}300}{52{,}000}(100\%)=42\ \%$$

That is, almost half of the energy released in the electron transport process is conserved in the formation of high energy phosphate bonds.

**Storage of high-energy phosphate**

The ATP yield is a rather unstable compound, rapidly utilised in other physiological reactions of the body and is present in small amounts only in tissue. For storage, especially in liver and muscle, any surplus high-energy phosphate is rapidly transferred from ATP to creatine phosphate, the major form of storage in all domestic animals. The terminal pyrophosphate linkage of ATP is hydrolyzed and a bond of similar free energy of hydrolysis, a phosphoguanidine linkage, is created by transfer of the phosphate to creatine, forming phosphocreatine. Any increase in the concentration of ATP favours the synthesis of phosphocreatine. When ATP concentration falls, phosphocreatine returns the high energy phosphate to yield ATP from ADP.

**Efficiency of utilization of free energy in the body**

In order to measure the efficiency with which the free energy released in a particular reaction occurring within the body is utilized it is necessary to know not only how much free energy is released but also how much of that released is captured in the two pyrophosphate bonds of ATP. This can now be done for many of the catabolic (oxidative) reactions which occur within the body and also for some of the anabolic (synthetic) reactions. It is thus possible to calculate an efficiency of free-energy utilization for a particular substrate undergoing oxidation in the body as

$$\text{Efficiency} = \frac{\text{kcal. free energy captured in ATP per mole substrate oxidized}}{\text{kcal. free energy released per mole substrate oxidized}} \times 100$$

When 1 mol of glucose is combusted in a calorimeter in an atmosphere of $O_2$ will release $CO_2$, water and about 686,000 calories.

$$C_6H_{12}O_6 + 6O_2 \longrightarrow 6CO_2 + 6H_2O + 686{,}000 \text{ calories.}$$

In atmosphere this is liberated rapidly and explosively and is dissipated away as heat. If it were to be used for bringing about other chemical reactions in the tissues or for doing work, there should be methods available in the organism which prevent such explosive liberation of energy. This is, in fact, so. The oxidation of glucose does not proceed directly as depicted in the above reaction, but it is channelled through a stepwise process where the several steps in the exerogonic reaction are coupled to other synthetic reactions (enderogonic) which take up the energy of glucose oxidation and store it in themselves as chemical energy. Even so, nearly 60 per cent of the energy is still dissipated. The chemical energy released in glucose catabolism is mainly used in addition of phosphate to the nucleotide structure, ADP, by a pyrophosphate linkage to form ATP.

$$C_6H_{12}O_6 + 6O_2 + 38\ \text{ADP} + 38\ H_3PO_4 \longrightarrow 6\ CO_2 + 44\ H_2O + 38\ \text{ATP} + 408{,}600 \text{ calories.}$$

The 38 ATP can be subsequently hydrolysed, as required, to yield again 38 ADP and 38 phosphate molecules and energy of about 277,400 calories for various anabolic reactions.

*The process whereby ATP synthesis is linked to the consumption of oxygen in the respiratory chain is referred to as Oxidative phosphorylation or Respiratory-chain phosphorylation.*

**Table 119**

Generation of high-energy bonds in the catabolism of glucose.

| Pathway | Reaction Catalyzed By | Method of ~Ⓟ Production | Number of ~Ⓟ Formed per Mol of Glucose |
|---|---|---|---|
| Glycolysis | Glyceraldehyde-3-phosphate dehydrogenase | Respiratory chain oxidation of 2 NADH | 6* |
| | Phosphoglycerate kinase | Oxidation at substrate level | 2 |
| | Pyruvate kinase | Oxidation at substrate level | 2 |
| | | | 10 |
| Allow for consumption of ATP by reactions catalyzed by hexokinase and phosphofructokinase | | | −2 |
| | | | Net 8 |
| Citric acid cycle | Pyruvate dehydrogenase | Respiratory chain oxidation of 2 NADH | 6 |
| | Isocitrate dehydrogenase | Respiratory chain oxidation of 2 NADH | 6 |
| | α-Ketoglutarate dehydrogenase | Respiratory chain oxidation of 2 NADH | 6 |
| | Succinate thiokinase | Oxidation at substrate level | 2 |
| | Succinate dehydrogenase | Respiratory chain oxidation of 2 $FADH_2$ | 4 |
| | Malate dehydrogenase | Respiratory chain oxidation of 2 NADH | 6 |
| | | | Net 30 |
| Total per mol of glucose under aerobic conditions | | | 38 |
| Total per mol of glucose under anaerobic conditions | | | 2 |

*It is assumed that NADH formed in glycolysis is transported into mitochondria via the malate shuttle. If the glycerophosphate shuttle is used, only 2~Ⓟ would be formed per mol of NADH, the total net production being 36 instead of 38.

Recall that 7,300 calories are required for the conversion of 1 mole of ADP to ATP. Thus 38 ATP will conserve 38×7,300=277,000 calories. The rest of the free energy is lost in the system. It is to be noted that most of the ATP is formed as a consequence of oxidative phosphorylation resulting from the reoxidation of reduced coenzymes by the respiratory chain. The remainder is generated by phosphorylation at the substrate level.

The efficiency of conversion is thus :

$$\frac{(277,000)}{(686,000)}(100\%)=40 \text{ per cent}$$

From the point of view of relating data obtained in studies of the energetics of intermediary metabolism at the cellular level to those obtained in energy metabolism studies with the intact animal, however, it is of greater interest to calculate for particular nutrients the caloric requirements for the synthesis of ATP from ADP i.e. for the synthesis of a high energy phosphate bond. Calculations of these requirements when the synthesis of ATP from ADP arises from the oxidation of carbohydrates, of fats and of proteins are described as follows:

**A) Caloric requirement for the formation of ATP from ADP in glucose oxidation**

It can be seen in page 402 that 38 ATP are formed during the oxidation of each mole of glucose. The major proportion i.e., 24 ATP (63%) being produced in the reactions occurring in the tricarboxylic acid (TCA) cycle. The calorific value for glucose determined in the bomb calorimeter is 673 kcal. Therefore, the caloric requirement for the formation of 1 mole ATP from 1 mole ADP is 673÷38=17.7 kcal.

**B) Caloric requirement for the formation of ATP from ADP during oxidation of fat (palmitic)**

It can be seen in page 402 that 130 ATP are produced during the degradation of palmitic acid. Since the calorific value of 1 mole of palmitic acid is 2340 kcal, the caloric requirement per mole of ATP synthesized equals 2340÷130=18.0 kcal.

**C) Caloric requirement for the formation of ATP from ADP during oxidation of protein (Casein)**

Unlike carbohydrate and fat, there are a number of difficulties associated with estimating the caloric requirement for the synthesis of a high energy phosphate bond from protein oxidation. The difficulties are as follows:

(i) Protein does not undergo complete oxidation in the body, the process stopping at the oxidation level of ammonia. In the determination of the heat of combustion of protein in the bomb calorimeter the oxidation is carried through completely to nitrogen and water. It is thus necessary to make a correction to the gross energy of calorific value in order to obtain the energy, termed metabolisable energy, that becomes available when protein undergoes oxidation in the body. The eminent English Scientists, Blaxter and Martin have carried out a number of experiments in which casein was infused into the rumen or abomasum of sheep. The dry casein contained 14.9% nitrogen and had a calorific value of 5663 kcal per kg. If the calorific value of end product i.e. urea be taken as 5.41% kcal/g nitrogen, then the calorific value of the urea excreted following the ingestion of 1 kg casein would be 806 kcal. The metabolizable energy content of casein would then be 5663−806=4857 kcal per kg.

Table 120

**Yield of ATP from ADP (moles) resulting from the oxidation within the body of 100 g casein**

| Amino acid | Net yield of ATP[1] (moles ATP/mole amino acid) | Net yield of ATP[1] (moles ATP/100 g amino acid) | Contents of amino acids in casein[2] % | ATP yield (moles ATP/100g casein) |
|---|---|---|---|---|
| Alanine | 16 | 18.0 | 3.2 | 0.58 |
| Valine | 30[3] | 25.6 | 7.2 | 1.84 |
| Leucine | 40 | 30.5 | 9.2 | 2.81 |
| Isoleucine | 41 | 31.3 | 6.1 | 1.91 |
| Serine | 13 | 12.4 | 6.3 | 0.78 |
| Threonine | 21 | 17.6 | 4·9 | 0.86 |
| Phenylalanine | 39 | 23.6 | 5.0 | 1.18 |
| Tyrosine | 42 | 23.2 | 6.3 | 1.46 |
| Proline | 30 | 26.1 | 10.6 | 2.77 |
| Cysteine | 13 | 10,7 | 0.4[4](0.8) | 0.08 |
| Methionine | 18 | 12.1 | 2.8 | 0.34 |
| Arginine | 29[5] | 16.7 | 4.1 | 0.68 |
| Histidine | 21 | 13.5 | 3.1 | 0.42 |
| Lysine | 35 | 24.0 | 8.2 | 1.97 |
| Aspartic acid | 16 | 12.0 | 7.1 | 0.85 |
| Glutamic acid | 25 | 17.0 | 22.4 | 3.81 |
| Glycine | 13 | 17.3 | 2.0 | 0.35 |
| Tryptophan | — | — | 1.2 | 0 00 |
| | | | Total | 22.69 |

[1] The data given for all amino acids except glycine and tryptophan are those calculated by Krebs and represent the ATP yields (from ADP) after deduction of the ATP requirements of urea synthesis (2 moles ATP/amino group—see text). The value for glycine is that based upon the assumption that it reacts with methyltetrahydrofolic acid to form serine and terahydrofolic acid. Tryptophan is not completely oxidised in the body and the end-products excreted in the urine have high energy values. Accordingly no value has been attributed to tryptophan.

[2] The amino acid composition of casein is that given by Martin and Blaxter.

[3] The value of 20 for valine given by Krebs is a typographical error.

[4] The figure 0.4 refers to cystine and this has been taken as approximating to 0.8 per cent cysteine.

[5] One mole of urea formed from arginine does not involve an ATP cost.

(ii) The next difficulty is the necessity to take into account the energy cost of synthesizing the urea which is produced via the Ornithine cycle (see page 448). In the study of the energetics of this cycle, it has been observed that for each atom of nitrogen in the original protein, two high energy bonds are used in the synthesis of urea. The two energy consuming steps of the cycle are:

(a) $NH_3+CO_2+2ATP \longrightarrow Carbamylphosphate+2ADP+2P$

(b) $Citrulline+aspartate+ATP \longrightarrow Arginosuccinate+AMP+PP$

(iii) For the sake of calculating yields of ATP resulting from the degradation of the individual amino acids, there remains doubt firstly to what extent some of the initial degradative reactions which do yield reduced coenzymes such as NADH and $FADH_2$ are linked to oxidative phosphorylation and secondly, whether in certain oxidative steps where reduced coenzymes are not present there is any capture of the free energy released. Another complication is that glycine and tryptophan follow alternate pathways of metabolism.

With the exception of the amino acids, glycine and tryptophan the net yields of ATP for the individual amino acids have been calculated and are based on the assumptions that all

**Table 121**

**Yield of ATP from ADP (moles) resulting from the oxidation within the body of 1 mole quantities of the steam-volatile fatty acids**

**The symbol (~P) denotes a high-energy phosphate bond**

| | ATP | | NADH | | $FADH_2$ | | Total |
|---|---|---|---|---|---|---|---|
| | net moles formed | net gain of (~P) | net moles formed | net gain of (~P) | net moles formed | net gain of (~P) | gain of (~P) |
| **Acetic acid** | | | | | | | |
| **Acetic acid to acetyl CoA** | −2 | −2 | | | | | −2 |
| **Acetyl CoA to carbon dioxide and water** | +1 | +1 | +3 | +9 | +1 | +2 | +12 |
| | | | | | | | **Total +10** |
| **Propionic acid** | | | | | | | |
| **Propionic acid to propionyl CoA** | −2 | −2 | | | | | −2 |
| **Propionyl CoA to methyl malonyl CoA** | −1 | −1 | | | | | −1 |
| **Succinyl CoA to succinate** | +1[1] | +1 | | | | | +1 |
| **Succinate to fumarate** | | | | | +1 | +2 | +2 |
| **Malate to oxaloacetate** | | | +1 | +3 | | | +3 |
| **Pyruvate to acetyl CoA** | | | +1 | +3 | | | +3 |
| **Acetyl CoA to carbon dioxide and water** | +1 | +1 | +3 | +9 | +1 | +2 | +12 |
| | | | | | | | **Total +18** |
| **n-Butyric acid** | | | | | | | |
| **Butyric acid to butyryl CoA** | −2 | −2 | | | | | −2 |
| **Butyryl CoA to crotonyl CoA** | | | | | +1 | +2 | +2 |
| **β-hydroxybutyryl CoA to acetoacetyl CoA** | | | +1 | +3 | | | +3 |
| **2 acetyl CoA to carbon dioxide+water** | +2 | +2 | +6 | +18 | +2 | +4 | +24 |
| | | | | | | | **Total +27** |

**A+ve sign denotes ADP—→ATP i.e. a gain of one high-energy bond; a —ve sign indicates the reverse.**

[1] **A high-energy terminal pyrophosphate bond is fixed in the conversion of succinyl CoA to succinate when guanosine diphosphate (GDP) is converted to guanosine triphosphate (GTP).**

oxidative steps involving components of the cytochrome system are effectively coupled to phosphorylation. From the Table No.120 data suggest that when 100 gm casein are oxidized in the body there is a net formation of 22.7 moles of ATP from ADP. The metabolisable energy content of casein has been calculated to be 4857 kcal/kg and thus a theoretical caloric requirement per mole of ATP synthesis from protein amounts to 4857÷22.7=21.4 kcal.

**Caloric requirement for the formation of ATP from ADP during oxidation of the steam volatile fatty acids**

In ruminants tne extensive fermentation of foods in the rumen results in the degradation of carbohydrates to smaller molecules than glucose, mainly acetic, propionic and butyric acids. Small quantities of lactic acid may be produced and absorbed when ruminants are fed certain diets. These acids, absorbed into the portal blood stream via the rumen wall, provide the major energy yielding substrates within the body of the ruminant. The yields of the terminal pyrophosphate bonds resulting from the complete oxidation of these acids are tabulated in Table No. 121. It is assumed that the acetate after activation is metabolized via the tricarboxylic acid cycle, propionic acid after activation is converted to methyl malonyl CoA and then via succinate and pyruvate to acetyl CoA while n-butyric acid gives rise to acetoacetyl CoA via butyril CoA, crotonyl CoA and β-hydroxy butyryl CoA· the acetoacetyl CoA gives rise to 2 acetyl CoA.

**Theoretical efficiencies with which nutrients can be used to meet the maintenance requirement**

In the fasting animal, body fat is the tissue component that is catabolised to provide the major portion of the energy required to maintain the essential life processes. The great English Scientists, Armstrong and Blaxter have pointed out that it is reasonable to expect that in meeting the energy requirement of maintenance, nutrients replace body fat in direct proportion to the free energy which they yield to the body when they are dissimilated. The lower the energy cost per mole of ATP formed from ADP the more efficiently will the energy of that nutrient be utilized. For a particular nutrient the caloric requirement per mole of ATP synthesized relative to that for such synthesis when fat is oxidized provides a measure of the theoretical efficiency with which the nutrient will be used to spare body fat. Alternatively for any single nutrient the value is calculated as follows :

$$\frac{\textit{Caloric requirement/mole ATP from nutrient—caloric requirement/mole ATP from fat}}{\textit{Caloric requirement/mole ATP from fat}} \times 100$$

This value gives a measure of the theoretical increment in heat that would be expected to occur when the nutrient in question is used to replace body fat in providing the free energy essential to life. Theoretical heat increments for various nutrients when used as substrates for oxidative metabolism are given in Table No. 122. The caloric requirement from tristearin has been assumed to be equivalent to that of body fat. Although naturally occurring triglycerides of depot fat are mixed triglycerides, and particularly in the case of simple stomached animals, do contain appreciable quantities of unsaturated fatty acids, the errors involved in the assumption are of little consequence in the present context. The values in Table 122 illustrates that if glucose replaces body fat as the source of free energy, the heat production of the animal should be less by 2 per cent than the fasting heat production. If the free energy is provided by the catabolism of protein then the heat production of the animal should be some 20 per cent higher than that of the animal when fasting. For ruminant animals a theoretical consideration of energy metabolism at the cellular level would suggest that all three volatile fatty acids are used less efficiently than body fat in the provision of the necessary free energy with acetic acid being efficient than propionic acid and both inferior to butyric acid.

**Table 122**

**Theoretical heat increments for nutrients when used to replace body fat in providing free energy for maintenance**

| Nutrient | Caloric requirement/ mole ATP formed from ADP (kcal/mole) | Theoretical heat increment[1] % | Theoretical efficiency of utilization %[2] |
|---|---|---|---|
| Tristerain | 18.1 | 0 | 100 |
| Glucose | 17.7 | —2.2 | 102.2 |
| Casein | 21.4 | 18.2 | 81.8 |
| Acetic acid | 20.9 | 15.5 | 84.5 |
| Propionic acid | 20.4 | 12.7 | 87.3 |
| n-butyric acid | 19.4 | 7.2 | 92.8 |
| Mixure of propionic and n-butyric acids in molar proportions 6 : 4[3] | 19.9 | 9.9 | 90.1 |
| Mixture of acetic, propionic and n-butyric acids in molar proportions 2.5 : 4.5 : 3.0 | 20.1 | 11.0 | 89.0 |
| n-butyric acids in molar proportions 7.5 : 1.5 : 1.0 | 20.5 | 13.3 | 86.7 |
| Mixture of acetic, propionic and n-butyric acids in molar proportions 9.0 : 0.6 : 0.4 | 20.7 | 14.4 | 85.6 |

[1] Calculated as

$$\frac{\text{calories required/mole ATP from nutrient—calories required/mole ATP from fat}}{\text{Calories required/mole ATP from fat}} \times 100$$

[2] Calculated as 100—heat increment

[3] Values of mixtures calculated from data for individual acids

**The efficiency of lipogenesis from glucose**

It may be observed from the previous discussions on the synthesis of fatty acids (page 436-439) that in the two reductions which follow each condensation the source of hydrogen is provided by the reduced coenzyme, nicotinamide adenine dinucleotide phosphate (NADPH). The reduced form of this coenzyme is produced primarily by the extra mitochondrial oxidation of glucose via pentose phosphate pathway according to the following overall reaction.

$$C_6H_{12}O_6 + 6H_2O + 12\ NADP^+ \longrightarrow 6CO_2 + 12\ NADPH$$

The overall process whereby nine moles of acetyl CoA condense to form 1 mole stearic acid can be depicted as

$$\text{Acetyl CoA} + 8\ \text{malonyl CoA} + 16\ NADPH \longrightarrow \text{Stearly CoA} + 8\ CO_2 + 16\ NADP^+$$

While it has already been agreed that the above pathway of synthesis is followed in the formation of palmityl CoA from acetyl CoA, the conversion of palmityl CoA to Stearyl CoA may proceed via a different pathway. At present it will be assumed that the final condensation and reductions proceed as described.

Blaxter has pointed out a theoretical calorimetric efficiency for the process of lipogenesis which is

$$Efficiency = \frac{\textit{Calorific value of the fat formed}}{\textit{Calorific value of the nutrients used}} \times 100$$

From this the synthesis of tristearin (a specific fat) from glucose, the efficiency of the process may be written as:

$$Efficiency = \frac{\textit{Calorific value of 1 mole tristearin}}{\textit{Calorific value of 'n' moles of glucose}} \times 100$$

Where 'n' represents the number of moles of glucose used in yielding not only the necessary carbon framework but also the necessary supply of reduced coenzymes. Calculation of 'n' is made as below in three steps:

A. For every mole of stearic acid the requirement of NADPH as mentioned earlier is 16. Thus for three moles of stearic acid there would be a requirement of $3 \times 16 = 48$ moles of NADPH which would necessitate 4 moles of glucose being metabolized through pentose phosphate pathway.

B. For the sake of carbon framework for 3 moles of stearic acid, $3 \times 9 = 27$ moles of acetyl CoA would be required. Since each mole of glucose metabolized via Embden-Meyerhof pathway can yield two of acetyl CoA, the metabolism of 14 moles glucose via this pathway could provide the necessary 27 moles acetyl CoA plus 1 mole of glyceraldehyde-3-phosphate which could be used to synthesize the mole of glycerol required.

Considering the discussions as under A and B it is easy to understand that 18 moles of glucose would provide all the necessary carbon fragments for the synthesis of a mole of tristearin and sufficient of the specific reduced coenzyme. It is now important to consider future requirement of glucose for supply of ATP required for the synthesis of tristearin.

C. From the data given in pages 412 & 415 it can be calculated in the same way as in Table No.121 that from the metabolism of 14 moles of glucose to 27 moles acetyl CoA and 1 mole glyceraldehyde-3-phosphate there would be a net yield of 183 ATP. Three of these, in the form of the reduced coenzyme NADH would be used in the reduction of the glyceraldehyde phosphate to glycerophosphate, 4 would be required to activate the 4 moles glucose subsequently metabolised via pentose phosphate pathway while a further $3 \times 8 = 24$ ATP would be required to provide the energy for the formation of the carbon-dioxide-biotin-enzyme complex which catalyses the conversion acetyl CoA to malonyl CoA. Although further small amounts of ATP would be required in the final reactions linking the 3 moles of fatty acid and 1 mole of glycerol to give the triglyceride but still there remains always a considerable surplus of ATP.

A theoretical calorimetric efficiency for the synthesis of tristearin from glucose can thus be calculated as

$$\textit{Efficiency} = \frac{\textit{Calorific value of 1 mole tristcarin}}{\textit{Colorific value of 18 moles glucose}} \times 100$$

$$= \frac{8286}{673 \times 18} \times 100 = 68.5 \text{ per cent.}$$

100−68.5=31.5 per cent has been utilized for heat increment. Thus it suggests that the efficiency with which glucose is used for synthesis of fat is considerably less than that pertaining when it is used to spare body fat from oxidation.

**The efficiency of lipogenesis from the steam-volatile fatty acids (VFA)**

Armstrong and his colleagues carried out a number of experiments in which two mixtures of the volatile fatty acids, one containing a high proportion of acetic acid and the other a low

**Efficiencies of lipogenesis from steam-volatile fatty acids and mixture measures in experiments with mature sheep**

| *Infused* | *Proportion of steam-volatile fatty acids (m-equiv/100 m-equiv total acid)* *In the rumen* | *Efficiency of lipogenesis*[1] |
|---|---|---|
| 75 acetic: 15 propionic: 10 n-butyric | 68 acetic: 20 propionic: 12 n-butyric | 31.8 |
| 25 acetic: 45 propionic: 30 n-butyric | 54 acetic: 30 propionic: 16 n-butyric | 58.1 |

[1] Measured as increase in kcal in energy stored/100 kcal additional metabolizable energy

proportion, were infused separately into the rumens of mature sheep receiving a maintenance diet of dried grass. Increments in energy balance were measured and efficiencies of lipogenesis calculated as for the experiments with glucose.

If the assumption is made that the molar proportions of the individual acids present in the rumen resemble the proportions in which they are absorbed it can be said that as the molar proportion of acetic in the total acid metabolized rose from 54 per cent to 68 per cent the efficiency of lipogenesis fell from 58 to 32 per cent. While some doubt must be attached to the correctness of the assumption made above it is apparent from these *in vivo* experiments that the efficiency of lipogenesis from steam volatile fatty acids is lower than that from glucose and furthermore it declines with increasing levels of acetic acid.

It is very difficult to account for the low efficiency of lipogenesis associated with steam volatile fatty acid mixture containing high proportion of acetic acid. In this connection Armstrong and Blaxter, the two pioneer English Scientists observed that the efficiency of energy storage in the body of the adult ruminant is higher when the process is accompanied by the simultaneous secretion of energy in milk than when it occurs in the non-lactating animals.

The theoretical efficiency for lipogenesis from propionic acid, calculated on the same basis as for glucose is 62.7 per cent.

**The efficiency of protein synthesis**

Concerning protein synthesis there is incomplete understanding of the metabolic pathway involved and in particular of the requirements of high energy bonds and co-factors required for the various intermediate steps. It is postulated from theoretical consideration, that the high energy bond requirement for peptide linkage may lie in the range of 8 to 12 ATP.

# 15

# CARBOHYDRATE METABOLISM

Glucose enters the cell from the intestinal fluid in the free state and is then actively transported across most cell membranes under the influence of the hormone insulin. Intestinal mucosa and brain do not require insulin for glucose transport. Free glucose cannot enter into other cellular metabolic activities; thus upon entrance into the cell, it is immediately phosphorylated, a process which requires ATP and which results in the formation of glucose-6-phosphate. Three chief pathways are open to the phosphorylated glucose:

(1) Glycolysis, (2) Glycogenesis (formation of glycogen), (3) Metabolism by way of the pentose phosphate shunt. The pathway followed is determined by the metabolic condition existing within the cell; primarily, the available amounts of glucose, ATP, NADP and oxygen determine the pathway of glucose degradation.

## GLYCOLYSIS

The pathway of glycolysis was elucidated by G. Embden and O. Meyerhof during the period between 1920 and 1940 and thus the processes of glycolysis is also termed as Embden-Meyerhof glycolytic pathway. The principal reactions involved in glycolysis are shown in page 412. Reactions corresponding to numbers are described below:

**1. Free glucose is phosphorylated to form glucose-6-phosphate which requires ATP.**

**2. Glucose-6-phosphate is isomerised to fructose-6-phosphate.**

**3. Fructose-6-phosphate is further phosphorylated by ATP at the first carbon to form fructose-1, 6-diphosphate.**

4. **Fructose-1, 6-diphosphate** is split into two molecules of glyceraldehyde-3-phosphate, and dihydroxyacetone phosphate. From this point, carbohydrate metabolism proceeds from glyceraldehyde-3-phosphate, but, because this compound and dihydroxyacetone phosphate are interconvertible, in effect, two molecules of glyceraldehyde are formed from one hexose unit.

5 Glyceraldehyde-3-phosphate is then oxidised to glyceric acid-1, 3-diphosphate. The hydrogen thus released is taken up by NAD which may be reoxidised by the mitochondrial electron transport system leading to the synthesis of 3 moles of ATP. In the absence of oxygen (anaerobic glycolysis), NADH is utilised in the formation of lactic acid from pyruvic acid.

6. Glyceric acid-1, 3-diphosphate reacts directly with ADP to form ATP and glyceric acid-3-phosphate.

7. Glyceric acid-3-phosphate is converted to glyceric acid 2-phosphate, essentially migration of the phosphate group.

8. Glyceric acid-2-phosphate is dehydrated to form phosphoenol pyruvic acid.

9. Phosphoenol pyruvic acid reacts with ADP, to form pyruvic acid and ATP

**Embden-Meyerhof of Glycolysis**

Glucose 6-phosphate ⇌ (2) Fructose 6-phosphate; ATP → ADP (3) Fructose 1,6-diphosphate

Glucose; ATP → ADP (1) Glucose 6-phosphate

Fructose 1,6-diphosphate → Dihydroxyacetone phosphate ⇌ (4) Glyceraldehyde 3-phosphate

Glyceraldehyde 3-phosphate; $P_i$, $NAD^+$ → NADH (5) 1,3-Diphosphoglyceric acid

1,3-Diphosphoglyceric acid; ATP ADP (6) ⇌ 3-Phosphoglyceric acid ⇌ (7) 2-Phosphoglyceric acid ⇌ (8) Phosphoenolpyruvic acid

Phosphoenolpyruvic acid; ADP → ATP (9) Pyruvic acid

Lactic acid ⇌ (10) $NAD^+$ NADH Pyruvic acid; $CO_2$ (11) Acetaldehyde; NADH $NAD^+$ (12) Ethanol

**The enzymes required in various steps are in: 1. Glucokinase, 2. Phosphoglucose isomerase, 3. Phosphofructokinase, 4. Aldolase, 5. Phosphoglyceraldehyde dehydrogenase, 6. 3-phosphoglyceric acid kinase, 7. Phosphoglyceromutase, 8. Enolase, 9. Pyruvic acid kinase and 10. Lactic acid dehydrogenase.**

**Table 123**

**Yield of ATP from glucose in glycolysis**

| *Steps* | | *Moles of ATP gained (+) or loss (−) per initial glucose unit* — *Anaerobically* | *Aerobically* |
|---|---|---|---|
| 1. Glucose+ATP | Glucose 6-phosphate+ADP | −1 | −1 |
| 2. Fructose-6-phosphate+ATP | Fructose-1,-6-diphosphate+ADP | −1 | −1 |
| 3. Glyceraldehyde-3-phosphate (2 moles) | 1, 3-diphosphoglyceric acid | — | +6 |
| 4. 1, 3-diphosphoglyceric acid+ 2 ADP (2 moles) | 3 phosphoglyceric acid (2 moles) +2 ATP | +2 | +2 |
| 5. Phosphenol pyruvic acid+2 ADP (2 moles) | Pyruvic acid (2 moles)+2 ATP | +2 | +2 |
| Net gain in ATP via Glycolysis | | +2 | +8 |

*Note that Glycolysis can proceed in both aerobic and anaerobic conditions.*

***Metabolic fates of pyruvate.***

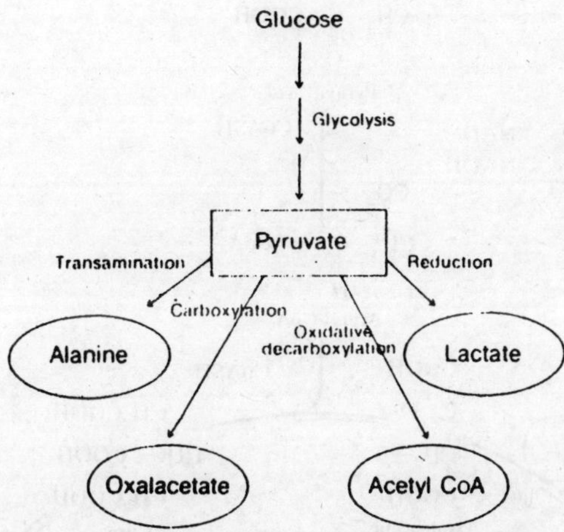


**10. Pyruvic acid, thus formed, enters the mitochondrion for further oxidation. When the oxygen supply is low, as in prolonged muscular activity, pyruvic acid may be used to oxidize NADH, forming NAD and lactic acid.**

$$\underset{\text{Glucose}}{C_6H_{12}O_6} \longrightarrow \longrightarrow \underset{\text{Pyruvic acid}}{2\,CH_3{-}\overset{\overset{\displaystyle O}{\|}}{C}{-}C{\genfrac{}{}{0pt}{}{\nearrow O}{\searrow OH}}} \xrightarrow{\text{without oxygen}}$$

$$\xrightarrow[\text{fermentation}]{\text{in yeast}} \underset{\text{Ethyl alcohol}}{2\,C_2H_5OH} + \underset{\text{Carbon dioxide}}{2\,CO_2} + \text{Energy}$$

$$\xrightarrow[\text{glycolysis}]{\text{in muscle}} \underset{\text{Lactic acid}}{2\,CH_3CHOHCOOH} + \text{Energy}$$

**Lactic acid, so produced in anaerobic condition, is transported to the liver for resynthesis to glycogen since there is no enzymatic mechanism in muscle cells for the conversion of lactic acid to glycogen.**

***Glycolysis may thus proceed in the presence or absence of oxygen. From the standpoint of energy yield to the cell, however, aerobic glycolysis is the more efficient mechanism.***

### The Tricarboxylic Acid Cycle

**The chemical energy that is not liberated when glucose is broken down anaerobically, to lactate, is released during the third stage of nutrient degradation when pyruvate is oxidised in the mitochondria to $CO_2$ and $H_2O$ via the tricarboxylic acid, TCA cycle. In a quantitative sense, this cycle is the most important phase in the oxidation of foodstuffs, since approximately 90 per cent of the energy released from food is the result of TCA cycle oxidation.**

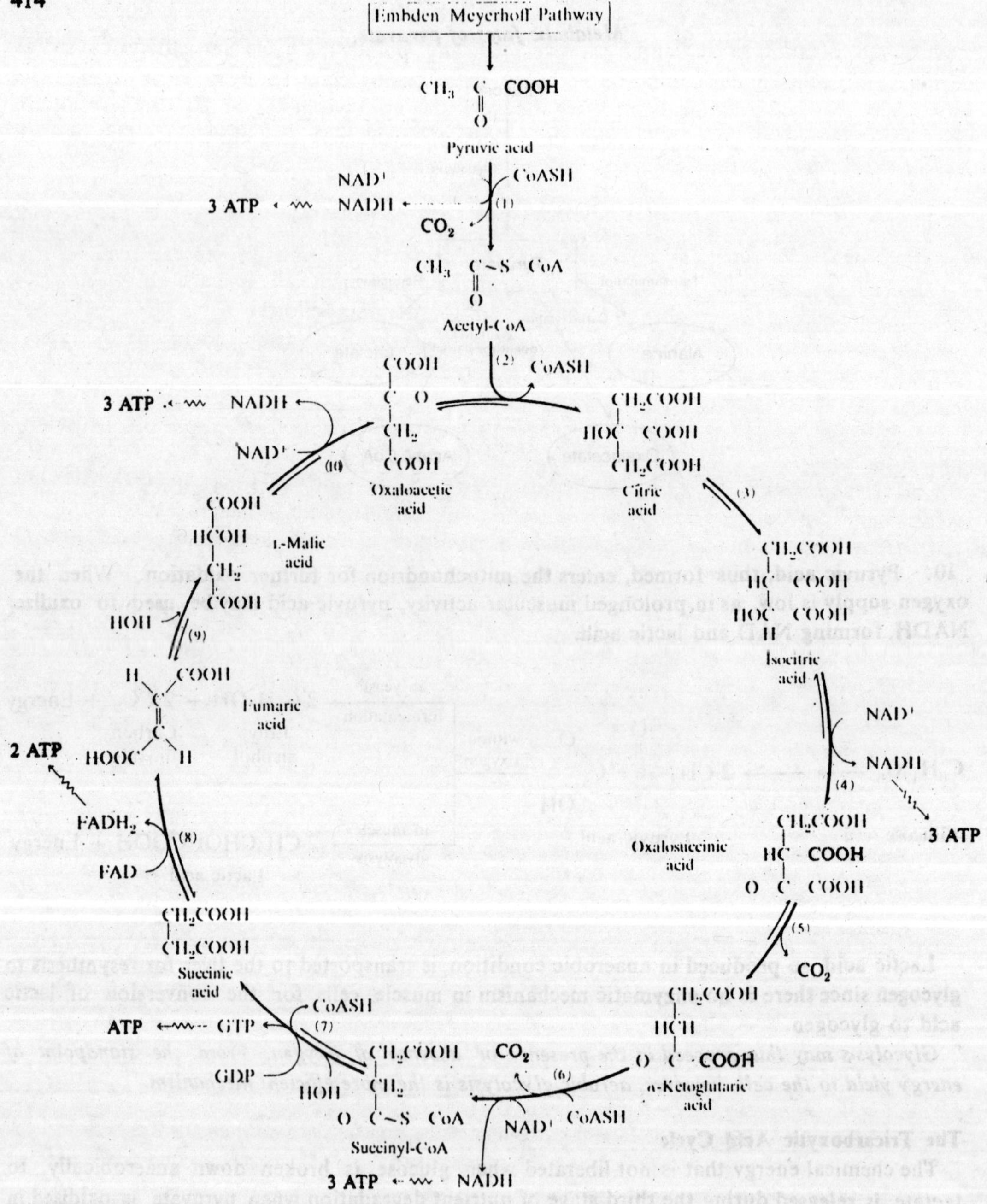


The Krebs cycle.

**Fig. 39 Enzymes required in various steps are in: 1. Pyruvate oxidase, 2. Citrate condensing enzyme, 3 and 4. Aconitase, 5. Isocitrate dehydrogenase. 6. α-keto glutarate dehydrogenase, 7. Succinyl thiokinase. 8. Succinate, dehydrogenase, 9. Fumerase, and 10. Malate dehydrogenase.**

Although metabolites may enter the cycle at any point, the cycle is usually visualised as beginning with the condensation of acetyl CoA with oxaloacetate to form citric acid. The subsequent series of reactions comprising the cycle uses up two moles of $H_2O$ and results in the release of two moles of $CO_2$ and four pairs of hydrogens and electrons. The over-all reaction in the degradation of acetate may be expressed as:

$$\underset{\text{Acetic acid.}}{CH_3COOH} + 2H_2O \longrightarrow 2CO_2 + 2H^+$$

The individual reactions of TCA cycle are depicted diagrammatically in page 414 A description of the reactions corresponding to numbers in the diagram follows:

1. Pyruvic acid is converted to an active form of acetic acid, acetyl coenzyme A (acetyl CoA). In the process of forming acetyl CoA, pyruvic acid is decarboxylated and two hydrogen ions are released and are picked up by $NAD^+$.

2. Condensation of oxaloacetate and acetyl CoA form citrate. CoA is split off hydrolytically in the process.

3 & 4. Isomerisation of citrate to yield isocitrate. *Cis*-aconitic acid may be formed as an intermediary. Water assists in the isomerisation but is not used up in the process.

5. Dehydrogenation and decarboxylation of isocitrate to form α-keto-glutaric acid NAD or NADP may serve as hydrogen acceptor.

Table 124

**Yield of ATP from pyruvic acid in TCA cycle**

| *Steps* | | *Moles ATP formed* |
|---|---|---|
| Pyruvic acid | acetyl CoA | 3 |
| Isocitric acid | α-keto-glutaric acid | 3 |
| α-keto-glutaric acid | succinyl CoA | 3 |
| Succinyl CoA | succinic acid | 1 |
| Succinic acid | fumeric acid | 2 |
| Malic acid | oxaloacetic acid | 3 |
| Total ATP per molecule | pyruvic acid | 15 |
| *Total from 2 mols of pyruvate* (15×2)= | | 30 |

The total ATP production from the oxidation of one mole of glucose aerobically is then:

| | Moles ATP |
|---|---|
| 1 mole of glucose to 2 moles of pyruvate | 8 |
| 2 moles of pyruvate to $CO_2$ and $H_2O$ | 30 |
| Total per mole of glucose | 38 |

6 & 7. Oxidative decarboxylation of α-keto-gluterate to form succinate. Succinyl CoA is an intermediary and both Thiamine pyrophosphate (TPP) and lipoic acid are required for this reaction. NAD is the hydrogen acceptor. The loss of a second $CO_2$ molecule results in a 4 carbon chain.

8. Dehydrogenation of succinate to form fumerate. FAD is the hydrogen acceptor.

9. Addition of water to fumerate to form malate.

10. Dehydrogenation of malate to form oxaloacetate.

Oxaloacetate now is available to condense with another mole of acetyl CoA and thus to repeat the cycle.

*Note: During the conversion of*

(*i*) NAD into NADH there is a genesis of 3 moles of ATP.

(*ii*) FAD into $FADH_2$ there is a genesis of 2 moles of ATP.

(*iii*) GDP into GTP there is a genesis of 1 mole of ATP.

***The entire process of citric acid cycle takes place inside the mitochondria under only aerobic condition.***

**Hexose Monophosphate Shunt of Glucose Catabolism**

The principal catabolic route for carbohydrates is the glycolysis pathway, followed under aerobic conditions, by the TCA pathway. The glycolytic enzymes are present in the soluble fraction of cell but the route from pyruvate is located in the mitochondria. There is however, an alternative route by which the oxidation of carbohydrates can take place. Quantitatively, it usually accounts for only a very small percentage of the oxygen taken up by the cell.

The discussion of this pathway is brief, for even indirectly it is not important for ATP production in skeletal muscle. It is, however, a way of converting glucose ultimately of $CO_2$ and $H_2O$ without going through the citric acid cycle. Its most important function is in generating NADPH, which is needed to furnish hydrogen for reduction steps whenever the body synthesises fatty acids and steroids.

Starting from glucose-6-phosphate, the balanced equation representing the net effect of this pathway is

$$6 \text{ glucose 6-phosphate} + 12 \text{ NADP}^+ \xrightarrow[\text{Shunt}]{\text{Hexose monophosphate}}$$

$$5 \text{ glucose 6-phosphate} + 6\, CO_2 + 12 \text{ NADPH} + 12\, H^+ + Pi$$

There are of course several intermediate steps, some of them using enzymes of the glycolysis pathway. Among the intermediates are certain 5-carbon sugars (e.g., ribose) needed by the body to make nucleotides and nucleic acids. We should remember that this shunt is an important way to produce NADPH for fat synthesis.

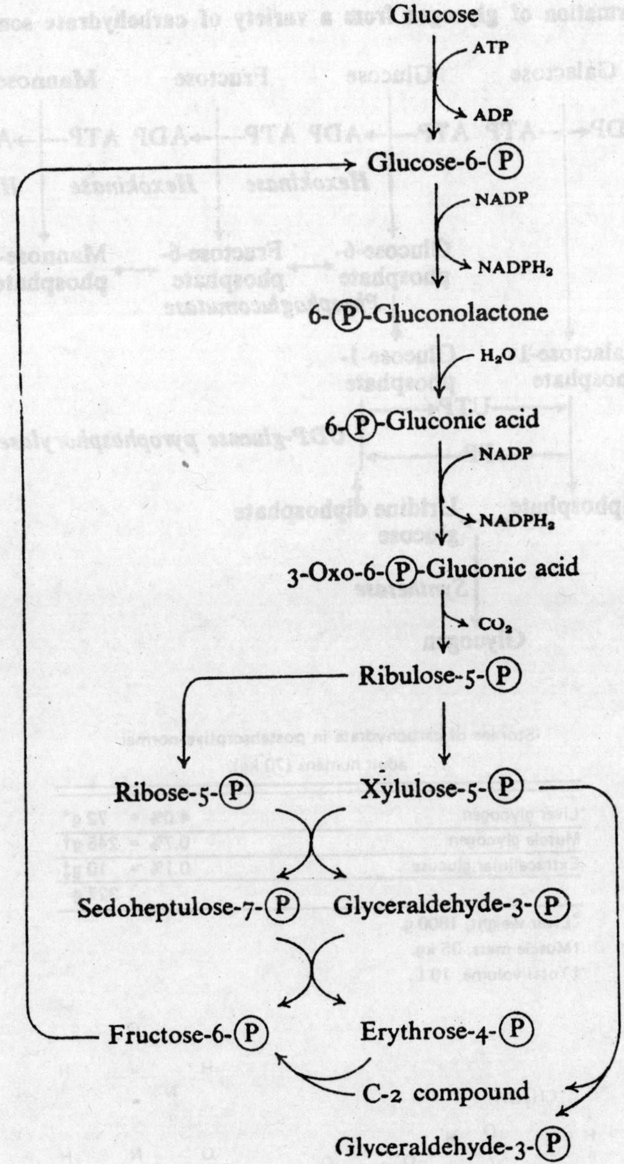


**Fig. 40 Reactions of the pentose phosphate pathway, sometimes called the hexose monophosphate shunt, or alternate pathway.**

## GLYCOGENESIS

The formation of glycogen occurs in practically every tissue of the body, but chiefly in liver and muscle. In man, the liver may contain as much as 5 per cent glycogen when analysed

**Formation of glycogen from a variety of carbohydrate sources**

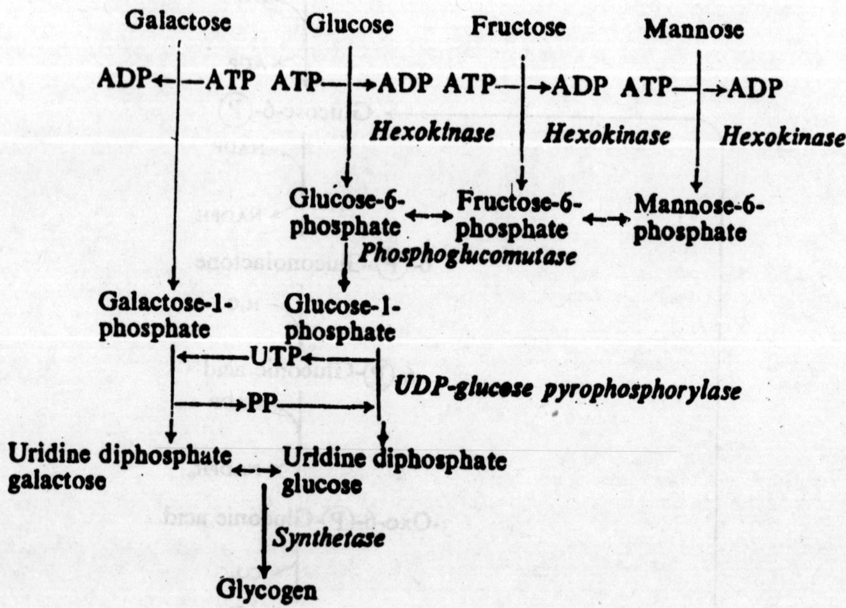


Storage of carbohydrate in postabsorptive normal adult humans (70 kg).

| | |
|---|---|
| Liver glycogen | 4.0% = 72 g* |
| Muscle glycogen | 0.7% = 245 g† |
| Extracellular glucose | 0.1% = 10 g‡ |
| | 327 g |

*Liver weight, 1800 g.
†Muscle mass, 35 kg.
‡Total volume, 10 L.

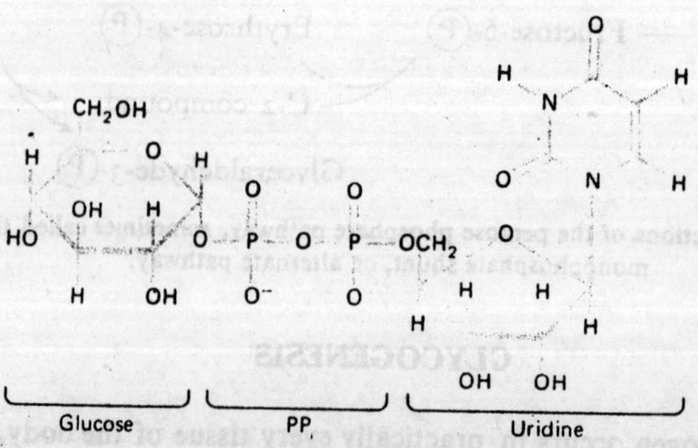


(a) Structure of UDP-glucose

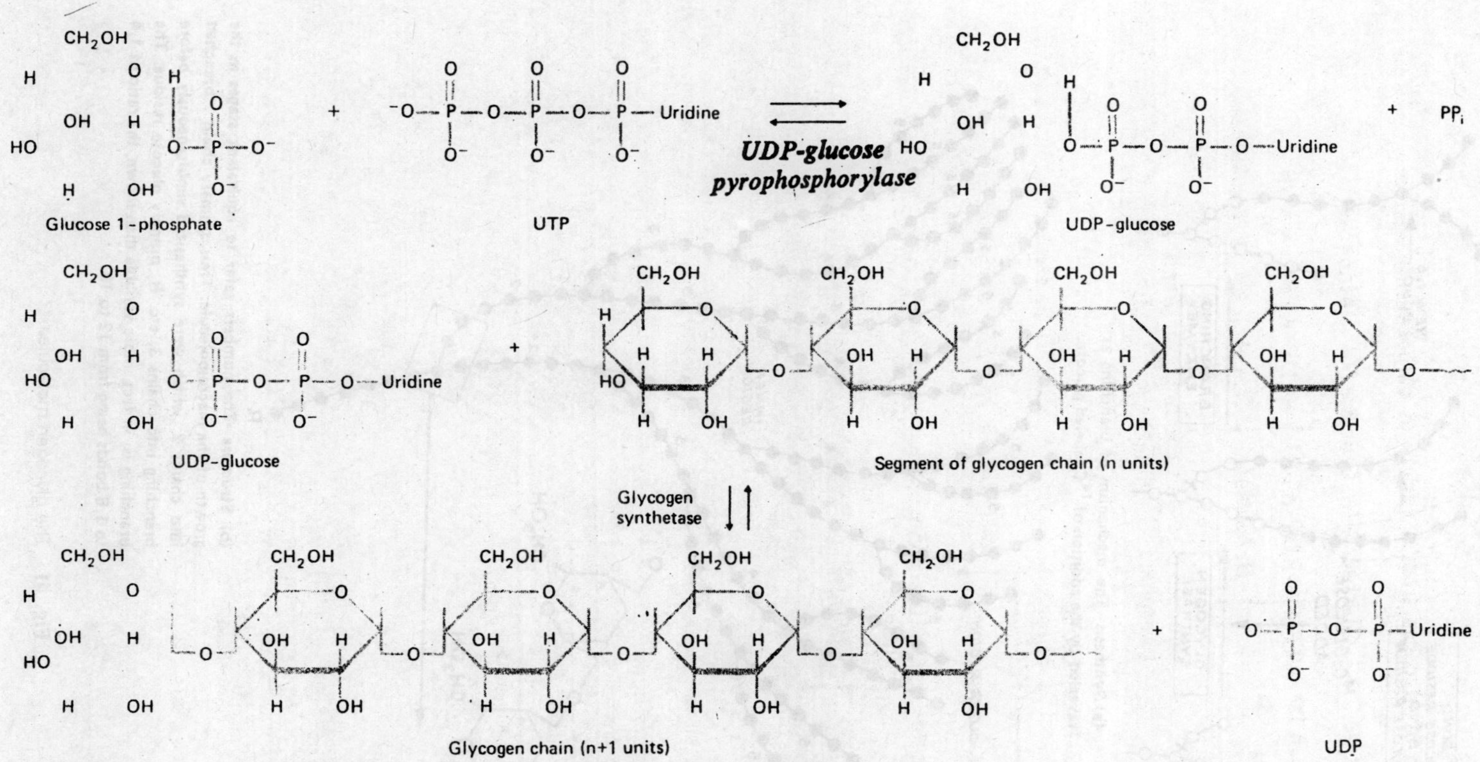

Glucose 1-phosphate + UTP $\rightleftharpoons$ (**UDP-glucose pyrophosphorylase**) UDP-glucose + $PP_i$

UDP-glucose + Segment of glycogen chain (n units)

Glycogen synthetase $\rightleftharpoons$

Glycogen chain (n+1 units) + UDP

(b) Glycogenesis

(a) The structure of UDP-glucose is composed of uridine, pyrophosphate, and glucose. Glucose is bonded to the pyrophosphate at carbon atom 1. (b) Glycogenesis is initiated by the formation of UDP-glucose from glucose 1-phosphate and UTP. Catalyzed by glycogen synthetase, UDP-glucose reacts with the —OH group on the fourth carbon atom of a terminal glucose unit in a glycogen molecule. The products of the reaction are UDP and a glycogen molecule with one additional glucose unit.

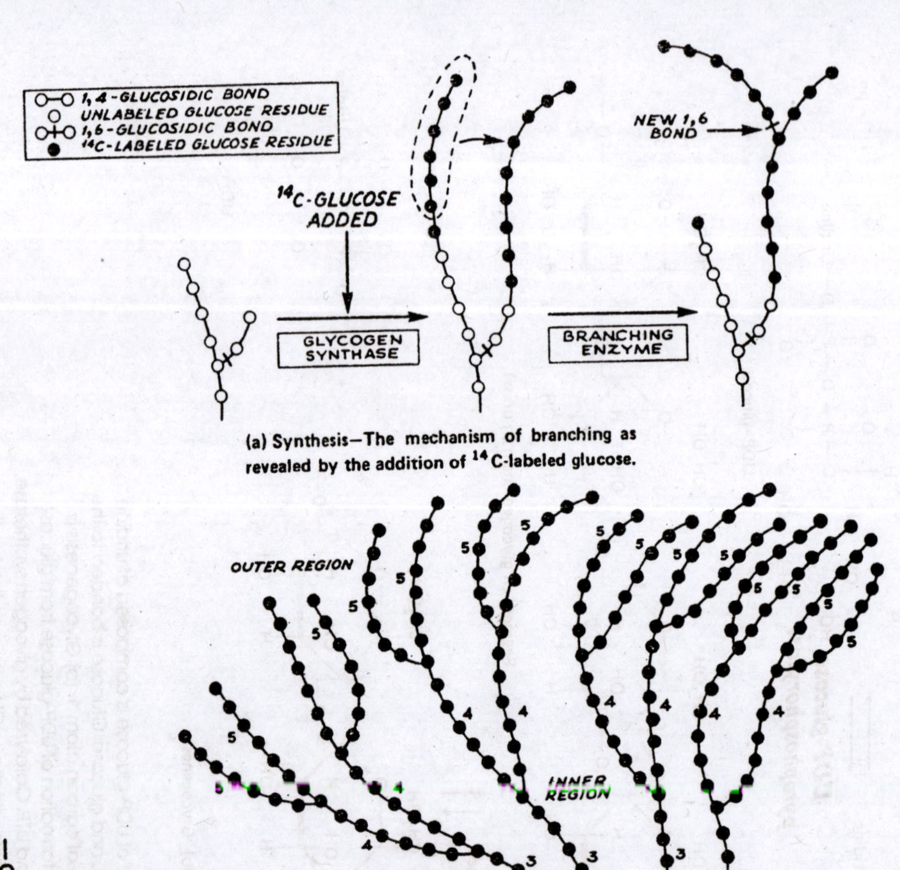


(a) Synthesis—The mechanism of branching as revealed by the addition of $^{14}$C-labeled glucose.

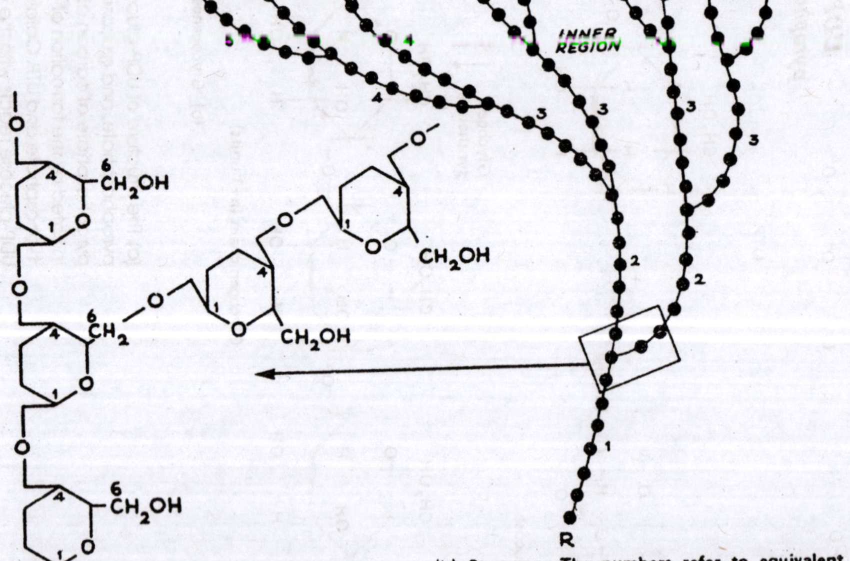


(b) Structure—The numbers refer to equivalent stages in the growth of the macromolecule. Thus, primary chain 1 branched into chains 2, which were synthesized simultaneously before branching into chains 3, etc. R, primary glucose residue. The branching is, in fact, more variable than shown, the ratio of 1,4 to 1,6 bonds being from 12 to 18.

(c) Enlargement of structure at a branch point.

**Fig. 41** The glycogen molecule.

shortly after a meal high in carbohydrate. Muscle glycogen is only rarely elevated above 1 per cent of the net weight of the tissue. Glycogen is a complex of polysaccharide made up of condensed glucose residues. The actual source material for glycogen formation is uridine diphosphate glucose (UDPG) which is produced from a variety of sources as shown in next page.

By the action of the enzymes glycogen synthetase and in the presence of a priming amount of polysaccharide the activated glucose units of UDPG are connected to one another by glucosidic linkages between the 1st and 4th carbons of adjacent glucosyl moieties. Uridine diphosphate (UDP) is liberated as a consequence.

The addition of a glucose residue to a pre-existing glycogen chain occurs at the non-reducing, outer end of the molecule so that the "branches" of the glycogen "tree" become elongated. As successiye-1, 4-linkages occur, when the chain has been lengthened to eight glucose residues,

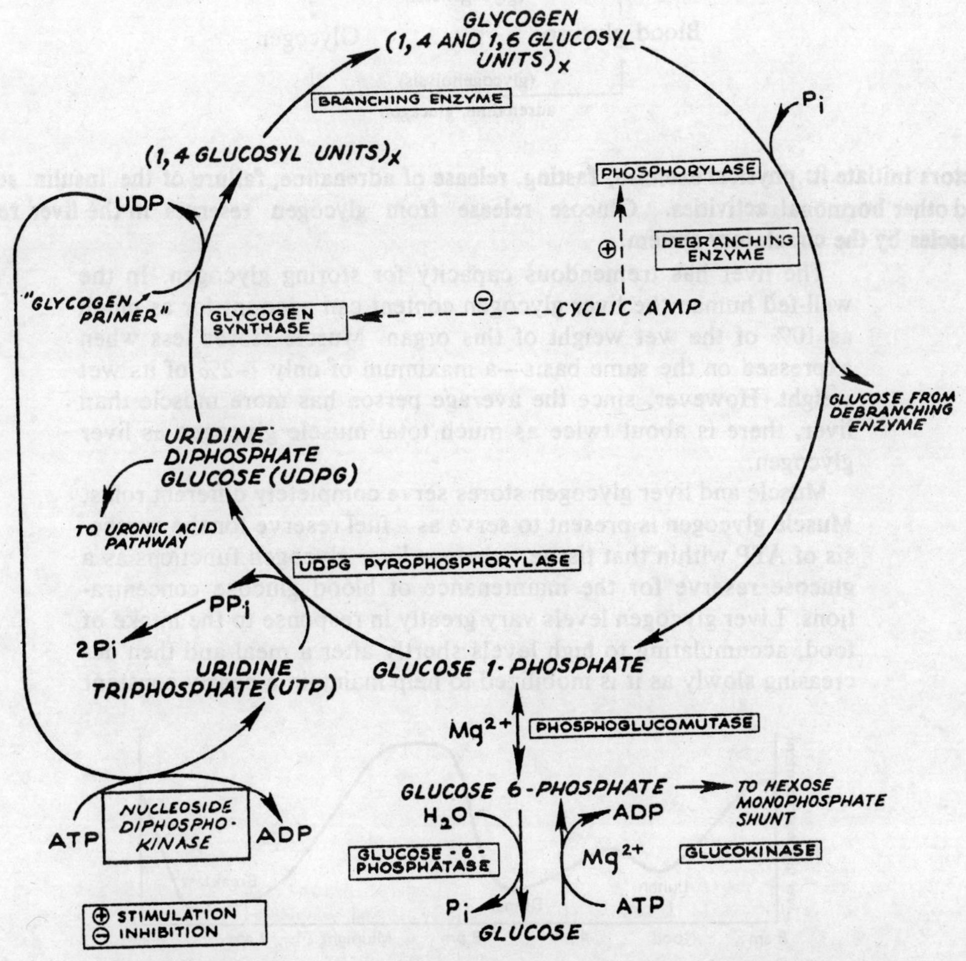


**Fig. 42** Pathway of glycogenesis and of glycogenolysis in the liver. Two high-energy phosphate bonds are used in the incorporation of 1 mol of glucose into glycogen.

**a second enzyme, the branching enzyme acts on the glycogen (Fig. 41). This enzyme transfers a part of the α-1, 4-chain to a neighbouring chain to form a α-1, 6-linkage, thus establishing a branch point in the molecule.**

## GLYCOGENOLYSIS

**When glycogen reserves are depleted because glycogen breaks down or is hydrolysed faster than glucose units are added, the process is called glycogenolysis. The glycogen content of muscles is rapidly used up in severe exercises, and fresh glucose molecules must be taken in from the blood stream. To replenish this supply, liver glycogen can break down. Several**

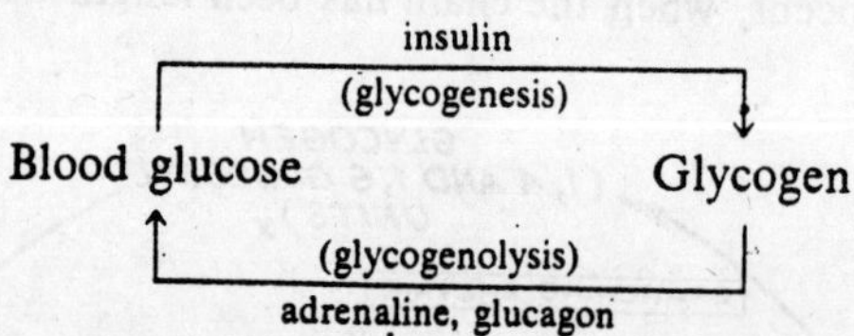


**factors initiate it: physical exercise, fasting, release of adrenaline, failure of the insulin supply, and other hormonal activities. Glucose release from glycogen reserves in the liver reaches muscles by the circulatory system.**

The liver has tremendous capacity for storing glycogen. In the well-fed human the liver glycogen content can account for as much as 10% of the wet weight of this organ. Muscle stores less when expressed on the same basis—a maximum of only 1–2% of its wet weight. However, since the average person has more muscle than liver, there is about twice as much total muscle glycogen as liver glycogen.

Muscle and liver glycogen stores serve completely different roles. Muscle glycogen is present to serve as a fuel reserve for the synthesis of ATP within that tissue, whereas liver glycogen functions as a glucose reserve for the maintenance of blood glucose concentrations. Liver glycogen levels vary greatly in response to the intake of food, accumulating to high levels shortly after a meal and then decreasing slowly as it is mobilized to help maintain a nearly constant

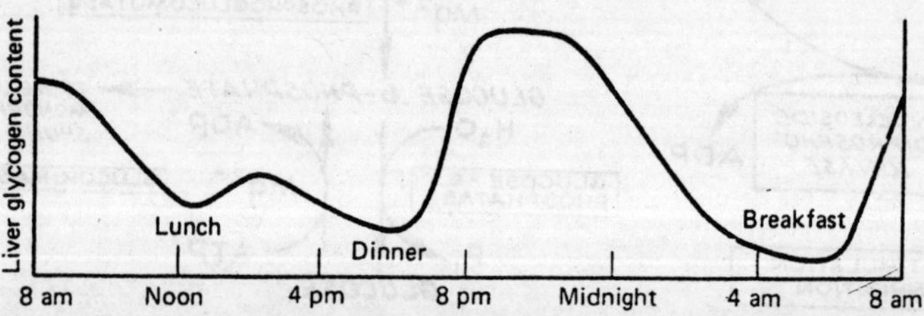


**Fig. 43** ***Variation of liver glycogen levels between meals and during the nocturnal fast.***

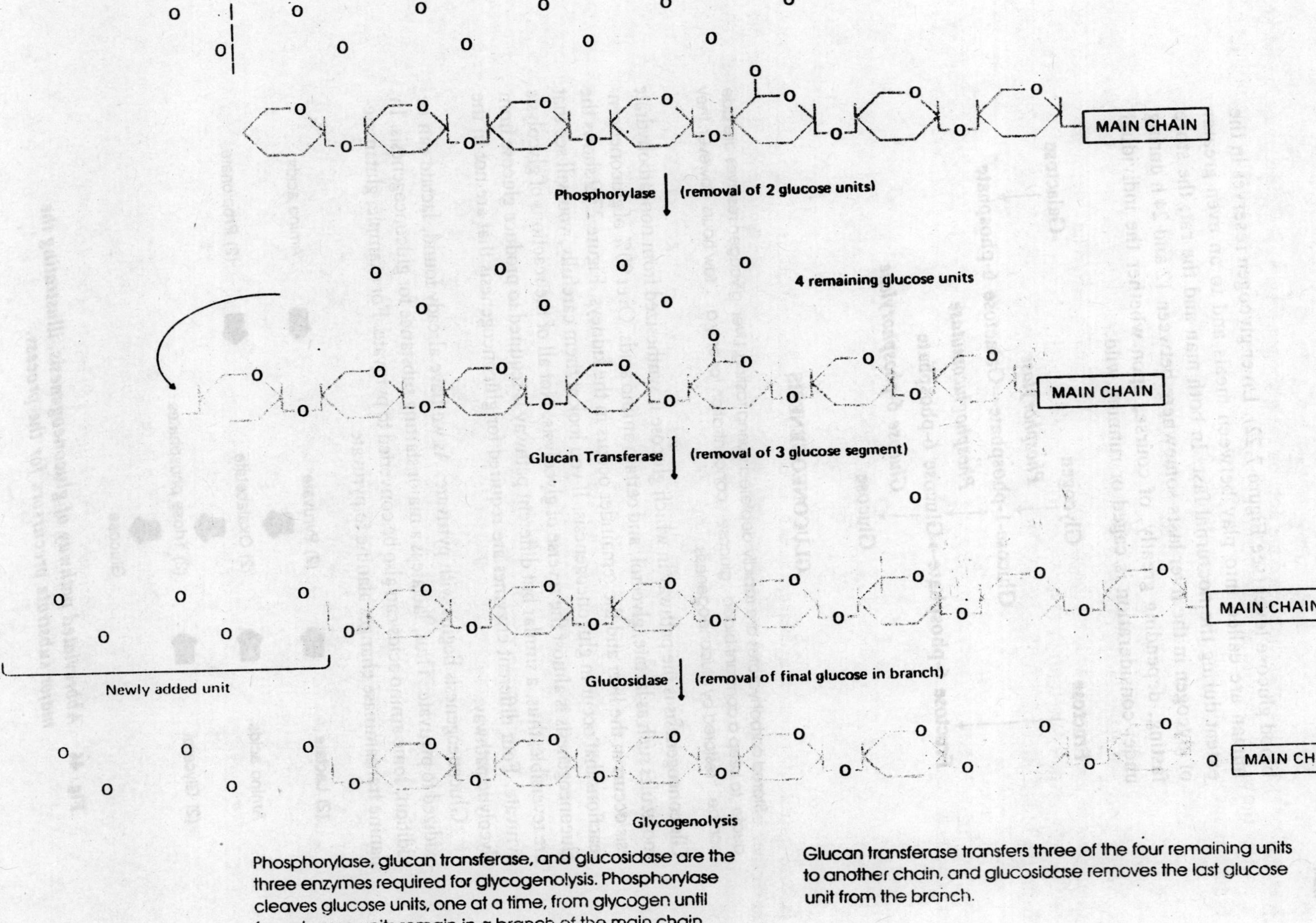


Phosphorylase, glucan transferase, and glucosidase are the three enzymes required for glycogenolysis. Phosphorylase cleaves glucose units, one at a time, from glycogen until four glucose units remain in a branch of the main chain.

Glucan transferase transfers three of the four remaining units to another chain, and glucosidase removes the last glucose unit from the branch.

blood glucose level (see Figure 7.22). Liver glycogen reserves in the human are called into play between meals and to an even greater extent during the nocturnal fast. In both man and the rat, the store of glycogen in the liver lasts somewhere between 12 and 24 h during fasting, depending greatly, of course, upon whether the individual under consideration is caged or running wild.

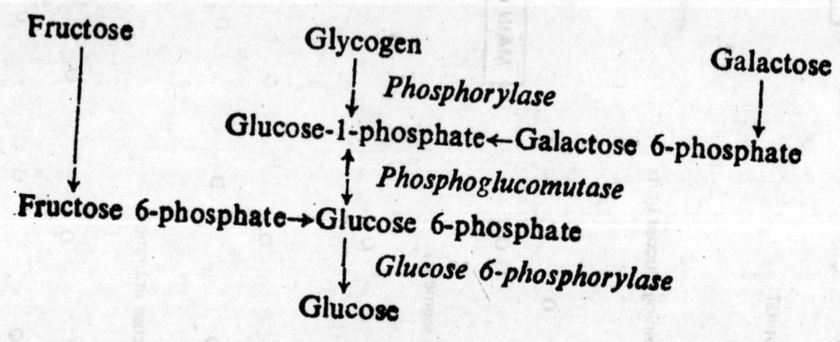


## GLUCONEOGENESIS

Stored carbohydrates are rapidly depleted auring tasting. Liver glycogen reserves are adequate to keep a constant blood glucose concentration for only a few hours. However, they can be restored by gluconeogenesis.

**Gluconeogenesis** is the pathway in which glucose is synthesized from noncarbohydrate molecules such as lactate, glycerol, and certain amino acids. Over 90% of gluconeogenesis occurs in the liver and the remainder occurs in the kidneys. Figure 27:9 shows the reactions that occur in gluconeogenesis. If you look at them carefully, you will see that gluconeogenesis is almost the reverse of glycolysis. Not all of the reactions of glycolysis are reversible; thus, a similar but different pathway is required to produce glucose from pyruvate. Four different enzymes are required for gluconeogenesis that are not in the glycolytic pathway.

Gluconeogenesis begins with pyruvate. As we have already found, lactate can be oxidized to pyruvate. Thus, lactate is a major starting substance for gluconeogenesis. In addition, some amino acids can also be converted to pyruvate. For example, glutamate-alanine transaminase changes alanine to pyruvate.

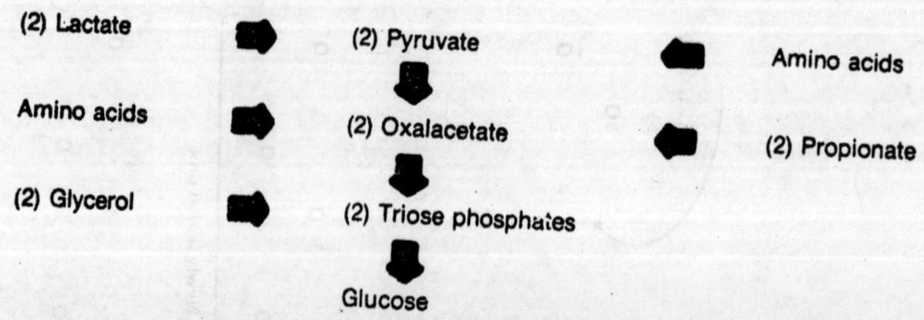


**Fig. 44** ***Abbreviated pathway of gluconeogenesis, illustrating the major substrate precursors for the process.***

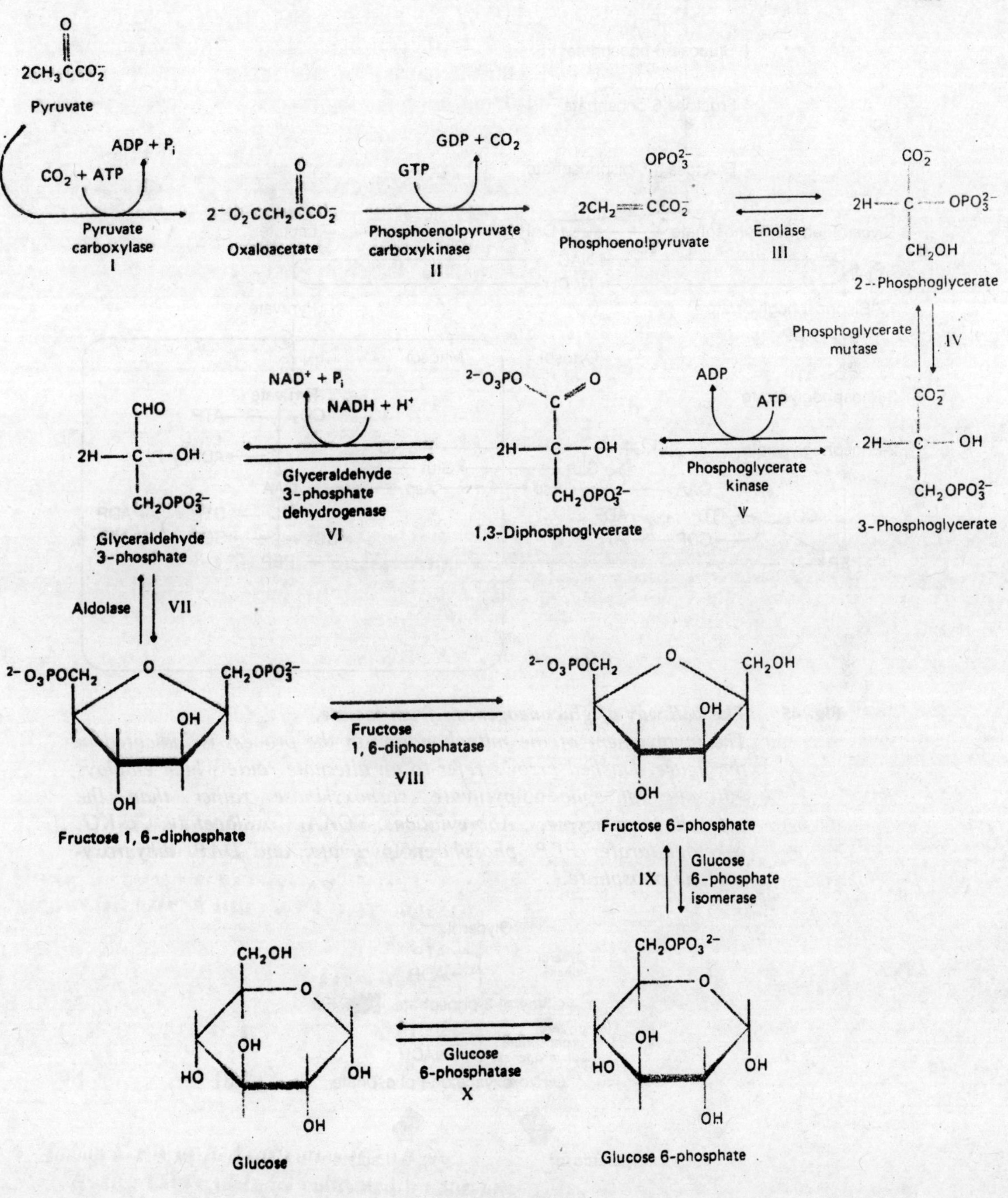


*The pathway of gluconeogenesis from pyruvate.*

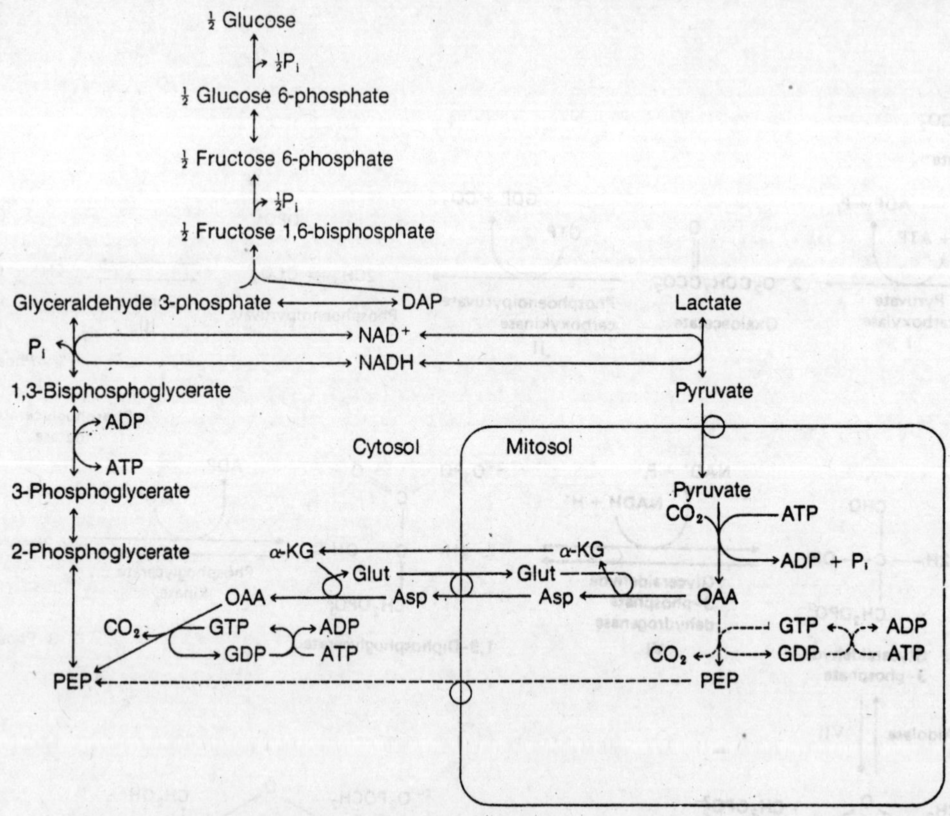


**Fig. 45** ***The pathway of gluconeogenesis from lactate.***
*The involvement of the mitochondrion in the process is indicated in the figure. Dashed arrows refer to an alternate route which employs mitosolic phospho*enol*pyruvate carboxykinase rather than the cytosolic isoenzyme. Abbreviations: OAA, oxalacetate; α-KG, α-ketoglutarate; PEP, phospho*enol*pyruvate; and DAP, dihydroxyacetone phosphate.*

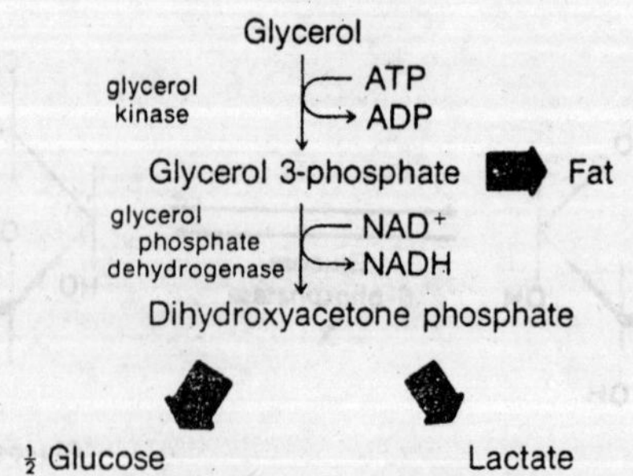


**Fig. 46** ***The pathway of gluconeogenesis from glycerol, along with competing pathways.***

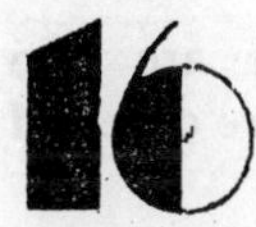

# LIPID METABOLISM

**Function of Body Lipids**

Animal systems contain a group of substances which are insoluble in water, but soluble in ether, chloroform, benzene are collectively known as lipids. The main groups of lipids of nutritional interest are the fatty acids, glycerides, phospholipids, cerebrosides, cholesterol and other alcohols which include vitamins A, D, E and K. From the stand point of the quantity present in the animal body and its food, the fatty acids are the most important lipid fraction. Some of the important characteristics of lipid are given below:

1. Much of the excess carbohydrate of the diet is converted to fat prior to its utilisation for supply of energy.
2. Some organs prefer fat as a fuel in preference to carbohydrate.
3. The calorific value of fat is about 2.25 times that of carbohydrate and protein i.e., 9.3 kcal per gram.
4. Lipids supply essential fatty acids, linolenic and linoleic acids and are carriers of fat soluble vitamins, A, D, E and K.
5. Phospholipids, cholesterol and glycolipids are essential components of various structural constituents of various organs in the body.
6. Amino acids can be synthesised from fatty acids and ammonia in the liver.
7. Being a poor heat conductor the subcutaneous fat helps in heat regulation.
8. The depot fats act mechanically in protecting the vital organs and also act as cushions and packing tissues.

**Fat Transport from Lymph to Tissues**

The main site of absorption of lipids by intestinal mucosa is the proximal jejunum. Investigation with electron microscope determined that the surface of the upper intestinal mucosal cell, which originally thought to be tiny pores, actually contains millions of small protoplasmic processes, termed micro-villi (Fig. 47). These are continuous with the intestinal epithelial cell and greatly increase the absorptive surface of each mucosal cell.

It is now believed that practically all of the triglycerides (with the exception of the very small amount of fatty acids of carbon atom less than 10-12 which are absorbed directly into the portal circulation), and other lipids as well, enter the lymph from these micro-villi of the intestine on their way to the liver and to other tissues. As mentioned earlier along with the discussion on absorption of fat digestion that triglycerides which are synthesised in the mucosa from dietary fatty acids appear in the lymph as *chylomicrons*. These are complex compounds containing triglycerides, phospholipid, cholesterol and its esters, and protein. Protein, free cholesterol and phospholipid (lecithin) form an outer coating for the triglyceride. Chylomicrons are formed in the smooth endoplasmic reticulum of the mucosal cell which are then discharged into the intercellular space and appear in the lacteals, from which they are collected into thoracic duct; and finally enter the blood system through the subclavian vein.*

The presence of large amounts of chylomicrons in blood makes the plasma milky (lipemic) in appearance for several hours following the ingestion of a fat-containing meal. Normally this alimentary hyperlipemia is moderate because very soon the rate of entry of chylomicron lipid into the plasma is balanced by its rate of exit—by uptake of the lipid by the tissues of the body.

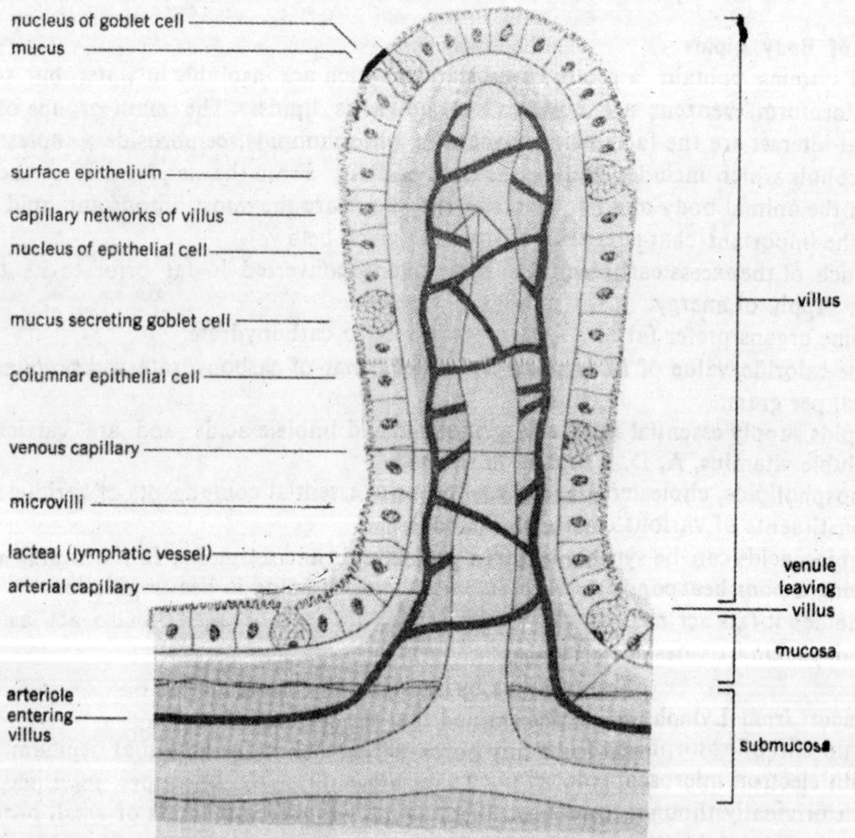


**Fig. 47** Structure of a villus, present throughout the small intestine. The centre is largely occupied by lacteal (lymphatic vessel) for absorption of fat and fat soluble materials (except fatty acids having less than 10–12 carbon atoms).

*Chylomicrons do not enter the portal blood directly because they are too large to pass through the endothelial membranes of blood capillaries. Therefore absorbed triglyceride, cholesterol, cholesterol ester, and phospholipid enter the body primarily through the lymph system.

Although most of the fatty acids in the chylomicron triglycerides are derived from the diet, endogenous fatty acids may be incorporated in significant amounts. In plasma the "triglycerides of chylomicrons" are quickly hydrolysed by the *lipoprotein lipase*, also known as clearing factor.

After the hydrolysis of chylomicrons with a concomitant clearance of blood serum from milky apperance, the lipid components, glyceride, phospholipid, cholesterol for the sake of solubility in water continues with a water soluble protein and forms *lipoproteins* in the liver which are then transported in the plasma. Lipoproteins are thus macromolecules with a central core of triglycerides surrounded by cholesterol and its esters, phospholipid, mainly phosphotidyl choline and sphingomyelin, and a little protein the apoproteins. The phosphate

**Table 125**

**Lipoproteins in plasma**

| *Lipoprotein* | *Electrophoretic mobility* | *Approx. conc. g/l* | *Density kg/l* | *Percentage composition (dry wt)* Protein and carbohydrate | TG | Total cholesterol | phospholipid |
|---|---|---|---|---|---|---|---|
| Chylomicrons | None | 0.5 | <0.96 | 2 | 83 | 9 | 7 |
| Very low density (VLDL) | pre-β | 1.5 | 0.96–1.006 | 9 | 50 | 22 | 18 |
| Low density (LDL) | β | 4.0 | 1.006–1.063 | 21 | 10 | 47 | 22 |
| High density (HDL) | α | 3.5 | >1.063 | 50 | 8 | 19 | 22 |

groups of phospholipids are in contact with the aqueous phase and their charge may stabilise the colloid. Lipoproteins then may be looked upon as transporters which carry triglycerides and cholesterol.

The three types of lipoprotein formed in the Golgi apparatus of the liver are designated as very low density lipoprotein (VLDL), low density (LDL) and high density (HDL) on the basis of their separation in ultra centrifuge. They are also classified as pre-β, β and α form in accordance to their mobility relative to the globulins during the electrophoresis of serum.. Each has its own structure and chemical composition.

## FAT STORAGE AND DYNAMIC STATE

In adult animals fat is stored mostly in adipose tissue. Approximately 5C per cent of the adipose tissue is found under the skin, the balance is located around certain organs, notably the kidneys, the membranes surrounding the intestines, in the muscles, etc. Adipose cells have the ability to store fat in a central vacuole surrounded by cytoplasm; other cells store only small amounts of fat as inclusions in their cytoplasm. The cells of the adipose tissue are equipped with a special enzyme system, which can take up fat from the tissue fluid and store it up in the cell and in time of necessity, the same enzyme system will help to mobilise the depot fats. In this connection it is noteworthy that adipose tissue forms 10–12 per cent of body weight, but

70–80 per cent of this is fat, mostly triglycerides. This tissue is known to be one of the most metabolically active body tissue. Fatty acids form the depots are being constantly mobilised and transported. Absorbed fatty acids merge with these form the depots. Some of the acids of this pool are constantly being converted into others. Some are degraded, while others are combined with glycerol and transported back to the depot. All of these reactions are so balanced that mixtures of fatty acids in the depots, blood, and organs tend to remain qualitatively and quantitatively constant.

## VOLATILE FATTY ACIDS AND ENERGY METABOLISM IN RUMINANTS

Energy metabolism involves a very large number of metabolites, many of which may be used by the body cells as fuel for respiratory oxidation.

Glucose is usually considered to be the main fuel. This is certainly true in the non-ruminants, and even in the ruminant where other metabolites may substitute : glucose still holds a central position and is vital for certain key functions such as brain metabolism, nourishment of foetus, requirement for lactation.

In non-ruminant only simple carbohydrates such as starch etc. are digested in the alimentary tract for releasing glucose as major end product. This simplifies energy metabolism as glucose is absorbed directly and is deposited in liver and in various tissues of the body as liver and muscle glycogen. The excess amount of course will be stored as depot fat. Under normal circumstances there is little need to synthesise glucose by gluconeogenesis until the animal needs to draw on its energy reserves.

In the ruminants the situation is entirely different. Ruminant species absorb very little glucose from the alimentary tract due to lack of production as end products of carbohydrate digestion. The rumen micro-organisms ferment greater part of dietary carbohydrates including soluble sugars, such as starches, insoluble carbohydrates as cellulose, hemicelluloses into short chain fatty acids (VFA) and they do this by means of microorganisms in the rumen which have powerful enzymes for converting all carbohydrates mostly into acetic, propionic and butyric acids and to some extent isobutyric, valeric, isovaleric with traces of various higher acids. Similarly during lipid digestion, a large portion of glycerol is fermented to propionic acid.

All these acids are absorbed directly through the rumen wall in the free form, apparently without active transport to the liver.

Only one of them, namely propionate, is capable of being converted into glucose, whereas acetate and butyrate serve as substrates for the production of energy (ATP) and acetate in particular may be used with glucose for the synthesis of fat in adipose tissue. *In ruminants glucose cannot be converted to fat as it lacks in necessary* two key enzymes. ATP citrate lyase (splitting citrate into oxaloacetate and malate) and NADP— malate dehydrogenase (converting malate to pyruvate, Thus the ruminant rely entirely on acetate or butyrate for fat synthesis

As mentioned earlier, glucose which is obtained mostly from propionate metabolism in ruminants are vital for the species for (i) lactose synthesis in milk production, (ii) for the supply of energy to the foetus, (iii) for the synthesis of triacylglycerides in adipose tissue. (iv) for the respiration of brain cells. Should a supply of glucose fail then a metabolic disorder known as *Ketosis* will occur.

On the other hand, an excess input of energy which might lead mearly to a transient hyperglycaemia in the non-ruminant can provoke a special condition in ruminant species. Excessive supplies of fermentable carbohydrate such as starch can upset the balance of fermentation in the rumen leading to the accumulation of lactic acid and a metabolic disorder known as *acidosis*.

Thus ketosis and acidosis are the result of imbalances between input and output of energy and are man-made problems imposed upon the ruminants.

## Normal Energy Metabolism

### Factors Controlling Input of Energy

1. *The Production of VFA*

As already stated, most carbohydrates eaten by ruminants are fermented to a mixture of volatile fatty acids (VFA's) by the rumen microbes. On roughage diets the most important VFA's are acetic, propionic and butyric acids produced in the approximate proportions of 65% acetic, 20% propionic and 15% butyric acids. Because the molecules are of different sizes, on a weight basis the proportions are closer to 50% for acetate, 25% propionate and 25% butyrate. The percentages depend on the nature of the feed. Those quoted above refer to a typical hay diet containing about 35% cellulose and 5% starch. In contrast ration, which contains 5% cellulose and 45% starch, given entirely different proportions of VFA's when fermented in the rumen. The predominant VFA then moves from acetic to propionic acid. Should the diet contain large quantities of starch appreciable quantities of lactic acid will also be produced and absorbed. This acid is normally found in low concentration within the rumen, but if it too is absorbed through the rumen wall it serves as a useful precursor of glucose in the liver. However, as mentioned earlier, excess is potentially toxic and may cause acidosis.

An exception to the general rule that ruminants do not absorb glucose as an end product of digestion needs mention. Some grain diets, specially those on ground maize, may partially escape fermentation within the rumen and pass through into the abomasum and small intestine for enzyme digestion with pancreatic amylase. Glucose, the end product of this digestive process is absorbed and metabolised in much the same way as in non-ruminants.

In spite of this exception the bulk of the digestible energy fed to the ruminant is fermented into VFA's. In fact the VFA contribution approximates 70% of the total energy input.

**A. Acetate :** This is the predominant VFA produced in the rumen by the fermentation of forage diets. It is absorbed through the rumen wall into the portal circulation, and although a little may be used for oxidation or fat synthesis in the liver most passes through and into the systemic circulation. It is also known that some acetate is synthesised within the liver so that in general circumastances the concentration of acetate in systemic blood is relatively high (about 10 mg/100 ml) compared with non-ruminants.

It is used by a wide variety of tissues as a source of energy. The initial reaction in this case is conversion of acetate to acetyl coenzyme A in the presence of acetyl-coenzyme synthetase.

$$CH_3COOH + H\text{–}S\text{–}CoA \xrightarrow[+ATP]{\textit{Acetyl-CoA Synthetase}} CH_3\text{–}CO{\sim}S\text{–}CoA + H_2O$$

Acetic acid   Coenzyme A   Acetyl CoA

**The acetyl-coenzyme A is then oxidised via the TCA cycle yielding 12 moles of ATP per mole. Since two high energy phosphate bonds are used in the initial Synthetase—mediated reaction the net yield of ATP is 10 moles per mole of acetate.**

**Acetate does not appear to contribute to the net synthesis of glucose although it serves as a component for fat synthesis both in adipose tissue and also in mammary gland.**

**B. Propionate :**

**It is the most important precursor of glucose, contributes as much as 30 – 54% of the total**

Propionate ($CO_2^-$–$CH_2$–$CH_3$) + CoA —propionyl CoA synthetase (ATP → AMP + $PP_i$)→ Propionyl CoA ($O=CSCoA$–$CH_2$–$CH_3$)

Propionyl CoA + $CO_2$ —propionyl CoA carboxylase (biotin) (ATP → ADP + $P_i$)→ (S)-Methylmalonyl CoA ($O=CSCoA$–$H\text{-}C\text{-}CO_2^-$–$CH_3$)

(S)-Methylmalonyl CoA —methylmalonyl CoA racemase→ (R)-Methylmalonyl CoA ($O=C\text{-}SCoA$–$H\text{-}C\text{-}CH_3$–$CO_2^-$)

(R)-Methylmalonyl CoA —methylmalonyl CoA mutase (vitamin $B_{12}$)→ Succinyl CoA ($O=CSCoA$–$CH_2$–$CH_2$–$CO_2^-$)

Succinyl CoA —succinyl CoA synthetase (GDP + $P_i$ → GTP; → CoA)→ Succinate ($CO_2^-$–$CH_2$–$CH_2$–$CO_2^-$)

Succinate —succinate dehydrogenase (FAD → $FADH_2$)→ Fumarate ($CO_2^-$–$CH$=$HC$–$CO_2^-$) ← CITRIC ACID CYCLE (Kreb's Cycle)

Fumarate + $H_2O$ —fumarase→ Malate ($CO_2$–$HCOH$–$CH_2$–$CO_2$)

Malate —malate dehydrogenase ($NAD^+$ → NADH)→ Oxalacetate ($CO_2^-$–$C{=}O$–$CH_2$–$CO_2^-$)

Oxalacetate → ½ Glucose *(By reversal of Embden – Meyerhof of Glycolysis)*

**body glucose. The acid after absorption through rumen wall is taken up to liver for the conversion. A small portion of propionate is changed into lactic acid in the rumen wall, which also later on converted into glucose in the liver.**

**An important factor affecting the rate at which propionate is utilised by the liver depends on the availability of vitamin $B_{12}$. Deficiency of this vitamin virtually elevates levels of propionic acid in the serum and contributes towards ketosis.**

**The metabolic route begins with conversion to propionyl-CoA and carboxylation to methylmalonyl – CoA followed by rearrangement of the carbon skeleton to *Succinyl – Co A*. The last step requires vitamin $B_{12}$. Propionate carbon enters the citric acid cycle in the form of succinic acid (see citric acid cycle) and in a few steps is converted to another important intermediate, *oxaloacetate*.**

**Oxaloacetic acid may also follow a third route to form glycogenic non-specific amino acids like aspertic acid, glutamic acid or alanine by reductive amination.**

**C. Butyrate :**

**Butyrate contributes relatively small proportion of total VFA and partly metabolised by rumen epithelium to ketone bodies principally acetoacetate and (D – ) β hydroxybutyrate which is interconverted in the liver.**

**In normal circumstances ketones are valuable metabolites. Although not used by the liver cells they are utilised almost preferentially by tissues such as cardiac and skeletal muscle as respiratory fuel for energy production. Net gain of ATP per mole of butyric acid is 25 ATP.**

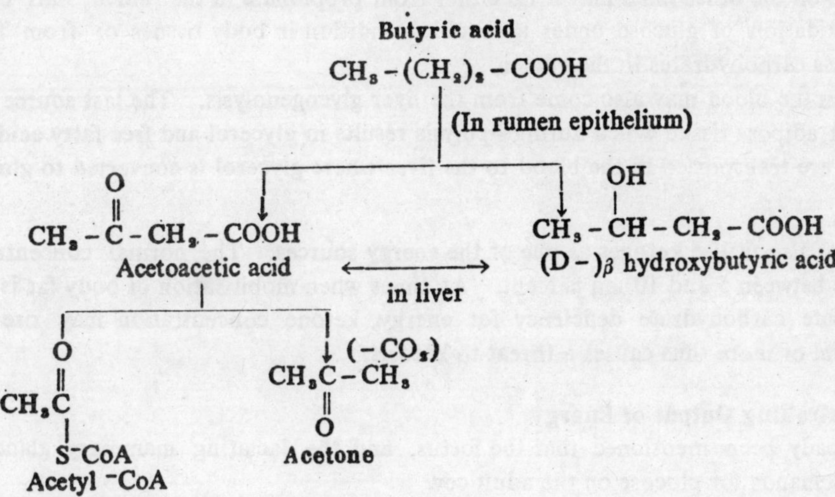


**Excess ketone bodies are excreted in the urine or may be recycled through the rumen. Acetoacetic acid is relatively unstable and is non-enzymetically decarboxylated to acetone, giving rise to the "*Sweet breath*" of ketotic ruminants. In rumen acetone can be reduced to isopropyl alcohol.**

**The absorption of all the VFA'S is facilitated by the papillae which consist of elongated**

projections from the rumen mucosa thus considerably increasing its surface area and absorptive capacity. This may be important as absorption of VFA's is not an active process but passive along a concentration gradient, the rate being proportional to concentration within the rumen. It is also pH dependent being specially rapid under acidic conditions within the rumen fluid. VFA's which have escaped absorption in the rumen may be absorbed in the reticulum, omasum, or even lower down the alimentary tract.

Another minor source of VFA's is the large intestine in ruminants. This receives feed materials and secretions which have escaped digestion and absorption higher up the alimentary tract. It contains microbes very similar to those found in the rumen. In horse, the main site of VFA production is the caecum.

It is clear that the VFA's are vital part of energy metabolism in the ruminant. They provide a source of energy to the rumen bacteria and also to the rumen wall and, although only propionate can be used to synthesise a supply of glucose, taken together they contribute the major part of total energy input of the ruminant.

*2. Gluconeogenesis*

Propionate produces 50% of glucose requirements while glucogenic amino acids contribute another 25%, and lactic acid 15%. The glucogenic amino acids may be derived either from the digestion of microbial protein in the intestines, or from the catabolism of body proteins. Alanine and the glutamine/glutamic acid couplet are said to be the most important amino acids.

Lactic acid on the other hand may arise either from propionate in the rumen wall or by incomplete oxidation of glucose under anaerobic condition in body tissues or from fermentation of excess carbohydrates in the rumen.

Glucose in the blood may also come from the liver glycogenolysis. The last source is from body fat in adipose tissue which during lipolysis results in glycerol and free fatty acids. Both compounds are transported in the blood to the liver where glycerol is converted to glucose.

*3. Ketones*

Ruminants also utilise ketones as one of the energy sources. The normal concentration in the blood is between 5 and 10 mg percent. At times when mobilisation of body fat is required to compensate carbohydrate deficiency for energy, ketone concentration may rise to some 50 mg/100 ml or more thus causes a threat to ketosis.

**Factors Controlling Output of Energy**

It has already been mentioned that the foetus, and the lactating mammary gland impose obligatory demands for glucose on the adult cow.

Glucose is the major source of energy supplied to the foetus *in utero*. In sheep on advanced stage of pregnancy requirement may range between 8-9 g glucose/kg body weight daily. A single foetus may require 32 g of glucose daily depending on the size. In certain circumstances the total glucose requirement may amount to 70% of the glucose entry rate for the mother cow.

Lactose may impose even large burdens on glucose supply. Fortunately, there is a *"fail safe"* mechanism i.e., as blood glucose falls milk yield tends to fall in parallel. However, mammary gland has no power of gluconeogenesis for lactose synthesis so it must be supplied with preformed glucose. Between 1 and 1.5 kg of lactose may be secreted in milk daily in early lactation. Glucose is also needed for the synthesis of glycerol which is a vital component of the milk fat and also for oxidative purposes in the mammary gland itself, so that in all 70-90% of the animals total glucose entry may be taken up by lactation.

### Endocrinological Control of Energy Metabolism

If the animal becomes hyperglycemic then the pancreas is stimulated to secrete insulin. This has several effects. It will tend to reduce blood sugar level by storing glucose in the liver and muscle as liver and muscle glycogen. *Insulin secretior in the ruminant is also stimulated by a rise in VFA concentration.* This is hardly surprising in view of the important part VFA's play in the energy metabolism in ruminants.

If the animal becomes hypoglycaemic, there will be increase in glucagon secretion. Moreover, hypoglycaemia will stimulate glucoreceptors in the hypothalamus to send impulses to the adrenal medulla for increased secretion of epinephrene. The combined effect of these will cause (1) more hepatic glycogenolysis, (2) will mobilise glycerol and FFA's from adipose tissue—the glycerol being used for gluconeogenesis and the FFA's as an alternative fuel for oxidation. In extreme cases it will also stimulate amino acid release from muscle for the production of glucose via gluconeogenesis.

## FAT SYNTHESIS

Fats are esters of fatty acids with the trihydric alcohol glycerol.

### Glycerol Synthesis

Glycerol is synthesised in the body from glucose. The latter is first broken down via Embden-Meyerhof pathway to dihydroxyacetone phosphate, which is then reduced to glycerol as below:

$$\text{Dihydroxyacetone phosphate} + \text{DPNH} + \text{H}^+ \underset{\textit{Phosphatase}}{\overset{\textit{Dehydrogenase}}{\rightleftharpoons}} \alpha\text{-glycerophosphate} + \text{DPN}^+$$

$$\alpha\text{—glycerophosphate} + \text{H}_2\text{O} \longrightarrow \text{glycerol} + \text{Pi.}$$

Glycerol enters the metabolic pathway through phosphorylation by ATP to α-glycerophopshate.

$$\text{Glycerol} + \text{ATP} \xrightarrow[\textit{Phosphokinase}]{\textit{Glycerol}} \alpha\text{-glycerophosphate} + \text{ADP}$$

### Biosynthesis of Fatty Acids

It would seem that a fatty acid can be made in the cell by simply reversing its degradation as will be discussed. But as we shall see in a moment, in the cell there are two independent pathways to produce fatty acids. One, localised in the mitochondria starts with an existing fatty acid and is simply elongated by condensations with acetyl-CoA. The other pathways, which is probably the major one, represents total synthesis of fatty acids in the cytoplasm, where soluble enzymes catalyse successive condensation starting with acetyl-CoA and malonyl-CoA.

*Cytoplasmic synthesis of fatty acids*

This system has been found in soluble fraction of many tissues, including liver, kidney, brain, lung, mammary gland and adipose tissue. Cofactors required are NADPH, ATP, $Mn^{+2}$ and $HCO_3^-$ ( as a source of $CO_2$ ). Acetyl-CoA is the substrate and Palmitic acid is the end product. These are some characters which contrast with those of beta-oxidation.

In non-ruminants acetyl-CoA is mostly formed in the mitochondria where pyruvate dehydrogenase is located. As because mitochondral membrane is impermeable to acetyl-CoA, thus it forms citric acid in combination with oxaloacetic acid. The compound is in a position to come out of mitochondrial wall and later on separated again into acetyl-CoA and oxaloacetate. In ruminants acetate becomes available by direct absorption from the gut and this may form acetyl-CoA in the presence of an enzyme, *acetyl-CoA synthetase* taking energy from ATP.

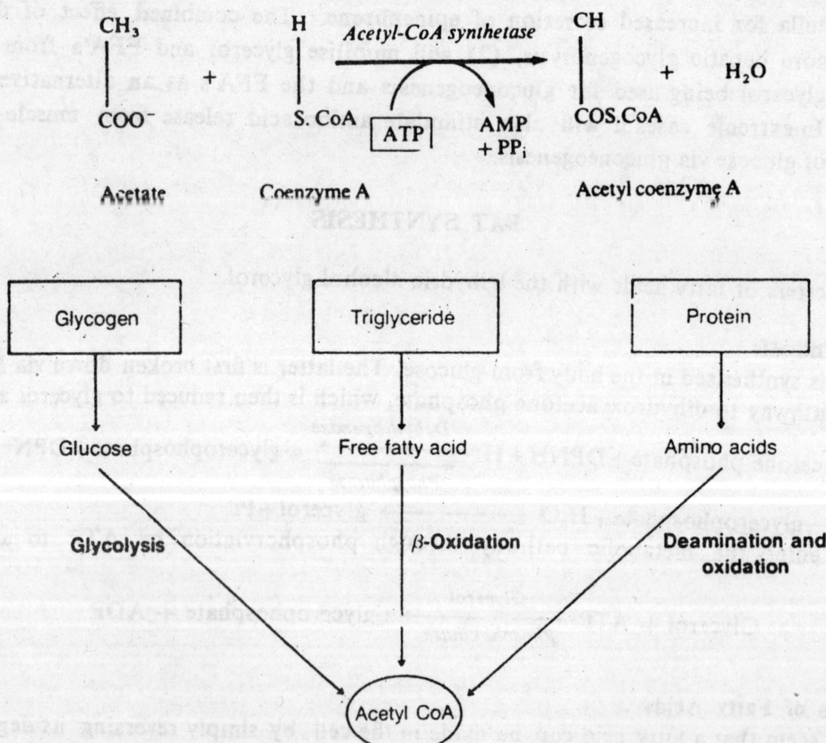


Bicarbonate as a source of $CO_2$ is required in the initial reaction for the carboxylation of acetyl-CoA to malonyl-CoA in the presence of ATP and acetyl-CoA carboxylase ( require a vitamin, *biotin* for activation ).

It is to be noted that once acetyl-CoA participates for conversion to palmitic acid, all subsequent intermediate compounds remain attached to an enzyme *fatty acid synthase*,

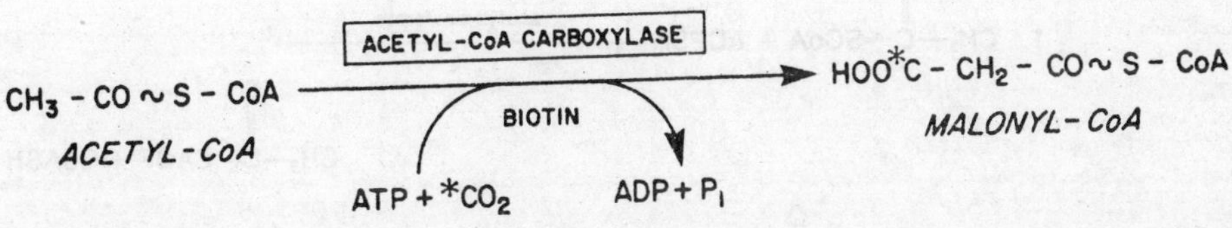


Biosynthesis of malonyl-CoA.

which itself is a multienzyme complex. The compounds remain as a part of enzyme complex.

In bacteria, plants and lower forms of life, the individual enzymes of synthase are separate and a special protein which binds the acyl intermediates during fatty acid synthesis is known as *acyl carrier protein* (ACR). However, in yeast, mammals and birds the synthase system is a multienzyme complex, that may not be subdivided without loss of activity and ACP is a part of this complex. The fatty acid synthase complex is a dimer, having two polypeptide chains, each consisting of one ACP and seven different enzyme

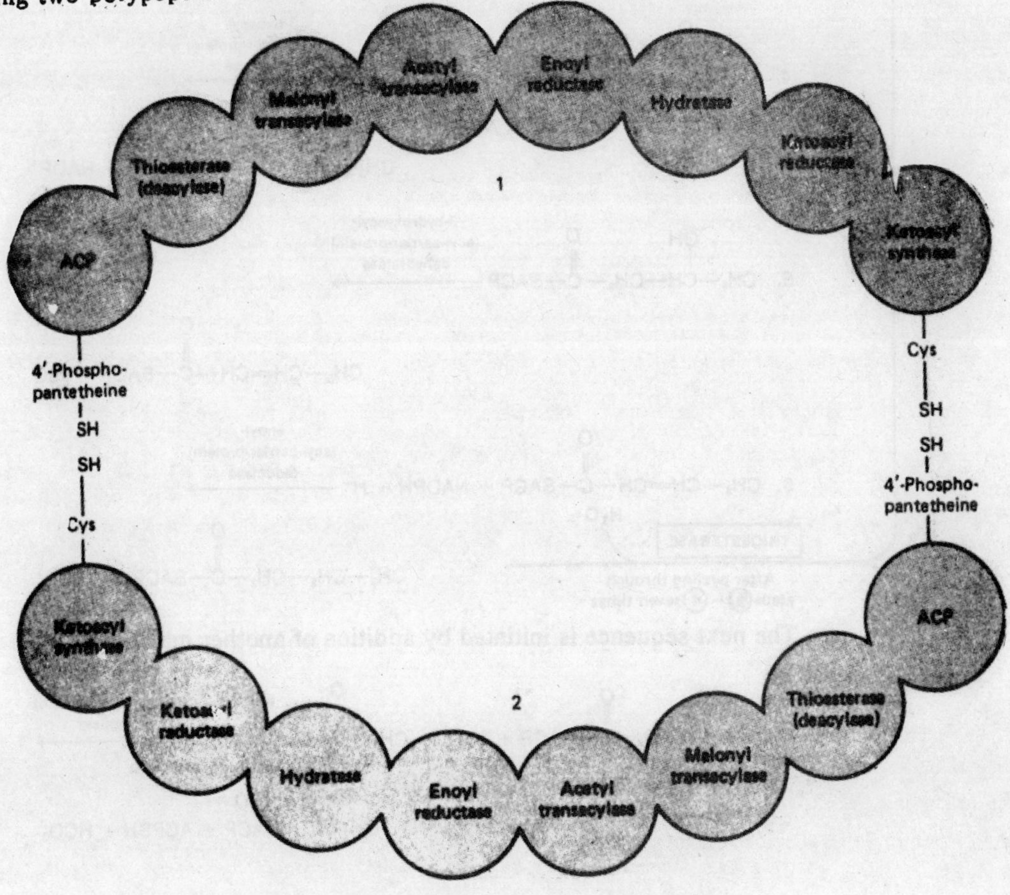

**Fig. 48** Fatty acid synthase multienzyme complex.

1. $$CH_3-\overset{O}{\overset{\|}{C}}-SCoA + ACPSH \xrightarrow[\text{acetyltransferase}]{\text{(acyl-carrier-protein)}} CH_3-\overset{O}{\overset{\|}{C}}-SACP + CoASH$$

2. $$^{-}OOC-CH_2-\overset{O}{\overset{\|}{C}}-SCoA + ACPSH \xrightarrow[\text{malonyltransferase}]{\text{(acyl-carrier-protein)}} {}^{-}OOC-CH_2-\overset{O}{\overset{\|}{C}}-SACP + CoASH$$

3. $$CH_3-\overset{O}{\overset{\|}{C}}-SACP + {}^{-}OOC-CH_2-\overset{O}{\overset{\|}{C}}-SACP + H_2O \xrightarrow[\text{synthase}]{\text{3-oxoacyl-(acyl-carrier-protein)}} CH_3-\overset{O}{\overset{\|}{C}}-CH_2-\overset{O}{\overset{\|}{C}}-SACP + ACPSH + HCO_3^-$$

4. $$CH_3-\overset{O}{\overset{\|}{C}}-CH_2-\overset{O}{\overset{\|}{C}}-SACP + NADPH + H^+ \xrightarrow[\text{reductase}]{\text{3-oxoacyl-(acyl-carrier-protein)}} CH_3-\overset{OH}{\overset{|}{C}H}-CH_2-\overset{O}{\overset{\|}{C}}-SACP + NADP^+$$

5. $$CH_3-\overset{OH}{\overset{|}{C}H}-CH_2-\overset{O}{\overset{\|}{C}}-SACP \xrightarrow[\text{dehydratase}]{\text{3-hydroxyacyl-(acyl-carrier-protein)}} CH_3-CH=CH-\overset{O}{\overset{\|}{C}}-SACP + H_2O$$

6. $$CH_3-CH=CH-\overset{O}{\overset{\|}{C}}-SACP + NADPH + H^+ \xrightarrow[\text{reductase}]{\text{enoyl-(acyl-carrier-protein)}} CH_3-CH_2-CH_2-\overset{O}{\overset{\|}{C}}-SACP + NADP^+$$

$H_2O$

THIOESTERASE

After cycling through steps (2)–(4) seven times

Palmitate

**The next sequence is initiated by addition of another malonyl ACP:**

$$CH_3-CH_2-CH_2-\overset{O}{\overset{\|}{C}}-SACP + {}^{-}OOC-CH_2-\overset{O}{\overset{\|}{C}}-SACP + H_2O \xrightarrow[\text{synthase}]{\text{3-oxoacyl-(acyl-carrier-protein)}} CH_3-CH_2-CH_2-\overset{O}{\overset{\|}{C}}-CH_2-\overset{O}{\overset{\|}{C}}-SACP + ACPSH + HCO_3^-$$

components. Each monomer is identical. The principal reactions involved shown below and are described as follows :

1. Initially an acetyl-CoA combines with the -SH group of ACP of one of the monomers, say monomer 1. The reaction is catalysed by *acetyl transferase*, an enzyme present in synthase multienzyme complex.

2. Malonyl-CoA similarly combines with the -SH group of ACP on monomer 2, catalysed by another enzyme of synthase complex known as malonyl transferase.

3. Acetyl-CoA from monomer 1 then reacts with malonyl-CoA on monomer 2 where acetoacetyl-S-ACP is formed and $CO_2$ is released in the form of bicarbonate. The ACP of monomer 1 is free. Subsequent reactions proceed on monomer 2 till the formation of butyryl-CoA.

4. There is a reduction of Acetoacetyl-S-ACP (enzyme) by *reductase* of synthase complex whereby $NADPH+H^+$ is utilised for the formation of beta-hydroxybutyryl-S-ACP. ( NADPH are generated from i) hexose monophosphate shunt, ii) malic enzyme and iii) isocitrate dehydrogenase ).

5 Water is then removed from the said compound by *hydratase* of synthase complex to form Crotonyl-S-ACP.

6. Crotonyl-S-ACP is then reduced by *reductase* of synthase complex whereby another molecule of $NADPH+H^+$ is utilised for the formation of butyryl-S-ACP.

7. Butyryl-S-ACP is then combines with another molecule of malonyl-S-ACP to form a $C_6$ fatty acid along with simultaneous liberation of $CO_2$ in the form of bicarbonate.

A stepwise condensation with further malonyl-S-ACP units occur until the final formation of Palmityl-S-ACP complex is produced, when it ceases. Palmitic acid may then be liberated by the action of *deacylase* enzyme of synthase multienzyme complex. We may write the overall reaction as follows

1 mole Acetyl-CoA + 7 moles Malonyl-CoA + 14 $NADPH+(H^+)$

$= \text{Palmitate} + 7CO_2 + 14\,NADP^+ + 6H_2O + 8H\text{-}S\text{-}CoA$

*Mitochondrial synthesis of fatty acids*

The synthesis is mostly restricted to lengthening of an existing fatty acid by a reversal of the beta-oxidation. This system requires, ATP, reduced $NAD^+$ and reduced $NADP^+$. It involves incorporation of acetyl-CoA into medium and long chain fatty acids.

The products of this system are saturated acids with 18, 20, 22 and 24 carbon atoms produced, usually from palmitic acid synthesised in the cytoplasmic system. The pathway is illustrated as shown below :

*Macrosomal synthesis of fatty acids*

Macrosome, a subcellular fraction that consists of ribosomes and endoplasmic reticulum is probably the main site for the elongation of existing long chain fatty acids. The pathway converts acyl-CoA compounds of fatty acids to acyl derivatives having 2 carbons more, using malonyl-CoA as a acetyl donor and NADPH as reductant. Intermediates in the process are the *CoA thioesters.* Fasting largely abolishes chain elongation. The principal reactions are shown below.

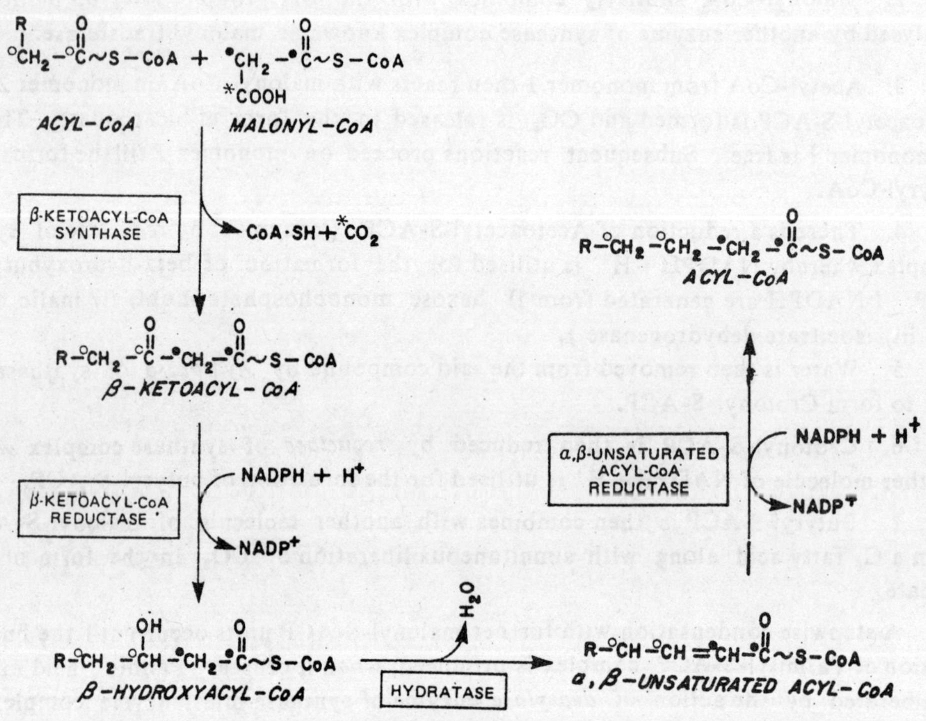


Microsomal system for chain elongation.

*Triglyceride synthesis.* The biosynthesis of triglycerides involves the reaction of L-α glycerophosphate with 2 moles of "activated" fatty acids (in the form of fatty acyl CoA) to form D-α-β-diglyceride. Addition of 1 mole of fatty acyl CoA results in a triglyceride.

## OXIDATION OF FATTY ACIDS

Knoop (1905) proposed that fatty acids were oxidised physiologically by β-oxidation. The catabolism of fatty acids to $CO_2$ and $H_2O$ occurs by means of the sequential combination of the multienzyme systems, the β-oxidation cycle and the TCA cycle. The β-oxidation cycle first converts the fatty acid into 2-carbon units, acetyl CoA. The TCA cycle then converts the acetyl moiety of acetyl CoA to $CO_2$ and $H_2O$. The steps in the oxidation of fatty acids are given

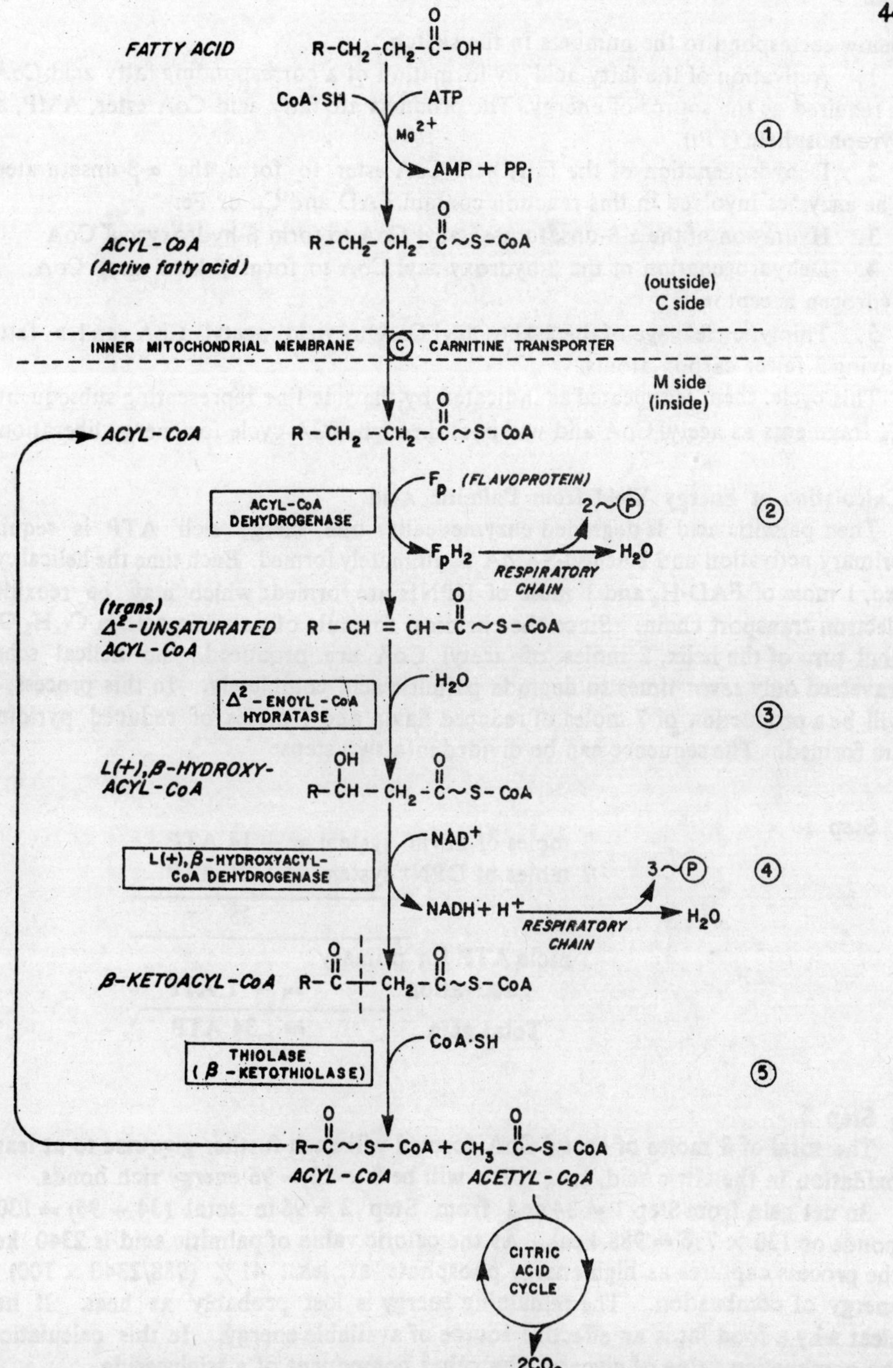


*β*-Oxidation of fatty acids. Long-chain acyl-CoA is cycled through reactions ② – ⑤, acetyl-CoA being split off each cycle by thiolase (reaction ⑤). When the acyl radical is only 4 carbon atoms in length, 2 acetyl-CoA molecules are formed in reaction ⑤.

below correspond to the numbers in the sketch.

1. Activation of the fatty acid by formation of a corresponding fatty acid-CoA ester. ATP is required as the source of energy. The products are fatty acid-CoA ester, AMP, and inorganic pyrophosphate (PPi).

2. Dehydrogenation of the fatty acid-CoA ester to form the α-β-unsaturated acyl CoA. The enzymes involved in this reaction contain FAD and Cu or Fe.

3. Hydration of the α-β-unsaturated acyl CoA to form β-hydroxyacyl CoA.

4. Dehydrogenation of the β-hydroxy-acyl CoA to form β-keto acyl CoA. NAD is the hydrogen acceptor.

5. Thiolytic cleavage of the β-keto-acyl CoA to yield acetyl CoA and a fatty acyl CoA having 2 fewer carbon atoms.

This cycle, then, is repeated as indicated by the side line representing subsequent removal of $C_2$ fragments as acetyl CoA and will pass through TCA cycle for energy liberation.

**Calculation of Energy Yield from Palmitic Acid**

Then palmitic acid is degraded enzymetically, one energy rich ATP is required for the primary activation and 8 acetyl-S-CoA is ultimately formed. Each time the helical cycle is traversed, 1 mole of FAD-$H_2$ and 1 mole of DPNH are formed: which may be reoxidised by the electron transport chain. Since the chemical formula of palmitic acid is $C_{16}H_{32}O_2$ and in the final turn of the helix, 2 moles of acetyl CoA are produced, the helical scheme must be traversed only *seven* times to degrade palmitic acid completely. In this process, in total there will be a production of 7 moles of reduced flavin and 7 moles of reduced pyridine nucleotide are formed. The sequence can be divided into two steps:

**Step 1**

| | |
|---|---|
| 7 moles of flavin system | = + 14 ATP |
| 7 moles of DPN⁺ system | = + 21 ATP |
| | 35 |
| 1 mole ATP for primary activation | = − 1 ATP |
| Total gain | = 34 ATP |

**Step 2**

The total of 8 moles of acetyl CoA formed will each further give rise to at least 12 ATP on oxidation in the citric acid, i.e., there will be 8 × 12 = 96 energy rich bonds.

So net gain from Step 1 = 34 and from Step 2 = 96 in total (34 + 96) = 130 energy rich bonds or 130 × 7.6 = 988 kcal. As the caloric value of palmitic acid is 2340 kcal per mole, the process captures as high energy phosphate at least 41% (988/2340 × 100) of the total energy of combustion. The remaining energy is lost probably as heat. It hence becomes clear why a food fat is an effective source of available energy. In this calculation we neglect the combustion value of glycerol, the other component of a triglyceride.

# 17

## PROTEIN METABOLISM

### Avenues through which Nitrogen is Excreted

1. FAECAL NITROGEN. The faecal nitrogen includes the undigested or unabsorbed feed nitrogen along with nitrogen from endogenous sources, called *metabolic faecal nitrogen* and comprises substances originating in the body, such as residues of the bile and other digestive juices, epithelial cells abraded from the alimentary tract by the feed materials passing through it and bacterial residues. Strictly speaking, the nitrogen in bacterial residues must be considered to have come, at least in part from the feed. The fact that the division of faecal nitrogen is made is due to the fact that the two components have their separate origins. When one is really interested to find out the amount of two fractions separately, it is customary to deduct the amount of metabolic faecal nitrogen from the total faecal nitrogen. The amount of metabolic faecal nitrogen in faeces is directly proportional to the dry matter consumption and the body size of the animal. Upon feeding a nitrogen free diet, it has been observed that animal excretes nitrogenous compounds through faeces. This amount is the metabolic faecal nitrogen. Using this procedure the amount of metabolic faecal nitrogen has beed found to be approximately 1 gram for rats, pigs and man per kg. of feed dry matter consumed, and 5 gram for ruminants. The latter figure is smaller with rations low in roughage, but greater where roughage alone is fed.

2. URINARY NITROGEN: Through urine a number of nitrogenous compounds are excreted originating from a variety of sources. These are discussed below:

(*i*) *Creatinine:* It is derived from the breakdown of creatine phosphate present in muscle brain and blood. Creatinine is the anhydride of creatine. It is formed largely in muscle by the irreversible and nonenzymatic removal of water from creatine phosphate.

```
        H                                       H ~ P
        |                                       |
HN=C—N                                  HN=C—N
   |    |          Non Enzymatic           |    |
   |   C=O   <——————————————————————       |   C=OOH
   |    |           in muscle              |    |
   N—CH₂              (—Pi)                N—CH₂
   |                                       |
   CH₃                                     CH₃
 Creatinine                          Creatine Phosphate
```

Excretion of creatinine is a constant physiological phenomenon. It is related to the muscle bulk and is higher in animals having more body weight. Amount of excretion is in no way related with the dietary intake.

(*ii*) *Urea* $CO(NH_2)_2$: More than 80 per cent of urinary nitrogen is excreted in the form of urea. The compound is derived mainly (*a*) from deamination of unused amino acids; (*b*) by conversion of absorbed ammonia from rumen fermentation; (*c*) from salts like ammonium carbonate, lactate, etc., (*d*) from the amino acid arginine—it breaks down into urea and ornithine, (*e*) from catabolism of pyrimidine bases. The end product of metabolism of these compounds in liver is urea. Urea formation helps to maintain the reaction of blood constant as in it one acid (carbonic acid) and two molecules of ammonia remain neutralised.

(*iii*) *Ammonia:* With a mixed diet in an adult animal, a small amount of ammonia is always excreted through urine as free ammonia. The compound is mainly formed (1) from deamination of amino acids, both exogenous and endogenous. Although deamination takes place chiefly in the liver, recent observations indicate that some free ammonia is also formed in the kidney largely from glutamine, which serves as a method of transfer of $NH_2^-$ groups in a non-toxic form between tissues, (2) Ammonia is also formed in large quantities in rumen part of which is directly diffused through the ruminal wall into the circulatory system.

(*iv*) *Uric acid and Allantoin:* The amount in urine depends partly on the purine content of the diet and rest on the rate of the turnover of purines in cellular nucleic acids. Uric acid is the catabolite of purines. Allantoin is the hydroliylic end product of uric acid which is highly water enzyme, *uricase* for cenversion of uric acid to Allantoin. So they excrete uric acid.

(*v*) *Amino acids:* Under normal conditions small amounts of amino acids are always excreted through urine.

(*vi*) *Other avenues of N loss:* Gaseous $NH_3$ losses from the alimentary tract can occur. Excretion and secretion from the skin contain urea and other N compounds. Protein is also lost through growth and removal of wool, feathers, horn, hair. During milk production a good amount of nitrogenous compounds are excreted and similarly faetal growth requires a good deposition of protein.

**Endogenous Urinary Nitrogen (EUN)**

From the discussions made so far under 'Urinary nitrogen', it may be observed that the total urinary nitrogen has got two sources: (*i*) the "inescapable" losses in tissues turnover of nitrogenous constituents: and (*ii*) the other highly variable contribution depending on effects of dietary protein level. Thus when the absorbed dietary protein is in excess of the requirement, it will exert pressure on kidney for a way out in the forms already discussed. Endogenous urinary nitrogen (EUN) comprises the first category. On protein free diets the animal will continue to excrete EUN and the amount of nitrogen in the urine may fall progressively for several days before stabilising at a lower level. This minimum nitrogen excretion is referred to as the *endogenous urinary nitrogen value* (EUN). At the time of conduction of experiments for obtaining EUN value, all care must be taken to feed the animals with diet balanced in all respects particularly the energy content because at lower level of energy, extra tissue will be broken down to meet the energy deficiency. Another important point that should be kept in mind that experimental animals will hardly continue to consume normal quantum of feed for a along time required for the experiment without any nitrogen (protein) in their ration. Thus it is very difficult to find out the EUN value although theoretically the procedure seems to be very simple. However, when the values are determined, the amount denotes the minimum amount of protein that should be put back (fed) to the system for filling up the daily loss of nitrogenous material. This is the amount that we say as the basal metabolism and in fact there is a relationship between the two conceptions (EUN and basal metabolism), viz., ·2 mg endogenous urinary nitrogen per kcal basal metabolic rate (BMR) for non-ruminants. The value is about 2.0 mg of nitrogen per kcal of BMR in ruminants. Brody and coworkers confirmed about a relationship between endogenous urinary nitrogen with that of body weight of the animal and accordingly a formula is also suggested by them which is as follows:

$$\text{EUN mg per day} = 146\ W_{kg}^{0.75}$$

Total nitrogen excreted through urine in excess of the endogenous portion is known as *exogenous urinary nitrogen*. This term implies that portion of nitrogen which is comming from dietary source alone and not from the body itself that might be resulting due to catabolism incident to the maintenance of the vital processes as already discussed.

**Interpretation of Nitrogen Balance Trial**

If all nitrogen losses are accounted for, and are debited against the nitrogen intake, the balance represents the amount of nitrogen retained by the animal. Whenever the nitrogen intake exceeds excretion, a *positive nitrogen balance* exists. Some of the conditions that cause this include (1) growth, (2) recovery from fasting, starving or extended illness and (3) pregnancy mostly related to foetus growth. *Negative nitrogen balance* is that condition in which the excretion of nitrogen exceeds the intake. An individual with a negative nitrogen balance is losing nitrogen from tissues more rapidly than it is being replaced—an undesirable state of affairs. Conditions that result include (1) fasting, (2) starvation, (3) high fever, (4) prolonged illness, (5) low protein diets, (6) diets optimum in protein per cent but the protein is of extremely poor quality or protein lacking in essential amino acids (affects all monogastric), (7) the caloric content of the diet if inadequate, the tissues will be broken down to supply energy, (8) injury, immobilisation etc., cause excessive breakdown of tissues. In all such conditions the liver is the major gland which is affected the most. As much as 50 per cent of its total nitrogen, and skeletal muscle may also lose considerable nitrogen. Some enzymes may decrease in activity while others may increase. In extreme protein restriction, certain peptide hormones may not be synthesised in adequate quantities and endocrine disorder may appear.

In case of animals where growth has ceased and no more protein is stored either in the form of growth, milk or foetus development, and the intake and output of nitrogen are the same, in that case the animal is in a state of *nitrogen equilibrium*. Established nitrogen equilibrium in any subject shows the following facts:

(1) That the animal is no more growing and therefore not storing any protein,
(2) That the protein in the diet is sufficient in quality and quantity,
(3) That the diet is adequate in energy,
(4) That the animal is not suffering from any wasting disease.

## PROTEIN RESERVE

Digestible carbohydrates when fed in excess are stored in the animal body either as liver or muscle glycogen or as fat. Similarly when dietary fat is more than what the body can immediately utilise, the extra amount will be deposited as depot fat either in the abdominal region or on vital organs like liver, heart, kidney etc. Fat soluble vitamins such as A, D, E and K are also stored in the similar fashion if the intake is in excess of the immediate requirement.

So far protein is concerned, although the body does not store in the sense that it stores carbohydrate, fat or fat soluble vitamins but certain "reserves" are available from practically all body tissues for the purpose of meeting emergent situations. It has been said earlier that when an animal is first placed on a nitrogen-free diet, the quantity of nitrogen in its urine may fall progressively for several days before stablising at a lower level, and when nitrogen is re-introduced into the diet there is a similar lag in the re-establishment of the previous status. This suggests that the animal possesses a protein reserve which can be drawn upon in times of emergency and restored in times of excess. In times of emergency, among all the tissues, liver is very much affected. Based upon the studies made so far with laboratory experimental animals, about one fourth of the body protein especially the liver followed by kidney, heart and skeletal muscles are depleted and repleted. Thus, due to this property, the vital functions may be protected upto 30-50 days of total starvation. It should be apparent that the use of these reserves eventually requires restoration of tissues of their normal protein composition.

## The Disposal of Excess Body Amino Acids

### Sources of Free Amino Acids

(1) As discussed earlier, body proteins are continually being broken down and reconstituted in the cells. The use of isotopically labelled compounds have made it abundantly clear about high rates of protein turnover in plasma protein, intestinal mucosa, pancreas, liver and kidney white muscle, brain, skin and connective tissue have low rates of turnover. On an average the half life of 'whole body' protein is 17-20 days.

(2) In the small intestine of all ruminants and non-ruminants the nitrogenous digestion products enter the blood stream mostly as amino acids along with small amounts of ammonia and simpler peptides.

Amino acid arising from cellular protein mix freely with those entering from outside the cells as absorbed through small intestines and this constitutes the *amino acid pool.* Eventually the amino acids are disposed of in one of the following ways:

### Disposal

1. A portion is utilised for the resynthesis of tissue proteins and other nitrogen containing tissue constituents. Such a synthesis includes the formation of the protein and other nitrogenous compounds of milk, replacement of tissues and nitrogenous compounds used up in the normal 'wear and tear' of body processes. Synthesis of essential body proteinous compounds always take a priority over deaminisation.

2. Some fraction of the pool of amino acids enters into other pathways either involving movement out of the cell or catabolism in the cell itself. Oxidative deamination and transamination methods result in a loss of amino acids to the system. Oxidative deamination in details will be explained along with discussions of protein digestion in ruminants, the other method of sorting out of amino group from amino acids is transamination, is discussed below.

### Transamination

A particular type of organic reaction catalysed by the enzyme transaminase. This is a process of combined deamination and amination according to which the amino group of one amino acid may be reversibly transferred to the keto acids forming another amino acid, thus affecting amino acid-keto acid interconversion.

In the catabolism of amino acids the first reaction is in most cases the removal of the α-amino group by transamination, the product being the corresponding keto acid. The amino group is thereby transferred to either oxaloaceate or α-ketoglutarate so producing aspartate or glutamate respectively.

$$\underset{\text{Glutamic acid}}{HOOC{-}CH(NH_2){-}CH_2{-}CH_2{-}COOH} + \underset{\text{Pyruvic acid}}{HOOC{-}C(=O){-}CH_3} \xrightleftharpoons[\text{GP transaminase}]{\text{pyridoxal phosphate,}} \underset{\alpha\text{-Ketoglutaric acid}}{HOOC{-}C(=O){-}CH_2{-}CH_2{-}COOH} + \underset{\text{Alanine}}{HOOC{-}CH(NH_2){-}CH_3}$$

$$\underset{\text{Glutamic acid}}{HOOC{-}CH(NH_2){-}CH_2{-}CH_2{-}COOH} + \underset{\text{Oxaloacetic acid}}{HOOC{-}C(=O){-}CH_2{-}COOH} \xrightleftharpoons[\text{GO transaminase}]{\text{pyridoxal phosphate.}} \underset{\alpha\text{-Ketoglutaric acid}}{HOOC{-}C(=O){-}CH_2{-}CH_2{-}COOH} + \underset{\text{Aspartic acid}}{HOOC{-}CH(NH_2){-}CH_2{-}COOH}$$

Aspartate can in turn, pass on the amino group to α-ketoglutarate. Much of the glutamic acid so formed is then oxidized by the action of the enzyme glutamate dehydrogenase, which is located in mitochondria. The result is that *ammonia* and NADH are produced, and α-keto glutarate is regenerated. The $NADH_2$ upon reoxidation by the mitochondrial electron transport system, yields ATP by oxidative phosphorylation.

$$\text{Glutamate} \xrightarrow{\textit{Glutamate dehydrogenase}} \alpha\text{-ketoglutarate} + NH_3$$

$$+$$

$$NAD \longleftarrow NADH + H^+$$

$2e + 2H^+$ by electron transport chain + 3 moles of ADP will produce 3 moles of ATP + $O_2$ + $H_2O$

**Method of Excretion of Circulatory $NH_3$ (Urea Cycle)**

In ruminants, urea is one of the main microbial fermentation products of proteinous feed formed inside rumen, the large quantum of which are utilised by the microbes for the synthesis of their body protein and a good amount enters in the circulation by diffusion through ruminal wall. Apart from this urea, the liver of all mammals synthesise urea out of the excess ammonia formed by deamination of amino acids on the liver, which if allowed to accumulate in the system by virtue of their toxic property could be fatal for the species concerned. However, a very small amount of ammonia is otherwise utilised for the formation of some non-essential amino acids, purines, pyramidines, creatine and to other non-protein nitrogenous substances. The major portion thus remains unutilised and that is why all mammals have evolved biochemical reactions to remove excess ammonia rapidly in the form of urea—a comparatively non-toxic substance finally excreted out through urine.

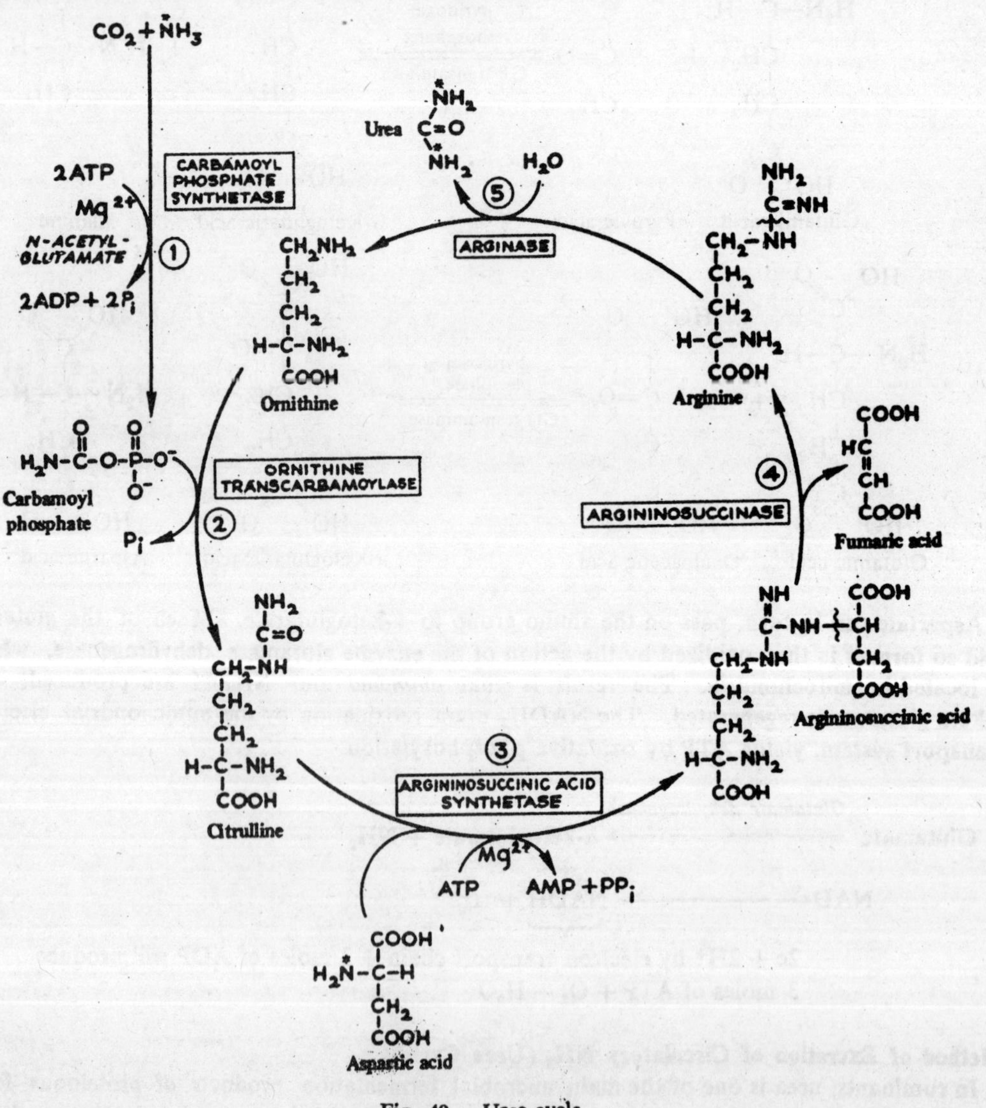

Fig. 49 Urea cycle.

**Technique**

The Krebs-Henseleit cycle (urea cycle) is a mechanism that explains the formation of urea. This is an energy requiring process. The ammonia combines with $CO_2$ (available from oxidation in the Kreb's cycle) and two molecules of ATP to form a *carbamyl phosphate*. (The compound provides the carbon atom and one of the two nitrogen atoms of the urea molecule at the final stage).

Carbamyl phosphate then reacts with a diamino acid *ornithine* in presence of an enzyme *ornithine transcarbamylase* resulting in the production of an amino acid *citrulline*, the other product being inorganic orthophosphate (Fig. 49).

A second amino group is then transferred from aspartic acid to carbamyl keto group of citrulline, to form the amino acid arginine.

In the presence of an enzyme, *arginase*, and magnesium, arginine yields one molecule of urea and of ornithine. Ornithine is thereby regenerated which can then participate in the next turn of the cycle

The urea so produced leaves the liver by the blood stream, which carries it to the kidney for excretion. The amount present in the body and the rate of its excretion depend largely on protein content of the diet.

## PROTEIN METABOLISM IN RUMINANTS

**Factors involved normal intake of Nitrogenous compounds**

The nitrogenous material ingested by the ruminant eating natural feeds consists of protein and nonprotein nitrogenous compounds such as free amino acids, peptides, amides, amines, ammonia, nucleic acids etc. These are broken down by the rumen microbes—mostly by the bacteria in two stages, firstly to free amino acids, and then very rapidly into ammonia.

It is known from work using radioisotope labelled amino acids that they are converted to ammonia at speeds measured only in minutes. In case of proteinous feeds it depends on the solubility of proteins, such as casein which is highly soluble, has a half life in the rumen of only 5.6-21.5 minutes, so that they become 90 per cent degraded before transit to the abomasum. On the other hand proteins such as zein from maize are only slowly degraded and a considerable proportion may pass unchanged into the abomasum and the small intestine where they are digested by enzymes mostly in the abomasum and rest in the small intestine. In general, however, about 50-80 per cent of proteinaceous material in feeds is degraded in the rumen and is converted into microbial nitrogenous compounds.

There are many species of bacteria in the rumen flora which have the property of secreting proteases capable of breaking down proteins to ammonia, which are utilised by those as a source of nitrogen for their nutrition in preference to amino acids. In one estimation 82 per cent of the bacterial strain isolated from rumen flora which grew with ammonia as their principal source of nitrogen. Thus, although ammonia may be considered as a potential hazard if present in harmful excess, it performs a vital function in maintaining the rumen flora.

It is known that cellulose digestion correlates with nitrogen intake in animals on low protein diets. In turn the synthesis of microbial proteins depends on the energy supplied to the microflora of the rumen by the products of carbohydrate fermentation. These compounds provide not only energy but also the necessary carbon skeletons for the synthesis of amino acids within the bacterial protoplasm.

*On the other hand, the protozoa within the rumen can hardly use ammonia as a source of nitrogen.* They require preformed amino acids for their growth. The protozoal species involved are ciliates which obtain their nutrient by engulfing and digesting bacteria together with fragments of plant material such as chloroplasts. *The protozoa form a readily available and high quality source of protein for subsequent digestion in the abomasum and small intestine.* Sudden access to highly soluble and rapidly fermentable feed will render the system unbalanced for the digestion of proteinaceous material in the rumen.

A limiting factor in the rumen digestion of protein is that much of the ammonia is lost and absorbed through the rumen mucosa before the micro-organisms have the chance to convert it into proteins. Some of the ammonia may be converted to urea in the rumen wall but most is carried by the portal blood circulation to the liver where ammonia is converted into urea by the enzymes of the Krebs-Hansleit cycle (urea cycle). In normal circumstances the uptake by the liver is highly efficient and very little ammonia is allowed to escape into the systemic circulation. Ammonia poisoning only occurs when the liver's capacity is overwhelmed.

Blood urea in the systemic circulation does not appear to have ill effects even in high concentration. As might be expected the concentration, which is normally between 10 and 20 mg of blood urea nitrogen/100 ml, depends on crude protein intake in the diet. On the introduction of low protein rations it falls dramatically to as low as 2 mg/100 ml, whereas on high intakes of protein it may rise to 30 mg/100 ml.

Blood urea may follow one of the two alternative routes. It may be excreted via the kidney and lost to the body in the urine. On the other hand it may also be returned to the rumen either by direct diffusion across the rumen wall down a concentration gradient, or by secretion through the saliva. Recycling to the rumen is correlated with blood urea concentration, increasing amounts being returned up to a critical concentration of about 18 mg/100 ml, but above this level proportionally greater amounts are excreted by the kidney. Urea returned to the rumen is hydrolysed to ammonia and made available again for the synthesis of bacterial protein, but that excreted from the kidney is lost and in a sense wasted as far as the animal is concerned. Potentially at least the urea cycle in ruminants has a protein sparing function especially on low protein diets when kidney excretion of urea will be at a minimum. It has also been claimed that the return of urea to the rumen assists in the support of the bacterial flora and in sparing protein resources during periods of feed deprivation. In these circumstances blood urea values tend to rise because of tissue catabolism and this will be recycled to the rumen for bacterial utilisation.

Blood urea diffuses not only into the rumen, but also into the lower ileum, caecum and colon. A total of 5.3 g blood urea/day was found to enter the digestive tract of sheep. Only 20 per cent of this was degraded in the rumen as compared to 25 per cent in the caecum, the remainder presumbly entering via the small intestine and colon. The fate of this urea is of great importance to the animal's nitrogen economy. Most that enters the large intestine will be built into bacterial protein which will be lost in faeces. In fact it is a relevant point that ruminants excrete faeces with a higher nitrogen content than most other mammals, nearly all of which are of microbial origin. This may appear to be wasteful but the value of the urea recycled into the large intestine is believed to be that it supports the bacterial fermentation of nutrients which have escaped digestion in the small intestine. This fermentation, resulting in the production of volatile fatty acids which are absorbed and used for energy production, is dependent on an active flora in the large intestine which, as in the case of the rumen microflora, is dependent on an adequate supply of nitrogen and available carbohydrates.

On diets containing high quality protein it may be a disadvantage because much of the nitrogen is lost as ammonia to be excreted as urea in the urine. Also, the conversion of high quality protein to bacterial proteinis not necessarily advantageous because there is doubt about the digestibility and availiblty of bacterial cell bodies lower down the digestive tract. One reason for a comparatively low availability is that bacterial protein is protected by cell walls which are resistant to enzymic action. A major chemical component of bacterial walls is a mucopeptide polymer which gives cellular rigidity. It is relatively insoluble and resists attack by trypsin. It contains a specific amino acid known as diaminopimalic acid which has been used as an index of bacterial nitrogen in the rumen. Also, at least 20 per cent of the bacterial nitrogen is in the form of nucleic acids which although about 80 per cent digestible in the small intestine may not have a high biological value. Limited evidence suggests 40-50 per cent of microbial nucleic acid nitrogen produced in the rumen is not absorbed, or if absorbed is excreted in the urine as *allantoin* and is therefore of little value to the animal.

Various methods have been proposed to improve the efficiency of protein utilisation. These nave usually involved the treatment of the feed protein in such a way that it is protected against bacterial attack in the rumen and is able to reach the abomasum and small intestine for direct degradation by the digestive juices. Some proteins such as zein do this naturally, but although relatively intact when they leave the rumen they are not highly digestible further down the alimentary tract. Alternative methods include treatment of the protein concentrate with heat, formalin, or tannin. However, caution is needed in this approach because if the rumen flora is deprived of its nitrogen support it may fail to ferment carbohydrate optimally. In other words it is arguable whether the economic benefit lies with taking advantage of the ruminant's ability to digest feeds unsuitable for other animals (including man), or with attempts to convert the ruminant into the equivalent of a single-stomached animal which can use high quality proteins and carbohydrates.

The nitrogenous compounds needed by the animal after it has completed the complex series of digestive processes are the amino acids. These are the vital components for the synthesis of protein whether it be in the form of meat or milk. Whilst the liver can synthesise some amino acids, others are known to be 'essential' in the sense that they must be supplied preformed from the alimentary tract. It seems clear that the rumen bacteria can synthesise all these essential amino acids, and indeed lactating cows have been kept successfully on diets where urea was the only source of nitrogen and where the only protein intake must have been derived from bacterial synthesis in the rumen. The problem is not so much that the essential amino acids have to be supplied, but that they must be in the optimal proportions for high production. This has been the subject of intensive investigation in recent years.

It seems clear that the amino acid composition of the rumen bacteria is reasonably constant whatever the amino acid composition of the ingested protein. Thus the rumen will tend to modify the protein available for digestion to a relatively common type. Slight differences can be provoked by altering the physical form of the diet and it also noteworthy that protozoa produce protein of a higher biological value with a high content of lysine so that diets which stimulate the proliferation of protozoa will affect the proportion of amino acid ultimately available for digestion.

Individual amino acids have specific functions. For instance, glycine which makes up a fifth of the amino acid nitrogen intake is used in the main for the detoxification of benzoic acid, and glutamate production is used largely as part of the process of detoxification of ammonia. The glucogenic amino acids and especially alanine are used for the production of glucose—*in fact between 11 and 30 per cent of glucose is produced from amino acids.* Methionine has certain important functions as far as lactation is concerned. It not only plays an important part in the synthesis of milk casein in the mammary gland where it appears to be a rate-limiting component, but it also acts as a methyl group donator in the synthesis of phospholipids and serves to bind lipids and proteins into lipoproteins for the transport of fats. It has been suggested that shortage of methionine may be associated with the pathogenesis of ketosis.

The concentration of amino acids in the blood plasma is very low—amounting to about 50-60 μg/ml—and the throughput is very rapid; many, and especially the glucogenic amino acids have a half life in the plasma of only two to five minutes. Thus, continuity of supply is vital.

The homeostasis of amino acid metabolism is complex. Attempts have been made to detect which are the limiting amino acids for various functions such as milk or wool production. Much depends on dietary intake, but methionine has frequently been implicated. The oral supplementation of the diet with a single amino acid such as methionine has little effect because of the degradation of all nitrogenous compounds in the rumen. However, direct infusion of the amino acid into the abomasum or blood where rumen degradation is avoided can be shown to promote wool growth or the extra milk production. In view of the fact that methionine may be a limiting factor efforts have been made to incorporate it into diets in such a way that it can bypass the rumen without degradation. One such attempt was the preparation of kaolin-saturated fat capsules which only in the presence of bile and pancreatin break down to release the amino acid. Another possibility is the use of an hydroxy analogue of methionine which escapes hydrolysis in the rumen. This has been shown to be capable of stimulating milk production.

## INTERCONVERSIONS OF THE MAJOR FOODSTUFFS

**Upon feeding of liberal amounts of carbohydrate diet along with sufficient rest, domestic animals may soon become fattened. The fact demonstrates the eases of conversion of carbohydrate into fat. A most significant reaction in this respect is the conversion of pyruvate to acetyl CoA, as acetyl CoA is the starting material for the synthesis of long chain fatty acid. However, the pyruvate dehydrogenase reaction is essentially nonreversible, which prevents the direct conversion of acetyl CoA, (formed from the oxidation of fatty acid) to pyruvates. As a result there is no net conversion of long chain fatty acids to carbohydrates. Only the terminal 3-carbon of a fatty acid having an odd number of carbon atoms is glycogenic, as this portion of the molecule will form propionate upon oxidation. Nevertheless, it is possible for levelled carbon atoms of all fatty acids to be found ultimately in glycogen after reversing the citric acid cycle; this is because oxaloacetate is an intermediate both in the citric acid cycle; and in the pathway of gluconeogenesis.**

**Many of the carbon skeleton of the non-essential amino acids can be produced from carbohydrate via the citric acid cycle. In it the amino group is added with the help of transamination reaction. By reversal of this processes, glycogenic amino acids yield carbon skeleton which are either members or precursors of the members of the citric acid cycle. They are**

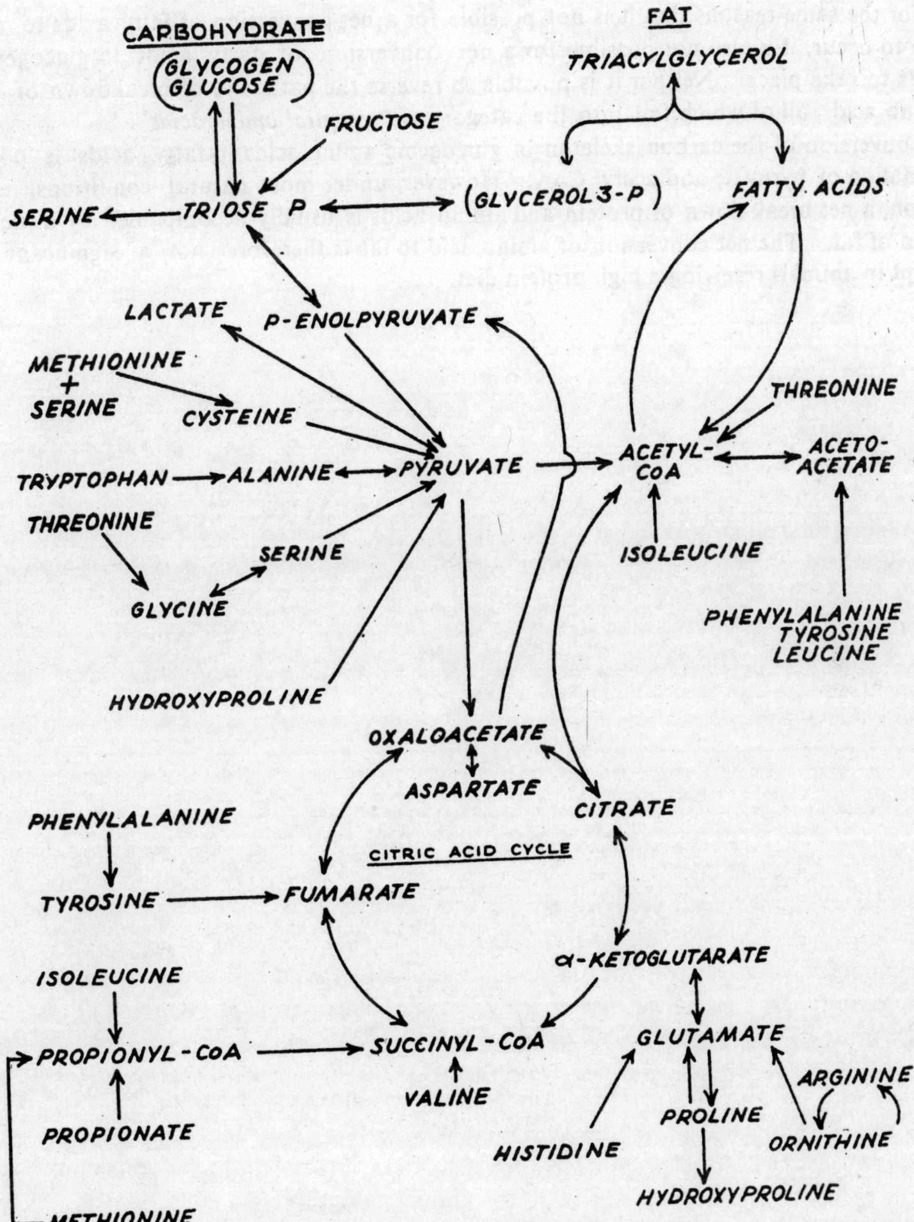


**Fig. 50** Interconversion of the major foodstuffs.

therefore readily converted by gluconeogenic pathway to glucose and glycogens. The ketogenic amino acids give rise to aceto acetate, which will in turn be metabolised as ketone bodies, forming acetyl CoA in extra hepatic tissues (Fig. 50).

For the same reasons that it is not possible for a net conversion of fatty acids to carbohydrate to occur, it is also not possible for a net conversion of fatty acids to glucogenic amino acids to take place. Neither it is possible to reverse the pathways of breakdown of ketogenic amino acids, all of which fall into the category of "*essential amino acids*".

Conversion of the carbon skeleton of glucogenic amino acids to fatty acids is possible by formation of pyruvate and acetyl CoA. However, under most natural conditions, e.g., starvation, a net break down of protein and amino acids is usually accompanied by a net breakdown of fat. The net conversion of amino acid to fat is therefore not a significant process except in animals receiving a high protein diet.

# DIGESTIVE ORGANS AND PROCESSES IN RUMINANTS AND NON-RUMINANTS

## DIGESTIVE ORGANS

This consists of the organs directly concerned in the reception, digestion and absorption of the food, its passage through the body and the expulsion of the unabsorbed portion. The system can be divided as (*A*) *Alimentary canal*—It runs from the lips to the anus. It has mouth, pharynx, oesophagus, stomach, small intestine, large intestine and rectum. (*B*) *Accessory digestive organs*—It includes teeth, tongue, salivary, liver glands and pancreas.

### Digestive Organs of Ruminants

A. ALIMENTARY CANAL

The alimentary canal of the ruminants is much more complex than that of the non-ruminants. It has four compartments in the stomach namely, (*i*) the *Rumen*, or paunch; (*ii*) the *Reticulum*, or honey comb; (*iii*) the *Omasum*, or many plies; and (*iv*) the *Abomasum*, or the true stomach. The intestine represents a long tubule approximately 180 feet long in average dairy cattle. The first three compartments of the compound stomach are considered to be the enlargements of the oesophagus or gullet. This peculiar feature of the stomach in ruminants seems to have developed under the stimulus of coarse feeds and feeding on them in a hurry without proper mastication.

### The Mouth

It is the organ of prehension, mastication, insalivation and rumination. The prehension (food gathering) is assisted by the rough tongue and teeth of a ruminant. It is followed by a preliminary chewing called mastication and mixing of the saliva. Enormous amount of saliva (100-200 lit. per day in a cow) is secreted by the three pairs of salivary glands located in the mouth region. It is rich in sodium bicarbonate and its amount increases with dry and acidic feeds like hay and silage. It lubricates the bolus and facilitates its passage through the pharynx and the oesophagus to the rumen. There is no ptyalin (a digestive enzyme present in some other species) in the saliva of the ruminants, therefore, no digestion takes place in the mouth of the ruminants.

After prehension is complete, the cow starts chewing her cud called rumination. The rough materials which escaped through grinding during preliminary mastication, and are stored and exposed to bacterial action in the rumen, are forced back into the mouth (regurgitation) for further mastication. This is also known as rumination. The regurgitated bolus weighing from 90–120 gm requires 3 seconds to ascend, about 50 seconds for rechewing and 105 seconds to descend. Rumination is therefore, a long process and occupies about 8 hours. If the animal is alarmed or disturbed or goes sick it ceases to ruminate.

After the bolus is thoroughly masticated and mixed with saliva it is swallowed again with the help of the throat muscle. This time it remains almost semisolid and goes into the ventral sac of the rumen wherefrom it finally passes to abomasum through reticulum and omasum. Water and other liquid drinks reach the omasum and/or abomasum directly. This is made possible by the oesophageal groove (Fig. 68).

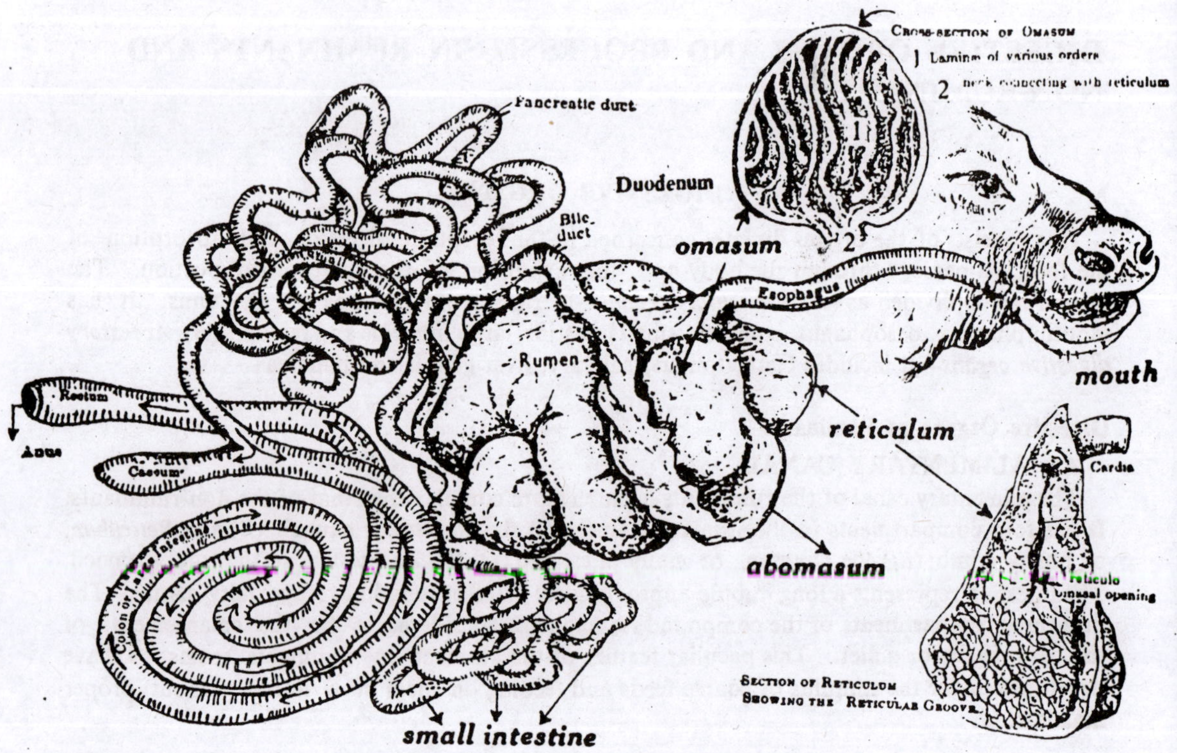


Fig. 51 The digestive tract of the ox (schematic).

**The Oesophagus**

The oesophagus, a direct continuation of the pharynx, is a muscular tube extending from the pharynx to the upper most part of the stomach known as *cardia* just caudal to the diaphragm. From the pharynx the oesophagus passes dorsal to the trachea and usually inclines somewhat to the left in the neck.

The muscular wall of the oesophagus consists of two layers that cross obliquely, then spiral and finally form an inner circular and outer longitudinal layer. The cardia is ordinarily tightly closed by contraction of a ring of muscle tissue, the *Cardiac sphincter*, but this muscle relaxes and the cardia relaxes and then cardia opens wide when boli are passing into or out of the rumen and when gas escapes.

**The Rumen**

It is the largest compartment of the stomach and has a very great significance in ruminant digestion and has several functions to perform. Even fifty years ago, the rumen action was a deep dark mystery. Today, thanks to scientific research, much more is known about the rumen processes than were known, 60 years ago.

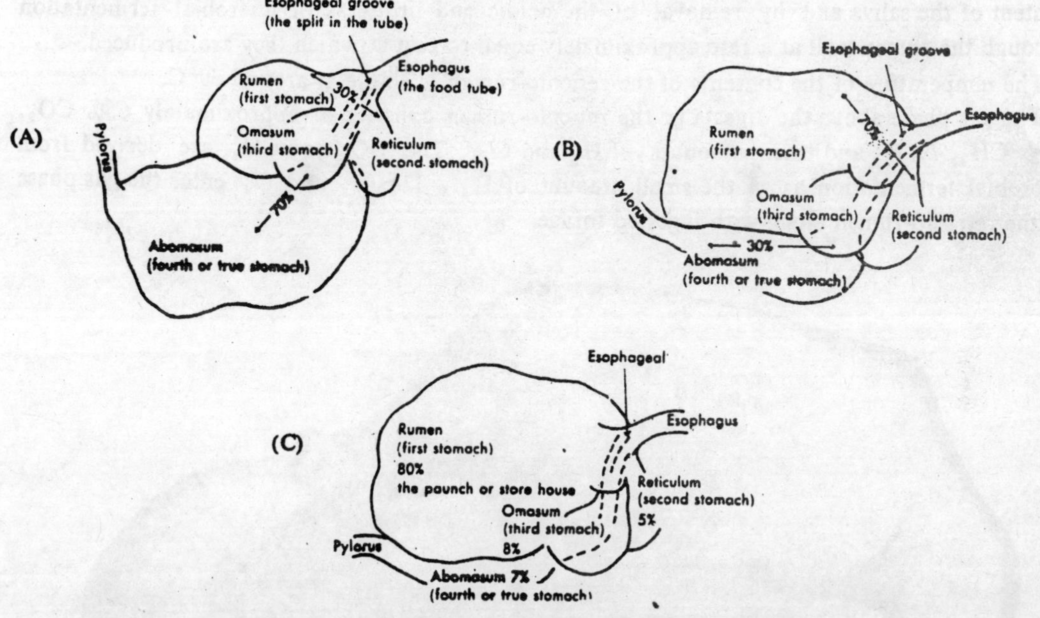


**Fig. 52** The development and relative capacities of the various stomach compartments of *(a)* the calf at birth, *(b)* the calf at 2 months, and *(c)* the mature cow.

This large voluminous sac which extends from the diaphragm to the pelvis almost entirely fills the left side of the abdominal cavity. The rumen is subdivided into sacs by thick muscular boundaries known as pillars, which appear from the exterior of the rumen as grooves. The dorsal and ventral sacs are separated by a nearly complete circle. The dorsal sac is the largest compartment. The dorsal sac overlaps the ventral sac and is continuous cranially with the reticulum over the *ruminoreticular* fold, which separates the floor of the rumen from the floor of the reticulum.

Caudally the dorsal sac is further subdivided by the dorsal coronary pillars, which form as incomplete circle bounding the dorsal blind sac. The caudal part of the ventral sac is a diverticulum separated from the rest of the ventral sac by the ventral coronary pillars.

The mucous membrane lining the rumen is glandless stratified squamous epithelium. The most ventral parts of both sacs of the rumen contain numerous papillae up to 1 cm. in length, but papillae are almost entirely absent on the dorsal part of the rumen.

*Rumen environment*

The liquid phase of the rumen contents contains about 10 – 20% by weight of organic matter and has a pH between 5.8 to 6.8. With large amounts of readily fermentable carbohydrate entering the rumen, however, the pH may fall to around pH 4.0. Conversely, on very poor forages, the pH may rise to pH 7.5 or more, but these are the extremes of the pH range.

The pH of the reticulo-rumen is maintained at a fairly constant level by the alkalanity of the large volumes of saliva (pH – 8.0) entering the rumen, by the buffering capacity of the $HCO_3$

content of the saliva and by removal of the acidic end products of microbial fermentation through the rumen wall at a rate approximately equal to that at which they are produced.

The temperature of the contents of the reticulo-rumen is stable at around 39°C.

The gas phase above the digesta in the reticulo-rumen consists of approximately 65% $CO_2$, 25% $CH_4$, 7% $N_2$ and trace amounts of $H_2$ and $O_2$. The $CO_2$ and $CH_4$ are derived from microbial fermentation as in the small amount of $H_2$. The $N_2$ and $O_2$ enter the gas phase of the reticulo-rumen along with ingested forage.

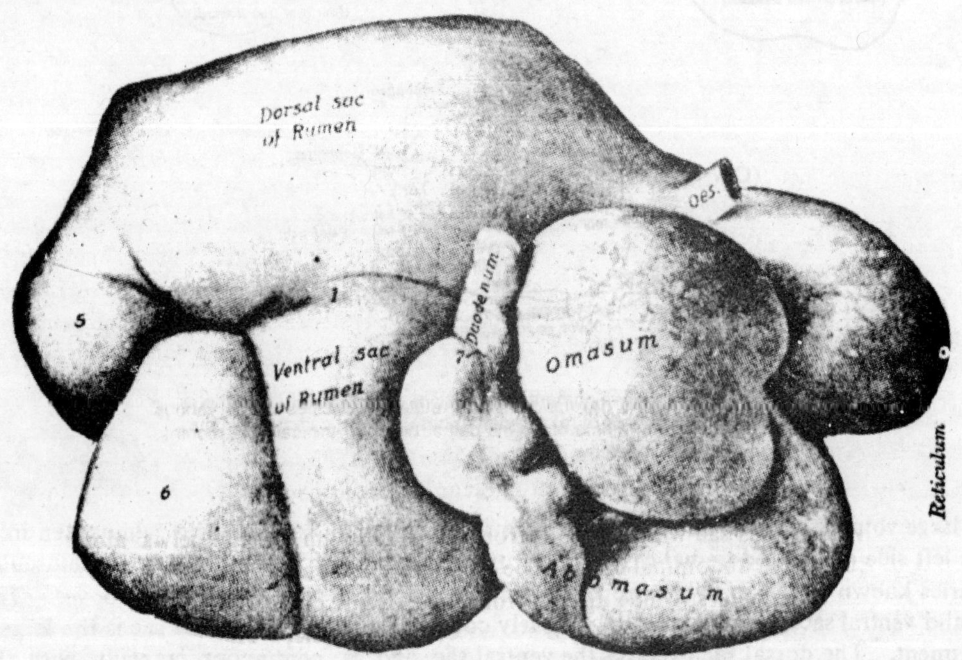


**Fig. 53** —Stomach of cow; right view. *Oes.*, Esophagus: *1*, right longitudinal groove of rumen; *2*, posterior groove of rumen; *3, 4*, coronary grooves; *5, 6*, posterior blind sacs of rumen; *7*, pylorus.

The liquid phase of reticulo-rumen has an oxidation-reduction potential of about − 350 mV, thus it is clear that reticulo-rumen environment is extremely reduced and almost devoid of oxygen.

The inorganic solutes present in the reticulo-rumen are derived from the saliva. Of the cations present in the rumen, only $Na^+$ is transported across reticulo-ruminal wall in gradient which occurs between the rumen and the blood stream. As a consequence of this, the ionic content of the rumen closely reflects that of the saliva.

### The Reticulum

The reticulum is the most cranial compartment. It is also called the honey comb, and as the names imply, it is lined with mucous membrane containing many intersecting ridges which subdivide the surface into honey comb like compartments. The surface is stratified squamous epithelium. The location of the reticulum immediately behind the diaphragm places it almost in opposition to heart, so any foreign objects such as wire or nails that may be swallowed tend to lodge in the reticulum and are in a very good position to penetrate into the heart. The reticular groove commonly referred to as the oesophageal groove, extend from the cardia to the omasum, and is formed by two muscular folds which can close to direct materials from the oesophagus into the omasum directly, or open and permit the materials to enter the rumen. The groove appears to be less functional in adult ruminants than in suckling animals. However, it has been demonstrated that in drenching sheep, the drench enters the abomasum directly.

**The Omasum**

The omasum is a spherical organ filled with muscular laminae, bearing pointed papillae arranged in such a manner that food is moved from the *reticulo-omasal* orifice between the laminae, and on to the *omaso-abomasal* orifice. Each lamina contains three layers of muscle, including a central layer continuous with the muscle wall of the omasum.

The floor of the omasum as well as the leaves are covered with stratified squamous epithelium. At the junction of the omasum and abomasum is an arrangement of folds of mucous membrane, the *vela terminalia*, derived from the omasum in the cow, but from the abomasum in the sheep.

**The large size of the reticulo-rumen has already been mentioned and, as the turnover rate of the reticulo-rumen is of the order of 1-1.5 volumes per day, it is clear that a very large volume of liquid enters the omasum from the reticulo-rumen. The material entering the omasum contains 90-95% water and the primary function of this organ is to remove water by about 50%.**

**In addition to removing water, the omasum also absorbs VFA.**

**The Abomasum**

The abomasum (true stomach) is the first glandular portion of the ruminant digestive system. It is located ventral to the omasum and extends caudally on the right side of the rumen. The pylorus (terminal part of the abomasum) is a sphincter (thickening of circular smooth muscle fibres) at the junction of the stomach and small intestine.

The epithelium of the abomasum changes abruptly from the stratified squamous epithelium of the omasum to a tall simple columnar epithelium capable of producing mucus. Presumably the mucus covering the stomach epithelium prevents the digestive juices from digesting the stomach cells.

**The abomasum corresponds in structure and function to the fundic region of the stomach of non-ruminants. The abomasal epithelium possesses cells which secrete electrolytes, specially HCl, pepsin and mucus. The pH of this section is in the range of pH 1.0 – 1.3 and overall pH of abomasal contents is about pH 2.0. The low pH of abomasal contents is responsible for the death of the microbes entering the abomasum ; it also provides optimum conditions for activity of the peptic enzymes responsible for the digestion of microbial protein in the abomasum.**

The acidity of stomach contents varies among the domestic animals, being highest in carnivores (pH 1 or less in dogs), and lowest in monogastric herbivores (pH 1.1-6.8 in horses). In carnivores the stomach will virtually empty it-self between each meal. In herbivores ingesta may remain within the stomach for several days.

The control of gastric secretion involves several regulatory phases as follows :

**(1) *Cephalic or Reflex phase***

Gastric secretion may be initiated by such things as the sight, smell or taste of food which may not enter the stomach. Stimuli reach the stomach by way of the vagus nerves to the myenteric plexus. (the nerve net work of the stomach wall). Herbivorous animals do not appear to have a cephalic phase of gastric stimulation.

**(2) *Gastric phase***

It accounts for about 75% of the total gastric juice secretion and occurs when food reaches the stomach. The distension of the stomach also results in a vasovagal reflex by which impulses are sent to the brain and then back to the stomach by way of the vagus nerves to

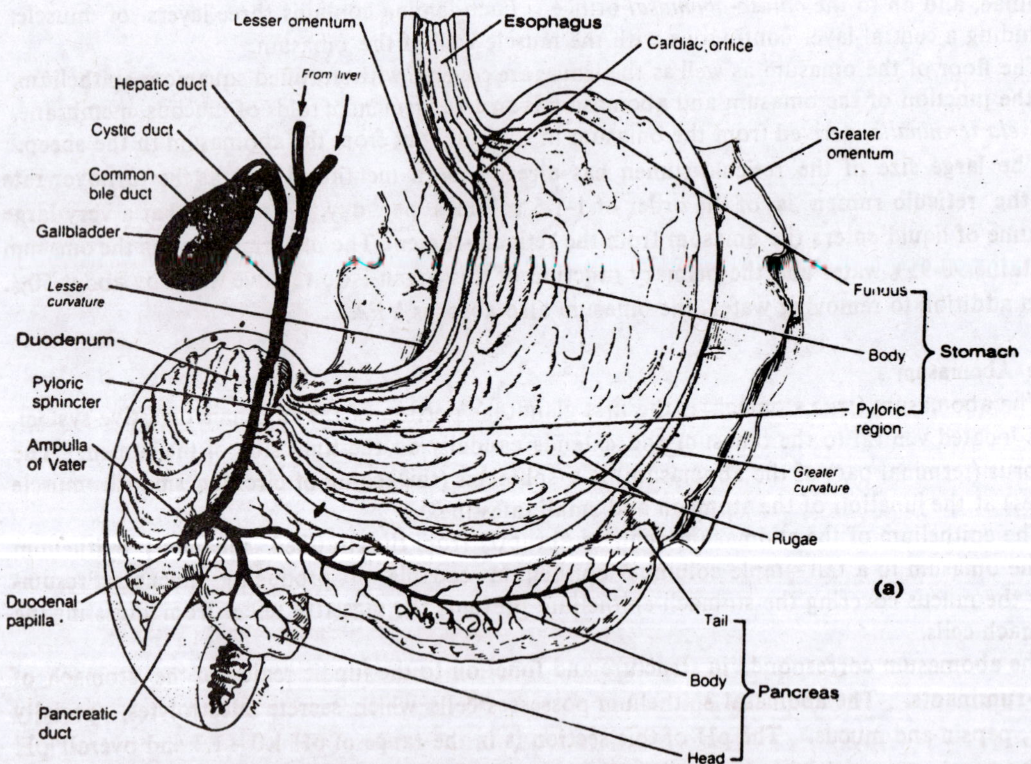


**Fig. 54** Frontal section of a typical mammalian monogastric stomach and duodenum showing the pancreatic and bile duct.

stimulate the flow of gastric juice and also release of the hormone gastrin.

The hormone is synthesised and released by the "G" cells in the antrum of the stomach. It causes the parietal cells to secrete HCl and intrinsic factor (IF), and the chief cell to secrete pepsinogen and stimulates gastric motility.

**(3) *Intestinal phase***

It involves small amount of gastric juice that continue to be secreted as lc .g as chyme remains in the small intestine, even though no food remains in the stomach.

Factors that inhibit gastric secretion are as follows :

(1) Feedback mechanism depends on the distention of the duodenum, fluidity of the chyme in the duodenum, and the concentration of amino acids and chyme acidity in the duodenum. As any of these substances increase in the duodenum, it also decreases the release of gastrin from the G cells, which in turn decreases the HCl secretion from the parietal cells.

(2) A second factor is involved in the control of gastric secretion. Two hormones, *secretin* and *cholecystokinin* (CCK) are synthesised by and secreted from mucosal cells in the duodenum in response to the same stimuli (i.e. chyme, pH, fluidity, digestive state). These hormones are secreted directly in the blood and are carried back to the stomach by the vascular system. In the stomach they decrease motility, inhibit the release of gastrin and thus inhibits HCl secretion.

(3) The stomach has a direct mechanism also, when the pH becomes low due to a high HCl concentration, this will inhibit the release of gastrin from the antral G cells, which in turn will inhibit the further secretion of HCl.

**The Small Intestine**

The small intestine is divided into three parts, duodenum, jejunum and ileum, because of

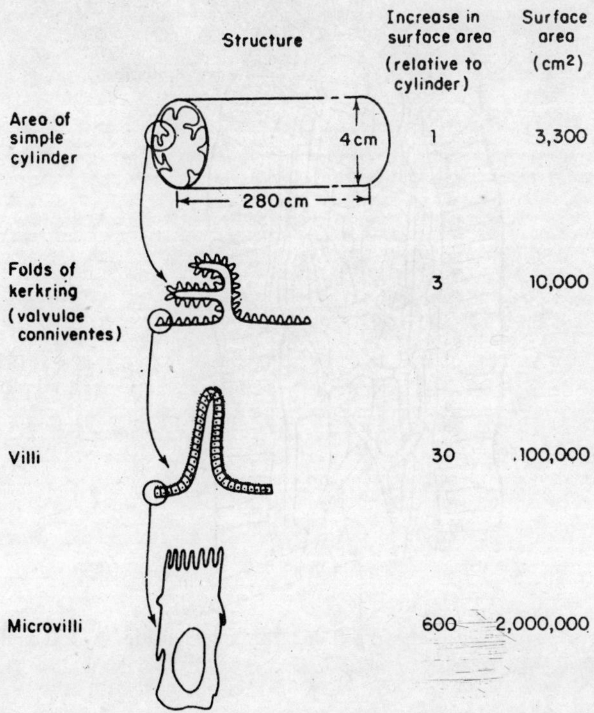


**Fig. 55** Mechanisms for increasing surface area of the small intestine.

histological or microscopic structural difference.

The *doudenum* is the first part of the small intestine. It is closely attached to the body wall by a short mesentery, the mesoduodenum. Ducts from the pancreas and liver enter the first part of the duodenum.

The *jejunum* is indistinctly separated from the duodenum. It begins approximately where the mesentery starts to become rather long. The jejunum and ileum are continuous, and there is no gross demarcation between them

The *ileum* is the last part of the small intestine. It enters the large intestine at the *ileo-ceco-colic junction.*

It is impossible to give a definite location for the jejunum and ileum, but they tend to be located toward the left ventral portion of the abdominal cavity in non-ruminants. The terminal part of the ileum, however, joins the *cecum* (horse) or cecum and colon (other animals) in the right caudal part of the abdominal cavity.

The small intestine is the chief site of absorption in most of the domestic animals. The mucus membrane of only the small intestine consists of numerous tiny finger like projections known as *villi.* Animals with the most rapid digestive and absorptive processes have a more highly developed system of villi to provide a greater surface area for absorption. Each villus is further surrounded by innumerable fingerlike projections known as *microvilli* for the sake

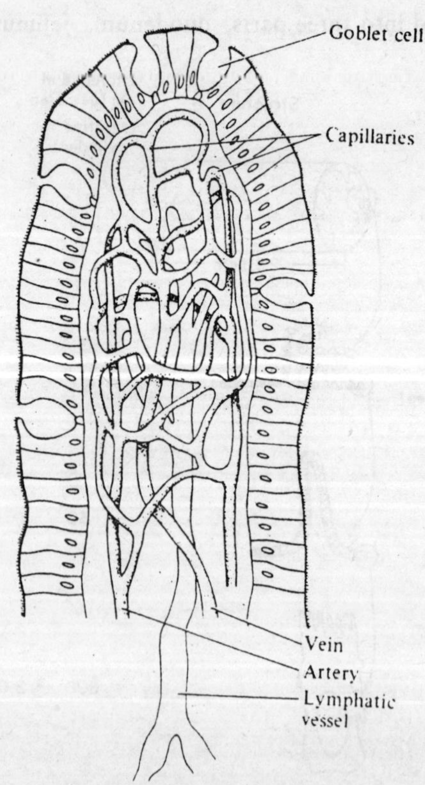


Fig. 56 Intestinal villus.

of unimaginable greater surface area for the absorption of nutrients. Villi undergo rhythmic (pumping) contractions, pendulum movements and tonic contractions and is controlled by a hormone, *villikinin* and thus aids in absorption.

The duodenum receives both bile from the gall-bladder and pancreatic secretions from the

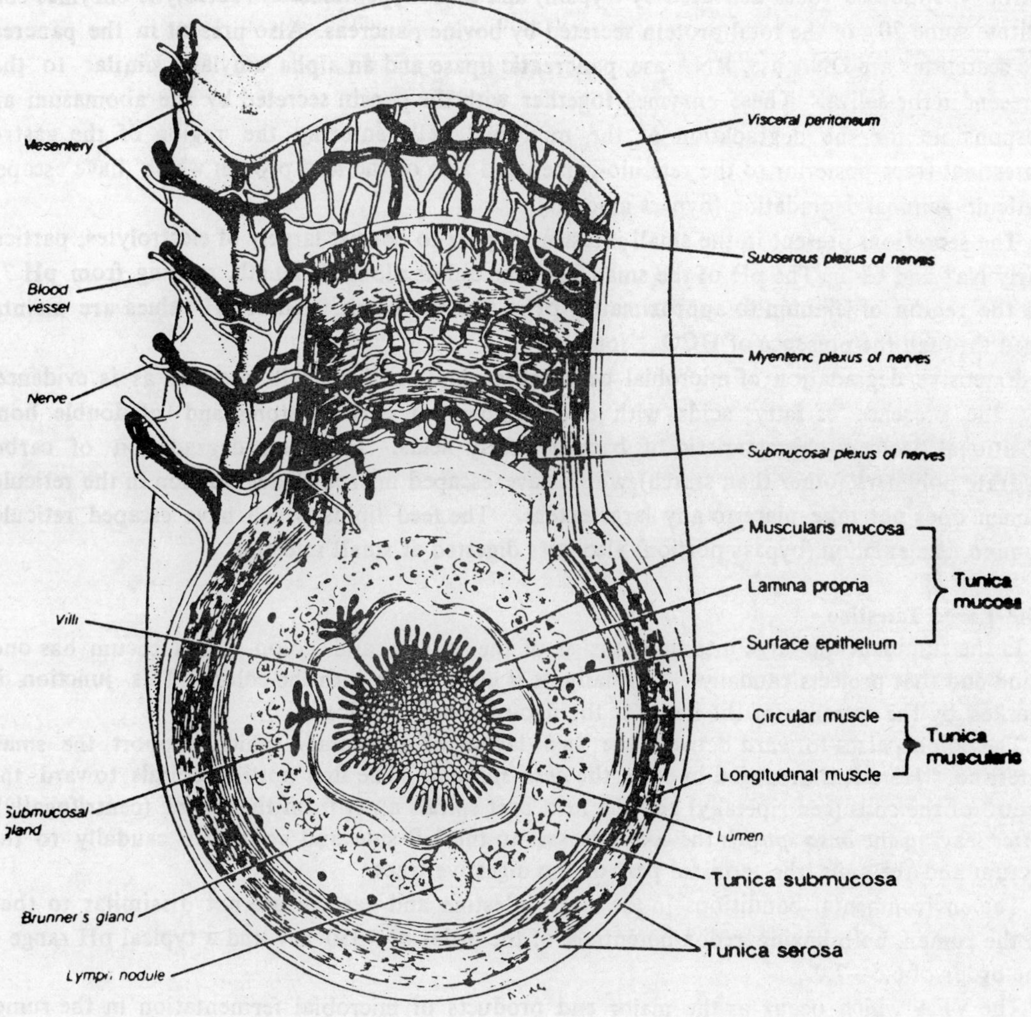


Fig. 57 Representing the layers of the wall of the stomach, small intestine and colon.

pancreas via a duct which at the point of entry into the duodenum is common to both organs since the bile duct and pancreatic duct fuse some 2-3 cm from this point.

Bile consists largely of bile acids and bile pigments, with small amounts of cholesterol, lecithin, electrolytes and protein. Bile acids before entering the duodenum conjugated of either glycine, giving glycocholic acid salt or taurine, giving taurocholic acid salts. Esterification takes place at the terminal carboxyl group of the parent acid.

The secretions of the pancreas include the proteolytic enzymes trypsinogen (converted to the active form, trypsin, by enterokinase secreted by the duodenum), chymotrypsinogens and procarboxypeptidases (both activated by trypsin) and carboxypeptidase. Proteolytic enzymes constitute some 70% of the total protein secreted by bovine pancreas. Also present in the pancreatic secretions are DNA ase, RNA ase, pancreatic lipase and an alpha amylase similar to that present in the saliva. These enzymes together with the pepsin secreted by the abomasum are responsible for the degradation of the microbial cells entering the region of the gastrointestinal tract posterior to the reticulo-rumen and also of the feed protein which have escaped reticulo-ruminal degradation (bypass amount).

The secretions present in the small intestine appear to consist largely of electrolytes, particularly $Na^+$ and $Cl^-$. The pH of the small intestine differs along its length, ranging from pH 7.1 in the region of jejunum to approximately pH 8.0 at the ileum. These pH values are maintained through the presence of $HCO_3^-$ ions.

Extensive degradation of microbial cells takes place in the small intestine as is evidenced by the presence of fatty acids with odd numbers of carbon atoms and of double bond positional isomers characteristic of bacterial fatty acids. However, degradation of carbohydrate polymers (other than starch) which have escaped microbial degradation in the reticulo-rumen does not take place to any large extent. The feed lipids which have escaped reticulo-rumino fermentation (bypass portion) also gets digested at small intestine.

### The Large Intestine

In the ruminant the large intestine consists of the cecum and colon. This cecum has one blind end that projects caudally. Cranially, it is continuous with the colon. This junction is marked by the entrance of the ileum at the ileo-ceco-colic orifice.

The colon passes forward between the two layers of mesentary which support the small intestine. Here it is arranged in coils, the *ansa spiralis*. The first portion spirals toward the centre of the coils (centripetally) and the next part spirals away from the centre (centrifugally). After leaving the *ansa spiralis* the colon crosses to the left side and continues caudally to the rectum and the anus, the terminal part of the digestive tract.

The environmental conditions in the large intestine and caecum are not dissimilar to these in the rumen, both having redox potentials of the order of—350 mV and a typical pH range of the order of 6.5—7.0

The VFA which occur as the major end products of microbial fermentation in the rumen are also found in large intestine and caecum due to microbial degradation of polysaccharides as well as other carbohydrates which have escaped digestion at a lower total concentration. (Rumen, 100—150mM ; Caecum, 60 mM and in large intestine 7 mM).

An important aspect of microbial fermentation in the large intestine and caecum from the host animal's point of view is that the microbial cells synthesised in these regions of the intestinal tract are not subjected to subsequent digestion, and therefore, are not available as potential sources of protein to the host animal.

It would not be unreasonable to suggest that the volatile fatty acids of hind gut and caecal origin contribute about 30% of the total VFA entering ruminant bloodstream, the remaining 70% being largely of ruminal origin. Water is also absorbed from the large intestine and caecum to the extent of 1.0—1.25 liters per day in sheep. Amino nitrogen @0.5—1.6 gram/day are also absorbed in sheep in the region of large intestine.

## B. ACCESSORY DIGESTIVE ORGANS

### The Salivary Glands

The main salivary glands consist of three pairs of well defined glands viz., *parotid, mandibular,* and *sublingual.* The other salivary glands include *labial, buccal, lingual* and *palatine* glands. The dog has also a zygomatic salivary gland near the eye. *The parotid salivary gland* is located ventral to each ear in relation to the caudal border of the mandible. The duct penetrates the mucous membrane of the cheek near the upper third or fourth cheek tooth. The *mandibular* or *submaxillary salivary gland* is located ventral to the parotid gland just caudal to the mandible. The mandibular salivary duct opens ventral to the tongue on a little papilla located in the fold that holds the tongue to the floor of the mouth. The *sublingual salivary gland* is located deep to the mucous membrane along the ventral side of the lateral surface of the tongue near the floor of the mouth. With the exception of the horse, the gland has a monostomatic portion that empties on to the floor of the mouth by way of major sublingual duct.

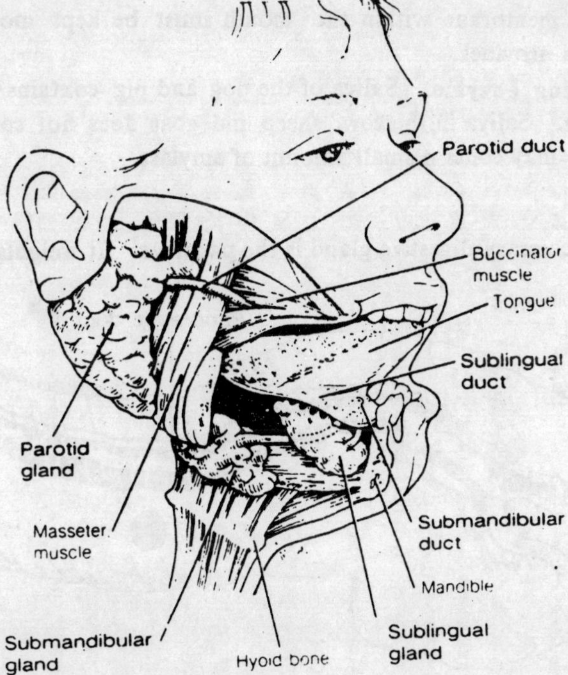


Fig. 58 The salivary glands. Glandular secretions are carried to the mouth through ducts.

The secretion of the saliva in ruminants is continuous, but the rate is greatly increased by stimuli associated with feeding, rumination and the presence of coarse feeds. An adult human may produce about 1.5—2 liters of saliva daily. In cattle total volume may range from 100—200 liters per day or sometimes equivalent to the volume of the rumen.

Paired parotid, inferior molar and buccal salivary glands produce thin watery secretions, highly alkaline having high concentration of $HCO_3^-$ ions with very little mucoprotein. Saliva from the paired submaxillary, sublingual, and labial salivary glands as well as the unpaired pharyngeal gland secrete a glycoprotein, mucin. The saliva of ruminants tends to be slightly alkaline (pH about 8). The uses of saliva in digestion are manyfold, including the following :

1. **Lubricant.** These secretions act as aids in mastication, formation of the bolus and swallowing.
2. **Buffering capacity.** A large quantity of bicarbonate is secreted in saliva, serving as a buffer in the ingesta.
3. **Nutrients for rumen microorganisms.** Saliva contains considerable amounts of urea, mucin, phosphorus, magnesium and chloride which all are utilised by rumen microbes.
4. **Prevention of frothing.** Gas can accumulate in the rumen and may cause bloat condition when eruction process is impaired. Saliva—acting as a surfactant—helps to prevent this problem.
5. **Taste.** Saliva solubilises a number of the chemicals in the feed which, once in solution, can be detected by the taste buds.
6. **Protection.** The membrane within the mouth must be kept moist in order to remain viable which saliva provides.
7. **Source of digesting enzyme.** Saliva of the dog and pig contains some amylase capable of digesting starch. Saliva in the cow, sheep and goat does not contain amylase, but the saliva of the horse may contain small amount of amylase.

## 2. The Pancreas

The second main accessary digestive gland is the pancreas. It weights 350 to 500 gram in

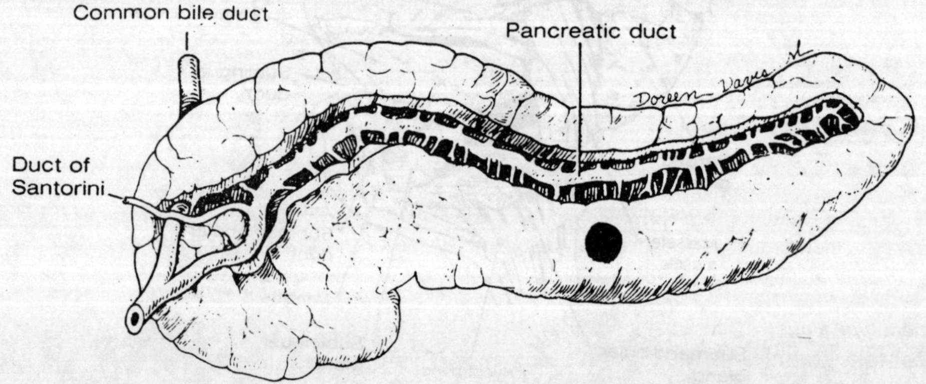


Fig. 59 The pancreas. The inset shows its microscopic structure

**the ox, and 50-70 gram in the sheep and goat. The pancreas is a dual organ. Its exocrine portion forms the great mass of the gland and secretes pancreatic juice into the duodenum. The endocrine tissue consists of the tiny spherical *islets of langerhans* which account for less than 1 per cent of the whole. The mixed exocrine and endocrine glands is elongated. The pancreas is a soft, lumpy organ with a large head, long body and tapering tail. The head lies within the concavity of the duodenum.**

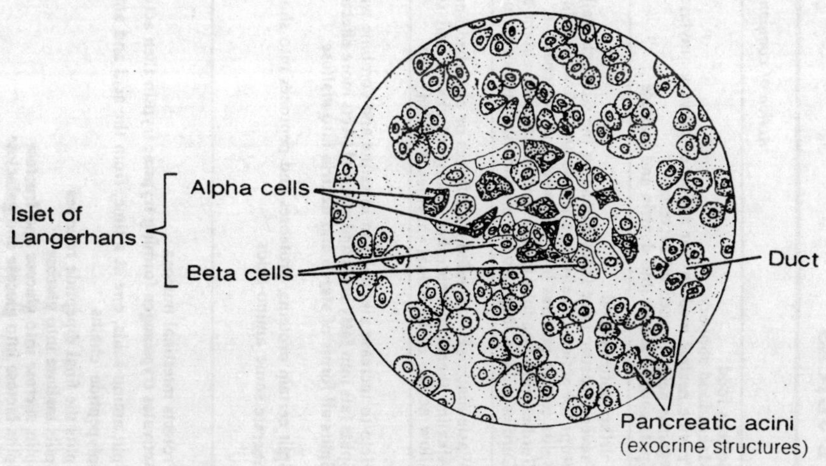


**Fig. 60** **(a)** Anterior view of the liver and its supporting ligaments.
**(b)** Superior (diaphragmatic) surface of the liver.

**Table 126**

**Composition of pancreatic juice**

| | | |
|---|---|---|
| Enzyme precursors | — | Trypsinogen, chymotrypsinogen |
| Active enzymes | — | Elastase, amylase, lipase |
| Cations | — | Sodium, potassium, calcium |
| Anions | — | Chloride, bicarbonate |
| pH | — | 7.5—8.0 |

N.B. : The inactive enzyme precursor *trypsinogen* is converted to the active *trypsin* by the enzyme *enterokinase*, which is liberated from unidentified cells of the duodenal mucosa. Trypsin also acts on the precursor *Chymotrypsinogen* to form the active chymotrypsin.

*Exocrine pancreas:* This is a compound tubulo-acinar gland, the acini are composed of cells which contain granules of the digestive enzymes (Zymogen granules). The acini are connected with excretory ducts which finally coalesce into a single duct which enters the duodenum.

FUNCTIONS OF PANCREATIC JUICE. (1) The alkalinity of the juice aids in the neutralisation

Table 127

## DIGESTIVE JUICES

| *Secretion* | *Where produced* | *Where effective* | *Principal components* | *Action of components* |
|---|---|---|---|---|
| Saliva | Salivary glands | Mouth (and temporarily in stomach) | Water<br>Mucus<br>Salts<br><br>SALIVARY AMYLASE | Softens food<br>Makes food slippery<br>Provide **neutral** medium for action of salivary amylase and help to preserve teeth against acids formed by bacteria<br>Splits cooked **starch** into **dextrin** and **maltose** |
| Gastric juice | Gastric glands | Stomach | Water<br>Mucus<br>Hydrochloric acid<br>PEPSIN (secreted as pepsinogen<br>RENNIN | Further softens food<br>Prevents gastric juice from damaging the stomach wall<br>Stops the action of salivary amylase and allows pepsin to work. Kills many germs.<br>Splits certain **proteins** into **proteoses** and **peptones,** i.e. shorter chain polypeptides<br>Curdles milk in adults (when rennin scarce or absent and in any case ineffective)<br>Curdles milk in many young mammals. Presence in man doubtful |
| Bile | Liver (stored in the gall bladder) | Small intestine | Water<br>Bile pigments<br>Bile salts | Waste materials—excreted with faeces or absorbed and re-excreted later<br>Alkaline therefore neutralise acidity of chyme and stop action of pepsin but allow action of Intestinal enzymes. Emulsify fats |
| Pancreatic juice | Pancreas | Small intestine | Water<br>Alkaline salts<br>PANCREATIC LIPASE<br>PANCREATIC AMYLASE<br>TRYPSIN (secreted as trypsinogen)<br>CHYMOTRYPSIN (secreted as chymotrypsinogen) | Help to increase alkalinity in intestine and combine with fatty acids to form soaps<br>Splits fats into **fatty acids** and **glycerol** (Acts more effectively than gastric lipase<br>Splits all forms of **starch** and **dextrin** into **maltose**<br>Split certain proteins, proteoses and peptones into shorter polypeptide chains and liberate some amino-acids |
| Intestinal juice | Duodenal glands and goblet cells throughout the small intestine | Small intestine | Water<br>Mucus<br>ENTEROKINASE<br>PEPTIDASES<br>Carboxypeptidase<br>Aminopeptidase<br>Dipeptidase<br>MALTASE<br>SUCRASE<br>LACTASE | Protects intestinal mucosa<br>Activates **trypsinogen** forming **trypsin;** trypsin then activates **chymotrysinogen**<br>Split amino-acids, one at a time, from the acid and amino ends, respectively, of the polypeptide chains<br>Splits the final dipeptide residues<br>Splits **maltose** into **glucose**<br>Splits **sucrose** into **glucose** and **fructose**<br>Splits **lactose** into **glucose** and **galactose** |

Table 128 Summary of digestive processes.

| Source of Secretion and Stimulus for Secretion | Enzyme | Method of Activation and Optimal Conditions for Activity | Substrate | End Products or Action |
|---|---|---|---|---|
| **Salivary glands of mouth:** Secrete saliva in reflex response to presence of food in mouth. | Salivary amylase | Chloride ion necessary. pH 6.6–6.8. | Starch<br>Glycogen | Maltose plus 1:6 glucosides (oligosaccharides) plus maltotriose |
| **Stomach glands:** Chief cells and parietal cells secrete gastric juice in response to reflex stimulation and chemical action of gastrin. | Pepsin A (fundus)<br>Pepsin B (pylorus) | Pepsinogen converted to active pepsin by HCl. pH 1.0–2.0. | Protein | Proteoses<br>Peptones |
| | Rennin | Calcium necessary for activity. pH 4.0. | Casein of milk | Coagulates milk |
| **Pancreas:** Presence of acid chyme from the stomach activates duodenum to produce (1) secretin, which hormonally stimulates flow of pancreatic juice; (2) cholecystokinin, which stimulates the production of enzymes. | Trypsin | Trypsinogen converted to active trypsin by enterokinase of intestine at pH 5.2–6.0. Autocatalytic at pH 7.9. | Protein<br>Proteoses<br>Peptones | Polypeptides<br>Dipeptides |
| | Chymotrypsin | Secreted as chymotrypsinogen and converted to active form by trypsin. pH 8.0. | Protein<br>Proteoses<br>Peptones | Same as trypsin. More coagulating power for milk. |
| | Carboxypeptidase | Secreted as procarboxypeptidase, activated by trypsin. | Polypeptides at the free carboxyl end of the chain | Lower peptides. Free amino acids. |
| | Pancreatic amylase | pH 7.1 | Starch<br>Glycogen | Maltose plus 1:6 glucosides (oligosaccharides) plus maltotriose. |
| | Lipase | Activated by bile salts, phospholipids, collpase. pH 8.0. | Primary ester linkages of triacylglycerol | Fatty acids, monoacylglycerols, diacylglycerols, glycerol |
| | Ribonuclease | | Ribonucleic acid | Nucleotides |
| | Deoxyribonuclease | | Deoxyribonucleic acids | Nucleotides |
| | Cholesteryl ester hydrolase | Activated by bile salts. | Cholesteryl esters | Free cholesterol plus fatty acids |
| | Phospholipase $A_2$ | | Phospholipids | Fatty acids, lysophospholipids |
| **Liver and gallbladder:** Cholecystokinin, a hormone from the intestinal mucosa—and possibly also gastrin and secretin—stimulate the gallbladder and secretion of bile by the liver. | (Bile salts and alkali) | | Fats—also neutralize acid chyme | Fatty acid-bile salt conjugates and finely emulsified neutral fat-bile salt micelles |
| **Small Intestine:** Secretions of Brunner's glands of the duodenum and glands of Lieberkühn. | Aminopeptidase | | Polypeptides at the free amino end of the chain | Lower peptides. Free amino acids. |
| | Dipeptidases | | Dipeptides | Amino acids |
| | Sucrase | pH 5.0–7.0 | Sucrose | Fructose, glucose |
| | Maltase | pH 5.8–6.2 | Maltose | Glucose |
| | Lactase | pH 5.4–6.0 | Lactose | Glucose, galactose |
| | Trehalase | | Trehalose | Glucose |
| | Phosphatase | pH 8.6 | Organic phosphates | Free phosphate |
| | Isomaltase or 1:6 glucosidase | | 1:6 glucosides | Glucose |
| | Polynucleotidase | | Nucleic acid | Nucleotides |
| | Nucleosidases (nucleoside phosphorylases) | | Purine or pyrimidine nucleosides | Purine or pyrimidine bases, pentose phosphate |

SOURCE: *Harper's Review of Biochemistry*, 19th Edition, 1983. D.W. Martin, P.A. Mayes and V.W. Rodwell; Maruzen Asian edition.

of the acid chyme passing into the duodenum from the stomach. This is an important function, since the enzymes of the pancreatic juice act optimally in an alkaline medium.

(2) Trypsin is formed from its precursor trypsinogen which hydrolyses the protein ingested to polypeptides and amino acids. The enzyme has its optimum pH at 8.0—9.7.

(3) Chymotrypsin, when formed from chymotrypsinogen has the action of curdling milk.

(4) The α-amylase converts all forms of starch rapidly into maltose.

(5) The pancreatic lipase converts neutral triglycerides to di-and monoglycerides and free fatty acids.

**Regulation of Pancreatic Secretion**

The exocrine secretory activities of the pancreas are controlled both hormonally and neurally. Two hormones, *secretin* and *cholecystokinin,* are released into the blood-stream from the mucosa of the duodenal and jejunal portions of the small intestine when gastric acid or chyme enters the intestine. Secretin which is released primarily in response to the presence of HCl, stimulates the release from the pancreas of a watery fluid that contains large amounts of bicarbonate ions. Secretin has little effect on the release of pancreatic enzymes.

*Cholecystokinin* (also known as pancreozymin), which is released principally in response to the presence of breakdown products of digestion protein of fats and carbohydrates in the duodenum mainly promotes the release of digestive enzymes from the pancreas—by circulating through blood. These two duodenal hormones also feed back to the stomach, as explained earlier, by decreasing secretion in the stomach and slowing the process of peristalsis.

Neurally, pancreatic secretion may be stimulated by way of the vagus nerves and the effect is mostly on enzymatic secretion. The response is specially evident during the cephalic and gastric phases of stomach secretion.

**3. The Liver and Biliary System**

The liver is the largest gland in the body. It is an important organ of intermediate metabolism. It has also an exocrine section, the bile, which is conveyed to the duodenum by the ducts of the liver, which convey bile from and within the liver to duodenum, and the gall bladder which stores and concentrates bile. All domestic animals except the horse have this gall bladder. Bile leaves the liver through the *hepatic duct,* which joins the *cystic duct* coming from the gall bladder to form the *common bile duct,* which then passes to the first part of the duodenum.

The composition and the role of bile will further be explained in connection with the digestion and absorption of lipids in non-ruminants in the later part of this chapter.

**Regulation of Bile secretion**

The rate of bile secretion is chemically, neurally and hormonally controlled.

Chemical substances that increase bile flow are called *Choleretics.* Bile salts present in the plasma as a result of enterohepatic circulation act as powerfull choleretics that stimulate bile flow.

Stimulation of the vagus nerves can also increase the rate of hepatic bile secretion.

In response to the presence of fat and protein breakdown products in the chyme, the hormone *Cholecystokinin* (CCK) previously known as *pancreozymin* is released from the duodenal mucosa which strongly stimulates gall bladder to contract. Secretin apart from its effect as stimulator for pancreatic bicarbonate also causes secretion of bile (not the rate of bile acid production).

**Table 129**

Gastrointestinal polypeptide hormones.*

| | Number of Amino Acid Residues | MW | Homologous Hormone | Cellular Location | Stimulus for Release | Actions as Gastrointestinal Hormones |
|---|---|---|---|---|---|---|
| **Established hormones** | | | | | | |
| Gastrin | 17 | 2100 | CCK(PZ) | G cells of antrum and duodenum, brain | Gastric distention and protein in the stomach | Stimulates acid and pepsin secretion; stimulates gastric mucosal growth; possibly stimulates lower esophageal sphincter. |
| Cholecystokinin (pancreozymin) (CCK[PZ]) | 33 | 3883 | Gastrin | Mucosa of entire small intestine, brain, islets, etc | Fat, protein, and their digestion products in the intestine | Stimulates gallbladder contraction; stimulates pancreatic enzyme secretion; stimulates pancreatic growth; inhibits gastric emptying. |
| Secretin | 27 | 3056 | Glucagon | Mucosa of duodenum and jejunum | Low pH in the duodenum; threshold pH 4.5 | Stimulates pancreatic and biliary $HCO_3^-$ secretion; augments action of CCK(PZ) on pancreatic enzyme secretion. |
| **Other hormones** | | | | | | |
| Gastric inhibitory polypeptide (GIP) | 43 | 5105 | Secretin, glucagon | Mucosa of duodenum and jejunum, brain | Glucose or fat in the duodenum | Stimulates release of insulin from pancreas; inhibits gastric $H^+$ secretion and gastric motility; antilipolytic. |
| Vasoactive intestinal polypeptide (VIP) | 28 | 3100 | Secretin | Mucosa of entire small intestine and colon, brain | ? | Inhibits gastric $H^+$ and pepsin secretion; stimulates pancreatic $HCO_3^-$ secretion and secretion from intestinal mucosa; inhibits gastric and gallbladder motility. |
| Motilin | 22 | 2700 | ? | Mucosa of duodenum and jejunum | Alkaline pH (8.2) in the duodenum | Stimulates gastric motility. |
| Enterogastrone | ? | ? | ? | Mucosa of small intestine | Fat in the intestine | Inhibits gastric $H^+$ secretion. |
| Entero-oxyntin (mediator of the "intestinal phase" of $H^+$ secretion) | ? | ? | ? | Mucosa of small intestine | Protein in the intestine | Stimulates gastric $H^+$ secretion. |
| Enteroglucagon | ? | 3500–7000 | Glucagon | Mucosa of small intestine | Glucose or fat in the intestine | Glycogenolysis. |
| Chymodenin | 43 | 4900 | ? | Mucosa of small intestine | Fat in the intestine | Specific stimulation of chymotrypsin secretion by the pancreas. |
| Bulbogastrone | ? | ? | ? | Duodenal bulb | Acid in the duodenal bulb | Inhibits gastric $H^+$ secretion. |

## Digestive Organs of Non-ruminants

The digestive organs of non-ruminants are much simpler. They differ from ruminant system mainly, in the structure of stomach and large intestine, and hence these two sections of the alimentary canal will be discussed here. The general description of other parts may be at present taken as more or less like ruminants.

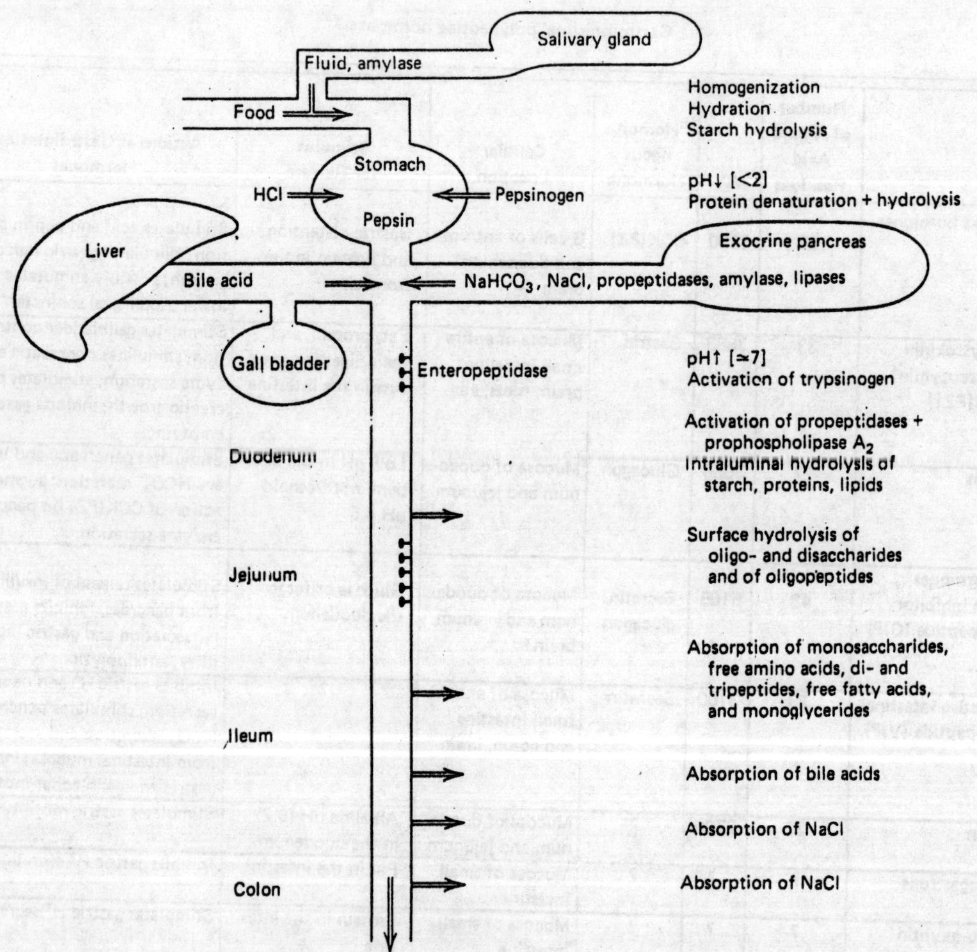


**Fig. 61** *Gastrointestinal organs and their functions.*

### The Non-ruminant stomach

The simple stomach is divided into three regions : *Cardiac, fundic* and *pyloric.* These vary considerably in size and shape between species. The fundic and pyloric regions are the principal centers of glandular activity.

The cardiac region is closest to the oesopageal region and contains the cardiac glands. They are mucous glands, and do not produce enzymes.

The body of the stomach is called the fundic region and contains the *fundic* or *gastric glands*. These are composed of three types of cells, (1) *body chief cells*, (2) *neck chief cells* and (3) *parietal cells*. Body chief cells are found in the body and deeper parts of the gastric

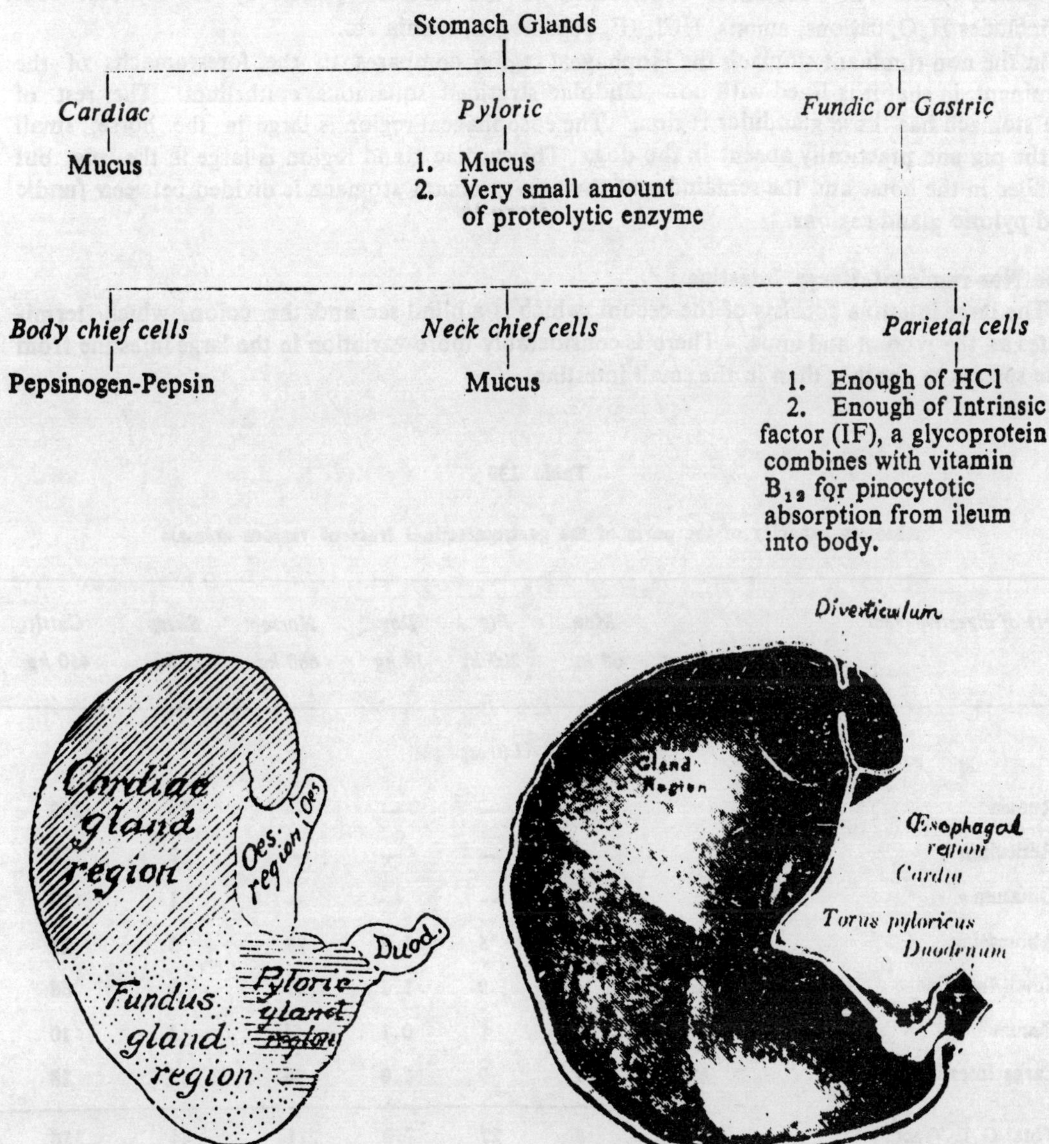


**Fig 62** Stomach of the pig

glands. They are enzyme producers and contain so called *zymogen granules* (substances from which gastric enzymes are derived), Neck chief cells line the gastric glands near their openings and are mucus secreting cells. Parietal or border cells produce HCl and "intrinsic factor".

The posterior part of the stomach is called the pyloric region and contains the pyloric glands. The products of their secretion are mucus and small amounts of proteolytic enzymes.

Gastric juice = All substances contributed to the stomach lumen by the mucosal cells. It includes $H_2O$, cations, anions, HCl, IF, pepsinogen, rennin etc.

In the non-ruminant stomach the esophageal region compares to the forestomachs of the ruminant, in that it is lined with non-glandular stratified squamous epithelium. The rest of the stomach has those glandular region. The eosophageal region is large in the horse, small in the pig and practically absent in the dog. The cardiac gland region is large in the pig but smaller in the horse and the remainder of the non-ruminant stomach is divided between fundic and pyloric gland regions.

**The Non-ruminant Large Intestine**

The large intestine consists of the cecum, which is a blind sac and the colon, which terminates as the rectum and anus. There is considerably more variation in the large intestine from one species to another than in the small intestine.

**Table 130**

**Absolute capacity of the parts of the gastrointestinal tract of various animals**

| *Parts of digestive tract* | | *Man* | *Pig* | *Dog* | *Horse* | *Sheep* | *Cattle* |
|---|---|---|---|---|---|---|---|
| | *Average body wt.* | *68 kg* | *200 kg* | *18 kg* | *680 kg* | *75 kg* | *450 kg* |
| | | *Capacity (Litres)* | | | | | |
| Rumen | | — | — | — | — | 23 | 202 |
| Reticulum | | — | — | — | — | 2 | 8 |
| Omasum | | — | — | — | — | 1 | 19 |
| Abomasum | | 1 | 8 | 4.3 | 18 | 3 | 23 |
| Small Intestine | | 4 | 9 | 1.6 | 53 | 9 | 66 |
| Cecum | | 0 | 1 | 0.1 | 44 | 1 | 10 |
| Large Intestine | | 1 | 9 | 1.0 | 96 | 5 | 28 |
| Total G.I. Tract | | 6 | 27 | 7.0 | 211 | 44 | 356 |

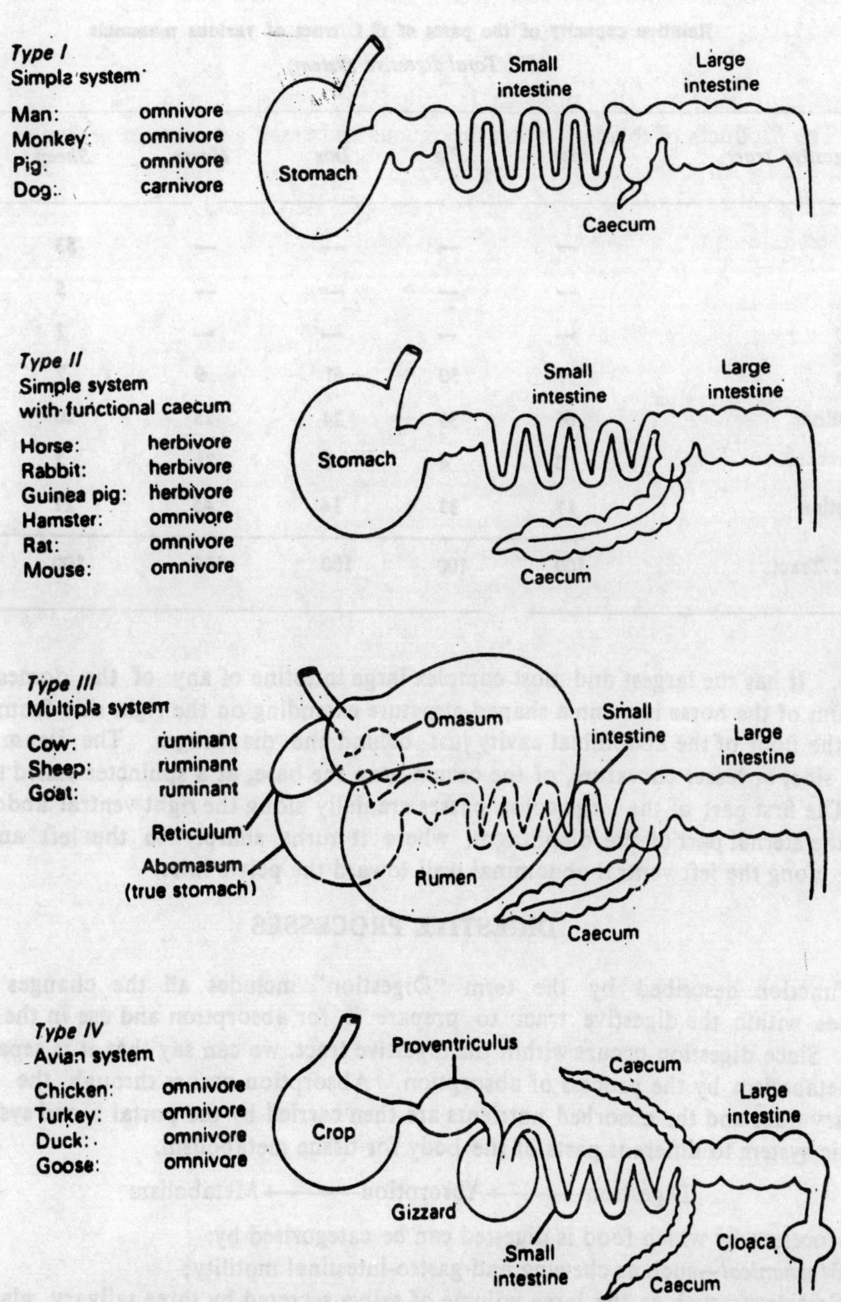
Type I
Simpla system
Man: omnivore
Monkey: omnivore
Pig: omnivore
Dog: carnivore
Stomach
Small intestine
Large intestine
Caecum
Type II
Simple system with functional caecum
Horse: herbivore
Rabbit: herbivore
Guinea pig: herbivore
Hamster: omnivore
Rat: omnivore
Mouse: omnivore
Stomach
Small intestine
Large intestine
Caecum
Type III
Multipla system
Cow: ruminant
Sheep: ruminant
Goat: ruminant
Reticulum
Abomasum (true stomach)
Omasum
Rumen
Small intestine
Large intestine
Caecum
Type IV
Avian system
Chicken: omnivore
Turkey: omnivore
Duck: omnivore
Goose: omnivore
Proventriculus
Crop
Gizzard
Caecum
Large intestine
Cloaca
Small intestine
Caecum

**Fig. 63** Classification of animals according to type of digestive system.

Table 131

**Relative capacity of the parts of G.I. tract of various mammals**
**(% *Total digestive system*)**

| *Parts of digestive tract* | *Man* | *Pig* | *Dog* | *Horse* | *Sheep* | *Cattle* |
|---|---|---|---|---|---|---|
| Rumen | — | — | — | — | 53 | 53 |
| Reticulum | — | — | — | — | 5 | 3 |
| Omasum | — | — | — | — | 2 | 5 |
| Abomasum | 17 | 30 | 61 | 9 | 7 | 6 |
| Small Intestine | 66 | 33 | 24 | 25 | 20 | 20 |
| Cecum | 0 | 4 | 1 | 21 | 2 | 2 |
| Large Intestine | 17 | 33 | 14 | 45 | 11 | 11 |
| Total G.I. Tract | 100 | 100 | 100 | 100 | 100 | 100 |

*Horse.* It has the largest and most complex large intestine of any of the domestic animals. The cecum of the horse is comma shaped structure extending on the right side from the pelvic inlet to the floor of the abdominal cavity just behind the diaphragm. The ileum enters the concave side, or lesser curvature, of the cecum near the base, at a sphincter called the *ileocecal valve.* The first part of the large colon passes cranially along the right ventral abdominal wall toward the sternal part of the diaphragm, where it turns sharply to the left and proceeds caudally along the left ventral abdominal wall toward the pelvic inlet.

## DIGESTIVE PROCESSES

The function described by the term "Digestion" includes all the changes which food undergoes within the digestive tract to prepare it for absorption and use in the body of an animal. Since digestion occurs within the digestive tract, we can say that it is separated from tissue metabolism by the process of absorption. Absorption occurs through the wall of the alimentary tract and the absorbed nutrients are then carried by the portal blood system and the lymphatic system to different parts of the body for tissue metabolism.

Digestion———→Absorption———→Metabolism

The processes by which food is digested can be categorised by:

(i) *Mechanical*—such as chewing and gastro-intestinal motility;

(ii) *Secretory*—such as the large volume of saliva secreted by three salivary glands of the mouth region; secretion of gastric juice by the stomach;

(iii) *Chemical*—such as hydrochloric acid in the true stomach; various digestive enzymes and the chemical activity of the rumen micro-organisms.

## DIGESTION AND ABSORPTION OF CARBOHYDRATES IN NON-RUMINANTS

When food is chewed, it is mixed with saliva, which contains the enzyme *ptyalin* (it is absent in the saliva of cat, dog, horse and all ruminant animals) secreted mainly by the parotid glands. The enzyme acts on the polysaccharides, starch and glycogen and certain of their derivatives, hydrolysing these to the disaccharide maltose, but the food remains in the mouth only for a short time and probably not more than 3 to 5 per cent of all the starches that are eaten will have become hydrolysed into maltose by the time the food is swallowed.

Even though food does not remain in mouth long enough for ptyalin to complete the breakdown of starches into maltose, the action of this enzyme continues long after the food has entered the stomach, until the contents are mixed well with stomach secretion. Then the activity of the salivary amylase is blocked by the acid of the gastric secretions. Nevertheless, before the food becomes completely mixed with the gastric secretions as much as 30 to 40 per cent of the starches will have been changed into maltose

Digestion of carbohydrates in the small intestine is mainly performed by the pancreatic secretion which like saliva, contains a large quantity of α-amylase capable of splitting starches into maltose and isomaltose. Also, a minute quantity of amylase is secreted in the intestinal juices. Therefore, immediately after the chyme empties from the stomach into the duodenum and mixes with pancreatic juice, the starches that have not already been split are digested by

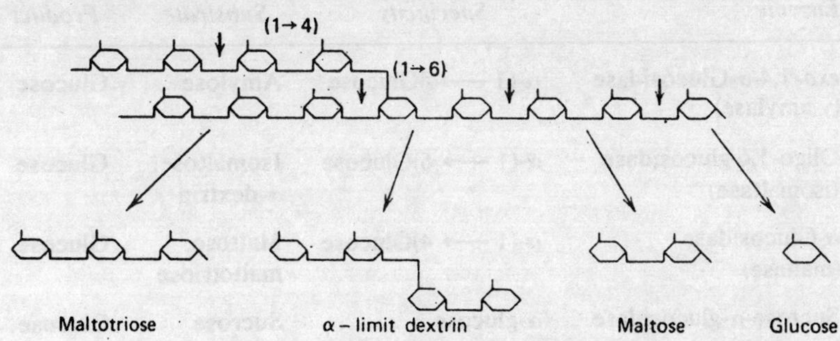


**Fig. 64** ***Digestion of amylopectin by salivary and pancreatic α-amylase.***

amylase. In general, the starches are almost totally converted into maltose and isomaltose before they have passed beyond jejunum. Indeed, pancreatic amylase is a more powerful enzyme than salivary amylase as the former can digest uncooked starch.

The epithelial cells of the small intestine contain four enzymes, *lactase*, *sucrase*, *maltase* and *isomaltase*, which are capable of splitting the disaccharides lactose, sucrose, maltose and isomaltose respectively, into their constituent monosaccharides. There is much reason to believe that these enzymes are located in the brush border of the cell lining, the lumen of the intestine and that the disaccharides are digested as they come in contact with this border. The digested products are then immediately absorbed into the portal blood. Lactose splits into a molecule of glucose and galactose. Sucrose spilts into a molecule of glucose and a molecule of fructose. Thus, the final products of carbohydrate digestion in non-ruminants are monosaccharides which are directly absorbed into the blood.

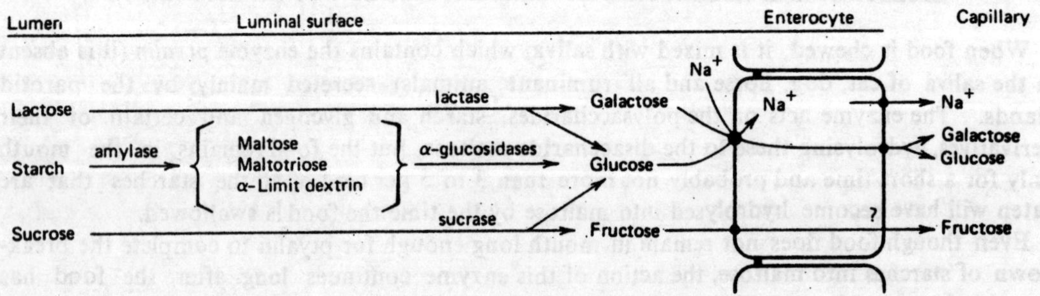


**Fig. 65** ***Digestion and absorption of carbohydrates.***

**Table 132**

**Di- and Oligosaccharidases of the Luminal Plasma Membrane in the Small Intestine**

| *Enzyme* | *Specificity* | *Natural Substrate* | *Product* |
|---|---|---|---|
| *exo*-1,4-α-Glucosidase (γ-amylase) | α-(1 ⟶4)Glucose | Amylose | Glucose |
| Oligo-1,6-glucosidase (isomaltase) | α-(1 ⟶ 6)Glucose | Isomaltose, α-dextrin | Glucose |
| α-Glucosidase (maltase) | α-(1 ⟶ 4)Glucose | Maltose, maltotriose | Glucose |
| Sucrose-α-glucosidase (sucrase) | α-glucose | Sucrose | Glucose, fructose |
| α,α-Trehalase | α-(1 ⟶ 1)Glucose | Trehalose | Glucose |
| β-Glucosidase | β-glucose | Glucosyl-ceramide | Glucose, ceramide |
| β-Galactosidase (lactase) | β-galactose | Lactose | Glucose, galactose |

SUGAR ABSORPTION. It has been known for over 60 years that the small intestine absorbs certain hexoses faster than others. If the rate of absorption of glucose is taken as 100, the absorption rate of certain other sugars are as follows (data from Cori, using the rat as experimental animal):

| | |
|---|---|
| Galactose—110 | Mannose—19 |
| Glucose—100 | Xylose—15 |
| Fructose—43 | Arabinose—9 |

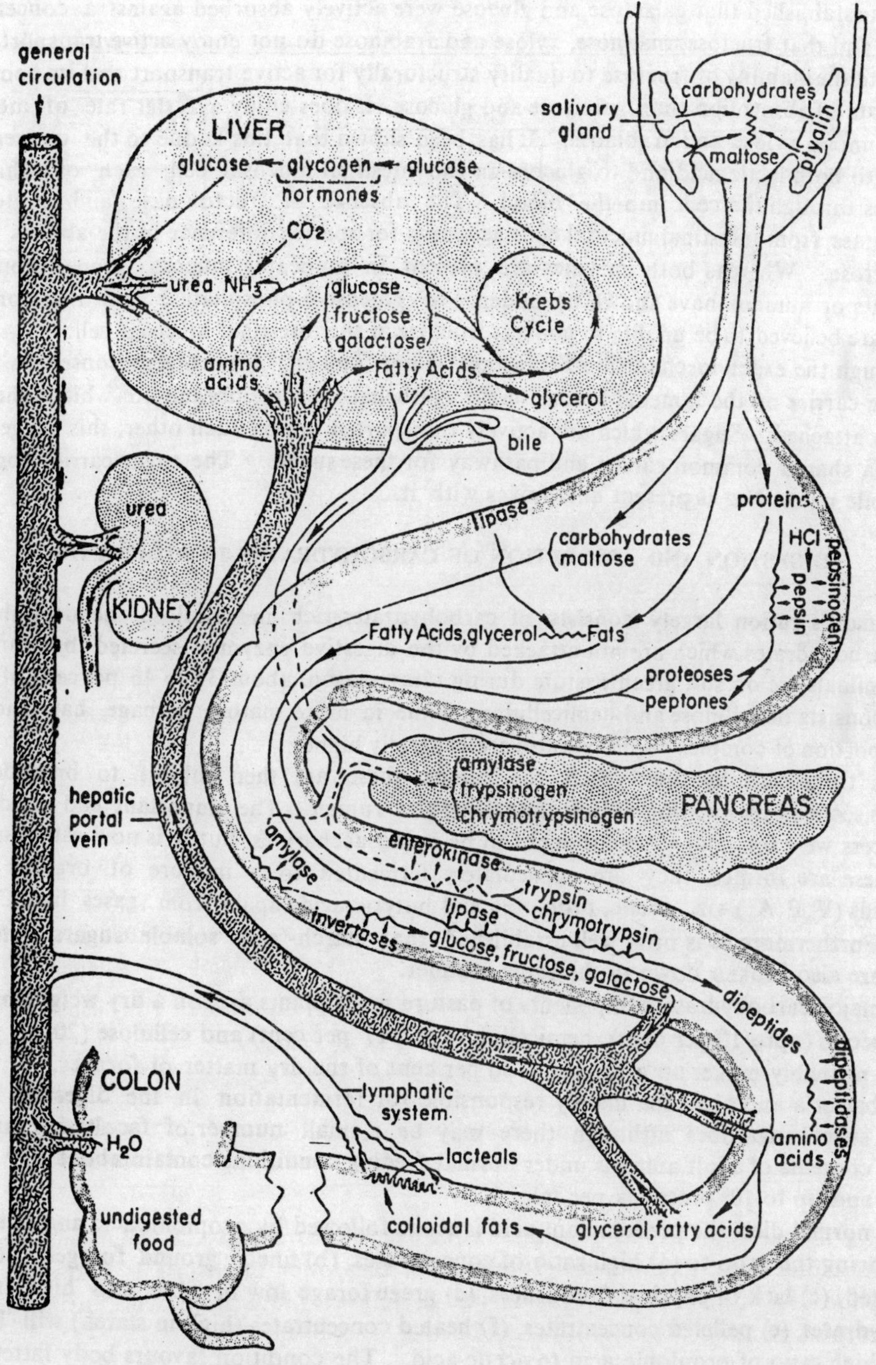


**Fig. 66** A partial history of food as it passes through the body in non-ruminants.

It was established that galactose and glucose were actively absorbed against a concentration gradient and that fructose, mannose, xylose and arabinose do not enjoy active transport.

Despite the inability of fructose to qualify structurally for active transport and its consequent slower rate of absorption than galactose and glucose, it does enjoy a faster rate of movement than mannose, xylose and arabinose. It has been shown that this is due to the conversion of fructose to both lactic acid and to glucose in the intestinal mucosal cell, each of which can then pass through the cell into the blood. The absence of fructokinase and/or glucose-6-phosphatase from intestinal mucosal cells accounts for species difference in the ability to convert fructose. Whereas both enzymes are present in guineapig mucosa, preparations from either rats or humans have shown no evidence of glucose-6-phosphatase and therefore these species are believed to be unable to convert fructose in the intestinal mucosal cell.

Although the exact mechanism of transport is not known, the current consensus is that there is a carrier on the lumenal border of the epithelial cell membrane to which the sugar becomes attached. Sugars which are actively transported inhibit each other; this suggests that there is a shared common carrier and pathway for these sugars. The sugar-carrier complex is not mobile unless $Na^+$ is present and moves with it.

## DIGESTION AND ABSORPTION OF CARBOHYDRATES IN RUMINANTS

Ruminant's ration largely consists of carbohydrates rich in cellulose, hemicellulose and other carbohydrates which are not attacked by the digestive enzymes secreted by ruminants. When animals are on soft green pasture during rainy season, about 35 to 46 per cent of the dry matter consists of cellulose and hemicellulose, while in more mature herbage, hay and straw, the proportion of complex carbohydrates are generally higher.

When these carbohydrates reach the rumen, these are then subject to breakdown by enzymes secreted by microorganisms inhabiting the rumen. The important end products of the process were for a long time thought to be monosaccharides, but it is now established that once these are formed they are immediately fermented to a mixture of organic volatile fatty acids (V.F.A.) viz., acetic, propionic and butyric acids apart from gases like $CO_2$ and $CH_4$. Furthermore it is now well established that starch and soluble sugars entering the rumen are also broken down in the same manner.

The major carbohydrate components of pasture grass plants are, on a dry weight basis consist of pectin (upto 10 per cent), hemicellulose (12–17 per cent) and cellulose (20–30 per cent). Protein probably makes up a further 1–30 per cent of the dry matter of forages.

The bacteria and protozoa mainly responsible for fermentation in the digestive tract are largely strict anaerobes although there may be a small number of facultative anaerobes. Rumen contents of adult animals under normal feeding conditions contain about $10^{11}$ bacteria per ml. and up to $10^6$ protozoa per ml.

With normal diets the predominant acid is acetic followed by propionic acid and butyric acid. By changing the ratio to (a) high ratio of concentrates, (b) finely ground forages, pelleted or unpelleted, (c) lack of physical fibrousness, (d) green forage low in fibre and high in soluble carbohydrates, (e) pelleted concentrates, (f) heated concentrates (high in starch) will bring relatively high ratio of propionic acid to acetic acid. The condition favours body fattening and lowers milk fat test. Propionic acid after reaching the liver is either oxidised or converted to glucose (ruminants can not utilise glucose for direct synthesis of fatty acids, mostly it is from

Table 133

**Types of common bacteria and protozoa involved in degradation of carbohydrate components of plants**

| *Organisms* | *Substrates* | *Products* |
|---|---|---|
| **A. Bacteria** | | |
| *Bacteroides succinogenes* | Cellulose, cellobiose, glucose, $CO_2$ | Succinate, acetate formate |
| *Ruminococcus* | Cellulose, cellubiose xylan, $CO_2$ | Succinate, lactate, acetate, ethanol, $H_2$ |
| *Butyrivibrio* | 10–12 carbohydrates, varying among strains including xylan | Butyrate, lactate, ethanol, formate, $CO_2$ and sometimes acetate and propionate. |
| *Eubacterium* | Glucose, cellobiose and 4–6 other sugars | Formate, lactate, acetate, butyrate, $CO_2$, $H_2$ |
| **B. Protozoa** | | |
| Holotrichs | | |
| *Isotricha prostoma I. intestinalis* | Many sugars bacteria. | Stored starch (?) $H_2$, $CO_2$, lactic, acetic, butyric |
| *Dasytricha ruminantium* | Many sugars, cellobiose | |
| Entodiniomorphs | | |
| *Entodinium spp.* | Starch, bacteria Protozoa (?) | Stored starch, $H_2$, $CO_2$, lactic, acetic and butyric acids |
| *Diplodinium spp.* | Starch, bacteria, cellulose, hemicellulose | |

acetic acid). Oxidation of acetic acid by liver tissue is less rapid, hence the body can utilise acetic acid either for milk formation or for other purposes. Butyric acid is mostly converted to ketone bodies in rumen epithelium and any butyric acid reaching the liver is also metabolised to ketone bodies or is oxidised in the TCA cycle after conversion to acetyl CoA.

The rate of gas production in the rumen is most rapid immediately after a meal and in the cow, may exceed 30 litres per hour. Carbon dioxide is produced partly as a byproduct of fermentation and partly by the reaction of organic acids with the bicarbonate present in the saliva. The major precursor of methane appears to be formic acid through carbon dioxide and hydrogen.

$$HCOOH \longrightarrow CO_2 + H_2$$

$$4H_2 + CO_2 \longrightarrow CH_4 + 2H_2O$$

About 4.5 g being formed for every 100 g. of carbohydrate digested by the ruminants.

The extent to which cellulose is digested in the rumen depends particularly on the degree of lignification of the plant material. Lignin is itself resistant to bacterial attack and appears to

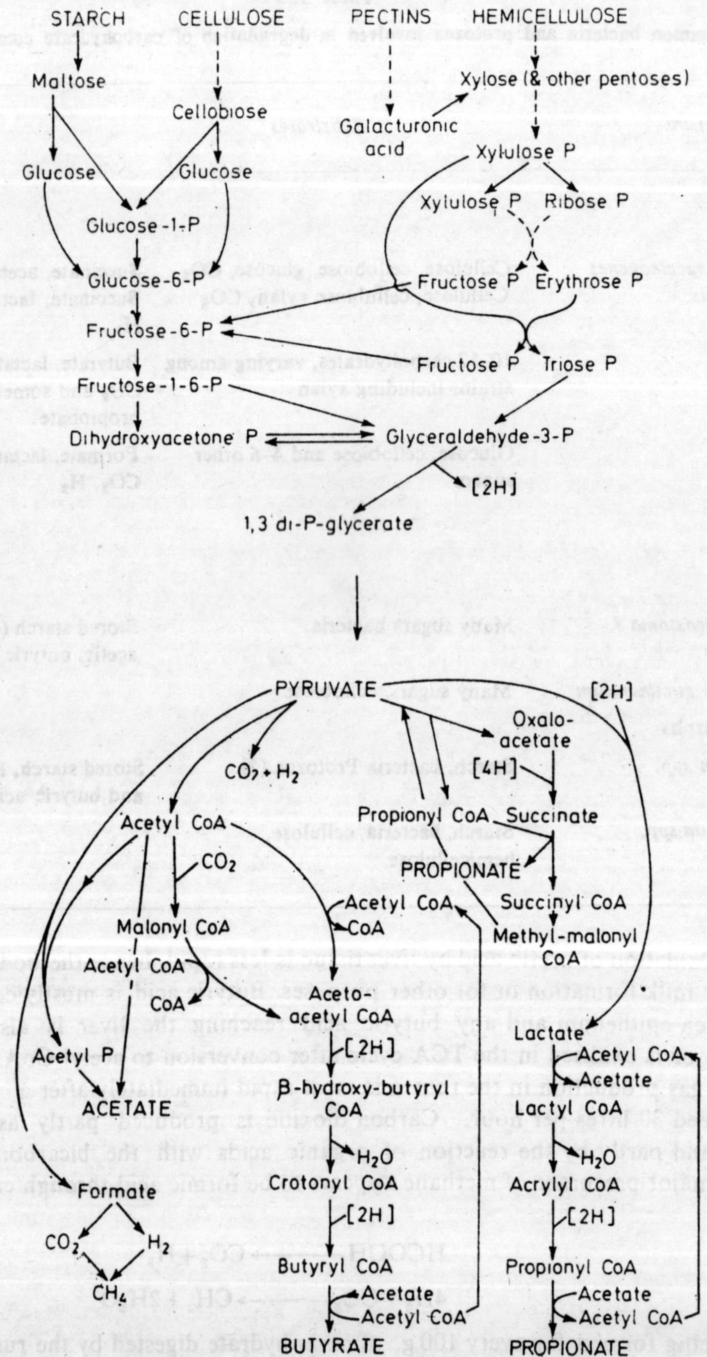


**Fig. 67:** *Pathway of carbohydrate metabolism in the rumen (adapted from Leng, 1970)*

hinder the breakdown of cellulose with which it is associated. Thus, in young pasture grass containing only 5 per cent lignin in the dry matter, 80 per cent of the cellulose may be digested but in older herbage with 12 per cent lignin the proportion of cellulose digested may be less than 50 per cent.

The fatty acids are absorbed into the portal blood system mainly through the rumen wall, but some of them may pass in the reticulum omasum or even in abomasum and from there the acids are absorbed. Small amounts of lactic acid may also be absorbed from the entire digestive tract. Present evidence indicates that little glucose is absorbed as such when the ration is very much rich in starch or other carbohydrates. Most of the gas produced is lost by erection; if gas accumulates it causes the condition known as bloat, in which the distention of the rumen may be so great that animal may die due to high pressure of the diaphragm towards heart.

## DIGESTION AND ABSORPTION OF PROTEINS IN NON-RUMINANTS

The dietary proteins are derived almost entirely from animal and vegetable portions of the diet You may recall that proteins are formed of long chains of amino acids bound together. The way each amino acid is linked with other amino acid is termed as *peptide linkage.* A typical linkage may be shown as follows:

Alanine + Leucine = Alanyleucine + Water

$$\underset{\text{(Alanine)}}{CH_3-CH(NH_2)-C(=O)-OH} + \underset{\text{(Leucine)}}{H-N(H)-CH(CH_2-CH_2-(CH_3)_2)-COOH} \longrightarrow \underset{\text{(Alanylleucine)}}{CH_3-CH(NH_2)-C(=O)-N(H)-CH(CH_2-CH_2-(CH_3)_2)-COOH} + \underset{\text{(Water)}}{H_2O}$$

The characteristics of each type of proteins are determined by the type of amino acids in the protein molecule and by the arrangement of these amino acids. When we talk of digestion of protein, we mean the sequential attack on protein by a series of hydrolytic enzymes and this renders the protein molecule into its unit structure, i.e., amino acids. We are to know the site of digestion of protein, what enzymes does that, in what condition it is performed, the way in which different enzymes attack the protein mole. This is what we will learn in protein digestion.

Digestion of protein starts in the stomach of the non-ruminants like man, pig, horse etc. In all non-ruminants, stomach functions as a reservoir, a place where a great mass of food may be received to be fed slowly into the intestine. It also possesses an important digestive function. The wall of the stomach is replete with glands. It has been estimated that there are about 350,000.000 such glands present in human stomach. The ducts of these gastric glands open into the stomach cavity.

Three types of cells have been described in the gastric gland. (1) Mucous neck cells secrete mucous; (2) chief cells secrete pepsin; (3) parietal cells liberate hydrochloric acid. Thus the gastric juice is composed of water, mucin, pepsin, hydrochloric acid and a gastric lipase.

Perhaps the most unusual component of the gastric secretion is the hydrochloric acid which has the following functions:

(a) Brings satisfactory pH for enzyme action
(b) Preliminary action on protein as swelling etc.
(c) Possibly renders some hydrolysis of protein
(d) Activates pepsinogen enzyme which after activation changes into active enzyme *Pepsin*
(e) Germicidal action on microbes
(f) Probably aids iron absorption.

The enzyme pepsin is capable of digesting any kind of protein of the diet. It does not complete the process of protein digestion all the way to amino acids but simply splits the polypeptide chain and converts protein into proteoses, peptones and some small polypeptide chains which then enters the small intestine.

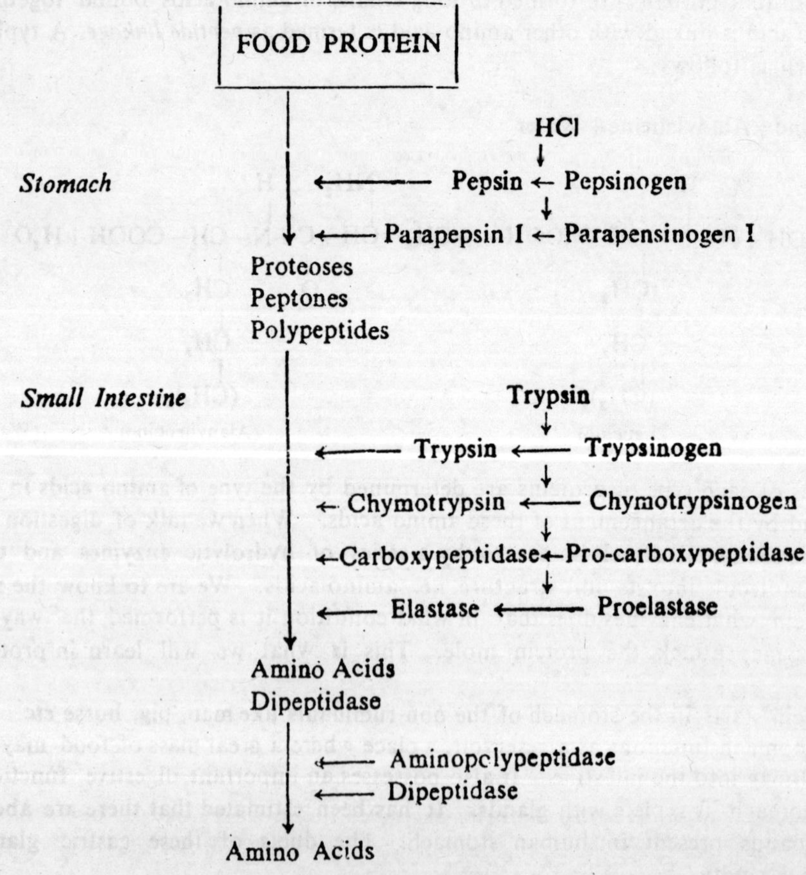


Note: In stomach, the main enzyme pepsin originates from pepsinogen and thus perapepsin I originates from parapepsinogen I and so on. In all cases, HCl cause these changes by activating the zymogen, i.e., precursor of these enzymes (here pepsinogen is the zymogen and pepsin is the active enzyme).

**In the small intestine all the zymogens are activated by trypsin.**

**Upon entering the small intestine these partial breakdown products of protein come in contact with pancreatic and bile secretion thereby in an alkaline environment the pancreatic enzymes complete the protein digestion.**

**The pancreatic juice contains apart from carbohydrate and fat digesting enzymes, inactive protein digesting enzymes (*trypsinogen*, *chymotrypsinogen*, and *procarboxypeptidases*). The juice is an aqueous, isotonic fluid with a high bicarbonate ion concentration and a basic pH (about 8.0). In the intestine trypsinogen is converted into active *trypsin* by a substance called**

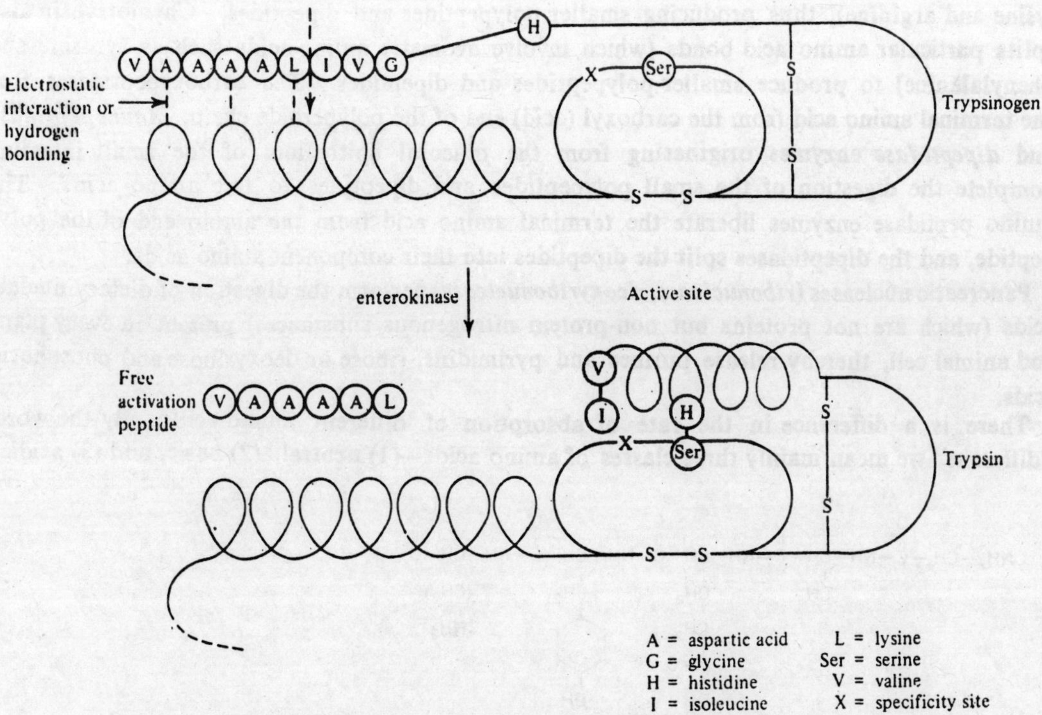


Fig. 68 Schematic representation of the structural changes involved in the activation of trypsinogen. Rupture of the lysyl–isoleucine bond in the N-terminal region (dashed arrow) leads to the liberation of the activation peptide and causes the newly formed N-terminal region of the polypeptide chain to assume a more nearly helical configuration. This in turn permits a histidine and serine side chain to come into juxtaposition so that these catalytic groups are properly aligned. The specificity site of the protein (X) is believed to be pre-existent in the zymogen molecule.

***enterokinase* from the intestinal mucosa and by previously formed trypsin. In turn trypsin is able to convert chymotrypsinogen to active *chymotrypsin*, and the procarboxypeptidases to active *carboxypeptidases*. These active enzymes continue the protein digestion begun in the stomach by pepsin. Trypsin splits bonds of the polypeptide chain next to basic amino acids (such as**

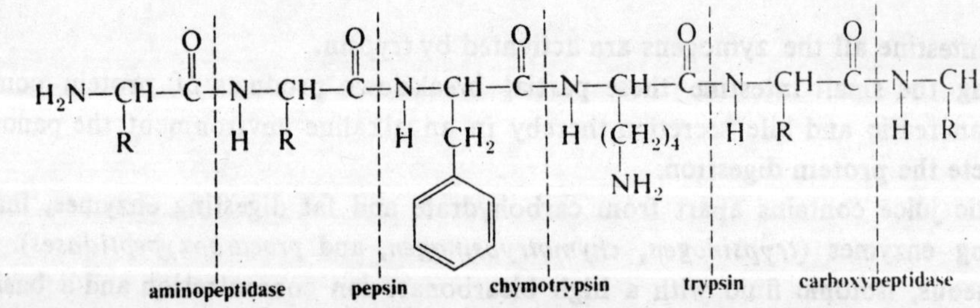

$$H_2N-CH(R)-CO \,|\, NH-CH(R)-CO \,|\, NH-CH(CH_2C_6H_5)-CO \,|\, NH-CH((CH_2)_4NH_2)-CO \,|\, NH-CH(R)-CO \,|\, NH-CH(R)-COOH$$

**aminopeptidase** **pepsin** **chymotrypsin** **trypsin** **carboxypeptidase**

Specificity of peptidase hydrolysis.

**lysine and arginine), thus producing smaller polypeptides and dipeptides. Chymotrypsin also splits particular amino acid bonds (which involve aromatic amino acids such as tyrosine and phenylalanine) to produce smaller polypeptides and dipeptides. The carboxypeptidases free the terminal amino acid from the carboxyl (acid) end of the polypeptide chain. *Aminopeptidase* and *dipeptidase* enzymes originating from the mucosal epithelium of the small intestine complete the digestion of the small polypeptides and dipeptides to free amino acids. The amino peptidase enzymes liberate the terminal amino acid from the amino end of the polypeptide, and the dipeptidases split the dipeptides into their component amino acids.**

**Pancreatic nucleases (*ribonuclease, deoxyribonuclease*) perform the digestion of dietary nucleic acids (which are not proteins but non-protein nitrogenous substances) present in every plant and animal cell, thereby release purines and pyrimidins, ribose or deoxyribose and phosphoric acids.**

**There is a difference in the rate of absorption of different amino acids. By the word "different" we mean mainly three classes of amino acids—(1) neutral, (2) basic, and (3) acidic.**

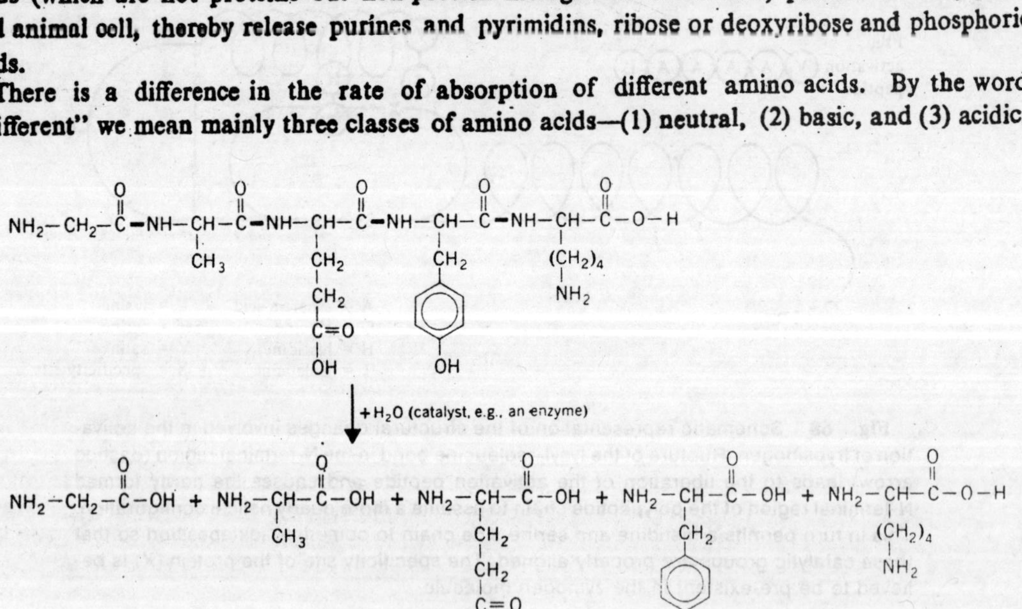

$$NH_2-CH_2-CO-NH-CH(CH_3)-CO-NH-CH(CH_2CH_2COOH)-CO-NH-CH(CH_2C_6H_4OH)-CO-NH-CH((CH_2)_4NH_2)-CO-O-H$$

$+H_2O$ (catalyst, e.g., an enzyme)

$$NH_2-CH_2-COOH + NH_2-CH(CH_3)-COOH + NH_2-CH(CH_2CH_2COOH)-COOH + NH_2-CH(CH_2C_6H_4OH)-COOH + NH_2-CH((CH_2)_4NH_2)-CO-O-H$$

Glycine Alanine Glutamic acid Tyrosine Lysine

**Fig. 69** The hydrolysis (or digestion) of a protein, illustrated here by the hydrolysis of a pentapeptide. Only peptide bonds break.

Table 134

The source and action of the proteolytic enzymes

| Enzyme | Source | Precursor | Activator | Action |
|---|---|---|---|---|
| *Endopeptidases (proteases)* | | | | |
| Pepsin | Stomach (chief cells) | Pepsinogen | $H^+$, pepsin | Hydrolyzes peptide bonds adjacent to aromatic amino acids and other bulky nonpolar residues |
| Trypsin | Pancreas | Trypsinogen | Enterokinase, trypsin | Hydrolyzes peptide bonds in which a dibasic acid (lysine or arginine) contributes the carboxyl group |
| Chymotrypsin | Pancreas | Chymotrypsinogen | Trypsin | Hydrolyzes peptide bonds in which an aromatic acid (or perhaps methionine) contributes the carboxyl group |
| *Exopeptidases* | | | | |
| Carboxypeptidase A | Pancreas | Procarboxypeptidase A | Trypsin | Hydrolyzes C-terminal aromatic residues |
| Carboxypeptidase B | Pancreas | Procarboxypeptidase B | Trypsin | Hydrolyzes C-terminal basic residues |
| Aminopeptidases | Intestine | | | Split off terminal amino acids with free $NH_2$ groups |
| Dipeptidases | Intestine | | | Split dipeptides to amino acids |

**You might have noticed the characteristics of 20 common amino acids which have previously been discussed. All neutral amino acids have one $-NH_2$ group but one $-COOH$ group, all basic have two or more $-NH_2$ groups but one $-COOH$ group, while acidic amino acids have two $-COOH$ groups with one $-NH_2$ group.**

**It has been postulated that these groups of acids utilise three different carrier systems (some unidentified compound which aids transferring amino acids from the lumen to the other side of the intestinal cell, imagined as a boat carrying passengers from one side of the canal to the other side).**

**Among all neutral amino acids, which utilises same carrier also has some competition, e.g., leucine is more inhibitor for glycine than others and so on. Like neutral, basic utilises a common carrier but they also have some competition among themselves, e.g., arginine or cystine inhibits lysine. Both neutral and basic amino acids are actively transported, i.e., they require extra energy for their transfer across the wall.**

**The absorption of acidic amino acids like glutamic and aspartic acid is still not entirely clear. It has been suggested that they are not actively transported since relatively small amounts were recoverable in the portal blood after feeding, but Wilson (1962) proposed that this might have been the result of transmission during absorption and that the system requires further investigation.**

**Some neutral acids compete with other basic or acidic acids but the reverse is not true.**

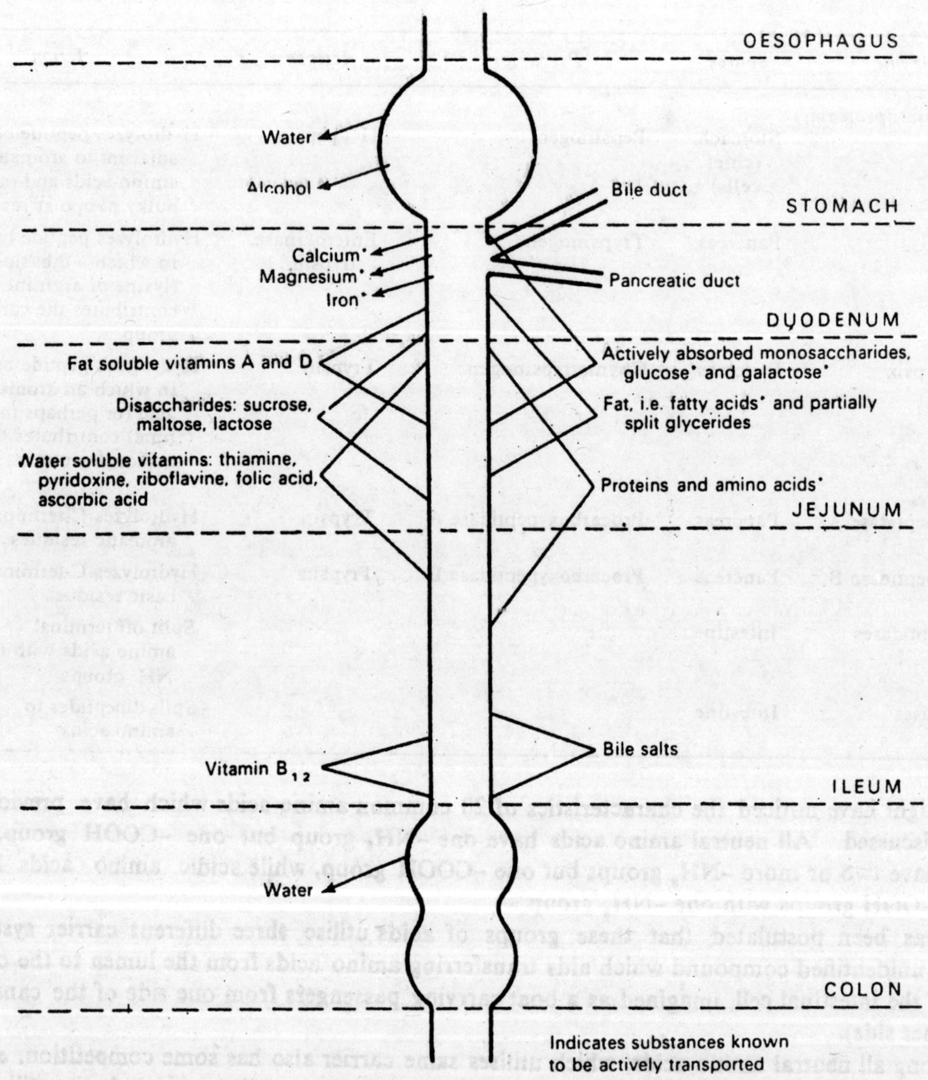


**Fig. 70 Site of absorption of foodstuffs in the Alimentary canal in non-ruminants.**

## DIGESTION AND METABOLISM OF PROTEINS AND NON-PROTEIN NITROGENOUS COMPOUNDS IN RUMEN

**Digestion and absorption of proteins in ruminants is unique by itself due to the presence of compound stomach. As early as 1938, it was recognised that microorganisms were responsible for proteolytic activity within the rumen, a fact subsequently confirmed by other workers.**

Unlike simple stomached animal, there is no free proteolytic enzyme source in the rumen wall. Microorganisms, which are normal inhabitants of the rumen, digest the dietary protein by releasing proteolytic enzymes which are mostly intracellular, associated with the cell wall fraction from which it is liberated. Thus all the proteins and non-protein nitrogenous compounds are hydrolysed by the rumen micro-organisms comprising both bacteria and protozoa.

**Proteolysis.** The bulk of the dietary nitrogen entering the rumen, under ordinary conditions of feeding, is in the form of protein. Since there is no extracellular, free proteolytic enzyme secreted by any part of the rumen, the feed proteins are entirely depended on rumen microbial enzyme for further simplification, i.e., proteolysis which involves at first conversion into free amino acids, followed by a change into ammonia. The rate of proteolysis being closely related to the solubility of the protein in the rumen fluid.

In spite of a strong proteolytic activity in the rumen, the amino acid concentration in the rumen fluid is low because of the presence of microbial deaminases, the activity of which increases with increasing protein content of the ration. The enzyme is directly responsible for the process of deamination. *Deamination* is the removal of the amino group from an amino acid which may be oxidative or non-oxidative as explained below:

**Oxidative Deamination.** A deamination reaction proceeds with a simultaneous oxidation as in the conversion of (1) an α-amino acid to an α-keto acid and (2) the amino group to ammonia. The reaction is catalysed by *amino acid oxidase*, an enzyme which contains the oxidising co-enzyme, FAD. The reduced coenzyme is further reoxidised by molecular oxygen (not by the respiratory chain) to form hydrogen peroxide ($H_2O_2$). Under the influence of *catalase*, $H_2O_2$ is then finally decomposed to water and oxygen.

1. $$\underset{\text{Alanine}}{\begin{matrix} CH_3 \\ | \\ CHNH_2 \\ | \\ COOH \end{matrix}} + FAD + H_2O \rightleftharpoons \underset{\text{Pyruvic acid}}{\begin{matrix} CH_3 \\ | \\ C=O \\ | \\ COOH \end{matrix}} + NH_3 + FADH_2$$

2. $$FADH_2 + O_2 \longrightarrow FAD + H_2O_2$$

3. $$H_2O_2 \xrightarrow{\textit{Catalase}} H_2O + 1/2O_2$$

**Non-oxidative Deamination.** By this process a significant contribution to the total ammonia production results in the rumen. The amino acids which are mostly affected are hydroxy amino acids, serine, threonine and homoserine. These acids are deaminated by a specific enzyme ***amino acid dehydrase***, which catalyse to form an intermediary unstable compound by primary dehydration. This unstable compound then reacts with water to produce an α-keto acid and ammonia as shown in page 261

The dietary nitrogenous compounds of the ruminants also contain appreciable amounts of nitrogenus materials other than the proteins (Fig. 72). Pasture plants, for example, contain about 20-30 per cent of their total nitrogen as non-protein nitrogen (NPN) and silage contains a much more greater proportion. Most of the compounds of the NPN fraction such as amino

$$HO-CH_2-CH(NH_2)-COOH \xrightarrow{-H_2O} CH_2=C(NH_2)-COOH$$

Serine

$$NH_3 + CH_3-\overset{O}{\overset{\|}{C}}-COOH \xleftarrow{+H_2O} CH_3-\underset{NH}{\underset{\|}{C}}-COOH$$

Ammonia + Pyruvic acid — Amino acid

acids and peptides, nucleic acids, nitrate and various amines are also rapidly degraded in the rumen and thus form mainly ammonia with less volatile fatty acids and other compounds. According to some recent studies, the volatile acids formed from the microbial breakdown of amino acids and other non-protein nitrogenous compounds appear to be $C_2$, $C_3$, $C_4$ and $C_5$ acids, the latter being principally branched chain acids which though absorbed, are probably not available for resynthesis of amino acids. This means that microbial action is wasteful of the carbon chains as well as of ammonia. Apart from NPN derived from natural feeds, various other ammonium compounds such as urea may be added to the diet of the ruminants upto a certain quantity. The strong *urease* activity of the rumen bacteria converts entire urea into ammonia. Thus for a wide variety of diets it appears that ammonia forms an important intermediate in the conversion of feed nitrogen to microbial nitrogen (Fig. 72).

Excessively high rates of ammonia production may result, particularly if large amounts of urea or proteins, such as casein, which are very soluble in rumen fluid, are eaten rapidly. The ingestion of rainy season grasses, particularly the leafy parts, also tends to cause rapid ammonia production in the rumen. If the rate of production exceeds the rate at which the bacteria can utilize the ammonia, the concentration of the ammonia in the rumen increases and thereby maximum amount will then be absorbed through portal blood and ultimately to liver where the excess ammonia will be converted into urea and finally excretion through urine will be the only way to get rid of ammonia toxicity. Thus excess ammonia production is definitely not only a great loss of the nitrogenous compounds of the feed material but also will exert an undue pressure on liver and kidney for the exit of the excess gas in the form of urea.

**Ammonia Production.** The preceding sections have shown that in the rumen, protein is rapidly hydrolyzed to amino acids which are then deaminated to ammonia. It has been further shown that more soluble proteins give rise to larger concentration of rumen ammonia. The rate of deamination is somewhat slower than proteolysis and thus immediately after feeding there may be increased concentration of amino acids and peptides in the rumen, but eventually, virtually all amino acids are deaminated; ammonia concentration being its maximum approximately three hours after feeding.

Ammonia may also be formed in the rumen from sources other than amino acids. Many proteins contain amide nitrogen and amidase activity is present in many proteolytic rumen bacteria. Many urea derivatives, for example, biuret and some amides such as guanidine acetate, are metabolised by rumen becteria but there is no evidence that ammonia is liberated. Rumen bacteria liberate ammonia from adenine, guanine, hypoxanthene, xanthene, uric acid,

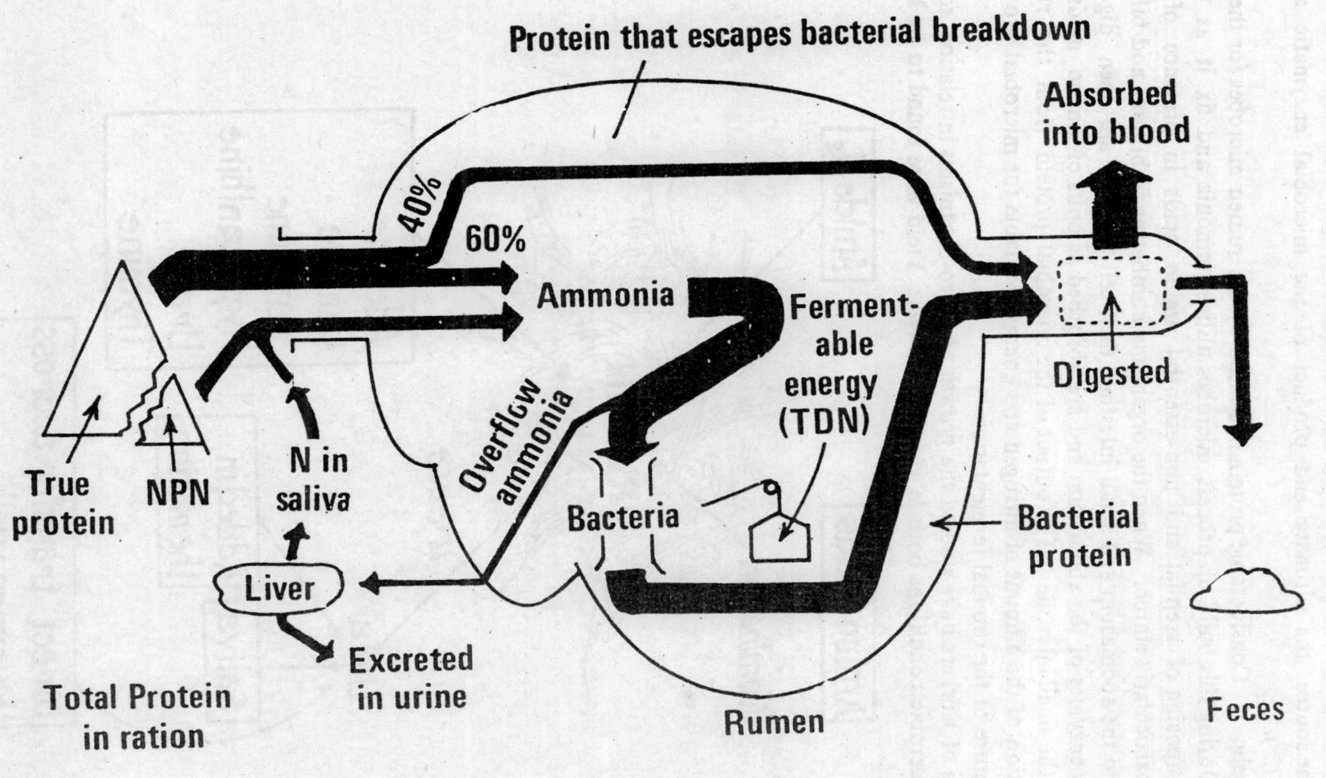


Fig. 71 Schematic summary of nitrogen utilization by the ruminant (adapted from Satter and Roffler, 1978).

uracil and thymine. Another source of ammonia in the rumen is urea from feed source or from saliva or back flow of ammonia through rumen wall directly inside the rumen. Whatsoever may be the source, the ultimate end product of the microbial enzymatic action is ammonia (Fig. 72).

**Fate of Ammonia.** 1. Considerable protein is utilised by the rumen microbes for their rapid proliferation. During this build up process, microbes utilise ammonia and fix it as excellent body protein composing of essential and non-essential amino acids in presence of soluble carbohydrates, particularly starch. When the organisms numbering in billions and billions are carried through to the abomasum and small intestine, their cell proteins are then digested by the usual gastric enzymes of the abomasum and are absorbed as units of amino acids mostly in the region of the small intestine. The output of the microbial protein from the rumen is, however, a function of the amount of nitrogen and energy available for microbial growth and the anaerobic nature of the ruminal fermentation.

Several groups of workers have studied the growth of micro-organisms in relation to energy supply under anaerobic conditions both *in vitro* and *in vivo*. Yield were found to be higher in

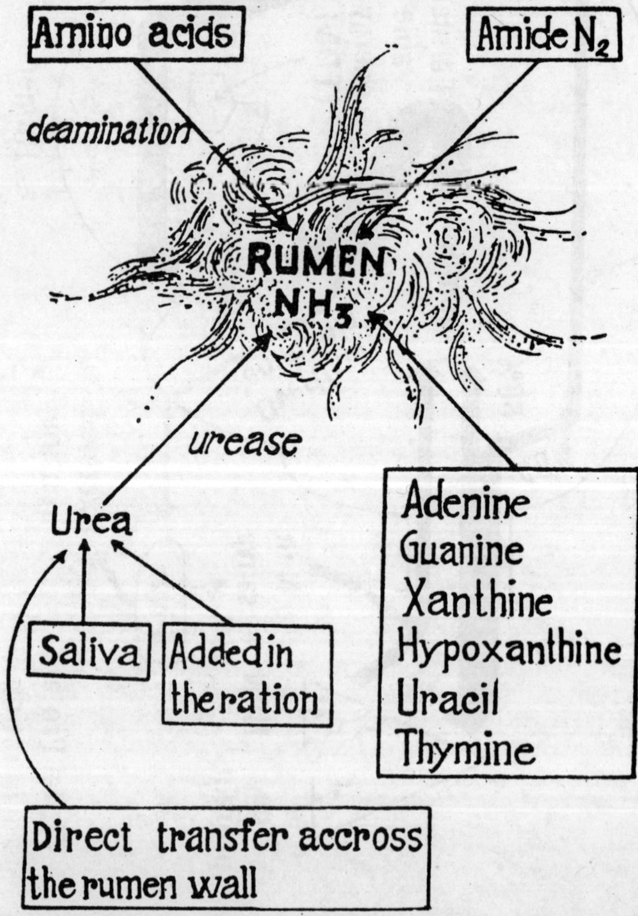


**Fig. 72** Schematic presentation of the possible ways and means of formation of $NH_3$ in rumen.

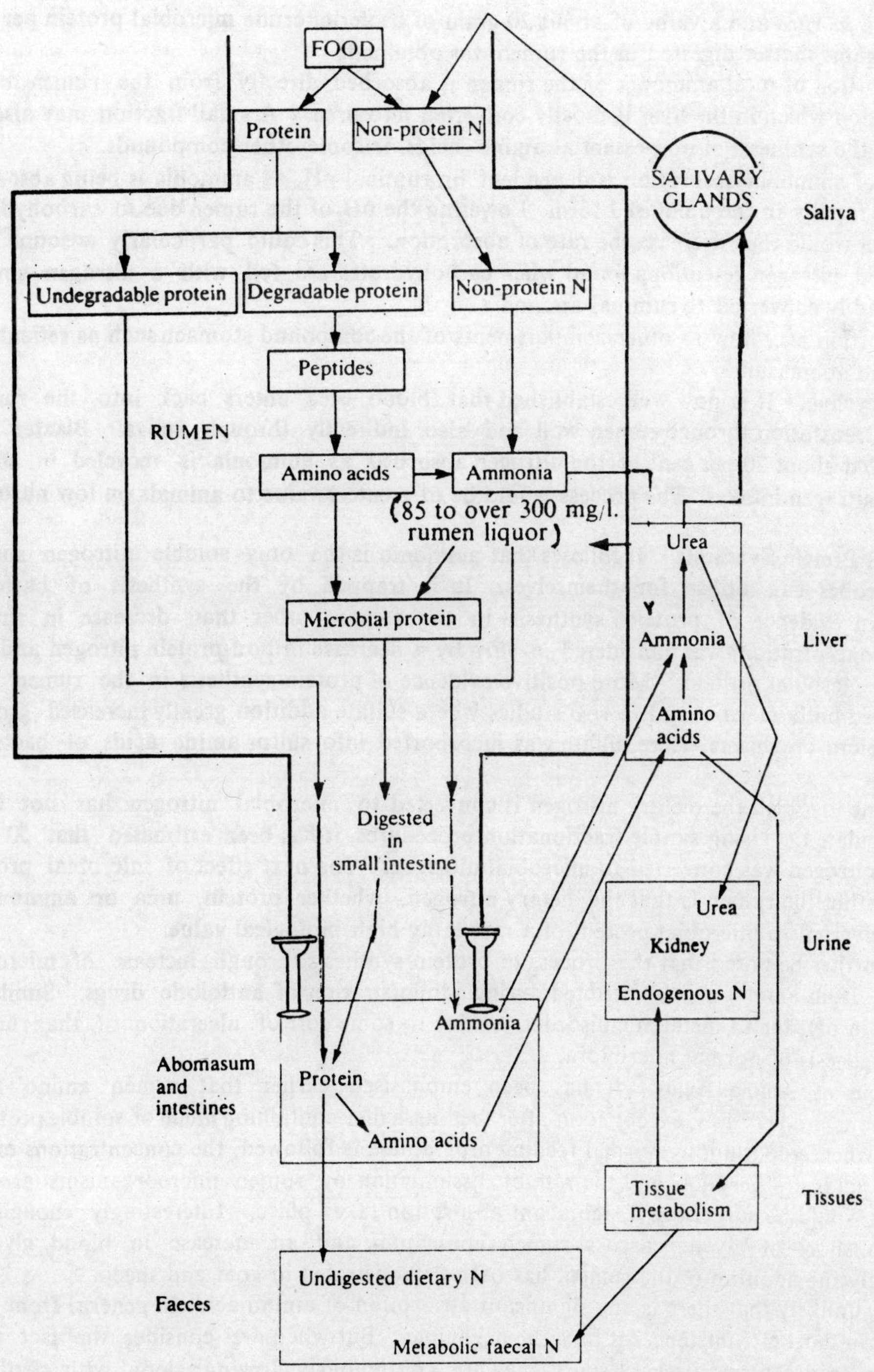


Fig. 73 A schematic representation of nitrogen metabolism in the ruminant.

*in vivo* than *in vitro* and a value of about 20 gram of bacterial crude microbial protein per 100 gram of organic matter digested in the rumen was obtained.

2. A portion of total ammonia of the rumen is absorbed directly from the rumen to the systemic blood which in the liver is mostly converted into urea. A small fraction may also be utilised for the synthesis of non-essential amino acids or some other compounds.

The rate of ammonia absorption is dependent on ruminal pH, as ammonia is being absorbed much more rapidly in the unionised form. Lowering the pH of the rumen due to carbohydrate fermentation would thus decrease the rate of absorption. This could particularly account for the increased, nitrogen retentions found when carbohydrates are fed with a nitrogen source which is readily converted to ruminal ammonia.

3. A portion may flow to other compartments of the compound stomach such as reticulum, omasum and abomasum.

**Urea Recycling.** It is now well established that blood urea enters back into the rumen directly by transfusion through rumen wall and also indirectly through saliva. Blaxter has estimated that about 20 per cent of the nitrogen absorbed as ammonia is recycled in sheep on normal nitrogen intakes. The process would be of greatest value to animals on low nitrogen intakes.

**Microbial Protein Synthesis.** It follows that ammonia is the only soluble nitrogen source which microbes can utilise for themselves. It is trapped by the synthesis of bacterial protein. An evidence of protein synthesis in the rumen, other than decrease in rumen ammonia concentration, was considered *in vitro* by a decrease in non-protein nitrogen and an increase in microbial protein. More positive evidence of protein synthesis in the rumen was demonstrated both *in vitro* and *in vivo* studies where sulfate addition greatly increased growth of rumen micro-organisms. Here sulfate was incorported into sulfur amino acids of bacterial protein.

The extent to which the dietary nitrogen is converted to microbial nitrogen has not been exactly calculated. Using simple fractionation procedures, it has been estimated that 50 per cent plant nitrogen was converted to microbial nitrogen. The next effect of microbial protein synthesis within the rumen is that the dietary nitrogen, whether protein, urea or ammonium salts, is converted to microbial protein of a resonably high biological value.

It may further be noted that the process of protein synthesis through increase of microbial population from ammonia is interrupted during administration of antibiotic drugs. Similarly, the change in pH due to metabolic disorders or due to some sort of ulceration of the rumen affects the genesis of normal microflora.

**Absorption of Amino Acids.** It has been emphasised earlier that rumen amino acid concentrations are very low, except soon after feeding a diet containing much of soluble protein. In general when a continuous normal feeding programme is followed, the concentrations of all free amino acids are very low and the rate of dissimilation by rumen microorganisms are so high that it would be surprising if significant absorption takes place. Interestingly enough, a definite transport of glycine across rumen epithelium and an increase in blood glycine following glycine addition to the rumen, has been demonstrated in goat and sheep.

It is very unlikely that there is any significant absorption of amino acids in general from the rumen and in most circumstances it must be negligible. But when we consider the fact that the life of microorganisms are very short, they are continuously flowing along with partially digested feeds through the gastro-intestinal tract in profuse amounts. In this way several billion dead microbes are brought to the abomasum, where like in monogastric animals, proteolytic enzymes are secreted by the numerous glands of abomasum, and as they reach the small intestine, pancreatic secretion and the proteolytic enzymes of the small intestine present in brush border of epithelial walls act on these dead microbes and bring about a complete protein digestion resulting in amino acids as end products. These amino acids are then absorbed through the microvilli of the small intestine for growth, tissue repair, maintenance of body protein reserves and for products like milk etc.

**Digestion of Nitrogenous Compounds in Small Intestine**

Apart from ammonia which is not present in any significant amount in the small intestine, the nitrogenous component entering the duodenum consists mainly of proteins which might have escaped digestion upto abomasum or may be the products resulted from partial digestion of protein in abomasum originally derived from microbial protein and partly from endogenous secretion into the abomasum (Fig. 73 ). Nucleic acids also account for an appreciable proportion of the nitrogen in the duodenal ingesta. In the small intestine the undigested protein is again digested to yield amino acids, some of which may also be deaminated to form ammonia. The ammonia thus formed is absorbed to the systemic blood through the epithelial lining of the small intestine. The enzymes required are secreted firstly by the pancreatic juices viz., trypsinogen, and chymotrypsinogen. The proteolytic enzyme *enterokinase* secreted by the unidentified cells of the duodenum catalyses the activation of trypsinogen to trypsin. Secondly several other proteolytic enzymes like amino *polypeptidase*, *dipeptidase* etc. are also released by the brush borders of the epithelial cells of the small intestine. These enzymes are responsible for final hydrolysis of the peptides into amino acids.

## USE OF UREA AS A PROTEIN REPLACER

J.K. Loosli and associates of Cornell University produced first time a specific evidence that microbial action in the rumen can synthesise all of the 10 essential amino acids required for rat growth from urea. Since than the non-protein nitrogen (NPN) utilisation is considered to be of great practical importance: several investigations have been made with ruminants receiving urea on the influence of rumen function, growth and nitrogen balance and now there are many excellent reviews on various aspects of NPN utilisation.

Several studies have shown that urea can replace satisfactorily upto about 30 per cent of the protein in practical rations for matured ruminants and lactating cows. This replacement has become possible since in practice, ruminants natural feed also contain about 30 per cent of the nitrogen as non-protein nitrogenous substances such as amino acids, amides and amines. This means that urea can be added at the rate of 3 per cent of the concentrate mixture. For the efficient utilisation of urea, simultaneous feeding of soluble carbohydrate, preferably of starch at the rate of 1 kg for every 100 gram of urea is a must for the sake of providing necessary energy requirement of the microbes.

**How Urea is Utilised by Ruminants?**

$$\text{Urea} \xrightarrow[\textit{from microbes}]{\textit{urease}} \text{ammonia } (NH_3) + CO_2 \qquad (1)$$

$$\text{Carbohydrate} \xrightarrow[\text{from rumen microbes}]{\text{enzymes}} \text{VFA + Keto acids} \qquad (2)$$

$$NH_3 + \text{Keto acids} \xrightarrow[\text{from microbes}]{\text{enzymes}} \text{amino acids} \qquad (3)$$

$$\text{Amino acids} \xrightarrow[\text{from microbes}]{\text{enzymes}} \text{microbial protein} \qquad (4)$$

$$\text{Microbial protein} \xrightarrow[\text{and small intestine}]{\text{enzymes in abomasum}} \text{free amino acids} \qquad (5)$$

Free amino acid absorbed from small intestine——→for building body protein in the ruminants (6)

Apart from these, addition of required amount of sulfur and phosphorus in the ration, containing urea will initiate in the synthesis of sulphur containing amino acids, so essential for the normal body components of the microbes.

Urea entering the rumen is rapidly hydrolysed by bacterial *urease* to ammonia which is then converted into amino acids (3) and finally utilised by the microbes for their synthetic activities.

Urea or any other NPN, if ever, has no technical advantage over feed protein of matured ruminants, and therefore, the use of such compounds has to be justified by economic considerations.

## DIGESTION AND ABSORPTION OF LIPIDS IN NON-RUMINANTS

In the usual diet, components of lipids comprises mostly of neutral fats but some phospholipid, cholesterol, cholesterol ester, and fat-soluble vitamins are also present. Almost no digestion of the lipid occurs in the mouth and stomach. Although gastric juice contains a lipase, there is very little hydrolysis of triglyceride in the lumen of the stomach because the pH optimum of *gastric lipase* ranges from 5.5 to 7.5 whereas the pH of the gastric contents is quite acidic.

However, as the amount of digestion in the stomach is mostly confined with the digestion of minute milk fat globules or of egg fat globules, the action is regarded as insignificant in adult animals.

The pre-requisite of fat digestion requires a drastic physical change which involves the conversion of water insoluble fats into partly water soluble forms. The principal steps include (1) emulsification, (2) enzymatic hydrolisation and formation of micelles, (3) absorption mostly in the forms of 2-monoacyl glycerides and free fatty acids in the intestinal epithelium, (4) resynthesis of fat molecules in the epithelium and finally (5) transportation of fat molecules mostly in the forms of chylomicrons and other low density lipoproteins through lymphatic channels.

Of the lipids being ingested are thus enter the duodenum from the stomach almost without any change at a slow rate (in human it is about 10 gm. of lipid per hour) along with the acid chyme. Mere presence of fats in the lumen of the duodenum stimulates the production of a digestive hormone, *Cholecystokinin* (previously termed as *pancreozymin*) which after originating from the duodenum reaches the gall bladder and pancreas through blood circulation and causes contraction of gall bladder as well as forces the pancreas to secrete pancreatic enzymes.

In the intestinal lumen under the influence of peristaltic action on the one hand and of the contact of bile, fat globules exist in the duodenum as a spherical coarse particle as emulsion in the semi-liquid intestinal contents. (*Emulsion is a colloidal dispersion of one liquid in another immiscible or partially miscible, liquid, size of the globules varies from* 300 – 1000 m $\mu$, *scatter light, require energy for formation.*)

As we know, the nonpolar compounds (compounds which have got no charge on the molecule) are insoluble in water and therefore no attraction for water molecules which are charged and thus polar, that is why fats are also totally insoluble in water. The important non-polar groups in lipids are primarily the hydrocarbon tails of the fatty acids, or fatty acyl moities, and the fused hydrocarbon rings of the steroids. However, lipids also contain polar groups, such as the three ester linkages of triacylglyceride, which because of a great mass of non-polar hydrocarbon, has lost the water soluble property. Similarly although cholesterol has got a polar carbinol group, it is highly insoluble in water because of the massive fused hydrocarbon ring. The carboxyl part of the bile salt is highly soluble in water, whereas rest of the fused hydrocarbon portion being non-polar is soluble in fats. These substances tend to occupy the inter-face between water and the non-polar lipid droplet and inhibit coalescence because of the repulsion forces of approaching polar groups. These stabilised dispersions of non-polar lipids in aqueous solutions are the *emulsions.*

***Bile***

The secretory and excretory activities of the liver continually produce bile which is stored in

**Table 135**

Composition of Hepatic and of Gall bladder bile
(Percent of Total bile)

| | Hepatic Bile (as secreted) | Bladder Bile |
|---|---|---|
| Water | 97.00 | 85.92 |
| Bile acid | 1.93 | 9.14 |
| Mucin and pigments | 0.53 | 2.98 |
| Cholesterol | 0.06 | 0.26 |
| Fatty acids and fats | 0.14 | 0.32 |
| Inorganic salts | 0.84 | 0.65 |
| pH | 7.1 – 7.3 | 6.9 – 7.7 |

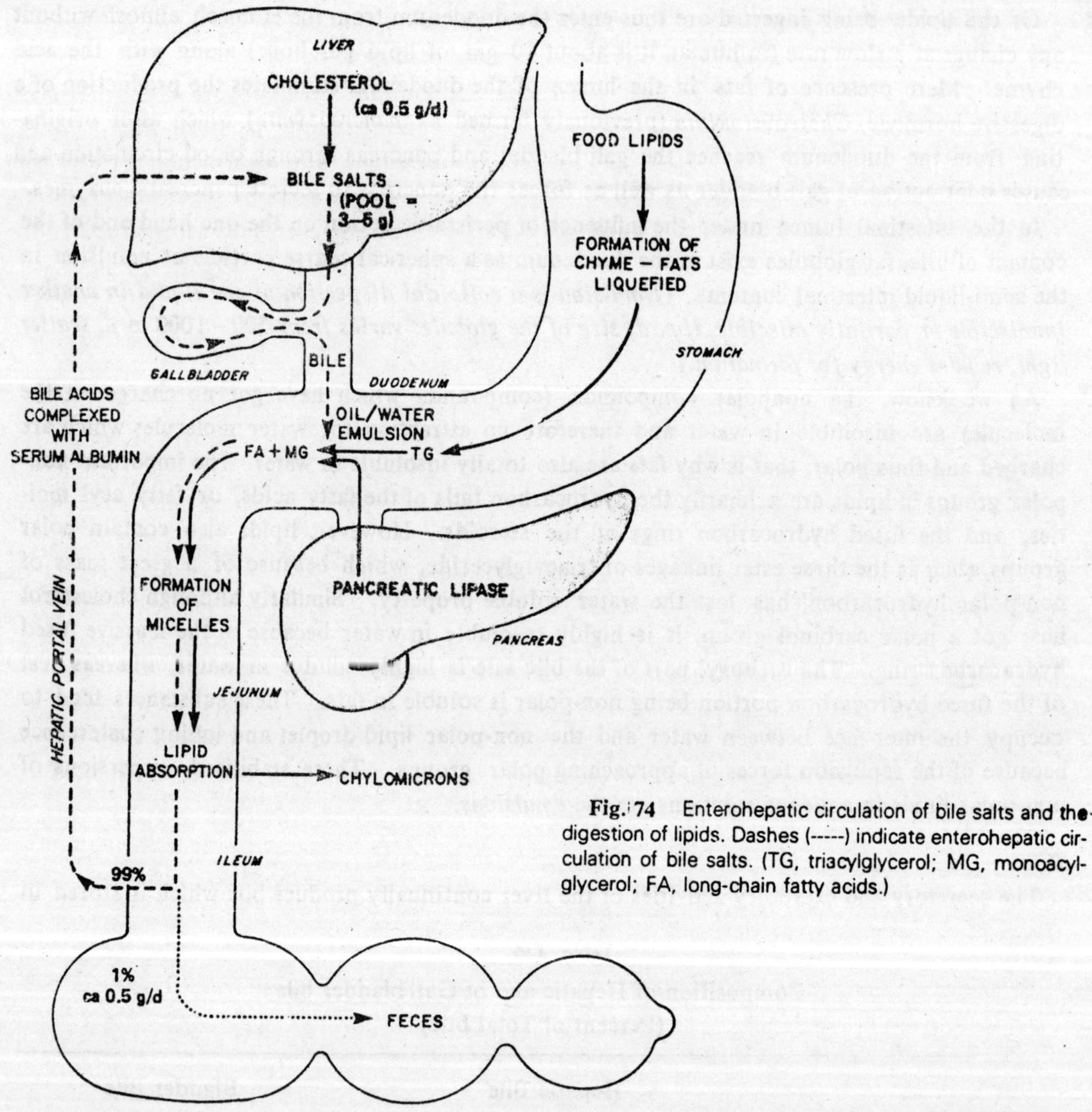


**Fig. 74** Enterohepatic circulation of bile salts and the digestion of lipids. Dashes (-----) indicate enterohepatic circulation of bile salts. (TG, triacylglycerol; MG, monoacylglycerol; FA, long-chain fatty acids.)

gall bladder and also travels directly through hepatic ducts. Bile from gall bladder is drained by the cystic duct, which joins with the hepatic duct to form the common bile duct.

Bile is an aqueous solution, greenish, or greenish yellow in colour with bitter taste. It contains no enzyme but electrolytes such as sodium and bicarbonate that contains bile salts. The acid side chains of the sodium salts are conjugated with taurine or glycine to form taurocholic or glycocholic acids, bile pigments, cholesterol, neutral fats and lecithin. Approximately 94 percent of the bile salts that are released into the duodenum are reabsorbed in the ileum. They may then be returned to the liver by the blood stream and resecreted. This cycle is known as *enterohepatic circulation.*

The rate of bile secretion is chemically, neurally and hormonally controlled. Chemical substances that increase bile flow are called *Choleretics.* Shortly after ingestion of a meal, the gall bladder contracts and bile is released into the duodenum. The contraction of the gall bladder is stimulated primarily by the hormone *Cholecystokinin*, which is released from the duodenal mucosa in response to the presence of fat and protein breakdown products in the chyme. Vagal stimulation may also cause weak contractions of the gall bladder.

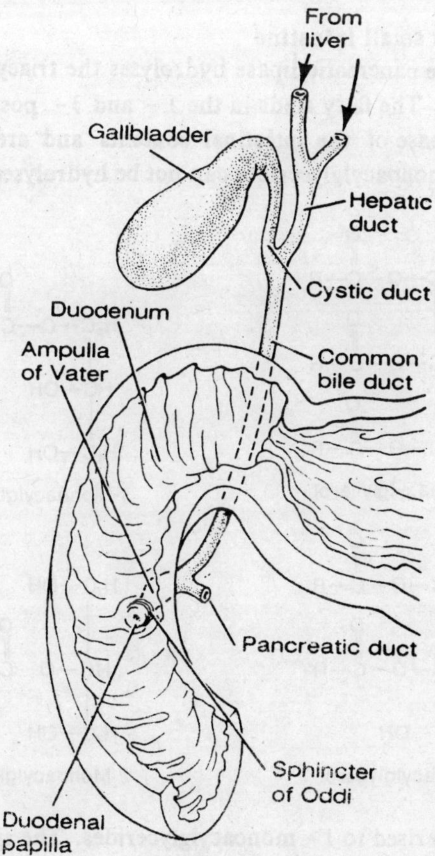


**Fig. 75** The gallbladder and bile ducts.

**Functions served by Bile**

1. It emulsifies fat thus by increasing number of fat globules it increases surface area to be acted upon by lypolytic enzymes.
2. Provides optimum pH for the enzymes to hydrolyse.
3. Activates the enzyme lipase.

4. An important vehicle of excretion. It removes many drugs, toxins, bile pigments and various inorganic substances such as copper, zinc and murcury.

**Pancreatic secretion**

Pancreas secrete its various digestive enzymes almost entirely by means of hormonal stimulation such as (1) *secretin*, which stimulates the production of watery fluid, high in bicarbonate but low in enzyme content & (2) *pancreozymin*, stimulates the production of secretion high in enzymes and low in bicarbonates.

So far lipid digestion is concerned, pancreatic lipase is the most significant contribution of pancreas.

**Hydrolysis of lipids in the small intestine**

In the presence of bile, the pancreatic lipase hydrolyses the triacylglyceride droplets into fatty acids and monoglycerides. The fatty acids in the 1 – and 3 – positions of the triacylglycerides project into the aqueous phase of the intestinal contents and are readily acted upon by the pancreatic lipase. The 2 – monoacylglycerides can not be hydrolysed as such, but may be broken

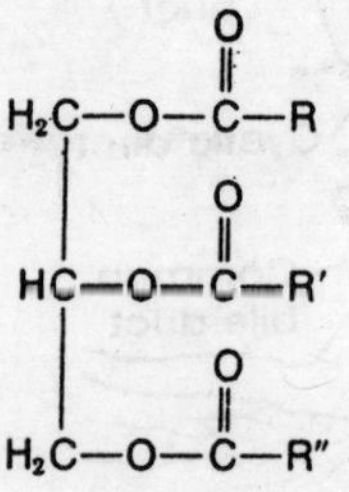

```
           O
           ‖
H2C—O—C—R
 |         O
 |         ‖
HC—O—C—R'
 |         O
 |         ‖
H2C—O—C—R"
```

Triacylglycerol

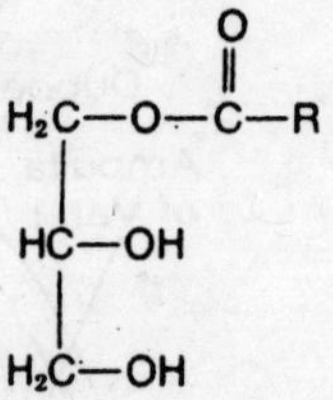

```
           O
           ‖
H2C—O—C—R
 |
HC—OH
 |
H2C—OH
```

1-Monoacylglycerol

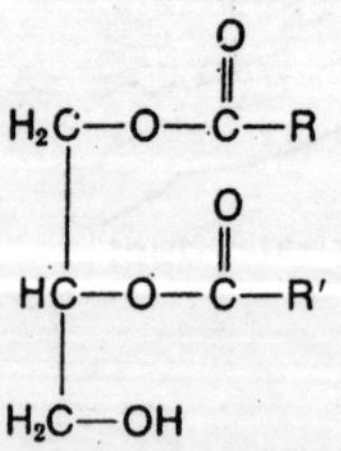

```
           O
           ‖
H2C—O—C—R
 |         O
 |         ‖
HC—O—C—R'
 |
H2C—OH
```

Diacylglycerol

```
H2C—OH
 |         O
 |         ‖
HC—O—C—R
 |
H2C—OH
```

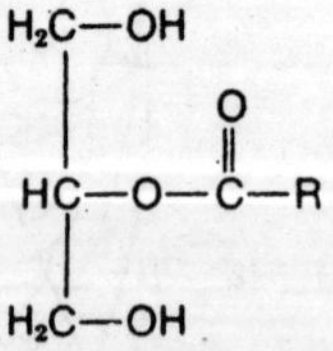

2-Monoacylglycerol

down only if they are isomerised to 1 – monoacylglycerides. The specificity of *pancreatic lipase* for the primary ester linkages of glycerides is not altered by the degree of unsaturation or chain length of the fatty acids involved. Using isotopically-labelled monoglycerides, it has been shown that unhydrolised monoacylglycerides are absorbed intact. 50-78% of the dietary triacylglyceride molecules are hydrolised to 2 – monoacylglycerides and absorbed in this form. A portion of the released monoacylglycerides and the unsaturated fatty acids aid in the formation and stabilisation of smaller emulsion droplets while most of the monoacylglycerides and unsaturated fatty acids, together with the conjugated bile salts, sponteniously form *mixed micelles*. It is estimated that each emulsion particle gives rise to nearly 1 million micelles.

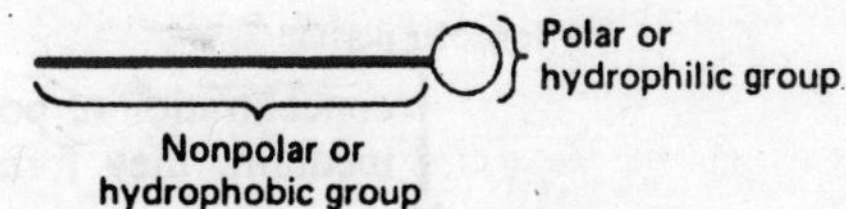


NONPOLAR PHASE — POLAR PHASE

$$CH_3CH_2CH_2CH_2CH_2CH_2CH_2CH_2CH_2CH_2CH_2CH_2CH_2CH_2CH_2CH_2CH_2{-}C{\begin{smallmatrix}{=}O\\ {-}O^{-}Na^{+}\end{smallmatrix}}$$

Hydrophobic (Lipophilic) — Hydrophilic (Lipophobic)

Sodium stearate

**Polar group in the water phase and the nonpolar group in the oil phase.**

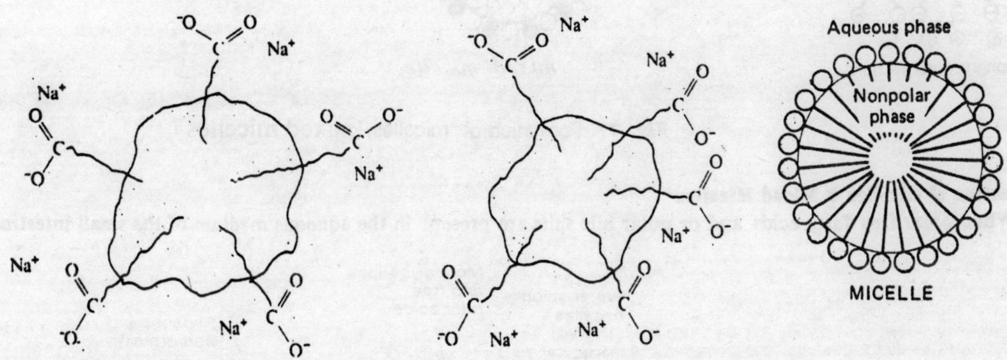


Two micelles will not coalesce because of the repulsions between their surrounding carboxylate groups.



(a) The formation of a thin film (a monolayer) on the surface of water. (b) A schematic representation.

**Fig. 76**

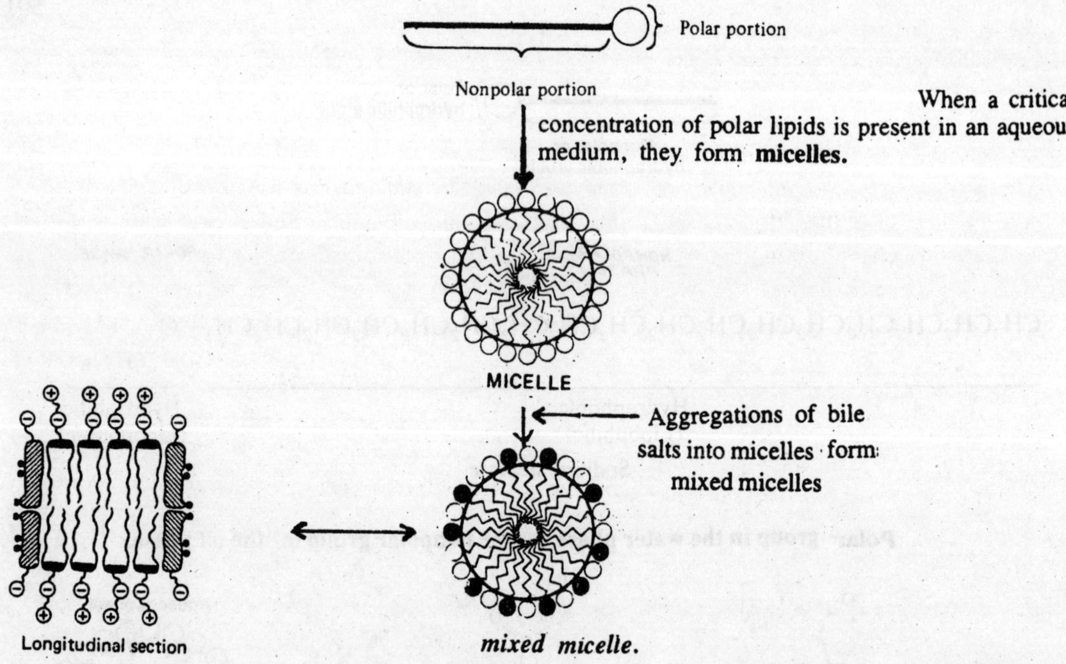


**Fig. 77** Formation of micelles, mixed micelles

**Formation of Micelles & Mixed Micelles**

**When polar free fatty acids and or polar bile salts are present in the aqueous medium of the small intestine,**

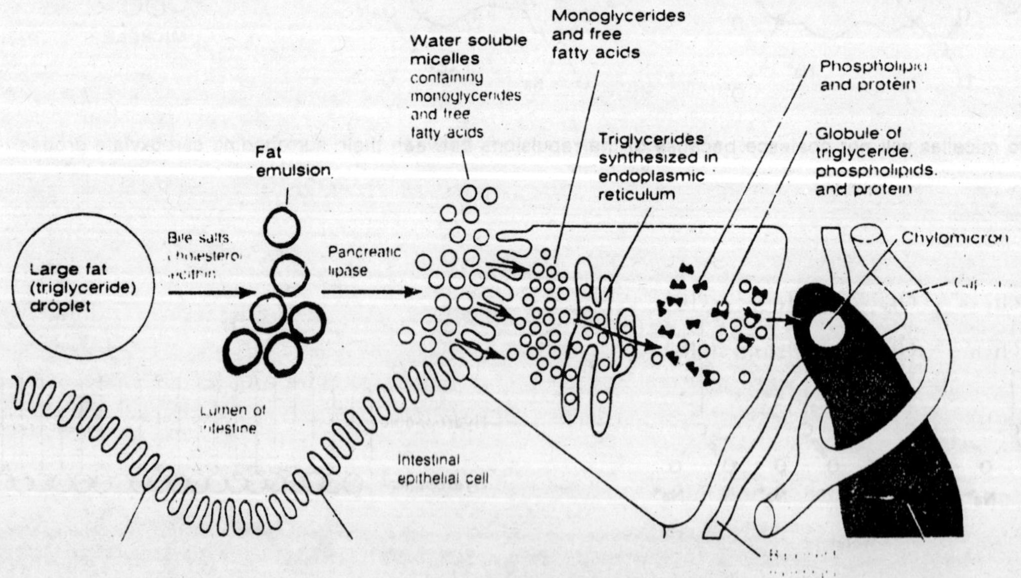


Fig. 78 Processes of fat digestion, absorption and chylomicron formation.

these will dissolve into small extent monomerically in water. When larger quantities of these polar compounds (20-50 bile salt molecules) are introduced at a characteristic concentration known as *critical miceller concentration* (CMC), they will form *micelles* of the size between 30 to 100 Å in diameter. Upon incorporation of some other polar lipids, the same micelles become *mixed micelles*.

These tiny mixed micelles become highly dispersed in the aqueous medium of the intestinal lumen. They solubilise the non-polar fatty acids such as palmitic and stearic acids. In this form the fatty acids and the monoglycerides are readily brought into contact with the microvilli. Each intestinal epithelial cell contains approximately 1000 microvilli which increase the surface area of the intestinal epithelial membrane by 15 to 25 fold. Monoacylglyceride and fatty acids

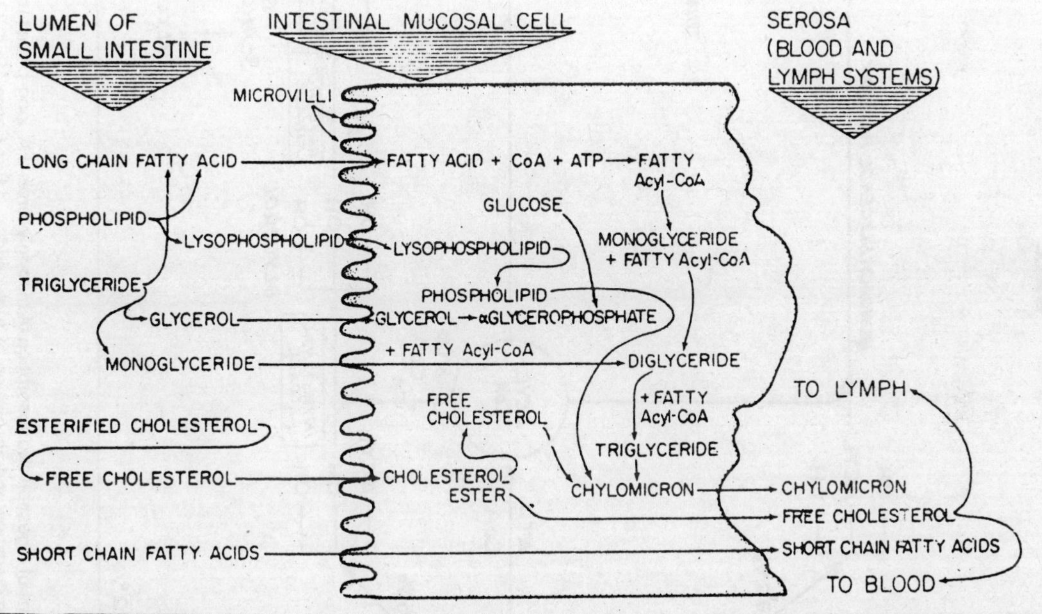


**Fig. 79** Schematic diagram of the major conversions that occur in transport of lipids across the intestinal mucosal cell during absorption.

enter the epithelial cells probably by simple diffusion. The bile salt micelles return to the intestinal lumen and are continuously re-utilised for subsequent micell formation. Ultimately, bile salts are absorbed in the ileum as part of the enterohepatic circulation process.

Within the intestinal epithelial cells, many of the monoglycerides are further digested to glycerol and fatty acids by the *lipase* of the epithelial cells. Within the endoplasmic reticulum of the epithelial cells, the free fatty acids are combined with newly synthesised glycerol and form various types of triacylglycerides. In addition the epithelial cells synthesise phospholipids and proteins.

Small globules of triacylglycerides, phospholipids, and protein (together with some free fatty acids and absorbed cholesterol) leave the epithelial cells and enter the lacteals of the lymphatic system as minute droplets known as *Chylomicrons* or very low density lipoprotein (VLDL)

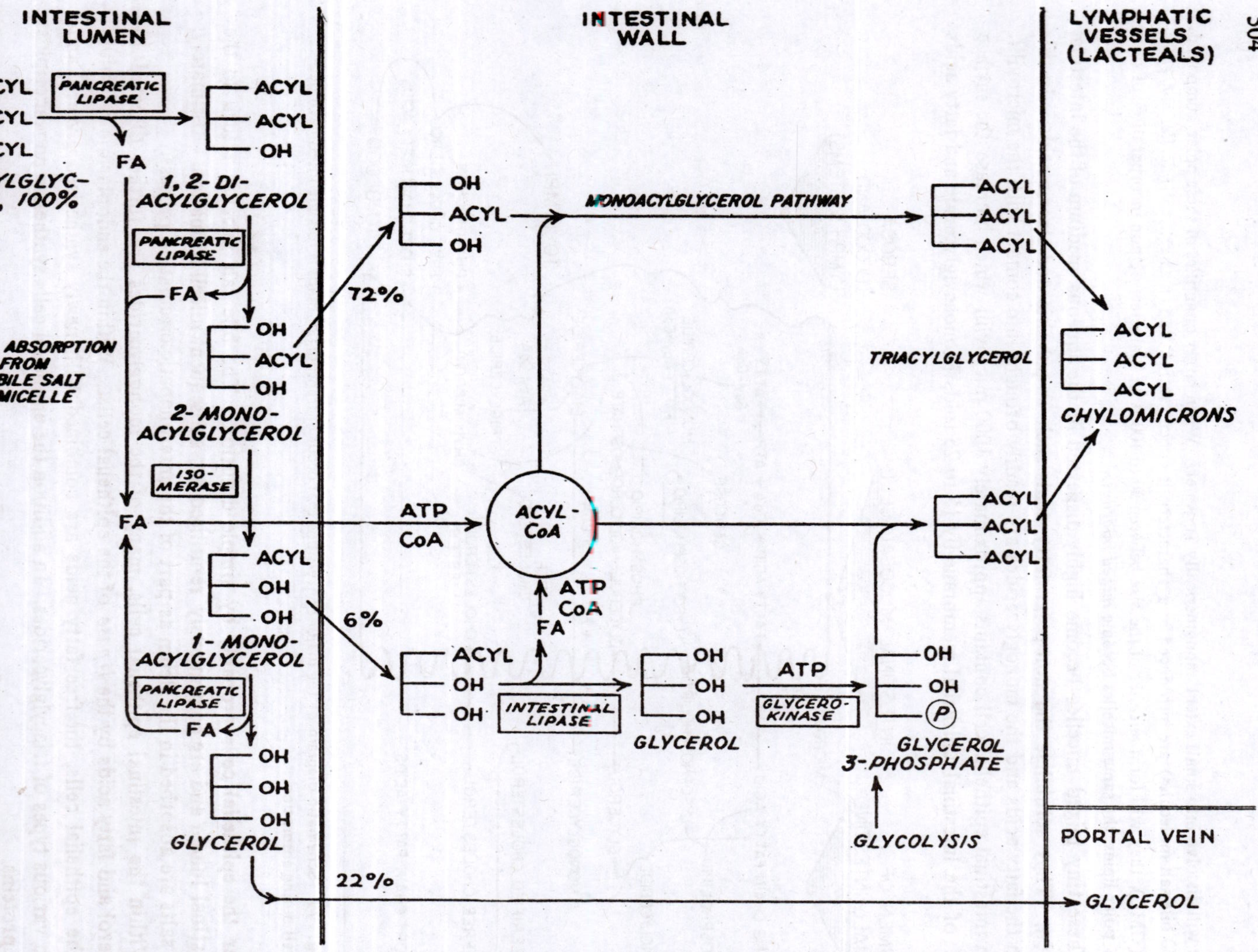


**Fig. 80** Chemical mechanisms of digestion and absorption of triacylglycerols. FA, long-chain fatty acid. (Modified from Mattson FH, Volpenheim RA: The digestion and absorption of triglycerides. *J Biol Chem* 1964;239:2772.)

particles. The composition of these and other lipid transport particles are shown in Table 79. While free glycerol (about 22-50 percent) by virtue of being soluble in water, is easily absorbed into the portal blood system and carried to the liver. Similarly unesterified fatty acids, shorter than 10-12 carbons are also directly absorbed into the portal vein and carried to the liver.

## DIGESTION AND ABSORPTION OF LIPIDS IN RUMINANTS

Until recently, little was known about the metabolism of lipids in ruminants. It is however recognised that this group of animal differed from other mammals and in particular from other herbivores in that (1) the depot fat of ruminant animals contain high levels of stearic and oleic acids, (2) presence of branched chain and odd numbered fatty acids in tissues and milk of ruminants, (3) dietary unsaturated fatty acids known to be readily assimilated into their depot fats by non-ruminants did not appear to be similarly incorporated into ruminant tissue lipids.

These observations tended to imply that the endogenous metabolism of fatty acids in ruminants differ in some fundamental ways from that in other mammals. However, when one considers that it had been known for sometime that carbohydrates and proteins are subjected to drastic bacterial fermentative changes in the highly modified stomach of the ruminants, it is perhaps a little surprising that only within the last decade or so the effects of the rumen bateria and protozoa on ingested lipids have been extensively investigated. These investigations have indicated that the aforementioned peculiar features of ruminant lipid composition are associated with the assimilation of the products of microbial modification of dietary lipids.

### DIGESTION OF LIPIDS IN THE RUMEN

**Dietary Lipids**

The diet of the grazing ruminant animal usually consists of pasture grasses and legumes which may also be consumed in a preserved form like hay or silage at the time of fodder scarcity or when the animals are housed indoors. In addition, ruminant animals are often given dietary supplements of cereals, oil cakes or meals, usually referred to as 'concentrates'. The lipid content of forage crops is low (5-10 g lipid per 100 g dry plant tissue). A grazing cow of 550 kg live weight consumes about 15 kg of forage dry matter per day and thereby ingests between 750 and 1500 g lipid per day.

The lipids of forage plants are normally concentrated in the leaf chloroplast which contains about 22 g lipid per 100 g dry tissue and consist mainly of glycosyl-diacylglycerols and phospholipids. Linolenic acid (53 per cent), linoleic acid (13 per cent) and oleic acid (10 per cent) together account for a high proportion of the total fatty acids of forage crops. In hay and silage although some changes occur during drying and ensiling, the lipids are similar in composition to those of fresh grass.

**The Sources and Composition of Lipids in the Rumen**

In cows given a diet of hay, for example, the concentration of total lipids in the contents of the rumen remains relatively constant during the day and amounts to about 500 mg per 100 g fresh material; approximately 80 per cent of this lipid is associated with feed particles, 16 per cent with protozoa and 4 per cent with bacteria.

*Lipids associated with feed particles.* The acyl ester bonds of dietary lipids are rapidly hydrolysed in the rumen and the resulting unesterified acids are adsorbed (deposition on the surface) on to a particular matter. Since most of the vegetable lipids are unsaturated and moreover after hydrolysis these fatty acids become unesterified, they are all exposed to rapid biohydrogenation.

*Bacterial lipids.* The proportion of lipid fractions in rumen bacteria have been accepted that they contain : (1) unesterified fatty acids, (2) cephalin, (3) phosphatidyl, serine (4) lecithin, (5) spingolipids and some glycolipids. The composition of the total fatty acids in mixed rumen bacteria is myristic 3.9 per cent; pentadecanoic 80 per cent; palmitic 31 per cent; margeric 1.6 per cent; stearic 1.5 per cent; oleic 6.0 per cent; linoleic 2.7 per cent and branched chain fatty acids 15.8 per cent.

*Protozoal lipids.* Protozoal composition of lipids consists of : (1) unesterified fatty acids, (2) monoacylglycerols, (3) diacylglycerols, (4) triacylglycerols, (5) phospholipids, and (6) sterol esters. Phospholipid accounts for about 80 per cent of the total protozoal lipids. The principal phospholipids are : (a) lecithin, (b) cephalin, (c) diacylglycerol aminoethylphosphonate, (d) ethanolamine plasmalogen which accounts for 36.3, 18.7, 11.0 and 9.5 per cent respectively of the total. The composition of the total fatty acids in mixed rumen protozoa is pentadecanoic 3.4 per cent; palmitic 43.1 per cent; stearic 9.3 per cent; oleic 18.4 per cent; linoleic 16.1 per cent and branched chain fatty acids 4.9 per cent.

## Lypolysis

The acylester linkages in triacylglycerols, phospholipids, galactosyl glycerides, sterol esters, methyl and ethyl esters are all rapidly hydrolysed in the rumen. The rumen bacterium, *Anaerovibrio lipolytica*, was shown to secrete a lipase that hydrolysed triacylglycerols containing medium and long-chain fatty acids. The intermediary formation of di- and monoacylglycerols are also hydrolysed at a very rapid rate. On the other hand, the lipase of *A. lipolytica* does not hydrolyse the acyl ester bonds in galactosylglycerides. The latter of plant choloroplasts are hydrolysed by mixed rumen micro-organisms to fatty acids, galactose and glycerol. Some rumen bacteria, including *Butyrivibrio fibrisolvens*, are able to hydrolyse cephalin, lecithin, lysolecithin (lysophosphatidylcholine) to fatty acids and glycerolecithin or glycerolphosphorylethanolamine. Protozoa play an insignificant role in the hydrolysis of phospholipids in the rumen. There remains a possibility that lipases and phospholipases from dietary herbage might contribute to the hydrolysis of the acyl bonds in the rumen.

The capacity of rumen microorganisms to digest lipids is strictly limited. The lipid content of average ruminant diets is 3-5 per cent on dry matter basis, if it is increased above 10 per cent, the activities of rumen microbes are reduced, the fermentation of carboydrate is also retarded, and feed intake falls through the suppression of methane forming bacteria. Upsetting of methane fermentation produces excess of hydrogen with the resultant alteration in ruman fermentation balance.

## Biohydrogenation

Before discussing the mechanism of biohydrogenation of unsaturated fatty acid released from ester combination, it will probably be helpful to refresh with some elementary idea about isomers. *Compounds that have the same molecular formula but different structural formulas are isomers* (Greek, *isos*, equal; *meros*, part).

Geometrical isomers are compounds that have different configurations because of the presence of a rigid structure in the molecule. In general geometrical isomerism occurs in the alkenes (having double bonds) when each carbon atom of a double bond bears two different substituents. When two identical substituents are on the same side of the double bond, the compound is the *cis* isomer; the *trans* isomer is the one in which similar groups are on opposite sides of the double bond. The following is an example of geometric isomers:

$$\begin{array}{c} H \quad H \\ C{=}C \\ H \quad CH_2CH_3 \end{array} \quad \text{is identical to} \quad \begin{array}{c} H \quad CH_2CH_3 \\ C{=}C \\ H \quad H \end{array}$$

$$\begin{array}{c} CH_3 \quad H \\ C{=}C \\ CH_3 \quad H \end{array} \quad \text{is identical to} \quad \begin{array}{c} H \quad CH_3 \\ C{=}C \\ H \quad CH_3 \end{array}$$

In general, geometric isomerism occurs in the alkenes when each carbon atom of a double bond bears two different substituents. When two identical (or nearly identical) substituents are on the same side of the double bond, the compound is the *cis* isomer; the *trans* isomer is the one in which similar groups are on opposite sides of the double bond. Following are some examples of geometric isomers.

$$\begin{array}{c} Cl \quad Cl \\ C{=}C \\ H \quad H \end{array} \qquad \begin{array}{c} Cl \quad H \\ C{=}C \\ H \quad Cl \end{array}$$

*cis*-1,2-Dichloroethene
mp −80°C
bp 60°C

*trans*-1,2-Dichloroethene
mp −50°C
bp 48°C

$$\begin{array}{c} H \quad CH_2CH_3 \\ C{=}C \\ CH_3 \quad CH_3 \end{array} \qquad \begin{array}{c} CH_3 \quad CH_2CH_3 \\ C{=}C \\ H \quad CH_3 \end{array}$$

*cis*-3-Methyl-2-pentene

*trans*-3-Methyl-2-pentene

Linoleic acid has two double bonds at carbon 9 and 12. In both cases the carbon atoms of double bonds bear identical substituents on the same side. Thus it is *cis*-9, *cis*-12. It is also 18 : 2 that is, it has 18 carbons and only double bonds at two places. Likewise linolenic acid is *cis*-9, *cis*-12, *cis*-15 and is 18 : 3 which means, it has three double bonds at carbon 9,12 and 15 places. All unsaturated double bonds are *cis*, and linolenic acid has a total of 18 carbons.

The intraruminal environment is a highly reduced one where liberated fatty acids are also neutralised at rumen pH probably mainly as calcium salts which have a low solubility. Hence these fatty acids remain adhered to the surfaces of bacteria and feed particles. Hydrogenation of unsaturated fatty acids are conducted by certain rumen bacterial strains. In particular, the anaerobic bacterium, *Butyrivibrio fibrisolvens*, contains a number of enzymes of importance in the biohydrogenation of linoleic acid resulting in the formation of saturated stearic acid 18 : 0 (18 carbon and no double bond). The metabolic pathways involved in the biohydrogenation of linolenic and linoleic acids in the rumen are as shown below:

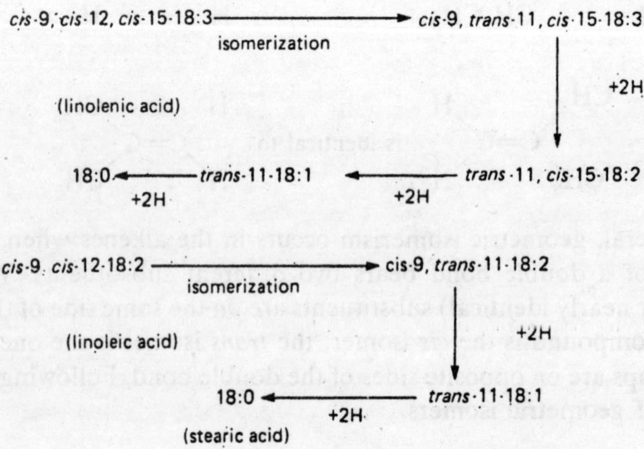


Biohydrogenation of linolenic and linoleic acids

The source of hydrogen is not yet confirmed. It is possible that the required hydrogen is obtained from water by the enzymatic action of *B. fibrisolvens*, while the electrons could be supplied by NADH, α-tochoperolquinol or deoxy-α-tochopherolquinol.

Both linoleic and linolenic acids have *cis* double bonds, but before they are fully hydrogenated one double bond in each is converted to the *trans* configuration; thus *trans* acids are hydrogenated with greater difficulty, and there is an accumulation of *trans* forms relative to *cis*. Some portion of trans unsaturated acids which have higher melting points than their *cis* relatives, are transferred and absorbed by the animal contributing to the generally higher melting point of ruminant fats.

**Biosynthesis of fatty acids**

There is enough evidence that rumen microbes also synthesise considerable quantities of mono-unsaturated, long chain saturated and some unusual fatty acids for example branched-chain fatty acids probably through the incorporation of propionyl Co-A into the carbon skeletons are synthesised. A number of rumen bacteria requires n-valeric acid for biosynthesis of odd-carbon fatty acids such as *Bacteroides succinogenes*, *Tiponema* and *Selenomonas*. The 15 carbon linear and branched acids are major components of microbial lipids. Apart from utilisation of these fatty acids for incorporation into the cellular complex of the microbes themselves, these are also incorporated into a range of neutral and polar lipid classes which are eventually distributed in the body fats of ruminants and in milk.

**Table 136**

Synthesis of long chain acids from VFA.

| Acid substrate | Organisms[a] | Products |
|---|---|---|
| Propionic | *Bacillus subtillis* | C15:0 |
| Butyric | *B. subtillis* | C14:0 iso, C16:0 iso |
| Isobutyric | *Ruminococcus albus* | C14 br, C15 br, aldehydes |
| | *Borellia* | C14 iso, C15 iso, aldehydes |
| | *Bacteroides succinogenes* | C14 iso, C15 iso, aldehydes |
| | Mixed rumen bacteria | C13:0, C13:0 br, C14:0 br, C15:0 br |
| | *B. subtillis* | C14 iso, C16 iso |
| 2-Methylbutyric | *B. subtillis* | 12-methyl C14:0, 14-methyl C16:0 |
| n-Valeric | *B. succinogenes* | C13, C15, aldehydes |
| | *Borellia* | C15, C17 |
| | *Selenomonas ruminantium* | C13, C15, C17 |
| | Mixed organisms | C18:1 |
| Isovaleric | *R. flavefaciens* | C15 br, C17, aldehydes |
| | *B. subtillis* | C15:0 iso, C17:0 iso |
| n-Caproic | *B. succinogenes* | C14, C16 |
| | *S. ruminantium* | C12, C14, C16 |

[a] *Bacillus subtillis* is included along with the various rumen species for comparative purposes.

This process could account for the appreciable concentrations of linolenic and linoleic acids that are found in the phospholipids of rumen protozoa. It seems more likely that these fatty acids originate from intact choloroplasts ingested by the protozoa. Polyunsaturated fatty acids in plant choroplasts would be largely in the esterified form and would thus be protected from hydrogenation in the rumen.

**Fermentation of Glycerol and Galactose** Both glycerol and galactose released from lipids in the rumen are readily fermented to yield voltatile fatty acids of which propionic acid is the main product of glycerol fermentation. Glycerol-fermenting bacteria isolated from sheep rumen contents were identified as *Selenomonas ruminantium* var *lactilyticus*; they did not show lipolytic activity. Galactose can be fermented by various rumen microorganisms including several bacterial species and the protozoan *Dasytricha ruminantium*. The main changes in the principal dietary lipids which are effected by microorganisms in the rumen are summarised as shown below.

All short chain fatty acids and volatile fatty acids produced from the hydrolysis and fermentation of lipids are largely absorbed through the rumen wall. Long chain fatty acids, mostly saturated are not absorbed in the rumen, so they pass along with rumen contents more or less continuously through the omasum into the true stomach or abomasum where also the dead bodies of million microorganisms reach and disintegrate before the digesta enters the small intestine. The extent of microbial lipids is not known though rough calculation indicate that the microbial lipids may provide upto 25 per cent of the total amount of fatty acids (about 12 grams per day in sheep) reaching the small intestine of sheep fed on hay and concentrates

**Fate of Dietary Lipids in the Rumen**

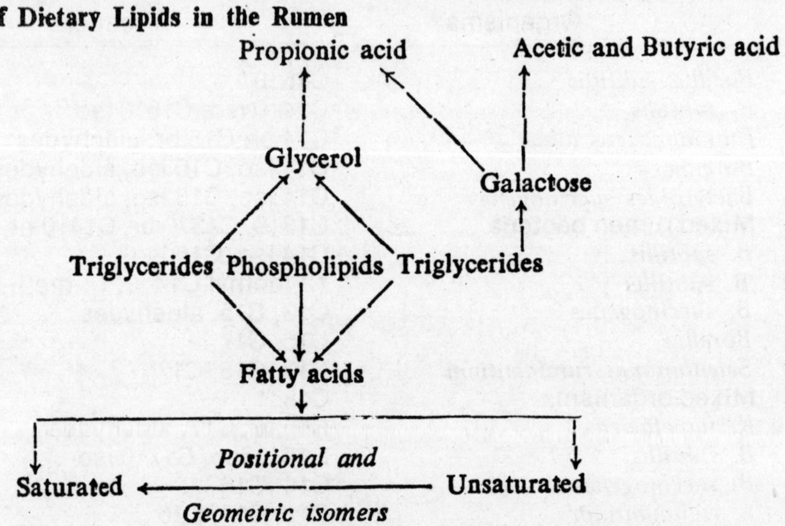


and it has also been concluded that at least 140 grams of microbial lipid per 24 hours are available for intestinal digestion by an adult cow.

## AMOUNT AND COMPOSITION OF LIPIDS ENTERING DUODENUM

The digestion and absorption of fatty acids by ruminants differs from the non-ruminant in that lipolysis occurs much further up the tract in the rumen. In the non-ruminant it occurs primarily in the small intestine near the site of absorption. Further, in contrast to the extensive absorption of short chain volatile fatty acids that occurs in the rumen, virtually no long chain fatty acids mostly saturated are absorbed from the digesta before they rich the small intestine of the ruminant through the omasum and abomasum where also the dead bodies of a million microbes reach and disintegrate for further absorption.

The synthesis of the various types of fatty acids including unsaturated linoleic, linolenic and branched chain fatty acids is utilised for a microbial body, and since little or no degradation of microbial fatty acids occurs in the rumen, the amount of total lipid passing through the omasum and abomasum into the duodenum is always greater than what is ingested.

Little or no change occurs in the composition of the lipids in the digesta as it passes through the omasum and abomasum. It has to be noted that most of the long chain fatty acids are neutralised at rumen pH and reach the small intestine as potassium soaps. But the admixture with the gastric secretions of the abomasum causes the disintegration of any intact bacterial and protozoal cells that are transported from the rumen. Thus the lipid entering the duodenum consists mainly of unesterified saturated fatty acids absorbed into the particulate matter and a small but variable proportion of the lipid is composed of phospholipids and other complex lipids released from the intact microbial cells that enter the abomasum from the rumen. The extent of microbial lipids is not known, though a rough calculation indicates that the microbial lipids may provide up to 25 per cent of the total amount of fatty acids (about 12 gm per day in sheep) reaching the small intestine of sheep fed on hay and concentrates, and it has also been concluded that at least 140 gm of microbial lipid per 24 hours are available for intestinal digestion by an adult cow.

Of the total fatty acids entering the duodenum and jejunum of ruminants, the *proportion* of free fatty acids is lower than the corresponding value of rumen contents and this is accompanied by an increase in the proportion of $C_{18}$ unsaturated compounds in an esterified condition. Such lipids could derive from the phospholipids of the bile, tissue fluid lipoprotein, shed epithelial cells and other secretion entering the intestinal lumen.

## BILE AND PANCREATIC SECRETION

In ruminant animals, the pancreatic duct joins the bile duct 5 to 10 cm from the point of entry of the common duct into the duodenum. The flow rate of biliary secretion is much greater than that of the pancreatic secretions; in ruminants. flow rates of 1.45 and 0.33 ml/hour/kg body weight have been observed.

### Biliary lipids

The concentration of total lipid in ruminant bile is of the order of 1400 mg per 100 ml : Lecithin accounts for about 80 per cent of this lipid whereas lyso-lecithin, cephalin, cholesterol and cholesterol esters amount to about 6.3 per cent, 2.7 per cent, 4.7 per cent and 2 per cent respectively. The molar percentages of the principal fatty acids present in lecithin of sheep bile are as follows: palmitic 36.0; stearic 9.2; oleic 27.9; linoleic 6.6; linolenic 4.9.

The concentration of bile acids in ruminant bile varies between 5000 mg and 8000 mg per 100 ml. The composition (gm per 100 gm) of ruminant bile salt is as follows : taurocholate, 54; glycocholate, 21; tauro-deoxycholate, 11; glycodeoxycholate, 6; taurocheno-deoxycholate, 4; cholate, 2; glycocheno-deoxycholate, 2.

### Pancreatic lipase

Pancreatic juice contains lipase and phospholipase $A_1$ and $A_2$. Optimum activity for the last two enzymes was found to be at pH 5.6. The phospholipase $A_1$ hydrolyses the acylester linkage in position 1 of lecithin or cephalin and thus releases mainly saturated fatty acids, whereas in phospholipase $A_2$ hydrolyses the acylester linkage is in position 2 and thus releases mainly unsaturated fatty acids. Another enzyme, *glycolipase* has been found to catalyze the hydrolysis of the acylester bonds in plant galactosyl diacylglycerols. However, whether the enzyme is distinct from pancreatic lipase is yet to be confirmed.

### Absorption

Ruminant animals absorb fats with a high degree of efficiency. Digestion coefficient varies between 80-90 per cent even when the dietary intake of fatty acids are marginally in excess. The lipid composition of the digesta changes markedly as it passes the point of entry of the common bile/pancreatic duct. The principal change is an increased proportion of lecithin, and this is maintained as the digesta pass through the remainder of the duodenum and the proximal jejunum. The activities of pancreatic phospholipases $A_1$ and $A_2$ would certainly be inhibited by the acidic conditions of the duodenum (pH 2-3.5) and the proximal jejunum (pH 3.6-4.2). Thus appreciable hydrolysis of phospholipids, mainly of lecithin begins only when the digesta reaches the mid-jejunum (pH 4.7-6.0) and continues throughout the distal jejunum (pH 6-7.6).

These conditions mean that there is little or no triacylglycerols available to be converted to mono-acylglycerol (a potent emulsifying agent) which play an important role in the formation of mixed micelles in non-ruminants. Furthermore, the pancreatic lipase will also be less active due to the acidic condition of the duodenum and upper jejunum.

Nonetheless, the active micelle formations of the long chain fatty acids (which when they reach the small intestine are saturated and unesterified) do occur in the upper tract under the influence of bile salts (ruminant bile is characterised by an excess of taurine over glycine conjugated bile acids which is more active in an acid media, even at pH 2.5, taurine conjugated bile acids are soluble and partly ionised). In contrast to non-ruminants, the *micelle of ruminants is ormed comprising saturated long chain of fatty acids, lecithin of feed and bile and bile salts* and not by monoglycerides as observed in non-ruminants.

It may thus be concluded that about 15-25 per cent of the total lipids are absorbed through the upper jejunum while the balance are absorbed in the lower three quarters of the jejunum. The pancreatic phospholipases hydrolyse lecithin into a fatty acid and the highly polar lysolecithin participate in micelle formation and aid absorption. There is evidence at a high level of feeding that calcium soaps (much less soluble) may escape absorption and appear in the faeces. Saturated fatty acids are absorbed more slowly than unsaturated acids, the ease of absorption decreases with increasing chain length. Similar to non-ruminants, the long chain fatty acids are absorbed into the lymphatic system. Since the flow of fatty acids is more or less continuous with rumen outflow, the lymph draining the intestine is perpetually milky. The particles are made up of about 75 per cent in the very-low-density-lipoprotein (VLDL density 0.93-1.006 g/ml; diameter 25-75 nm) fraction and 25 per cent of chylomicrons which is about the reverse for the non-ruminant. Chylomicrons of bovine plasma contain about 87 per cent triacyl-phospholipid 4 per cent; cholesterol 4 per cent; cholesterol ester 2 per cent; protein 3 per cent of the total. Similarly bovine VLDL are composed of triacylglycerols 74 per cent; phospholipids 7 per cent; cholesterol 7 per cent; cholesterol esters 5 per cent; protein 8 per cent.

Unlike non-ruminants, where it is possible to vary the fatty acid composition of body fats by altering the composition of dietary fats, in ruminants, this is not the case, and the predominating fatty acids of ruminant depot fats is the stearic acid resulting from hydrogenation in the rumen.

The lipid in the form of chylomicrons and VLDL is carried by the capillaries to the adipose tissue situated under the skin (50 per cent), kidneys, in the membranes surrounding the intestines, in the muscle and elsewhere. The adipose tissue is extremely dynamic, has blood and nerve supply whereby fats in the body are in a state of flux.

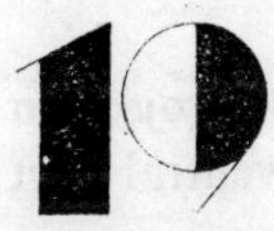

# PHYSIOLOGY AND MICROBIOLOGY OF RUMEN

## GROWTH AND DEVELOPMENT OF RUMINANT STOMACH

### Foetal Development

The stomach develops from a long spindle-shaped dilation of the primitive gut which gives rise to differential development of the various stomach compartments. In the case of bovine embryos (9.5 mm), the stomach becomes apparent in 28 days. Definite segments are observed by about 56 days of the embryo. By about five months of foetal age the abomasum becomes more in size than other compartments and at birth it weighs about half (47 per cent) of the total four stomachs. The honeycomb structure of the reticulum develops between 72 and 100 days of the foetal life. In terms of relative capacities of the various stomach compartments at the time of birth, the rumen and reticulum together hold only 30 per cent of the total stomach capacity while abomasum which is the largest compartment along with omasum hold 70 per cent of the total stomach capacity.

### Postnatal Development

After birth the differential development continues for some period of time and is modified by factors like type of diet, nutritional stress and species differences. The section of the complex stomach develops more or less in the order of its functional importance. Since the calf immediately after birth depends on suckling whereby liquid passes through the reticular groove omasum and abomasum, these two compartments remain more active and occupy about 30 per cent of the total stomach capacity. The fourth stomach (abomasum) is by far the largest of the compartments. Thus digestion in the young calf is more like that of a simple-stomached animal. As the calf begins to eat solid food the first two compartments (often considered together as the reticulo-rumen) enlarge greatly, until in the adult stage they occupy 85 per cent of the total capacity of the stomach. (Fig . 52. . .) In adults, the oesophageal grooves do not function under normal feeding conditions, and both feed and water pass into the reticulo-rumen. However, the reflex closure of the groove to form a channel can be stimulated even in adults, particularly if they are allowed to drink. Under normal conditions, the calf rumen becomes functional in about six to eight weeks. Evidence of a functional rumen is based on : (1) rumen odour, which is indicative of fermentation; (2) a decline in blood glucose; and (3) the production of volatile fatty acids. As soon as the animal starts to ingest dry feed the size of the reticulum and rumen undergoes a very rapid increase in size. The abomasum gradually regresses in relative size, although not in absolute size and the omasum develops slowly taking a longer time to reach a relative mature size than the reticulum or rumen which undergoes a rapid relative growth prior to eight weeks of age and the relative mature size probably is attained by 12 to 24 weeks. Variances of this type are related partially to different feeding regimens, such as, ingestion of roughage is stimulatory in terms of weight and thickness of the tissue along with the development of normal papillae (small nipple-shaped projection up to 1 cm in length located on the interior of the rumen wall particularly on the ventral part of both sacs).

Relative mature size of the stomach is reached in about eight weeks in sheep and goats, in three to four months in deer and in five to six months in cattle.

### Passage of Feed Through the Ruminant Stomach

Ruminants, in common with other large herbivores, require a large bulk of feed in order to satisfy their demands for nutrient and energy needs of the body. A cow on an average spends eight hours each time for grazing, ruminating and resting. However, a proportion of the time spent in the ingestion of feed is markedly less under conditions in which the animals are fed concentrates as ground or pelleted forms.

#### Prehension

The term prehension means the seizing (the act of binding) and conveying of feed to the mouth. In ruminant species the lips, teeth and tongue are the principal prehensile organs. One peculiarity of ruminant animals is that they do not have upper incisor teeth. Rather the upper incisors are replaced by tough dental pads, which provide a surface against which the lower incisors can put pressure. The tongue in cattle is the chief prehensile structure. It is elongated and covered with rough papillae, making it adapted to wrapping around grass and other forages, whereas the upper lip performs that function in a horse.

#### Mastication

Mastication or chewing is the mechanical reduction of feed to a smaller particle size. In non-herbivore animals including man mastication is done by movement of the mandible in a vertical plane. In herbivores, well developed lateral movements greatly facilitate the grinding action required to reduce fibrous plant material to a size or shape that may be swallowed. In addition, the upper jaw is wider than the lower jaw making it possible for the animal to use the molars on only one side at a time. Furthermore, the grinding surfaces of the molars are in different planes, thus increasing efficiency of mastication.

Even though ruminants are well equipped to thoroughly masticate fibrous feed material, it is not their custom to do so while ingesting feed. To meet the great demand of feed, the only means by which animals can satisfy their requirements is by quick swallowing and later on by regurgitation. It has been noted that dairy cows on an average make 94 jaw movements per minute when eating grain and silage and 78 per minute when eating hay. In 24 hours thus a cow requires about 4,700 bites for eating grain and silage and 10,530 bites for eating hay. In addition, the animal bites about 24,600 during rumination. This makes a total bite of 42,000 per day. The rate of mastication varies with hunger (less bite) and nature of the feed.

#### Feed Bolus

After brief mastication, the feed is mixed with saliva to form a bolus. The bolus is propelled down the oesophagus by peristaltic contractions with such considerable force that it falls in the anterior rumen. This rapid propulsion of the bolus is achieved through the action of striated muscles in the oesophageal wall of the ruminant.

In cattle, bolus weighs about 100 gram. When eating first begins, the weight of the forage boli tends to be smallest (70-80 g); it increases to a peak by the time one-third to two-third of the total forages required have been consumed.

**Salivary Production and Function**

Saliva is produced in copious amounts by five sets of paired glands namely; (1) parotid; (2) inferior molar; (3) submaxillary or mandibular; (4) sublingual; and (5) buccal salivary glands. Among these the parotid accounts for 40-50 per cent of total saliva production. In cattle there are also three unpaired salivary glands which are : (1) palatine gland; (2) labial gland; and (3) pharyngeal gland.

On the basis of the type of salivary secretion, ruminant glands may be grouped into two:

**1. Alkaligenic glands**

These comprise the paired parotid, inferior molar and buccal salivary glands. They secrete a fluid containing a high concentration of $HCO^{-}_{3}$ ions with little mucoprotein.

**2. Mucogenic glands**

They comprise the paired submaxillary, sublingual and labial salivary glands as well as

**Table 137**

Summary of characteristics of the salivary glands of sheep.

| Glands | Mean weight | Weight relative to parotids (%) | Cell type | Factors governing rate of flow | Estimated saliva volume (l./24 hr) | Saliva type |
|---|---|---|---|---|---|---|
| Both parotid | 23.5 | 100 | Serous | Continuous flow when denervated. Respond to stimulation of mouth, esphagus and reticulo-rumen | 3-8 | Fluid and isotonic. Strongly buffered with $HCO_3$ and $HPO_4$ |
| Both inferior molar | 5.9 | 25 | Serous | Continuous flow when denervated. Responds to stimulation of mouth, esophagus and reticulo-rumen | 0.7-2.0 | Fluid and isotonic or nearly so. Strongly buffered with $HCO_3$ and $HPO_4$ |
| Palatine, buccal and pharyngeal | 20.7 | 88 | Mucus | Very slow continuous flow when not stimulated. Respond to stimulation of mouth, esophagus and reticulo-rumen | 2-6 | Very mucus and isotonic or nearly so. Strongly buffered with $HCO_3$ and $HPO_4$ |
| Both submaxillary | 18.2 | 77 | Mixed | No flow when denervated. Strongly stimulated by feeding. Little or no response to stimulation of esophagus or reticulo-rumen | 0.4-0.8 | Variably mucus and hypotonic. Weakly buffered |
| Both sublingual | 1.3 | 6 | Mixed | Continuous flow when not stimulated. Moderately stimulated from esophagus; other reflexes not studied | 0.1 (?) | Very mucus and hypotonic. Weakly buffered |
| Labial | 10.9 | 46 | Mixed | Little or no flow when not stimulated. Little or no response to stimulation of esophagus and reticulo-rumen; other reflexes not studied. | ? | Very mucus and hypotonic. Weakly buffered |

the unpaired pharyngeal gland and the numerous other glands in the buccal epithelium. The secretion of the mucogenic glands are predominantly mucoprotein.

Table 138

Composition of saliva

| Gland | Nature of secretion | Ion content | | | | | | | |
|---|---|---|---|---|---|---|---|---|---|
| | | $Na^+$ | $K^+$ | $Ca^{++}$ | $Mg^{++}$ | P | $Cl^-$ | $HCO_3^-$ | $HPO_4^=$ |
| | | mg% [a] | | | | | | | |
| Mixed | from mouth | 370-462 | 16-46 | 1.6-3.0 | 0.6-1.0 | 37-72 | | 25-43 | |
| Parotid | fistula | 352-447 | 12-45 | 0.1-2.0 | 0.4-1.1 | 19-129 | | 19-238 | |
| | | meq/l.[b] | | | | | | | |
| Parotid | from anesthetized sheep | 182-189 | 5 | | | | 9-16 | 91-99 | 71-79 |
| Inferior molar | from anesthetized sheep | 175 | 7-10 | | | | 7-12 | 97-110 | 44-51 |
| Palatine | from anesthetized sheep | 179 | 4 | | | | 25 | 109 | 25 |
| Submaxillary | from anesthetized sheep | 3-66 | 15-51 | | | | 2-9 | 1-9 | 14-175 |
| Sublingual | from anesthetized sheep | 16-47 | 6-25 | | | | 16-40 | 8-18 | 0.3-2.0 |
| Labial | from anesthetized sheep | 29-47 | 3-9 | | | | 34 | 2-4 | 2-10 |

[a] From McDougall (1948)
[b] From Kay (1960a); Kay's values represent collections from resting or stimulated glands.

**Secretion**

During the period when the animal is not feeding, there is a basal level of secretion of alkaline saliva but little secretion of mucoproteins. Feeding stimulates secretion of alkaline saliva and greatly stimulates that of mucoproteins. This stimulation was greatest with coarse fibrous feed, and appeared to result from reflexes initiated by stimulation of the walls of the rumen by coarse feed particles, especially those in the vicinity of the rumino-reticular fold. To a lesser extent, salivation is stimulated by pressures within the rumen.

The more or less continuous secretion of alkaline saliva by the parotid glands is responsible for the large volume of saliva secreted by the ruminants. In cattle, the total volume may range from 100 to 200 litres per day or sometimes equivalent to the volume of the rumen. The volume is affected by the physical nature of feed, dry matter content, volume of fluid in the gut and psychological stimulation.

## Factors Affecting Total Feed Intake

The total feed intake in ruminants is controlled by a number of factors which are not necessarily the same as in non-ruminants. The various major factors are described as below:

1. The capacious gastro-intestinal volume when filled, leads to distension in the reticulo-rumen and restricts further intake.
2. Gastrin, the digestive hormone secreted from the antral portion of gastric mucosa and pancreatic islets, stimulates the motility of omasum and inhibits the motility of rumeno-reticulum leading to low feed intake.
3. Roughages high in lignin have poor palatability and there is less feed intake (may be as low as 2 per cent of body weight) than fodders having low lignin content. With certain good quality green fodders the intake may go as high as 3.5 per cent of live weight.
4. Shift in hormonal balance during pregnancy restricts the energy regulatory system and foetal displacement of the reticulo-rumen affect feed intake.
5. The palatability, small size of feed particles, feeds having higher digestibility contribute towards high intake.
6. Certain blood components such as glucose, absorbed VFA from the walls of rumen, reticulum and omasum (production of which may be as high as 4.0 kg per day per cow) suppress feed intake by affecting the reception centre in the hypothalamus.
7. High environmental temperature decreases feed intake and low temperature stimulates the eating centres (located in the lateral hypothalamus) for increase in feed intake.

## Mixing of Digesta in the Reticulo-Rumen

Development of the forestomach (rumen, reticulum and omasum) enabled the animal to consume a large amount of feed very rapidly with a minimum of chewing before swallowing to the rumen and reticulum and then move to a resting place to rechew the feed. In fact most of these (ruminants) animals fearful of their enemies have little time to devote to feeding. In consequence, they consume suitable forage as quickly as possible and they hide or rest like all domestic animals, and ruminate at their ease the feed which has undergone a little alteration or digestion.

Ingested feed is thoroughly mixed in the reticulo-rumen by means of an orderly and synchronised cycle of events involving both reticulum and rumen. The cycle can be considered to start with *two contractions* of the reticulum.

The *first contraction* lasts approximately 2 to 3 seconds and at its maximum the réticular volume is reduced by about half. This contraction is succeeded by a brief period of relaxation in cattle.

The *second contraction* begins immediately after relaxation which has the effect of forcing most of the reticular contents over the reticulo-ruminal fold into the rumen after which the reticulum again relaxes.

The pair of contractions is often referred to as the *byphasic contraction* of the reticulum and takes some 10 seconds from start to finish. It is repeated at intervals of roughly one minute in the resting or ruminating animal, and rather more frequently while feeding.

During the second part of the biphasic contraction, some parts of the rumen also contract and thereby the volume of digesta in the ruminal dorsai sac moves to the ventral sac of the

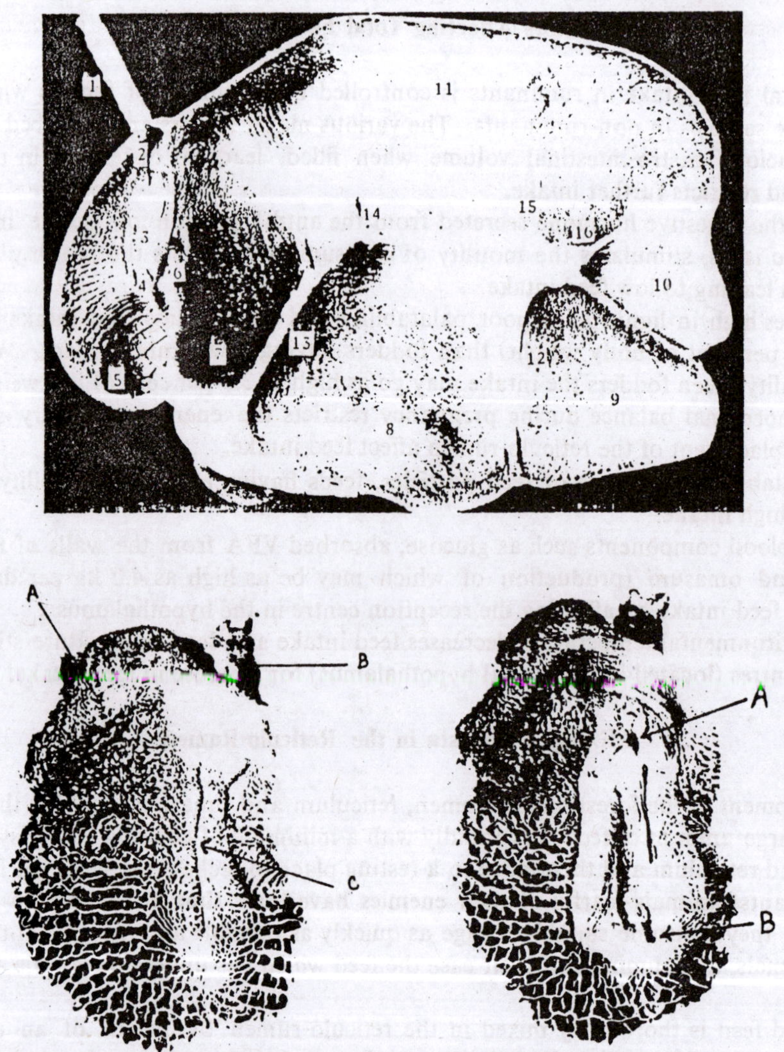


**Fig. 81** A dried bovine stomach which illustrates oesophagus,1; cardia,2; reticular groove,3; reticulomasal opening,4; reticular groove,5; rumino-reticular fold,6; cranial sac,7; ventral anterior sac,8; ventral posterior blind sac,9; caudal blind sac,10; dorsal sac,11; ventral coronary pillars,12; cranial pillar,13; pillar between dorsal and ventral sac,14; longitudinal pillar,15; dorsal coronary pillars,16.

The reticulum and reticular groove of bovine. Left. A, the dorsal aspect of the reticuloruminal fold ; B, the oesophagus : C, the reticular groove in a closed position. Right. The groove is pinned in an open position to show its interior, the opening into the oesophagus. A : and the reticulo-omasal orifice, B.

rumen and thus mixing of the rumen contents goes on vigorously. Mixing aids in inoculating the fresh ingesta with microbes, spreads saliva throughout the reticulum. and enhances absorption of the products of digestion.

## Rumination

The phenomenon of "Chewing the cud" or rechewing rumen content ingested at some earlier time is one of the features most characteristic of ruminant animals. Briefly rumination involves regurgitation of ingesta from the reticulo-rumen, swallowing of regurgitated liquids, remastication of the solids accompanied by resalivation and reswallowing of the bolus.

During rumination, these occur as an additional contraction of the reticulum which precedes the normal biphasic contraction. This contraction raises the level of the contents of the reticulum above the level of the *cardia* (the area comprising the terminal end of the oesophagus and upper opening of the stomach and the rumen). The cardia relaxes, thereby enlarging the opening of the rumen to the oesophagus. The changes in pressure within the rumen and reticulum during the mixing cycle described above are sufficient to propel digesta into the oesophagus.

Movement of digesta (during rumination) from the distal portion of the oesophagus to the mouth is also aided by a wave of antiperistaltic (reverse peristalsis) contraction of the oesophagus about 107 cm per second in cows. This rapid movement of the oesophageal muscle is possible due to the fact that in ruminants the muscle is striated.

There is evidence that the animal also contracts the diaphragm and closes the glottis, (the opening between the vocal cords in the larynx) reducing the pressure in the thorax to less than atmospheric, thus producing a pressure gradient in the oesophagus. Once in the oesophagus, the bolus is carried to the mouth by reverse peristalsis. Rumination also appears to be stimulated by the presence of coarse material in the stomach.

Although the time spent in ruminating depends, among other factors, on the type of feed, typically it involves about eight hours per day or about equal to the time spent in grazing.

During remastication that occurs while ruminating, the bolus is reinsalivated. However, the salivary secretion is of a different nature than that which occurs during eating. Parotid glands secrete more saliva rich in bicarbonates.

The ruminated bolus is swallowed, enters the rumen and is mixed with the rumen contents in the same manner as ingested feed. Immediately after the entry of a ruminated bolus into the rumen, a second bolus is regurgitated and, since regurgitation precedes the mixing cycle of the reticulo-rumen, rumination is synchronous with mixing, one bolus being ruminated per mixing cycle.

## Eruction
### (*Belching of Gas*)

Substantially more gas is produced during ruminant digestion than by simple stomached animals. Among microbial gases, $CO_2$ and $CH_4$ are produced in large amounts, which must be eliminated; otherwise bloating results. Normally, these gases are expelled quite freely by eructation and to a lesser extent by absorption into the blood draining from the rumen, from which they are eliminated through exhaled air from the lungs.

The average volume of gas produced in the reticulo-rumen of cattle may be expected to be in the order of two litres per minute for an adult animal. The period of peak production of gas is 30 minutes to two hours after feeding.

The events of the eructation mechanism have been shown to be associated with secondary rumen contraction for the most part. Tension (stretch) receptors in the cardial area of the rumen have a stimulatory action on eructation. It may be noted that regurgitation occurs in association with an extra-reticular contraction, while eructation is associated with secondary rumen contraction.

## Rumen Environment

Rumen is the first and largest stomach of the four stomachs viz., rumen, reticulum omasum and abomasum possessed by a group of cud chewing animals like cattle, buffalo, bison, sheep, goat, deer, antelope and giraffe. In camels, llamas, alpacas and vicunas which are also ruminants (cud chewing animals), the omasum is missing. Thus they have three compartments of stomach namely, rumen, reticulum and abomasum. Surprisingly, in such animals the reticulum is glandular.

The reticulo-rumen system of all ruminants is extremely capacious, occupying a large part of the body cavity—a cow, for instance, has a volume of about 100 litres and a sheep about 8 litres. The food is held in this region for a comparatively long period and is subject to microbial action and to the additional maceration due to rumination.

Rumen is an exceptional habitat, in providing constant conditions of moisture, pH, temperature and finally anaerobic atmosphere for a large number of desirable strains of microorganisms. The temperature of rumen varies from 38-42°C with an average of 39°C.

The liquid phase of the rumen contents are about 10-20 per cent by weight of organic matter and has a pH generally within the range of pH 5.8 to 6.8. With large amounts of readily fermentable carbohydrate entering the rumen, the pH may fall around pH 4.0 Conversely, on very poor forages the pH may rise to pH 7.5 or more but these are the extremes of the pH range. The pH of the reticulo-rumen is maintained at a fairly constant level by the alkalinity (pH=8.0) of the large volumes of saliva entering the rumen, by the buffering capacity of the $HCO_3^-$ content of saliva. The maintenance of a constant level of pH is also aided by the rapid removal of acidic end products of microbial fermentation through the rumen wall at a rate approximately equal to that at which they are produced. The usual pH of the rumen is about 6.5, and this is about the optimum growth pH for rumen bacteria and protozoa.

Osmotic pressure in rumen is fairly close to that in the blood stream. As the liquid phase of the reticulo-rumen has an oxidation-reduction potential of about —350 mv, it is clear that the reticulo-rumen environment is extremely reduced and is almost devoid of oxygen. However, its stability is such that it will tolerate an addition of considerable amounts of oxygen without marked or prolonged changes in oxidation reduction potential or in microbial fermentation.

The gas phase above the digesta inside reticulo-rumen in percentage consists of aproximately 65 $CO_2$, 25 $CH_4$, 7 $N_2$, 0.6 $O_2$, 0.2 $H_2$ and 0.01 $H_2S$. The $N_2$ and $O_2$ enter the gas phase of the reticulo-rumen along with ingested forage.

The inorganic solutes such as $HCO_3^-$, $HPO_4^-$, $Cl^-$, $Na^+$, $K^+$ and $Ca^+$ are derived from the saliva. Of the cations present in the rumen only $Na^+$ is transported across the reticulo-ruminal wall in appreciable amounts against the concentration gradient which occurs between the rumen and the blood stream. As a consequence of this, the ionic content of the rumen closely reflects that of saliva.

The major organic solutes present in the reticulo-rumen are the short-chain ($C_2$—$C_5$) monocarboxylic acids produced as a result of microbial fermentation from about 50 mM to 150 mM concentrations of these acids. This is again roughly proportional to the extent of feeding. Although the proportion of fatty acids varies with the type of feed, as a very rough approximation, in rumen, concentration of short chain fatty acids is about 100 mM and the molar proportions of individual acids as a percentage of the total are acetic 65; propionic 20; *n*-butyric 12; *iso*-butyric 1; *n*-valeric 1; *iso*-valeric and 2-methyl-butyric 1 (compiled from a range of values given by Hungate in his book "The Rumen and Its Microbes").

Due to the high rates of turnover resulting from rapid microbial metabolism, soluble sugars, amino acids and $NH_4^+$ are present in solution in the reticulo-rumen at low concentrations. A rough estimate indicates the concentration of free dissolved amino acids and dissolved ammonia in order of 25 mM each.

## Microbial Population of the Reticulo-Rumen

The rumen provides an environment that is very favourable for microbial growth. The pH ranges between 5.8 and 6.8 for the most part and the temperature is (38-42°C) near optimum for many enzyme systems. The food supply is provided in a more or less continuous manner. Contractions of the stomach help to bring the microorganisms in contact with freshly ingested or ruminated feed and the ever-moist conditions of the rumino-reticulum are favourable for many organisms. End products of fermentation, which may be inhibitory, are removed by absorption and pass out of the stomach. Lastly the complete anaerobic condition creates a favourable environment for the growth of microbes both anaerobic and facultative anaerobes. They include bacteria, protozoa, oscillospira, yeast, moulds and bacteriophages.

**Table – 139**

**Average number of various types of micro-organisms in rumen liquor**

| Type of organisms | Buffalo | Cow | Sheep |
|---|---|---|---|
| 1. Total bacterial count × $10^{10}$ (Direct microscopic) | 6.9 to 32.70 | 5.4 to 31.4 | 18.0 to 88.0 |
| 2. Protozoa × $10^6$ | 1.8 to 13.8 | 0.3 to 19.7 | 1.4 to 7.8 |
| 3. Oscillospira × $10^4$ | 4.7 to 16.7 | 6.1 to 8.5 | |
| 4. Yeast × $10^3$ | 6.4 to 18.0 | 0.0 to 10.0 | 8.0 to 13.0 |
| 5. Bacteriophages | Exceeds bacteria in the ratio of 2:1 to 10:1 in all ruminants. | | |

## Rumen Bacteria

The bacterial flora of the reticulo-rumen is around × $10^{10}$ per ml of rumen liquor and over 60 species have so far been identified. Most are non-spore forming anaerobes, Gram negative or weakly Gram positive.

The different groups of bacteria present in the rumen have been classified:

A. On the basis of their biochemical activities.

B. Oxygen requirement.
C. Morphology.

A. **On the basis of biochemical activities**

1. *Cellulolytic* (*cellulose digesting*) *bacteria*: Bacteria attacking cellulose may be either rod shaped or cocci.

This group of bacteria is mainly responsible for the digestion of cellulose of the feed. They also ferment glucose, celloboise cellulose, pectin, starch, D-xylose, maltose, sucrose, fructose, L-xylose with the production of acetic, succinic, formic, butyric, lactic, propionic, diaminopimelic acids, ethanol, carbon-dioxide and hydrogen.

Rod shaped cellulolytic bacteria which are abundant in the rumen comprises : *Baceriodes succinogenes, Butyrivibrio fibrisolvens* and *Clostridium lochheadii, Clostridium longisoporum, Cillobacterium cellulosolvens, Cellulomonas fimi*.

Amongst cocci shaped are *Ruminococcus albus, Ruminococcus flavefaciens.*

The cellulose decomposing bacteria varies from 3-7 per cent of the total microflora. The cellulose digested in the rumen constitutes as much as one-third of the total fermented substrate.

2. *Hemicellulose digesting bacteria*: Hemicellulose differs from cellulose in that it contains pentose as well as hexose sugars and usually uronic acids. Hemicellulose is an important plant constituent, and organisms which are capable of hydrolysing cellulose are usually capable of utilising hemicellulose. However, a number which can utilise hemicellulose cannot utilise cellulose. Some of the species which digest hemicellulose include: *Butyrivibrio fibrisolvens, Lachnospira multiparus, Bacteroides ruminicola.*

3. *Amylolytic bacteria* (*starch digesters*): They mainly hydrolyse starch in the presence of amylolytic enzyme which is found in the rumen ($\alpha$-amylase) due to microbial secretion by some typical microbes. Some cellulolytic bacteria are also amylolytic in nature. The fermentation products are lactic, formic, acetic, succinic and propionic acids and even butyric acid.

The cellulolytic species which are also amylolytic are *Clostridium lochheadii, Bacteroides succinogenes, Butyrivibrio fibrisolvens*, and amongst non-cellulolytic species are *Bacteroides amylophilus, Bacteroids ruminicola, Butyrivibrio fibrisolvens, Streptococcus bovis, Succinimonas amylolytica, Selenomonas ruminantium.*

Amylolytic organisms are found in much larger percentages of the total microbial population when rations high in starch are fed.

4. *Bacteria utilising sugars*: Most of the bacteria which are capable of utilising polysaccharides are also capable of utilising disaccharides or monosaccharides. Plant material, particularly from young plants, contains a relatively large amount of water soluble carbohydrates and these would be available to bacteria. Presumably, sugars from dead and lysing bacterial cells or from capsular material of bacterial cells would also be available, otherwise, the rapid fermentation of soluble carbohydrates would make survival difficult for organisms that depend on sugars for their energy source. Cellobiose may be a source of energy for some of these

organisms since it has been demonstrated that many noncellulolytic organisms have the β-glucosidase enzyme required to hydrolyse cellobiose. High concentrations of organisms utilising lactose are found in the rumen of young ruminants.

5. *Bacteria utilising acids*: A number of organisms are known to utilise lactic acid although it is not normally present in appreciable amounts in the rumen in abnormal situations. Others utilise succinic acid or similar acids such as malic or fumaric. Some species which utilise lactic acid include: *Veillonella gazogenes*, *V. alacalescens*, *Peptostreptococcus elsdenii*, *Propioni bacterium* sp., *Desulphovibrio* and *Selenomonas lactilytica.*

6. *Proteolytic bacteria*: They digest feed or plant protein from which microbial protein is synthesised which is ultimately used by the host. These bacteria do utilise ammonia and sugars as energy. They live on other bacteria in the absence or shortage of substrates. The increased concentration of $NH_3$ before feeding is due to the action of these cytoclastic types.

The organisms involved are nonspore forming *Proteus* spp. Corny bacterium and Micrococcus and amongst spore formers *Lachnospira multiparus*, *Bacteroides succinogenes*, *B. amilophilus*, *Bacillus licheniformis*, *Eubacterium ruminantium*, *Aerobactor aerogenes*, *Bacteroides ruminicola*, *Lactobacillus fermenti*, *Streptococcus elsdenii*, *Peptostreptococcus elsdenii*, *Clostridium sporogenes* are notworthy.

7. *Ammonia producing organisms*: This class may be a duplication to some extent of No. 6. However, a number of organisms are known to produce ammonia from various sources. These are: *Bacteroides ruminicola*, *Selenomonas ruminantium*, *Peptostreptococcus elsdenii* and some strains of *Butyrivibrio.*

8. *Methanogenic bacteria*: Being very difficult to culture bacteria producing methane *in vitro*, very little is known about such organisms with respect to their specific requirements, even though the rumen must harbour a large number of this group of bacteria to produce 25 per cent of the total gas as methane. Methanogenic bacteria that have been identified include: *Methanobacterium ruminantium*, *M. formicicum* which grow with hydrogen and $CO_2$ as energy source and convert these to $CH_4$ and $H_2O$. Species believed to be of lesser importance include: *M. sohngenii*, *M. suboxydans* and *Methosarcina* sp.

9. *Lipolytic bacteria*: This group is associated with the hydrolysis of fat into glycerol and fatty acids. The fermentation products are acetic, propionic, butyric and succinic acids with large quantities of other gases including hydrogen sulphide. Among sugars, glycerol, ribose and fructose are fermented.

The bacterial species concerned with the fermentation of fat are *Anaerovibrio lipolytica.*

10. *Ureolytic bacteria*: These organisms mostly utilise ammonia and urea nitrogen which come through saliva from blood and also from nonprotein nitrogenous substances of the feed. The dead microbial cells are utilised by the host. The organisms concerned with this are *Lactobacillus bificlus*, *Bacteroides amylophilus*, *Proteus mirabillis.*

11. *Sulphate utilising bacteria*: The rumen microorganisms which decompose cellulose

and utilise urea nitrogen have a requirement for sulphur which can be met by sulphate. The sulphate present in the rumen is reduced to sulphide (a compound of sulphur with another element or a radical) and the sulphite (a salt of sulphurous acid) incorporated into amino acids.

This is done by *Clostridium nigrificans. Lachnospira multiparus, Butyrivibrio fibrisolvens* and *Bacteroides* species.

**B. On the basis of oxygen requirement**

i) *Facultative anaerobes*

Many species of facultatively anaerobic bacteria have been isolated from the rumen. However, in many cases, little evidence has been presented to indicate that these bacteria were of numerical importance. These organisms include number of the genera *Flavebacterium, Pseudomonao, Proteus* and *Micrococcus* which comprise the following types:

1. *Coliform* bacteria
2. *Bacillus* group
3. *Propionibacteria*
4. *Lactobacillus*
5. *Streptococci*

ii) *Anaerobes*:

1. *Spore forming rods*:
   (a) *Clostridium*
2. *Nonspore forming rods*
   (a) *Lactobacilli*
   (b) *Ramibaeteria*
   (c) *Eubacteria*
   (d) *Methanobacteria*
   (e) *Lachnospirae*
   (f) *Cillobacteria*
   (g) Succinic acid-producing bacteroides
   (h) *Amylophilus*
   (i) *Butyrivibrio*
   (j) Bytyric acid-producing bacteroides
   (k) *Fusobacteria*
   (l) *Succinivibrio*
   (m) *Desulfovibrio*
   (n) *Selenomonas*
   (o) *Bo*ı*elia*
   (p) *Succinimonas*
3. *Cocci*
   (a) *Peptostreptococci*
   (b) *Ruminococci*
   (c) *Veillonellae*

**C. On the basis of bacterial morphology**

The different groups of bacteria which are found in the rumen, morphologically they may be classified as rods, cocci, spirillum and vibrio. The population of cocci is predominant 50-89 per cent, followed by the rods 45-70 per cent, the spirillum 0-5 per cent and the vibrio 0-4 per cent. Variation in numbers mostly depend on the type of feed. Inclusion of more proteinous feed and high concentrates results in the increase of rods and absence of spirillum. Feeding of legume feeds results in an increase of rods and cocci while there is a simultaneous decrease of spirillum along with complete disappearance of vibrio.

Table 140

Characteristic of some rumen bacteria

| Organism | Shape of cells | Gram stain | Substrate utilised | Major end-products of fermentation |
|---|---|---|---|---|
| **Cellulose degradation** | | | | |
| *Bacteroides succinogenes* | Rods to Coccoid | — | Cellulose, cellobiose, glucose, $CO_2$ | Succinate, acetate, formate |
| *Ruminococcus flavefaciens* | Cocci, mostly in chain | ± | Cellulose, cellobiose, xylose, $CO_2$ | Succinate, lactate, acetate, formate, $H_2$ |
| *Ruminococcus albus* | Cocci | ± | Cellulose, cellobiose, xylose, $CO_2$ | |
| *Clostridium lochheadii* | Rods | — | Cellulose, glucose, starch, fructose, Hemicellulose | Acetate, formate |
| *Butyrivibrio fibrisolvens* | Curved rod | — | Cellulose, wide range of sugars | Butyrate, lactate, formate, $CO_2$ |
| *Cillobacterium cellulasovens* | Coccoid to rod | | Cellulose, glucose | Volatile fatty acids |
| **Starch degradation** | | | | |
| *Bacteroides amylophilus* | Rods to coccoid | — | Starch, maltose, $CO_2$ | Succinate, acetate, lactate |
| *Streptococcus bovis* | Cocci | + | Starch, wide range of sugars | Lactate |
| **Pectin degradation** | | | | |
| *Lachnospira multiparus* | Curved rod | ± | Pectin, cellobiose, hemicellulose | Formate, lactate, acetate, $CO_2$, $H_2$ |
| *Succinivibrio dextrinosolvens* | Spinal | — | Pectin, dextrin, maltose, xylose | Acetate, succinate, lactate |
| **Methane production** | | | | |
| *Methanobacterium ruminantium* | Curved rod | + | $CO_2$, $H_2$, formate, acetate | $CH_4$ production |
| *Methanobacterium formicicum* | Curved rod | + | $CO_2$, $H_2$, formate, acetate | $CH_4$ production |
| **Lipolytic** | | | | |
| *Anaerovibrio lipolytica* | Rods | | Glycerol, fats and oils | Volatile fatty acids |
| **Proteolytic** | | | | |
| *Bacteroides amylophilus* | Rods to coccoid | — | | Ammonia, VFA, $CO_2$ |
| *Selenomonas ruminantium* | Crescentic | — | Protein and NPN plant component | |
| *Bacteroides ruminicola* | Rods to coccoid | — | Glucose, xylen, starch | |
| **Urolytic** | | | | |
| *Lactobacillus bifidus* | Rods | — | Protein, urea | Ammonia, VFA, $CO_2$ |
| *Bacteroides amylophilus* | Rods to coccoid | | Protein, urea, starch, maltose | Ammonia, VFA lactic acid |

## Rumen Protozoa

Protozoa are present in much smaller numbers ($10^6$/ml) than bacteria but being larger may equal the latter in total mass. Rumen protozoa constitutes mostly of ciliates and a few species of small flagillates. The ciliate protozoa of the reticulo-rumen are of two types generally referred to as *Holotrichs* and *Entodiniomorphs.*

The holotrichs are characterised by the possession of cillia over the whole body surface. These are paramaecium-like cells having two distinct sizes for its two genera : (1) *Isotricha*—are large ($65\mu \times 130\mu$), whereas (2) *Dasytricha*—are small ($35\mu \times 65\mu$). The holotrichs metabolise soluble sugars as sources of carbon and energy, generally polymerising hexoses to amylopectin. The major fermentation products of the holotrichs are acetic, butyric and lactic acids together with gases of $CO_2$ and $H_2$.

They keep motility longer in the presence of oxygen. In young animals holotrich establishes first. The species belonging to this order are as follows:

*Blepharoconus cervicalis*
*Blepharocory bovis*
*Blepharoprosthium pirem*
*Blitschlia parva*
*Dasytricha ruminantium*
*Didesmis quadrata*
*Holophryoides ovalis*
*Blepharosphaera intestinalis*
*Blepharozoum zonatum*
*Bundleia postciliata*
*Isotricha intestinalis*
*Isotricha prostoma*
*Polymorpha ampulla*
*Prorodonopsis coli*

The entodiniomorphs are represented by many genera, chief among them being *Entodinium, Epidinium, Eudiplodinium, Diplodinium, Polyplastron* and *Ophryoscolex*. The distribution and proportions of these genera in the reticulo-rumen are greatly influenced by the diet of the animal.

The entodiniomorphs are characterised by their cilia being confined to specific regions of the body surface, usually at the anterior end. They are predominantly particle feeders, ingesting both plant and bacterial cells and starch grains; soluble carbohydrates are only used as sources of carbon and energy when particulate food is unavailable. Fermentation products of entodiniomorphs are similar to those of holotrichs that is, $CO_2$, $H_2$, various volatile fatty acids and lactic acid.

*Unlike rumen bacteria, most of which appear to use $NH_4^+$ as a source of nitrogen for protein biosynthesis, the entodiniomorphs utilise amino acids of plant and bacterial origin without prior deamination.*

With respect to nitrogen metabolism, they rapidly hydrolyse a variety of different proteins, producing ammonia from amide groups along with liberation of amino acids and peptides.

From the point of view of lipid metabolism in the rumen, the entodiniomorphs ingest particulate material of plant origin, including chloroplasts and could potentially protect the unsaturated fatty acids of these from hydrogenation by rumen bacteria.

The species belonging to this order observed are :

*Galoscolex cuspidatus*
*Cochliatoxum periachtum*
*Cunhaia curvata*
*Eodinium lobatum*
*Epidinium caudatum*
*Eremoplastron bovis*

*Cycloposthium bipalmatum*
*Cycloposthium dentiferum*
*Diplodinium dentatum*
*Diploplastron affine*
*Ditoxum funinucleum*
*Elytroplastron hegneri*
*Entodinium brusa*
*Entodinium caudatum*
*Enoplastron triloricatum*
*Eudiplodinium maggii*
*Metadinium medium*
*Ophisthotrichum janus*
*Ophryoscolex bicoronatus*
*Ophryoscolex caudatus*
*Ophryscolex quadricoronatus*
*Ostracodinium dentatum*
*Polyplastron multivesiculatum*
*Tripalmariado gieli*

## Oscillospira

Ine organism is motile and iodophilic in nature. In comparison with bacteria it is large in size. The cell structure shows filaments filled transversely making partitions in the cell. It could not be cultured outside the rumen. Till recently it was considered to be a yeast. But it possesses similar cell wall structure and composition as in Gram negative bacteria. This depicts that this organism is a higher form of bacteria. *Oscillospira guilleromondii* has been found only in the rumen.

## Rumen Yeast

The role of yeast is not clear as yet but it is understood that they are normal inhabitants, in small numbers, of the rumen and intestines of herbivores. They are also found in the faeces of humans. They may be concerned with sugar fermentation and cellulose digestion as well. Under certain conditions they may also suppress the growth of pathogens, synthesise B-complex vitamins and also may help in stabilising normal rumen flora.

Nine species of yeasts belong to four genera namely, *Candida*, *Trichosporon*, *Rhodtoirula* and *Saccharomyces* have so far commonly observed in the rumen.

## Rumen Moulds

Presence of moulds in the rumen have been reported very recently. The function, if any, is not known as yet. Moreover the moulds are not commonly found. The moulds that have been identified belong to *Mucor*, *Rhizopus* and *Aspergillus* species.

## Rumen Bacteriophages

The information about the normal existence of bacteriophages in the rumen is of much more recent origin. During the last 10 years, identification of more than 125 morphologically distinct types have been made. Further, the phages were found in more than 65 distinct rumen bacteria as intracellular phage. Counts indicated that bacteriophages exceeded bacteria in the ratio of 2 : 1 to 10 : 1.

## Digestion in the Rumen

### 1. Digestion of carbohydrates

The vigorous fermentation of carbohydrate is perhaps the outstanding feature of the whole rumen process. A wide variety of substances, ranging from the simple soluble sugars of plant juices to the physically tough and chemically resistant cellulose fibre, is converted here into a group of common products. All the commonly known monosaccharides (D-ribose, D and L-arabinose, D-xylose, D-glucose, D-mannose, D-galactose and D-fructose), as well as some of their derivatives such as sugar alcohols and uronic acids, are fermented. Most of the naturally occurring oligo- and polysaccharides are built from one or more of the above sugars, so that the ability of the rumen contents to ferment them depends on the synthesis of the necessary hydrolytic enzymes by at least a few of the microorganisms present. The different organisms of the microflora and fauna can muster between them an impressive array of carbohydrases; the following have been detected either in the mixed rumen organisms or in pure cultures: a number of α- and β-D-glucosidases of varying specificity, α- and β-D-galactosidase, α-D-mannosidase, β-D-glucuronidase, invertase, β-D-xylosidase, L-arabinosidase, α-amylase, cellulase, dextranase, laminarinase, xylanase, polygalacturonase and pectin methyl esterase. With the aid of these enzymes almost all of the oligo- and polysaccharides which normally enter the rumen may be hydrolysed, but a few polysaccharides seem to be quite unaffected. The principal ones are some of the polysaccharides of seaweeds, some plant gums and the capsular polysaccharide of *Streptococcus bovis*.

#### (i) Cellulose

It comprises the most abundant organic substance in the world. In cattle eating green forages, most of the cellulose will be digested in the rumen, and the rest will be in the caecum and colon.

To digest cellulose, which comprises the bulk of ruminant feed, there is an absolute need of cellulase enzyme. Cellulase is absent from the entire gastrointestinal secretions of most of the animals and so the digestion of the cellulosic material of plants is brought about only by the enzyme secreted by the microorganisms of the digestive tract.

The vigorous fermentation of cellulose is perhaps the most outstanding feature of the whole rumen process. The component in the rumen is fermented by microbial enzyme-cellulase to volatile fatty acids through the initial formation of glucose; but whether acetic or propionic acid is the major products ultimately formed from glucose is a matter of controversy. Some are of the opinion that the molar ratio of propionic acid : acetic acid as found in sheep rumen liquor varies between 1.5 and 2.0 in *in vitro* experiments but others, who added radioactive cellulose to rumen liquor in which hay and grass were already being fermented, found that this ratio was less than one. In the whole animal, the fibrous diets lead to a high proportion of acetic acid in the ruminal volatile fatty acids. In spite of being subject to attack at more than one site in the gut, cellulose is never digested completely. It rarely exceeds 70 per cent what is eaten and the rest is voided out through faeces. The most important factor influencing cellulose digestibility is the extent to which cellulose is lignified. Cellulose digestibility is further depressed if more readily fermented materials such as starch or casein are also present and also by the products of cellulose fermentation. Among stimulatory agents of cellulose fermentation, valeric acid and to a lesser extent butyric acid and the presence of minerals are important.

CELLULOSE (a complex polysaccharide)

CELLULASE — an enzyme synthesized by some bacteria and protozoa but not by animals

CELLOBIOSE (1,4' β glucoside)

CELLOBIOSASE β glucosidase

D-GLUCOSE

The breakdown of cellulose in the rumen are brought by both bacterial and protozoal enzymes. Most of the cellulolytic bacteria of the rumen are strictly anaerobic in nature. As discussed earlier, the most common cellulolytic bacteria of the rumen fall in the genera *Ruminococcus, Bacteroides, Butyrivibrio*; of next importance are *Cillobacterium* and *Clostridium.*

In sheep it has been determined that approximately 70 per cent of the digestible cellulose in the feed is fermented in the rumen, 17 per cent in the caecum and 15 per cent in the colon. Apparently, no cellulose digestion takes place in the abomasum or in the small intestine.

The end products of cellulose digestion in the rumen are acetic and propionic acid together with $CO_2$ and methane. Certain strains produce free hydrogen which is utilised for other reactions like methane formation or for hydrogenation of free unsaturated fatty acids in the rumen.

Among the protozoa of the rumen, a number of protozoa such as *Polyplastron multiresienlatum* and *Ophryoscolex tricoronatus* have active cellulase activity. The protozoa digest cellulose to liberate mostly cellobiose and glucose. The members of protozoa Oligotrich ingest cellulose but Holotrichs do not have this property and are excellent in digesting starch due to strong α-amylase activity.

**(ii) Digestion of pentose**

The pentosans occur in the feed of ruminants to a large extent in close association with cellulose, and their disappearance during digestion closely parallels the disappearance of the cellulose.

*In vitro*, rumen contents or washed suspensions of rumen bacteria ferment pentosans mainly to acetic acid and propionic acid. Butyric acid is formed only in small amounts, and lactic acid hardly at all. Similar products are formed when the rumen contents ferment xylose or glucuronic acid, both of which are constituent sugars of pentosans.

The bacteria which are of importance in ruminal fermentation of pentosan are all strict anaerobes and belong mainly to the genera *Ruminococcus*, *Bacteroides* and *Butyrivibrio*.

Enzymes hydrolysing pentosan in the rumen have attracted some more attention. From two pure cultures of rumen bacteria three enzymes were separated : (i) a *xylanase* which hydrolyses xylan at random as far as xylobiose, (ii) a β-*xylosidase* which hydrolyses xylobiose, and (iii) an *arabinosidase*, which removes arabinose side-chains from pentosans.

Of the rumen protozoa, *Epidinium ecaudatum*, mixed *Entodinium* species and *Polyplastron multivesiculatum* are able to hydrolyse pentosans.

**(iii) Digestion of starch**

The compound is unnatural for ruminants and probably that is why feeding of large amounts of starchy feed to ruminants can often lead to digestive disturbances. The presence of rumen bacteria and protozoa have been identified which can decompose starch. Among bacteria, *Streptococcus bovis*, a facultative anaerobe digests starch rapidly, yielding a mixture of acetic acid and lactic acid as products of digestion. More recently, a group of strictly anaerobic rod has been found to be involved in starch fermentation in rumen. These include *Butyrivibrio*; *Bacteroides amylophilus*, which ferment only starch and maltose, producing succinic acid and smaller amounts of formic acid and acetic acid. Some strains of *Bacteroides ruminicola*, and a number of strains of *Selenomonas ruminantium*, yield succinic acid as the main fermentation product, and others propionic acid, probably according to their ability to synthesise the appropriate decarboxylase. *Succinivibrio dextrinosolvens* can not ferment starch, but it can ferment dextrin, maltose and glucose.

A high proportion of the ciliate protozoa of the rumen can ferment starch. Swallowing of the starch grains by the protozoa appears to be essential for this fermentation to occur. There is considerable agreement in the pattern of fermentation products among these organisms. Acetic acid and butyric acid are the main products in all cases; propionic acid is a minor product; and formic acid and lactic acid are formed only in traces. The protozoa also produce hydrogen and carbon dioxide in molar ratios between 1 : 1 and 2 : 1.

Of the protozoa, *Entodinum caudatum*, *Epidinium ecaudatum*, *Ophryoscolex purkynei*, *O. caudatus*, *Eudiplodinium maggii* and *Polyplastron multivesiculatum*, which are all starch digesting protozoa of the rumen possess α-amylase and they swallow starch grains.

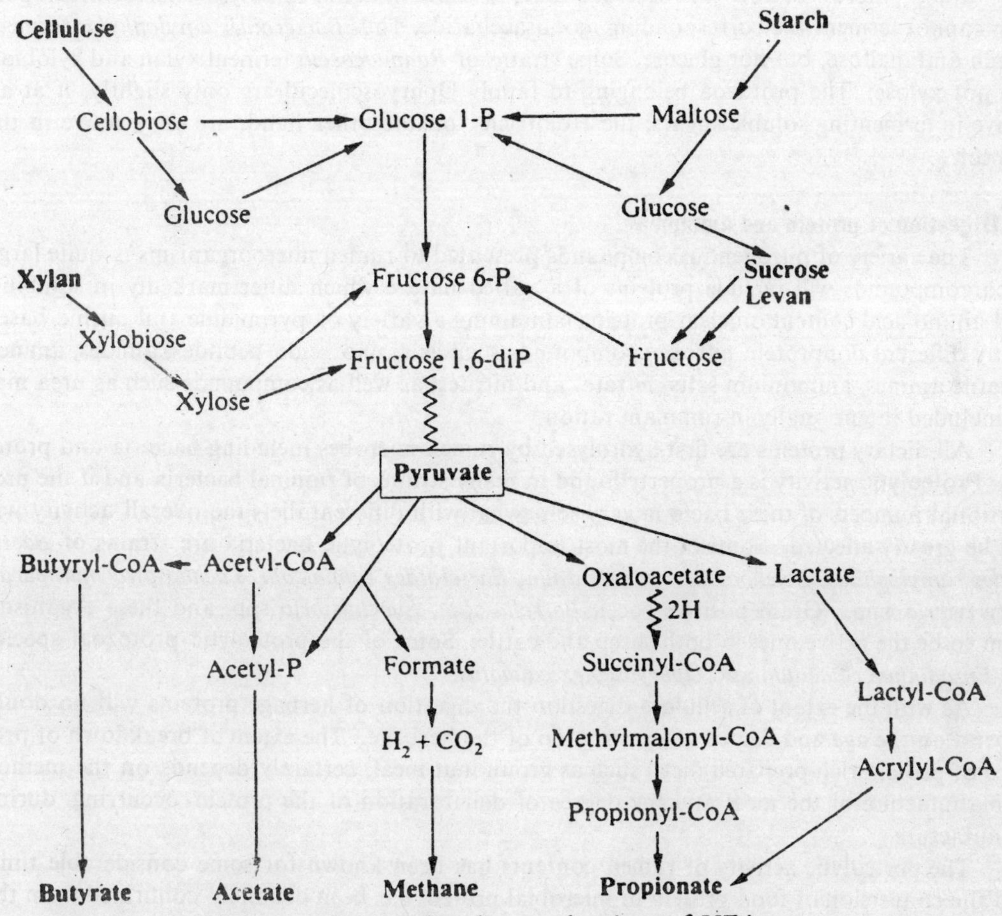


**Fig. 82** Metabolic pathways for the production of VFA

**(iv) Fermentation of soluble sugars**

It will be convenient to consider not only mono and di-saccharides under this heading but also those soluble polysaccharides known as fructosans. Usually the plants just before flowering contain these compounds at over 25 per cent of the dry matter.

Some bacteria, osciollospira and protozoa (Holotrichs) are capable of fermenting fodder sugars. The result is that the ruminant absorbs little or none of the soluble sugar of the ration but instead obtains the short chain fatty acids mainly as acetic and propionic acids. Lactic acids may appear temporarily in the rumen when a large amount of sugar is fed. Lactic acid, however, is not stable in the rumen as the bacteria are capable of fermenting it further to acetic and propionic acids.

Less is known about the pentose sugar. Mixed rumen organisms are known to ferment xylose and pentose. The products of xylose fermentation are also mainly acetic and propionic acids with less of butyric and traces of formic acid.

It is of interest to note that several strains of bacteria active in polysaccharide decomposition cannot ferment the corresponding monosaccharide. Thus *Bacteroides amylophylus* ferments starch and maltose, but not glucose. Some strains of *Ruminococcus* ferment xylan and xylobiose but not xylose. The protozoa belonging to family Ophryoscolecid are only slightly, if at all, active in fermenting soluble sugars; the Holotrichs, on the other hand, are very active in this respect.

**2. Digestion of protein and ammonia**

The variety of nitrogenous compounds presented to rumen microorganisms is quite large. Such compounds will include proteins of a varied nature which differ markedly in solubility and amino acid content, nuclear proteins containing a variety of pyrimidine and purine bases, many different nonprotein nitrogen compounds such as amino acids, peptides, amides, amines, votatile amines, ammonium salts, nitrates and nitrites, as well as compounds such as urea may be included intentionally in ruminant ration.

All dietary proteins are first hydrolysed by rumen microbes including bacteria and protozoa. Proteolytic activity is a property found in many strains of ruminal bacteria and if the proportional numbers of these bacteria vary somewhat with different diets the overall activity will not be greatly affected. Some of the most important proteolytic bacteria are strains of *Bacteroides amylophilus*, *Selenomonas ruminantium*, *Bacteroides ruminicola*, *Lachnospira multiparus*, *Butyrivibrio* spp., Gram positive cocci, *Borrelia* spp., *Succinivibrio* spp. and these organisms seem to be the active ones in both sheep and cattle. Some of the proteolytic protozoal species are *Entodinium caudatum* and *Ophryoscolex caudatus*.

As with the extent of cellulose digestion the digestion of herbage proteins will no doubt depend on the age and degree of lignification of the herbage. The extent of breakdown of proteins of protein rich prepared diets, such as groundnut meal, certainly depends on the method of manufacture of the meal and the degree of denaturation of the protein occurring during manufacture.

The proteolytic activity of rumen contents has been known for some considerable time, and the conversion of food protein to microbial protein has been definitely confirmed from the work of John K. Loosli (teacher of the author) of Cornell University who fed sheep and goats on a synthetic diet of sugar, starch, cellophane, minerals, lard, urea and vitamins A and D and found that the animals gained weight on this diet over a three month experimental period. The diet did contain traces of amino acids, probably from a protein contamination of maize starch, but the rumen contents contained 9 to 20 times more amino acids than the diet.

The amino acids are produced by the microbes during their extensive proliferation by utilising rumen ammonia originating from protein and nonprotein nitrogenous compounds of the feed. Microbial yield of protein is variable but ranges between 90 and 230 g per kilogramme of organic matter digested. This amount is adequate to provide the protein for growing animals over about 100 kg and to maintain levels of milk production up to 10 kg per day. Feed protein *per se* obviously must be provided for high producing cows. The microbial protein is of good digestibility (true digestibility of protozoa is about 88 per cent and of bacteria it is 66 per cent) and has an amino acid content similar to that of a good pasture protein. The protozoal protein is much better than bacterial protein particularly as because protozoal protein is rich in essential amino acids, notably lysine. The protozoal protein may make up some 20 per cent of the total microbial protein. Thus the ammonia nitrogen is utilised along with the available carbon skeletons, plus energy and minerals particularly sulphur and phosphorus, to build up huge quantities of bacterial and protozoal protein which pass into rest of the G.I. tract to be digested for releasing all essential amino acids to the host. At the same time, if there is sufficient protein in the diet to result in a surplus in the rumen, this proportion will not be degraded and so will pass to the abomasum and small intestine for digestion. Thus there is rumen *degradable* and *nondegradable protein.*

Any nonprotein nitrogen, which will include any urea given in the diet, will be degraded first. The more soluble proteins, such as casein in milk will be degraded before less soluble feed proteins, such as maize protein. The latter stand a better chance of avoiding deamination by the rumen micro-organisms.

The disappearance of the initial protein hydrolysis products from the rumen takes place in two ways, as there is little absorption of amino acid through the rumen epithelium. Firstly, the amino acids are incorporated into microbial protein and some peptides may be preferentially utilised for microbial growth. Secondly, the amino acids are deaminated. Unlike proteolytic activity the deaminative activity of rumen microbes appears to depend to some extent on the diet.

A diet containing a soluble protein will undergo more of deaminative activity. The final products are principally ammonia, $CO_2$ and VFA. *Deamination* of amino acids is probably the principal source of the branched-chain fatty acids utilised during the growth of some rumen bacteria. Deaminative activity appears less frequently in rumen bacterial strains than in proteolytic activity. Strains of *Bacteroides ruminocola*, *Butyrivibrio* and *Selenomonas ruminantium* are amongst the more active deaminating bacteria. The rate of deamination is usually slower than proteolysis. Rumen microbes also liberate ammonia from adenine, guanine, hypoxanthine, xanthene, uric acid, uracil and thymine at a slow rate. Hence there is a greater concentration of amino acids and peptides, followed by ammonia concentration approximately three hours after feeding. Valine, leucine and isoleucine are degraded and decarboxylated to liberate isobutyric, isovaleric and β-methyl butyric acids respectively. The amino acids which are degraded through oxidative decarboxylation or deamination are as follows :

| | |
|---|---|
| Glycine | —Acetic acid+$NH_3$ |
| L-serine | —Acetic acid+$CO_2$+$NH_3$ |
| L-threonine | —Propionic acid+$CO_2$+$NH_3$ |
| L-aspertic acid | —Fumeric acid+$NH_3$ |
| L-glutamic acid | —L-ketoglutaric acid+$NH_3$ |
| L-lysine | —Cadavarine* +$NH_3$ |
| L-arginine | —Ornithine+$NH_3$ |
| L-ornithine | —Putrescine* +$NH_3$ |
| L-histidine | —Urocanic acid+$NH_3$ |
| L-phenylalanine | —Phenylacetic acid+$NH_3$ |
| L-tyrosine | —Phenyl propionic acid+$NH_3$ |
| L-tryptophan | —Indol-zyl- acetic acid+$NH_3$ |

*(Polyamines that contains two amino groups).

Deamidation, an activity which has been demonstrated in some strains of *B. ruminicola, Butyrivibrio, S. ruminantium, Eubacterium* and other rumen bacteria will release ammonia from amides.

Urea is always present in the saliva and may also be introduced into the rumen as a nitrogenous supplement. The urea from the saliva may have its origin from ammonia absorbed into the blood stream through the rumen epithelium. Thus although absorption of ammonia formed by the rumen bacteria can lead to loss of nitrogen in the urine of the ruminant, its reappearance as salivary urea (or in secretions from the rumen epithelium) can also provide a second opportunity for bacteria to utilise it and convert it into valuable protein of use to the animal. *Lactobacillus bifidus*, the only anaerobic ureolytic bacterium has so far been isolated.

The activities of urease and deaminating and deamidating mechanisms produce enough ammonia which vary widely from 85 to over 300 mg per litre. It has been confirmed that many of the rumen bacteria, whether supplied with exogenous amino acids or not, will synthesise their body protein from the nitrogen of ammonia and the carbon of volatile fatty acids including branched-chain butyric and valeric acids.

Sulphur is also needed for the formation of sulphur-containing amino acids such as for cystine and methionine. Supply of elemental sulphur or sulphide is acceptable to microorganisms but for sulphate, it has to be reduced as sulphide before being incorporated in a microbial body. The only true sulphate reducing bacterium so far isolated from the rumen has been a strain of organism known as *Clostridium nigrificans.* Protozoa instead of utilising sulphur, utilise the preformed amino acids of ingested bacteria. It may be noted that *ciliate protozoa (both holotrichs and entodiniomorphs) are unable to utilise $NH_3$ as such and hence they feed mostly upon bacteria to derive their nutrients.* In fact protozoa have got very little ability to synthesise amino acids and B-complex vitamins. They obtain these two groups of nutrients from bacteria, and may hydrogenate unsaturated fatty acids to liberate saturated fatty acids.

**Amino acid composition of rumen microbial protein**

The gross amino acid composition of the microbial fraction entering the duodenum is

**Table 141**

**The Amino acid composition of bacterial and protozoal protein isolated from rumen of sheep**

| Amino acids (AA) | Bacterial protein (g AA/16 g N) | Protozoal-protein (g AA/16 g N) |
|---|---|---|
| Threonine | 5.37 ± 0.39 | 5.07 ± 0.48 |
| Valine | 5.49 ± 0.35 | 5.24 ± 0.60 |
| Isoleucine | 4.68 ± 0.20 | 5.80 ± 0.54 |
| Leucine | 6.47 ± 0.30 | 7.18 ± 0.66 |
| Phenylalanine | 3.98 ± 0.18 | 5.29 ± 0.51 |
| Histidine | 1.49 ± 0.11 | 1.79 ± 0.15 |
| Lysine | 6.99 ± 0.37 | 10.14 ± 0.60 |
| Arginine | 4.09 ± 0.25 | 4.58 ± 0.31 |
| Methionine | 1.78 ± 0.09 | 1.65 ± 0.16 |
| Aspertic acid | 12.10 ± 0.56 | 12.62 ± 1.24 |
| Serine | 4.24 ± 0.23 | 4.10 ± 0.37 |
| Glutamic acid | 11.18 ± 0.59 | 13.81 ± 1.62 |
| Glycine | 4.85 ± 0.34 | 3.61 ± 0.46 |
| Alanine | 6.12 ± 0.37 | 3.48 ± 0.40 |
| Tyrosine | 3.90 ± 0.19 | 4.49 ± 0.48 |

Source : Ling, J.R. (1976) Ph.D. Thesis, University of Nottingham quoted by P.J. Buttery and A.N Foulds, Recent Advances in Animal Nutrition, 1985, Butterworths Publication, London.

not markedly influenced by the diet of the animal. Bacteria make up the major component of this fraction and even changes in the ratios of individual species of bacteria are unlikely to influence the amino acid pattern of the combined bacterial fraction.

The amino acid composition of different strains of protozoa does differ but this is thought to be of little significance. While the amino acid composition of either the protozoal fraction or the bacterial fraction are unlikely to differ much with variation in the diet, there are marked differences in the composition of bacterial and protozoal protein. *The differences in the proportions of lysine (higher in protozoa) and methionine (higher in bacteria) are potentially of significance.*

It has further been observed that the true digestibility of rumen microorganism nitrogen is 0.81, and the absorbed nitrogen from rumen microorganisms is used with an efficiency of 0.67. Under most dietary conditions, microbial protein synthesised in the forestomach (rumen, reticulum and omasum) of the ruminant accounts for 60-80 per cent of the total amino acid nitrogen entering the small intestine.

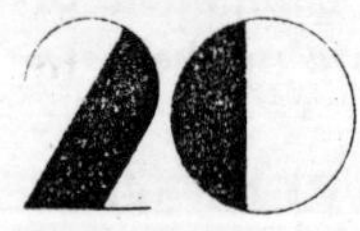

# FACTORS AFFECTING DIGESTIBILITY

For convenience, the factors affecting digestion may be discussed as follows:

**A. Animal Effects**

1. AGE. Very young or very old animals are usually less efficient in their digestion of feeds. The young can neither eat nor digest very much roughage until their digestive tracts, specially their rumens are developed. In case of old animals their ability to digest feed is often impaired by poor teeth, which makes adequate chewing of their feed very difficult. Declining health might further adversely affect digestibility at an advanced age.

2. WORK. Light exercise seems to improve digestibility of feeds while heavy exercise depresses it.

3. INDIVIDUALITY. Animals have been shown to differ in their digestion of the same kind of feed as much as 25 per cent. However, most animals vary about 4-5 per cent.

**B. Plant Effect**

1. VARIETY. Differences have been reported between varieties within the same species, i.e., two varieties of lucerne. However, there may be more actual difference in the feeding value of the two lots of the same variety of hay than there is between hay of two entirely different kinds. Thus, other factors such as soil fertility, method of harvesting, etc., are much more important than the variety.

2. STAGE OF MATURITY. Hay that is cut late has considerably lower digestibility than that which is cut early, if the early-cut hay is cured well. The percentage of protein, digestibility and the content of minerals and vitamins all decrease as hay crops advance in maturity.

3. SOIL FERTILITY BALANCE. The supply of mineral nutrients in the soil affects both the yield and the composition of forages.

4. HARVESTING. Loss of leaves, fermentation, bleaching and leaching all contribute to a lower value of hay.

**C. Preparation of Feed**

1. DEGREE OF FINENESS

(*a*) *Roughage.* If particle size becomes too fine, digestibility is decreased while total consumption will probably rise. The results of feeding roughage, which is of small particle size, are changes in the concentration of acetic and propionic acid produced in the rumen, as shown by consequent decreases in milk-fat percentages; probably due to increased rate of passage.

(*b*) *Grain.* If the particle size is too small, the feed is less digestible and less palatable.

2. LEVEL OF FEEDING. Increased levels of feeding result in decreased digestibility. However, in the case of animals which are kept for meat, milk or work, levels of feeding well above the requirements for maintenance are needed for production.

3. NUTRIENT BALANCE. When several feeds are fed in a ration, one feed may influence the digestibility of the other, or it gives "associative effects". For example, protein may increase the breakdown of the higher, more complex carbohydrates because of its favourable effect upon the rumen micro-organisms.

4. EFFECT OF PELLETING. Pellets or cubes are made by grinding, pressing and extruding concentrates consist of finely ground feed and/or hay or other roughage in special machines. This process reduces the bulkiness of feeds. Since a given weight of pelleted feed takes up less space, animals may eat more pelleted feed than ground feed Review of the literature shows that the feeding of pelleted roughage does not increase digestibility. What actually happens upon consumption of ground and pelleted feed by the ruminants may be summarised as below:

1. Reduced time of prehension and mastication,
2. Less of saliva secretion,
3. Decrease in rumination,
4. Increase in rate of fermentation in the rumen,
5. Decreased in pH in the rumen,
6. Increase rate of passage of feed particles from the rumen,
7. Decrease in ratio of acetate to propionate in rumen,
8. Increase in concentration of rumen VFA one to 4 hours after feeding,
9. Increased dry matter intake,
10. Decrease in dry matter and crude fibre digestibility,
11. The finer the grinding of the forage prior to pelleting, the greater the effect.

5. TREATMENT OF STRAWS, HULLS, SAWDUST, etc., TO INCREASE DIGESTIBILITY. Products having very poor feeding value when treated by soaking, cooking, boiling, steaming with and without pressure, roasting, fermenting with yeast, hydrolysing and treating with chemicals such as NaOH, Ca $(OH)_2$, HCl, $Na_2S$, $NaHCO_4$ and $H_2SO_4$ followed by washing and drying did not appear to influence digestibility.

6. MOLASSES. May improve the palatibility of the ration, but large amounts tend to depress cellulose digestion. Levels above 7 per cent seem to depress digestibility while lower levels improve it. Most benefits will be received with lower amounts of molasses.

7. SALT AND WATER. Adequate amounts tend to favourably improve digestibility.

8. ADDITION OF ANTIBIOTICS. Feeding antibiotics to farm animals have been found to stimulate growth. The benefits have been postulated to be caused by: (*i*) the inhibition of toxin producing bacteria, (*ii*) the reduction in total numbers of intestinal bacteria and lowering of competition between host and micro flora for nutrients, and (*iii*) the selective inhibition of micro-flora permits increased growth of other micro-organisms that synthesise unidentified essential nutrients, promote digestion or detract from it. The antibiotics have not been found to exert any effect on the digestibility of dry matter, the ether extract, crude fibre or nitrogen-free extract.

**D. The Following Factors, while of Less Practical Importance Have Been Observed in Laboratory Work to Affect the Digestion of Cellulose Which Comprises a Large Per Cent of Roughages**

1. Ash from lucerne crops improves cellulose digestion; probably due to the presence of cobalt in the lucerne which is needed for vitamin $B_{12}$ synthesis.

2. Many minerals in varying amounts are needed for optimum cellulose digestion, especially cobalt, phosphorus, calcium, chlorine, magnesium, sodium, potassium, sulfur and others in trace amounts.

3. Protein, in quantities up to 15 per cent of the ration, increases cellulose digestion.

4. Rumen fluid has properties which cannot be substituted in the laboratory; it improves cellulose digestion.

5. Plant enzymes, when included in the substrate, improve cellulose digestion.

6. Other factors such as urea and maize extract, stilbesterol and others have shown to be beneficial to rumen micro-organisms in the breakdown of cellulose.

**What Can Be Done to Improve Digestion of Feed in the Dairy Herd?**

The following ten points are suggestions which might be made to improve the quality of the feed and its digestibility, thus improving the efficiency of production on the farm. Undoubtedly there are other factors which have been overlooked.

1. The basis of selection of dairy cows should include their efficiency of digestion; however, a practical method of doing this is not readily available. If a cow is a high producer, she should provide ample profits, although she might not be quite as efficient in feed digestibility as another cow of slightly lower production.

2. Providing feed of the highest nutritive value is probably the best means of improving digestibility. One should try to:

(*a*) Test soil prior to seeding pastures and forage crops; provide the mineral balance needed by the soil.

(*b*) Use only the highest quality seed for establishing the stand: use recommended varieties and certified seed.

(*c*) Cut hay crops early when possible; while less tonnage may be received, more digestible dry matter will probably be obtained.

(*d*) Avoid excess exposure of hay to rain and sun to keep leaching, bleaching and shattering to a minimum.

(*e*) Provide adequate storage of high quality hay; keep it out of the weather.

3. If finely ground roughage is fed, such as dehydrated alfalfa pellets, it is advisable to provide at least 3–4 kg of coarse roughage to the milking cow in order to avoid butterfat depression.

4. Evaluate the quality of roughage available to the milking herd and determine the approximate amount of energy needed, which should be provided through concentrates.

5. Avoid unnecessary fine grinding of concentrates which are unpalatable and costly to grind.

6. When feeding increases amount of grain (probably 10 kg or more), observe cows individually to avoid throwing.

7. **Provide ample salt and plenty of fresh water.**
8. **Avoid prolonged exposure of animals to adverse weather; provide shade and shelter.**
9. **Feed, milk and care for the herd on schedule with a reasonably qulte atmosphere.**
10. **Use good common sense in the application of the above recommendations.**

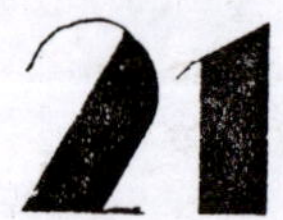

# EVALUATION OF ANIMAL FEED QUALITY

The evaluation of feeds used for the nutrition of our domestic animals is a matter of very great importance. This problem, therefore, is given much emphasis in all textbooks on animal nutrition. The estimation of livestock requirements and the extent to which different feeding stuffs supply those needs are essential to the efficient feeding of millions of cattle and other animals. The criteria by which the relative values of different feeds may be assessed are

A. *Chemical Analysis*
   1. Proximate analysis (Weende system of feed analysis)
   2. The Van Soest method of analysis.

B. *Digestibility trials*
   1. Conventional type of digestion trial
   2. In-vivo digestibility methods.

C. *Estimation of energy content*
   1. Carbon Nitrogen balance technique
   2. By bomb calorimeter
   3. By calculating TDN from digestion trial
   4. From chemical composition.

D. *Evaluation of protein quality*

   (a) *For non-ruminants*
   1. Protein efficiency ratio
   2. Biological value (BV)
   3. Net protein utilisation (NPU)
   4. Nitrogen balance
   5. Nitrogen balance index
   6. Net protein ratio
   7. Crude protein
   8. True protein

   (b) *For ruminants*
   1. D.C.P. estimation by digestion trial
   2. Nitrogen balance experiment.

## A. CHEMICAL ANALYSIS

Chemical analysis is the starting point for determining the nutritive value of any feed. The methods of chemical analysis that have been described have a history of more than 100 years.

Millions of feed samples have been analysed by these methods. Thus, much data has been published on feeds expressed as crude protein, ether extract, crude fibre, ash and nitrogen-free-extract. By these methods we can have first hand information about the potentiality of the feed to fulfil the required nutrients. The procedure is simple, economic and rapid. From the results of analysis we can merely know the gross chemical composition of a feeding stuff without any idea of its efficiency of being utilised in animal system.

## 1. Proximate Analysis

The methods used in the analysis are called feed analysis, agricultural analysis or proximate analysis. Also since many of the techniques were first worked out at Weende, a village near the University of Goettingen in Germany, where early research in animal nutrition was conducted, it is also called Weende system.

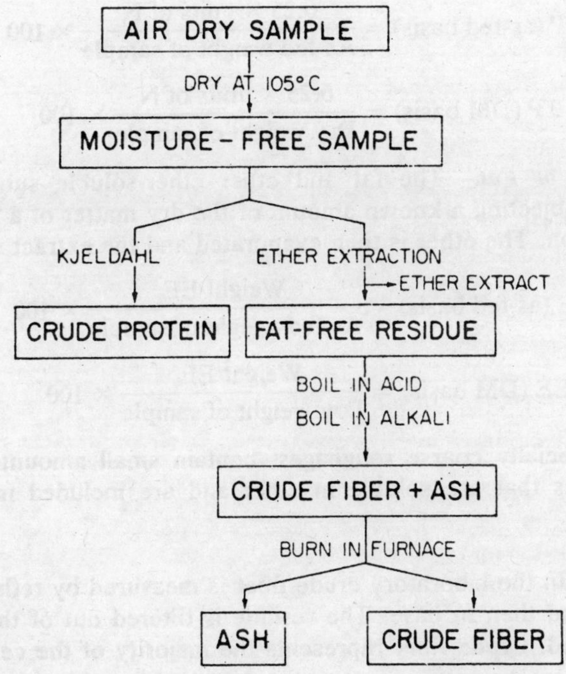


Flow diagram for the proximate analysis.

Proximate analysis is a system for approximating the nutritive value of a feed or material for feeding purposes without actually using the feed in a feeding trial and was developed at Weende in the middle of 1800 A.D. The principle of the analysis is to separate the feed components into groups or fractions in accordance with their feeding value. The various fractions are:

*1. Dry Matter.* That material remaining after drying a feed sample at 100°C for a given period of time.

$$\% \text{ DM} = \frac{\text{Dry weight}}{\text{Wet weight}} \times 100$$

$$\% \text{ Moisture} = \frac{\text{Wet weight} - \text{dry weight}}{\text{Wet weight}} \times 100$$

*2. Total Protein.* The percentage of nitrogen (N) of a sample of feed is multiplied by the factor 6.25. The factor 6.25 is used because average protein contains 16% nitrogen.

$$100 \text{ units of protein} \div 16 \text{ units of nitrogen} = 6.25$$

$$\% \text{ TP (as-fed basis)} = \frac{6.25 \times \text{units of N}}{\text{As-fed weight of sample}} \times 100$$

$$\% \text{ TP (DM basis)} = \frac{6.25 \times \text{units of N}}{\text{Dry weight of sample}} \times 100$$

*3. Ether Extract or Fat.* The fat and other ether-soluble substances are determined by subjecting a known amount of the dry matter of a feedstuff to an ether extraction. The ether is then evaporated and the extract weighed.

$$\% \text{ EE (as-fed basis)} = \frac{\text{Weight EE}}{\text{As-fed weight of sample}} \times 100$$

$$\% \text{ EE (DM basis)} = \frac{\text{Weight EE}}{\text{Dry weight of sample}} \times 100$$

Some feeds, especially coarse roughages, contain small amounts of gums, resins, and waxes that are soluble in ether and are included in the ether extract.

*4. Crude Fiber.* In the laboratory crude fiber is measured by refluxing a dry sample in acid and then in base. The residue is filtered out of the solution, dried, and weighed. Crude fiber represents the majority of the cellulose and lignin in the feed.

$$\% \text{ CF (as-fed basis)} = \frac{\text{Weight of fiber residue}}{\text{As-fed weight of sample}} \times 100$$

$$\% \text{ CF (DM basis)} = \frac{\text{Weight of fiber residue}}{\text{Dry weight of sample}} \times 100$$

*5. Ash.* This represents the mineral components of a feed. A dry sample is placed in a crucible and completely combusted in a furnace at 650°C. The residue is the ash.

**Table 142**

**Makeup of the proximate principles of the Weende food analysis**

| | | | | |
|---|---|---|---|---|
| Organic | Nitrogenous | Protein | Dispensable amino acids | Glutamic acid, aspartic acid, alanine, serine, hydroxyproline |
| | | | Semidispensable amino acids | Arginine, glycine, histidine, cystine, tyrosine, proline |
| | | | Indispensable amino acids | Lysine, tryptophan, phenylalanine, methionine, threonine, leucine, isoleucine, valine |
| | | Non-protein | Nucleic acids, amines, etc. | |
| | Lipid | Neutral | Acylglycerols | Triglycerides |
| | | | Sterols | Cholesterol, vitamin D, etc. |
| | | | Terpenoids | Carotene, vitamin A, xanthophylls, etc. |
| | | Phospholipids | Phosphoglycerides | Lecithin |
| | | | Sphingolipids | Sphingomyelin |
| | Carbohydrate | Nitrogen-free extract | Water-soluble vitamins | Thiamin, riboflavin, niacin, vitamin $B_6$, pantothenic acid, biotin, folacin, vitamin $B_{12}$, ascorbic acid |
| | | | Monosaccharides | Simple pentose or hexose sugars |
| | | | Oligosaccharides | Compound sugars |
| | | | Polysaccharides ("soluble") | Starches |
| | | Crude fiber | Polysaccharides ("insoluble") | Celluloses<br>Hemicelluloses |
| Inorganic | Ash | Essential elements | Macro | Ca, Mg, Na, K, P, Cl, S |
| | | | Micro | Mn, Fe, Cu, I, Zn, Co, Mo, Se, Cr, Sn, F, Ni, V, Si |
| | | Possibly essential elements | | As, Ba, Br, Cd, Sr |
| | | Potentially toxic elements | | Cu, Mo, Se, As, Cd, F, Pb, Hg, Si |
| | | Nonessential elements | | Al, Sb, Bi, B, Ge, Au, Pb, Hg, Rb, Ag, Ti |

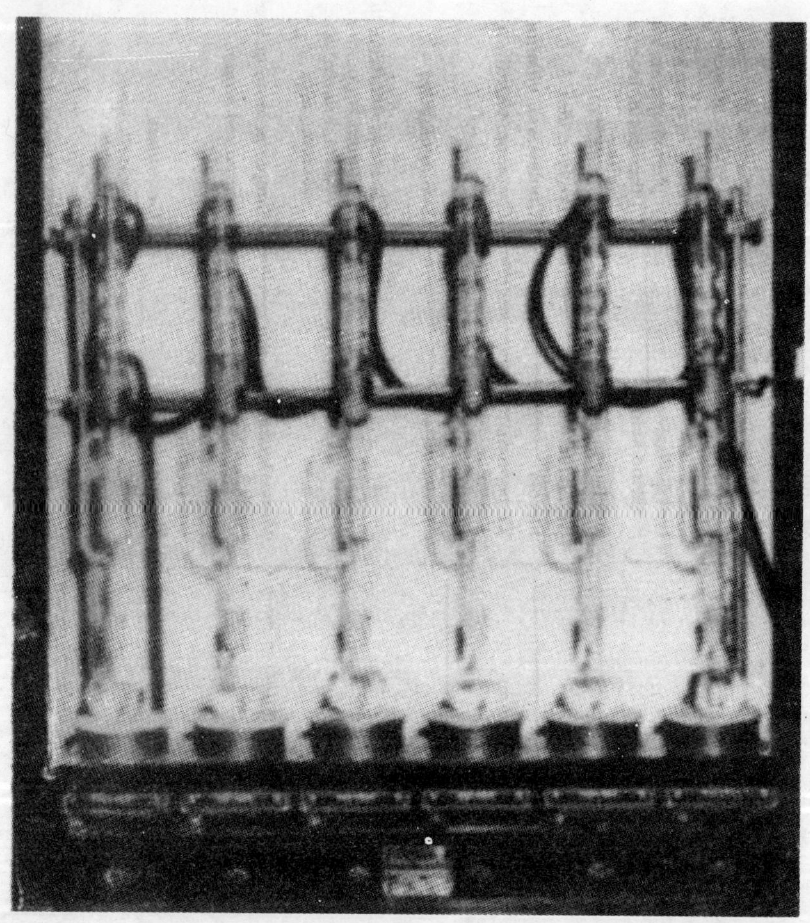

Figure 83 The Soxhlet apparatus to determine the ether extract (fat) in 6 samples, showing the condenser at the top, the extractor with the 2 side arms in the middle and the flask at the bottom, resting on an electric heating element.

$$\% \text{ ash (as-fed basis)} = \frac{\text{Weight of ash}}{\text{As-fed weight of sample}} \times 100$$

$$\% \text{ ash (DM basis)} = \frac{\text{Weight of ash}}{\text{Dry weight of sample}} \times 100$$

***6. Nitrogen-Free Extract.*** This represents the more soluble carbohydrates such as starches and sugars. The nitrogen-free extract is determined mathematically by difference and not by actual analysis.

$$\% \text{ NFE} = 100 - (\% \text{ } H_2O + \% \text{ ash} + \% \text{ EE} + \% \text{ TP} + \% \text{ CF})$$

The coefficient of digestibility for any of the nutrients may be calculated as follows.

$$\frac{\text{Weight of the nutrient in the feed} - \text{Weight of the nutrient in the feces}}{\text{Weight of the nutrient in the feed}}$$

The basis of the scheme is that the feedstuff contain organic and inorganic constituents. The former comprises of carbohydrates, crude fibre and nitrogen free extract, fats and oils, proteins and other nitrogenous compounds along with other numerous organic compounds.

The inorganic matter comprises ash composed of various minerals but the proximate analysis gives no indication about the kinds of minerals present. Rice straw contains about 16 per cent ash, but 85 per cent of this ash is silica which is of no value to the animal. On the other hand, meat and bone meals have about 30 per cent ash mainly of calcium and phosphorus

**Table 143**

**The fractions of proximate analysis**

| *Procedure* | *Fraction* | *Major components* |
|---|---|---|
| Drying at approximately 100°C to constant weight | Moisture | Water and any other volatile compounds |
| Ignite at 500°C to 600°C | Ash | Mineral elements |
| $N_2$ by Kjeldhal digestion | Crude protein | Proteins, amino acids, Non-protein $N_2$ |
| Extraction with pet. ether | Ether extract | Fats, oils, waxes |
| Residue after boiling with acid and alkali | Crude fibre | Cellulose, hemicellulose, lignin |
| Remainder; i.e., 100 minus sum of the other fractions | N-free extract | Starch, sugars, some cellulose, hemicellulose and some lignin. |

which are so essential for animal body. It was originally assumed that crude fibre represented the indigestible portion of the feed material and as such was considered as non-nutritive residue. But since the crude fibre is partially digestible in herbivora, this assumption has been proved to be wrong.

Further, the nitrogen-free-extract includes pentosans and small amount of other complex polysaccharides along with some soluble lignin which are by no means completely digestible, thus overestimates the digestibility of nitrogen-free-extract.

**Table 144**

**Limitations of the proximate analysis (Harris, 1970)**

| *Component* | *Supposed to contain* | *Contains* | *Missing* | *Excess* |
|---|---|---|---|---|
| Crude Fibe | Fibrous matter | Cellulose, part of lignin | Hemicellulose, part of Lignin and acid insoluble ash | None |
| Nitrogen-free-extract | Soluble carbo-hydrates | Soluble carbo-hydrates, hemi-cellulose, part of lignin and acid insoluble ash | None | Hemicellulose, Lignin and Acid insoluble ash |
| Ether extract | Crude fat (fats, oils and fatty acids) | Free fats, oils and fatty acids, chloro-phyll, sterols, antho-cyanin, carotinoids | Protein, Protein bound lipid | Chlorophyll, Sterol, Anatho-Cyamins, waxes etc. |

Another reason the so-called proximate analysis is not adequate as it does not incluae many chemical factors that are important in feeding to-day. The ash gives no indication of the chemical elements in it, yet the chemical elements in the ash must be known as the deficiency of any essential mineral element will cause failure in proper animal feeding. The method also does not include vitamins. Some of the vitamins can be determined chemically, rest biologically by microbiological assay.

Because of such limitations of Weende system or proximate analysis, numerous workers over the past several years have been suggested various other procedures particularly for a logical separation of feed carbohydrates. Among them in 1938 Crampton and Maynard suggested a procedure for grouping carbohydrates of feed into cellulose, pentosans and lignin. In 1953 Ely *et al.*, proposed that the grouping of cellulose and hemicellulose as holocellulose would provide a useful parameter of digestibility. None of the above modifications were successful in predicting the total carbohydrate digestibility than the crude fibre originally suggested in Weende system.

The procedure which has recently received wide consideration as a possible substitute for the conventional crude fibre determination is that of P. J. Van Soest of Cornell in U.S.A.

**2. Van Soest Method**

Dr. P.J. Van Soest in 1965 developed a method which makes use of the concept that the dry matter of plant origin consists of two principal parts: *Cell wall* and *Cell contents.* Thus the method has become highly efficient to take care of the defects in the principle of estimating crude fibre and NFE by proximate analysis.

**Table 145**

*Division of Forage Organic Matter by System of Analysis Using Detergents.* (*Van Soest, 1966*)

| *Fraction* | *Components* | *Nutritional available* | |
|---|---|---|---|
| | | *Ruminant* | *Non-ruminant* |
| CELL CONTENTS (*soluble in neutral detergent*) | Lipids | Virtually complete | Highly available |
| | Sugars, organic acids, and water soluble matters | ,, | ,, |
| | Starch | ,, | ,, |
| | Non-protein nitrogen | ,, | ,, |
| | Soluble protein | ,, | ,, |
| | Pectin | ,, | ,, |
| CELL WALL (Fibre insoluble in in neutral detergent) | | | |
| (1) *Soluble in acid detergent* | Hemicellulose | Partial | Very low |
| (2) *Insoluble in acid detergent* (acid detergent fibre) | Cellulose | ,, | ,, |
| | Lignin | Indigestible | Indigestible |
| | Lignified nitrogen compounds | ,, | ,, |
| | Heat damaged protein | ,, | ,, |
| | Silica | ,, | ,, |

Plant cell contents consist of sugars, starch, soluble carbohydrates, pectin, non-protein nitrogen, protein, lipids and miscellaneous other water-soluble materials, including minerals and several vitamins. True digestibility is almost complete, averaging 98 per cent.

The cell walls of feeds of plant origin are not uniformly nutritious, in the sense that their principal components consist of cellulose, hemicellulose, silica, lignin, etc., singly or in such combinations as nitrogen-hemicellulose or lignocellulose and differ widely in nutrition availability depending on the kind and maturity of the plant as well as on the age and species of the animal fed. Nitrogen-hemicellulose are not at all digestible.

## B. DIGESTIBILITY TRIAL

### 1. Conventional Type of Digestion Trial

A digestion trial involves an experiment by which the amount of nutrients actually digested and absorbed from a measured amount of feed consumed by an animal is determined.

The accurate feeding of weighed amounts of thoroughly mixed rations or individual feeds and the collection of the excreta of farm animals without any loss are important in conducting digestion trials.

Digestibility trials are conducted with animals in specially designed stalls and the series of operations may be compared roughly with the keeping of a banking account. It is obviously not possible to measure directly the amount of food that is digested, and the method adopted, therefore, is to measure the amount of food materials which the animal eats on the one hand and the excreta purged out on the other hand. The difference between the two tells us how much of the different parts of the food have been digested for further utilisation of the animal body.

The ability to utilise the nutrients of different feed varies in different species of animals because of their anatomical and physiological differences in the digestive tract. This is more pronounced in case of roughages. The ruminants have great power of utilising roughages while omnivorous and carnivorous have less of such power.

In animal nutrition when we speak of digestible nutrients, we mean the difference between the amounts of each nutrient in the feed and the faeces, that is the portion of a nutrient which is digested and taken into the body. The term is usually applied only to proteins, carbohydrates and fats. The digestion coefficient of a nutrient may then be defined as the percentage consumed in the ration which does not appear in the faeces. It is an expression of how much of each nutrient has disappeared during the passage of the feed through the digestive tract as a result of chemical reactions between feed ingredients, action of enzymes and other chemicals secreted from the animal body or by micro-organisms, and the physical action.

Digestibility of ash is not usually determined as it does not contribute to the energy content of a feed. Moreover, much of the ash in faeces is not undigested feed ash. The faeces are a pathway for the excretion of minerals from the body—minerals that have already been absorbed and which may already have served a purpose within the body. A digestion coefficient for ash, therefore, has no real meaning.

#### Techniques

#### Total Collection Method

*(A) Direct Method*

By this method, experimental animals are generally fed one type of feed stuff of roughage to know the amount of digestible nutrients present in it. The accurate feeding of weighed amount of thoroughly mixed individual feed and the collection of the excreta of farm animals without loss are vital for the conduction of such digestion experiments. In this regard there are eleven salient points which a beginner should know before taking up the experiment.

**1. Work to do Before the Experiment.** The first essential step in properly outlining an investigation is to acquire as complete a knowledge as possible of the previous research on the specific subject by a thorough study of the literature. It would be desirable after reading the literature to discuss it with others who might have got experience in this field.

After having a good background for the work to be done, one should prepare clear, accurate, comprehensive and detailed plans of the specific investigation which has been selected and may include (1) the precise descriptive name of the research project that is to be done, (2) location or locations of the work, (3) co-operating institutions or departments, (4) objective of the research, (5) names of persons participating, (6) introduction or justification for doing these experiments including a brief review of the literature, (7) the procedure: a description in simple, direct anguage of precisely what is proposed to be done.

**2. Selection of Experimental Animals.** In determining the digestibility of a feed of any class of livestock, the usual procedure is to select several animals (depending upon the species) for digestion trial. It is usually desirable that all experimental animals should be of similar breed, type, size or weight condition and age. It is preferable if they are of the same sex and that all animals used in the same experiment should have been produced in the same herd as by this they will probably have had the same pre-experimental treatment.

It is advantageous to have the animals which are castrated males except for those involving in milk production or in other female functions.

It is important that the animals for digestion experiments should be thriving, vigorous and with good appetites. So far as age is concerned, it is recommended that young adult animals or growing animals approaching maturity be used because they usually eat and perform better than those of other ages. Regarding number of experimental animals, it may be assumed that smaller the species, (sheep, goat, poultry) larger may be included for each treatment but for cattle this is not practically possible and it is said that not less than three animals should be used in each lot. If possible six animals should be used as a general convention for each treatment.

After selecting the animals, they should be clipped, dipped, drenched for internal parasites, vaccinated against such contagious diseases as may be necessary, have their feet trimmed, be ear tagged or otherwise marked, and individually weighed before they are put on experiment. It is believed that infestation with internal parasites often tends to decrease digestibility in sheep.

**3. Preparation of Apparatus.** The strictest attention is essential to such matters as the cleanliness of all apparatus and equipment and the sanitary conditions of the stall, surroundings and animals before and during the progress of the experiment. Scales and balances, in particular, should be checked up thoroughly. The following steps should be taken regarding balances.

1. On the day prior to weighing, remove any water that may have collected in the scale pit.
2. Clean all moving parts on the underside of the scale. Check weight marker bar and sliding indicator.
3. By placing exact weight on platform balances, check the accuracy of the balance. During the weighing operation, balance scale (set scale at zero) before each animal enters the scale box.

**4. Metabolic Stall or Crate.** A metabolism crate is actually a specially designed stall or box large enough for the experimental animal to house in controlled condition during experimental period. Here the animal enjoys freedom of movement, particularly as regards lying down and getting up. It is so designed to permit the collection of faeces and urine separately under it. In older type, the bottom is a metal grid or mesh of metal rods through which both the faeces and urine pass, the faeces being caught on a screen underneath and below the latter is a metal hopper or funnel like subfloor to catch the urine. In the type now more commonly used, the animal is confined so that he cannot turn around, and the length of the cage is adjusted to the size of the animal in such a way that the faeces fall into a properly placed container. The feed box is attached to the front, so constructed and placed as to prevent scattering. In order to avoid feed lodging at the corners of the feed trough, the bottoms of the metal boxes should be rounded at the sides; the side toward the steer (a young castrated ox) being set at a slight angle with the vertical and the edges of the box flanged to extend just beyond the wooden framework, if any. The bottom of each feed box, if of metal, should be made of one continuous piece of smooth sheet metal to eliminate joints or corners where feed may accumulate. Thus very little or no feed may be lost.

The crate may be made more portable by putting it on large castors or on 4 wheels.

In absence of any metabolic stall or crate, ordinary barn may be adapted to use for digestion experiments with minor modifications in relation to manger and faeces collection arrangement. Regarding manger, it may be mentioned that these are much larger than is common in dairy barns, made to hold large amounts of bulky feeds without spilling. The floor of the manger is sloped so that the last traces of feed remain within reach of even dwarf type of cattle. Care should be taken to prevent crevices on which feed might collect. The high cement walls between stall, 1.8 meters high in front at the mangers, prevents cows from stealing feed from their neighbours. So far as the faeces collection is concerned, it may be done either manually, whereby watchman or attendants collect the faeces behind the animals throughout the collection period. For this, at least 3 persons are to be engaged @ 8 hours per day to look after six animals for each 24 hours. Alternatively, faeces collection can also be made by using a faeces collection bag specially made for this purpose.

**5. Animal Comfort.** The comfort of the animal should be one of the factors to be considered in deciding the method to be followed for collection of faeces. One must decide which makes an animal uncomfortable: a harness strapped here and there to hold a faeces bag and then supporting the weight of the faeces bag as it fills during the day, or small stall limiting the cow's movement enough so that the faeces will fall into a pan or box placed behind it.

An essential feature of metabolism cages is that the animal must have some freedom of movement, particularly with regard to lying down and getting up. If a stanchion or a stall is so rigid as to make it difficult for cattle to lie down and get up, fatigue may result.

Good ventilation is a must for the animals. Although giving cows exercise has not been shown to influence the digestibility of feed nutrients directly by giving an opportunity to stretch the muscles during confinement at the stall will definitely lead to comfort of the animals and thereby normal metabolism will be maintained. Of course, for animals used for digestion trial if exercise is given, all care must be taken to prevent the animals from grabbing a mouthful of grass from elsewhere and no excreta should be lost. During the time of exercise, watchmen should always accompany with pails to catch any excreta.

Care should always be taken to prevent animals from the botheration of excessive flies or mosquitoes. To prevent slipping, the floors if made of concrete should be roughened slightly during construction.

**6. Feed Consumption and Residual Feed.** Accurate control to obtain unvarying intake of feed from the preliminary period through the collection period is essential for the accuracy of digestion trials. When the animals refuse to eat part of the feed assigned to them, this introduces uncontrolled factors for variation in obtaining uniform results. There are various practices that may help to avoid residual feed, refused feed, weigh backs or orts, as they are called.

(i) Healthy, thrifty young animals that have good appetites are less likely to refuse feed.

(ii) Thorough mixing of moderate size, grinding and pelleting prevents animals from picking out and refusing the coarser portions of hays and other roughages.

(iii) Increasing molasses from 5-15% improves palatability (not in chicks).

(iv) Addition of selected antibiotics have shown to influence the palatability in some species. Similarly, certain natural and artificial flavour may increase feed intake of young pigs as much as 35 per cent.

Addition of any additives should depend on the type of technical programme.

One technique to get rid of most of the residual feed is that during the preliminary periods, feed intake should be regularised in such a way that very little or nothing is left as residual feed.

Inspite of all efforts, there remains always some residual feed in some animals during the collection period. A short guide line in respect to handling of orts is discussed below:

(i) In some investigations the waste from one feeding, either in its natural condition or after drying and grinding, are consumed by the experimental animals, if mixed with the next meal.

(ii) It has also been suggested that the waste feed that is unfit to be eaten should be added to the faeces to determine the digestible nutrients. From the strictly economic view point. this would certainly be correct, but if the purpose is to make a purely physiological study and to obtain the digestibility of the nutrients eaten, the usual method of deducting the nutrients in the feed refused from those in the feed offered to determine the amount of each nutrient actually eaten is to be preferred.

(iii) In most of the digestion experiments it is a common practice to clean out the feed through every day and any appreciable amount of orts removed before the next feed is offered. While removing the residual feed of individual animals is preserved in air dry condition for the entire collection period. At the end of this period, a representative sample from each individual collection is analysed for the nutritive value. Once it is known, the total amount of nutrients rejected by the individual animals can also be ascertained for the total quantity of the residual feed of individual animal. This is done as the residual feed mostly differs significantly from the feed offered by virtue of being more coarse or dirty. The individual nutrient content of the refused feed is deducted from the amount of the same nutrient in the feed offered. The refused feed is often higher in ash because of the dirt that the animal does not eat Refused feed may also contain more fibre because of uneaten stems. Also, it is often lower in protein and nitrogen free-extract than the portion consumed.

**7. Preliminary Periods.** It is essential that the collection period of a digestion experiment be preceeded by a preliminary period of several days in which the same feed to be investigated is fed in the same weighed amounts daily as in the collection period. This is for the purpose of removing all residues of the previous feed and also of establishing as uniform a rate of passage of feed products and excretion of faeces as practicable, relative to feed intake.

Kellner stated that a preliminary period of at least five days should be allowed for ruminants. Later workers specified that the experimental animals should be subjected to a preliminary feeding of 7 to 10 days for horses and swine while for ruminants it may vary between 10–12 days.

During this period feeding of the experimental feed must be of the same quantity as during the experimental period to follow.

It is known that the rumen microbial population are affected both in types and numbers by the kind of ration fed. At the time of drastic change in ration, consiberable time may be required for the kinds of micro-organisms to become stabilised to the new environment so that a more suitable microflora may develop for the efficient digestion of the experimental feed.

Maynard observed that when the amounts of hay and silage fed to dairy cows were generally identical in preliminary and collection periods as in transition periods and when the grain mixtures were little changed, short preliminary periods before collecting excreta were adequate. In experiments in which the ratio of roughage to concentrate is kept constant and only the amount of protein varies, a preliminary period of 7 days may be adequate.

Recent trend is in favour of three periods instead of the conventional two periods, one preliminary and the other for collection as follows:

*1. Period of adjustment.* This might also be termed as a preparatory, ad-libitum, adaptation, pre-experimental subperiod, change over period or period of acclimatisation. During this period the animals become accustomed to the feed, and the level at which each individual will eat is regulated. During the period the experimental animals may not be put into digestion stalls or metabolic crates, but the arrangement should be such that a careful record may be kept of the amount of feed eaten by each individual. The period may continue for 7 days or longer as needed.

*2. Preliminary period.* During this period amount of feed offered is important as it must be continued without any variation throughout this and the collection period which follows.

*3. Collection period.* The third and last period. The details in this period are discussed in the following section.

**8. Collection Periods.** After allowing the number of days that have been decided upon to continue as a preliminary period, the collection of the faeces is begun and continued throughout the collection period. The faeces obtained during the period is assumed to be from a uniform amount of feed consumed during the same number of days.

Using longer collection periods lengthens the risk period wherein accident, animal sickness, feed refusal or other disturbing circumstances may affect results significantly and might necessitate repeating the trial. Shortening the collection period, on the other hand, may also give rise to inaccuracies due to the inability to make faeces collections that are as correctly representative of the digestibility in quantity and/or chemical composition as might possibly be obtained from a longer collection period. While the brightest possible accuracy is the aim, the factors of time, labour, expense and other considerations are important in deciding the length of the collection period to obtain greater accuracy.

The length of collection periods necessary depends upon the species; longer periods being necessary in the case of herbivores, especially ruminants, than for other animals because of variability in daily faeces excretion. In general a collection period of 7–10 days for ruminants is acceptable to most.

Recently, some experts recommended that following adequate adjustment and preliminary periods, two one-week collection periods in succession, be conducted. Sample should be composited separately and chemical analysis done for each week. The data may then be calculated both by weeks and for a full 14–day collection period for the sake of comparison. Such a plan gives an excellent opportunity for checking one week against the other or the data from only the second week may be used if it appears that the first collection period should be considered as an additional preliminary period.

The days of each complete experiment may be numbered. For instance, days 1 to 14 may be designated as the adjustment period, days 15–21, the preliminary period and days 22 to 28 and 29 to 35 as collection periods.

**9. Faeces Markers.** With non-ruminants the time of first appearance of faeces resulting from the feeding of experimental feed can be detected if any marker is mixed-up with the feed. A good marker must have the following qualities, (1) distinctly mark the faeces resulting from the feed with which the marker was fed; (2) be insoluble and unable to be absorbed through intestine; (3) have no toxic, laxative, costive or other physiological effect on the experimental subject; (4) not contain or react with the nutrient or nutrients under investigation.

Lampblack (soot, carbon); carmine; methylene-blue; ferric oxide; chromic oxide; barium sulfates; copper sulfate; bismuth subcarbonate, purple green and yellow cellophane; all of which render colour to faeces have been tried. Some have been used more extensively than others. Carmine is in use for the longest time and is favoured by some workers because of its intense red colour. In powder form, 0.25 to 1.00 gram of carmine may be mixed with the first food of an experimental period to have a distinct colour of the faeces.

With ruminants the use of markers does not result in a clear separation of the faeces because there is no marking of the beginning and end of the period. The contents of the digestive tract of ruminants do not pass through its length in the same order in which they were consumed in the feed. Markers are thus not at all satisfactory with ruminants.

**10. Preparing Faeces Samples.** At the end of each 24 hour collection period, faeces from individual animals are first weighed and then sampled for analysis. A 5 per cent aliquot is the amount that is most frequently kept aside as sample. With pigs, sheep or other small animals, since there is less faeces than with cattle, all or major portion of the faeces may be stored until the end of the collection period.

Usually faeces are preserved in cans, polythelene bags or in wide mouth glass jars with air tight covers. The daily samples are then labelled and if possible, stored in quick-freeze at minus 16 to 20°C until needed for making composite samples for the entire period. At the end of collection period the daily samples of faeces are brought from the refrigerator and the temperature is raised up to laboratory temperature. After that the containers, each with either one day's full amount of faeces for one animal or with a given percentage of faeces, are removed from refrigeration, weighed and finally combined to make a single composite sample for one animal for one collection period and a composite sample representing the faeces for the entire collection period is taken for analysis. From the aliquot portions two samples are taken, one larger portion for drying and the other for analysis in the fresh condition, mainly for protein estimation.

Faeces to be preserved should be free from automicrobiat (including mould) fermentation. Also care should be taken to prevent or reduce the loss of nitrogen as ammonia in drying. For these two reasons when faeces are to be dried, a mixture of HCl and alcohol should be used for preservation of faeces. $H_2SO_4$ at 3 per cent concentration is also a common preservator. Among other reagents, toluene, formaldehyde, thymol are all in use. Approximately 5 g of finely-ground thymol is enough for preserving daily sample of faeces under ordinary condition.

If refrigeration facilities are limited, sample should straight away be put into drier. The evidence appears to favour quick drying at 90°C to 100°C instead of low temperature for longer times whereby nutrient losses tends to be greater. The dried samples should then be exposed to the open air (put the containers on laboratory working table covering them with net to prevent rats from stealing some of the sample) at the ordinary tempeature for 4-5 days.

After drying and equilibrating with air humidity, weigh the air dried sample. Grind them thoroughly; put the samples into tight receptacles and keep them in cold storage if possible.

It is always preferable to estimate the nitrogen content of the fresh faeces (composite sample for the entire collection period) before drying but do all other analvses on the usual air dry samples.

**11. Calculation of Digestibility.** In digestibility experiments, attempts are made to find out the digestibility coefficient of the food as a whole or some constituents of the food. The digestibility coefficient may be defined as the percentage of the total amount consumed which is digested and absorbed. The usual calculation of the digestion coefficient (DC) can be shown in an equation as follows.

$$\text{DC of Nutrient} = \frac{\text{kg. nutrient eaten} - \text{kg. in faeces}}{\text{kg. nutrient eaten}} \quad 100$$

The above formula is useful whenever there is no residual feed. The usual formula for the calculation of DC in which the nutrient in the residual feed is deducted from the feed offered is as follows:

$$\text{DC of nutrient} = \frac{(\text{kg. nutrient offered} - \text{kg. nutrient refused}) - \text{kg. nutrient in faeces}}{\text{kg. nutrient offered} - \text{kg. nutrient refused}} \times 100$$

Computations are made independently for each experimental animal and the average coefficient is then calculated. It has now become customary to report coefficient of the entire organic matter in the feed or ration along with usual coefficients of crude protein, crude fibre, nitrogen free extract and ether extract. Further, increasingly the digestion coefficient of the energy are being determined routinely whenever digestion experiments are conducted.

The data needed for calculating the DC are: (1) the chemical composition of feed eaten, (2) the chemical composition of the facces, (3) the weight of the feed eaten, and (4) the weight of the faeces excreted.

*Example No. 1*

A bullock was fed on an average 4.0 kg of hay per day for three weeks. Over the experimental period of 7 days the animal excreted an average weight of 5.8 kg. Samples of the hay and the faeces were found to contain the percentages of composition as in Table No. 68. Find out the digestible coefficient of each nutrient and also the TDN per cent.

Four kg of hay actually contain 3.36 kg of dry matter while 5.8 kg of faeces contain 1.45 kg of dry matter.

The difference 1910 gram, which did not appear in the faeces, is regarded as having been digested by the bullock. This amount is 56.84 per cent of the 3360 gm of the dry matter eaten. It is said, then, that the digestion coefficient of the dry matter of the hay was 56.84. In

Table 146

**Chemical composition of feed and faeces**

**(Fresh basis)**

| | *Hay (%)* | *Faeces (%)* |
|---|---|---|
| Moisture | 16.00 | 75.00 |
| Ash | 6.00 | 2.00 |
| Crude protein | 12.57 | 3.22 |
| Crude fibre | 27.78 | 9.50 |
| NFE | 35.15 | 9.74 |
| Ether extract | 2.50 | 0.54 |
| | 100.00 | 100.00 |

the same way the percentage digestibility of each nutrient may be computed as shown in Table 70 below.

Table 147

**Digestion trial with hay**

| *Daily average* | *Dry matter (gm)* | *Crude protein (gm)* | *Crude fibre (gm)* | *Nitrogen free extract (gm)* | *Ether extract (gm)* |
|---|---|---|---|---|---|
| a. 4.00 kg hay | 3360 | 502.80 | 1,111.2 | 1,406.00 | 100.00 |
| b. In faeces | 1450 | 186.76 | 551.0 | 564.92 | 31.32 |
| c. Digested | 1910 | 316.04 | 560.20 | 841.08 | 68.68 |
| d. Digestion coefficient | 56.84 | 62.85 | 50.41 | 59.82 | 68.68 |

**Computation of Digestible Nutrients and of TDN.** Digestible nutrients are also calculated on the fresh basis directly by multiplying the percentage of each nutrient by its digestion coefficient and as the result is expressed as the kilogram of digestible nutrient per 100 kg of feed, the entire equation is further divided by 100 as below:

$$\text{per cent Digestible Nutrient} = \text{per cent Nutrient} \times \frac{\text{Digestion coefficient of the Nutrient}}{100}$$

Using the data from the same digestion experiment with hay in bullocks, the digestible nutrients may be calculated as in Table 89.

**Table 148**

| | *Composition % on fresh* (*a*) | *Digestion coefficient* (*b*) | *Per cent digestible nutrients* $a \times \frac{b}{100}$ |
|---|---|---|---|
| Crude protein | 12.57 | 62.85 | 7.90 |
| Crude fibre | 27.78 | 50.41 | 14.00 |
| NFE | 35.15 | 59.82 | 21.02 |
| Ether extract | 2.50 | 68.68 | 1.71 |
| Dry matter | 84.00 | 56.84 | 47.74 |

The total digestible nutrients (TDN) express the relative energy values of feeds. The calculation of TDN can now easily be made from the above Table keeping in view one more factor that 2.25 is to be multiplied with the amount of digestible ether extract because of the greater caloric value of fat which is 2.25 times more than carbohydrates or protein on unit basis

T.D.N = per cent digestible protein + per cent digestible NFE + per cent digestible crude fibre + (per cent digestible ether extract × 2.25)

$$= 7.90 + 21.02 + 14.00 + 1.71 \times 2.25$$

$$= 46.76$$

**Digestibility by Difference.** The method described previously is the direct method of digestion trial. In it the digestibility of most of the roughages can be found out, but with concentrates, the above method is unsuitable as concentrates fail to supply the required bulk in ruminants. The digestibility of the concentrates in such cases is found out by the method of difference. In this method digestibility of a roughage is found out first and then the concentrate mixture is added to the roughage for a second trial. The coefficient of a digestibility of the concentrate is found out by subtracting the figures obtained for the roughage alone from the figures obtained in the combined ration. The figures thus obtained may not be very accurate, as the method does not eliminate the associate action of different feeds.

*Example No. 2*

Find out the digestible coefficient of maize when fed to the same bullock along with same hay in the example no. 1 given in the previous section. The bullock received 4.0 kg of same hap per day along with 4.2 kg of ground maize. The average daily excretion of faeces on this mixed ration was 8.5 kg. The composition of maize and the faeces are given in next page.

The digestible matter contained in the total ration, computed exactly like the previous example, as is shown in the first five lines (a to e) of Table 150. If it is assumed that the digestibility of hay (line f) was unaltered by the addition of the maize grain, it is possible to compute how much of each kind of digestible matter (protein, crude fibre, NFE and fat) in the total ration was derived from the hay, that is amount of per cent digestible nutrient in the feed. As suggested earlier, this is done by multiplying the digestion coefficient with per cent nutrient of the feed and then by dividing the entire result by 100. The remainder (line g), therefore, must have come from the maize grain (line b), and by comparison with the total amounts present in the later, the precentage digestibility (line h) or digestion coefficient of the maize is computed. The value of line f are deducted from the total digested (line e) to estimate the amount digested from the maize The later (line g) divided by the grams of each nutrient in the maize eaten (line b), expressed as a percentage is the digestion coefficient of each nutrient. These are shown in the last line (h).

*Computation of TDN of Maize*

For finding out TDN, it is necessary to first calculate the value of per cent digestible nutrients of maize as below:

$$\text{Per cent Digestible nutrient} = \frac{\text{Digestible coefficient} \times \text{per cent nutrient present in maize}}{100}$$

$$\text{Per cent Digestible Crude protein} = \frac{71.76}{100} \times 9.65 = 6.924 \text{ per cent}$$

$$\text{Per cent Digestible Crude fibre} = \frac{98.12}{100} \times 1.9 = 1.864 \text{ per cent}$$

**Table 149**

**Composition of Maize and Faeces (fresh basis)**

| | *Maize grain* | *Faeces* |
|---|---|---|
| Water | 12:75 | 80.95 |
| Ash | 1.20 | 1.75 |
| Crude protein | 9.65 | 3.55 |
| Crude fiber | 1.90 | 6.50 |
| NFE | 70.85 | 6·75 |
| Ether Extract | 3.65 | 0.50 |
| | 100.00 | 100·00 |

Table 150

**The digestibility of maize by difference**

| *Daily average* | *Dry matter (gm)* | *Crude protein (gm)* | *Crude fiber (gm)* | *N-free extract (gm)* | *Ether extract (gm)* |
|---|---|---|---|---|---|
| a. 4 kg hay | 3360.0 | 502.80 | 1111.2 | 1406.0 | 100.00 |
| b. 4.2 kg maize | 3664.5 | 405.30 | 79.8 | 2975.7 | 153.30 |
| c. Hay+Maize (a+b) | 7024.5 | 908.10 | 1191.0 | 4381.7 | 253.30 |
| d. Total faeces | 1619.25 | 301.75 | 552.5 | 573.75 | 42.50 |
| e. Total digested (c—d) | 5405.25 | 606.35 | 638.5 | 3807.95 | 210.80 |
| f. Estimated digested from hay based on % digestible nutrients* | 1910.00 | 315.50 | 560.20 | 841.08 | 68.68 |
| g. Calculated digested from maize (e—f) | 3495.25 | 290.85 | 78.30 | 2966.87 | 142.12 |
| h. Digestion coefficient of maize (g/b×100) | 95.38 | 71.76 | 98.12 | 99.70 | 92.70 |

*The % digestible dry matter along with other digestible nutrients have already worked in example 1 under Direct Method. Those data have been utilised here since the hay used in this case is the same.

$$\text{Per cent Digestible NFE} = \frac{99.70}{100} \times 70.85 = 70.64 \text{ per cent}$$

$$\text{Per cent Digestible Ether Extract} = \frac{92.70}{100} \times 3.65 = 3.38 \text{ per cent}$$

$$\text{Per cent TDN of Maize is} = 6.924 + 1.864 + 70.64 + (3.38 \times 2.25) = 87.03$$

**(B) Indicator Method**

In recent years an indirect method of digestion trial has been developed. It is less time consuming and the result obtained has a clear correspondence with that obtained in the conventional method. In this method an indicator is used alone with the feed to be tested. By determining the ratio of the concentration of the indicator to that of a given nutrient in the feed and the same ratio in the faeces resulting from feed, the digestibility of the nutrient can be obtained without measuring either the feed intake or faeces output. This is done as follows:

$$\text{Faecal Dry Matter (DM)} = \frac{\text{Amount of Indicator ingested (mg/day)}}{\text{Indicator in faeces (mg/gm DM)}}$$

The digestibility of the DM in a diet can be computed as follows:

$$\textit{Indigestibility of DM (per cent)} = 100\left[\frac{\text{Indicator in diet (per cent)}}{\text{Indicator in faeces (per cent)}}\right]$$

Then, digestibility of DM (per cent) = 100 − Per cent Indigestibility of DM.

The digestibility of a specific nutrient can be computed as follows:

*Digestibility per cent of a nutrient*

$$= 100 - \left(100 \times \frac{\text{per cent indicator in feed}}{\text{per cent indicator in faeces}} \times \frac{\text{per cent nutrient in faeces}}{\text{per cent nutrient in feed}}\right)$$

A variety of substances have been employed as indicators such as chromic oxide ($Cr_2O_3$), lignin, plant pigments, indigestible nitrogen, polyethylene, glycol etc.

An ideal indicator should have the following qualities:

1. Totally indigestible
2. Pass through the tract at a uniform rate
3. Readily determined chemically.

*The following criteria are expressions of digestibility:*

1. Digestible DM (gm.) = DM intake (gm.) − DM in faeces (gm.)

2. $\text{Digestible DM (per cent)} = \frac{\text{DM intake} - \text{DM in faeces}}{\text{DM intake}} \times 100$

3. TDN (gm.) = (DM intake × Chem. comp.) − (DM in faeces × Chem. comp.),

4. $\text{TDN (per cent)} = \frac{(\text{DM intake} \times \text{Chem. comp.}) - (\text{DM in faeces} \times \text{Chem. comp.})}{\text{DM intake}} \times 100$

5. DE (kcal) = Energy intake (kcal) − Energy in faeces (kcal)

6. $\text{DE (per cent)} = \frac{\text{Energy intake} - \text{Energy in faeces (kcal)}}{\text{Energy intake (kcal)}} \times 100$

Abbreviation used above: DM = dry matter; TDN = total digestible nutrients; DE = digestible energy; kcal = Kilocalorie.

**2. In Vivo Digestibility Methods**

(i) NYLON OR DACRON BAG TECHNIQUE. The nylon bag techniques require placing of dried samples in bags made of an indigestible material such as nylon, dacron or silk which are then tightly tied. These bags are placed inside the rumen through the opening of fistulae by a veriety of techniques and after incubating for a specific time are removed. The rate and extent of digestion are measured by the loss of dry matter or nutrient content from the sample.

Because of the simplicity of the procedure and requirement of small amount of laboratory equipment (analytical balance and drying oven) and small amount of substrate to be analyzed, the technique is quite useful for evaluating the rate of forage digestion or for measuring the effect of various ration treatments, such as supplementation, on the rate and extent of digestion within the rumen.

However, the method is subject to considerable variability and is difficult to standardise. Sources of variation include: size and type of bags; cloth mesh size; sample size and fineness of grind; number of samples per trial; diet of host animal; method of suspension in the rumen; location and time in the rumen; and the method of cleaning and rinsing the bags after removal from the rumen. Attempts have been made to reduce the variability by leaving the bags in the rumen for longer periods of time; and by use of a large sample size (10 gm), a large number of samples per trial (up to 48), and by allowing the bags to move about freely with the rumen contents.

It has been further suggested that the addition of a pepsin treatment of the remaining residue in the nylon bags after removal from the rumen may improve the reliability of the method. The treatment permits more effective washing and reduces variation among triplicates, which is attributed to the elimination of microorganisms.

(ii) IN VIVO ARTIFICIAL RUMEN (VIVAR) TECHNIQUE. The Vivar technique is for studying nutrient utilisation by rumen microorganisms under controlled conditions in the rumen. The system consists of a porcelain test tube or stainless steel or glass jars fitted with bacteriological membranes to provide controlled interchange of the Vivar and rumen contents. The Vivar containers are equipped with a gas escape outlet and suspended in the rumen of a fistulated animal for the desired period of incubation. The system, though developed to stimulate conditions occurring in the living animal, appears to be of little value in its present form for the quality evaluation of forages. However, the method is useful in studying the rate phenomena in the rumen and determining the effect of changes in ration treatments on digestion and volatile fatty acid production.

## C. ESTIMATION OF ENERGY CONTENT

1. CARBON-NITROGEN BALANCE TECHNIQUE. The main forms in which energy is stored by the growing and fattening animal are protein and fat since carbohydrate in the body is small in amount and fairly constant. The object of a nitrogen and carbon balance trial is to know the stored amount of protein and fat in the animal body. Once we obtain such information by estimating the amounts of these elements absorbed and living in the body and so, by difference, the amounts retained, the energy retained can then be calculated by multiplying the quantities of nutrients stored by their calorific values.

Let us take an example where a bullock was fed on an average 6,988 grams of hay and 400 grams of linseed meal. The amount of nitrogen and carbon intakes through feeding are recorded on the basis of the per cent composition of the feed ingredients and the loses of these two components through various avenues have been noted in Table 151. Systematic approach of calculation will ultimately lead to find out the *Net Energy gain or loss* by the bullock.

Determinations are made of the carbon and nitrogen in the food, faeces, urine, and of the carbon in the gaseous output. Thus we know the amount of carbon gained with a side by side nitrogen gain, we can easily find out the protein deposited. By subtracting the carbon of protein from the total carbon gain we can estimate the total fat stored from rest of the carbon.

**Table 151**

**Calculation of energy retention of a bullock from its Nitrogen and Carbon balance**

| | | *Nitrogen* | | *Carbon* | |
|---|---|---|---|---|---|
| *Material* | *Amount* | *Income (gm)* | *Outgo (gm)* | *Income (gm)* | *Outgo (gm)* |
| **Food:** | **6,988 gm hay** | **56.4** | **—** | **2831.7** | **—** |
| | **400 gm linseed (meal)** | **21.9** | | **172.6** | |
| **Excreta:** | **16,619 gm faeces** | **—** | **33.5** | | **1428.7** |
| | **4357 gm urine** | **—** | **32.4** | **—** | **124.2** |
| | **37 gm brushings** | **—** | **1.3** | **—** | **8.0** |
| | **4730 gm $CO_2$** | **—** | **—** | **—** | **1290.2** |
| | **142 gm methane** | **—** | **—** | **—** | **46.6** |
| **GAIN ⟶** | | **+11.1 gm** | | **+46.6 gm** | |

**On this ration the animal therefore, gained 11.1 gm nitrogen. Body protein contains 16.65 per cent nitrogen, hence gain of protein is:**

$$11.1 \times \frac{100}{16.65} = 66.66 \text{ gm.}$$

**But this protein is known to contain 52.54 per cent carbon therefore, the carbon used for this protein is:**

$$66.6 \times \frac{52.54}{100} = 35.0 \text{ gm.}$$

**The total gain of carbon was 46.6 gm therefore, the amount of carbon available after fulfilling the requirement of protein is:**

$$46.6 - 35.0 = 11.6 \text{ gm.}$$

**Fat contains 76.6 per cent carbon, therefore the fat gain is:**

$$11.6 \times \frac{100}{76.5} = 15.2 \text{ gm.}$$

**The final result is therefore:**

**A gain of 66.6 gm protein and 15.2 gm of fat energy retention.**

| | |
|---|---|
| **Energy stored as protein** | **(66.6 × 4.00) = 266.6 kcal** |
| **Energy stored as fat** | **(15.2 × 9.00) = 136.8 kcal** |
| **NET ENERGY GAIN** | **= 403.4 kcal** |

Once we know the net energy retained, we can find out the heat loss by deducting the net energy from metabolisable energy:

(a) ME—Energy of heat loss = Net energy, so
(b) ME—Net energy = Energy of heat loss
(c) ME = Gross energy—Energy loss in faeces, urine, gas as methane.

Gross energy of the feedstuff, faecal energy and urinary energy can be determined by usual bomb calorimeter technique (described earlier). For methane the estimation can be done by several ways as analysing the methane of the respiratory calorimeter (described afterwords), or by adopting some formula like Axelsson's formula which is:

Methane energy in kcal $= 1083X_2^{0.638}$
Where $X_2$ = digested carbohydrate in kg.

For general calculation, methane production can be estimated as 8 per cent of gross energy intake.

Thus by Nitrogen Carbon technique, we can not only know the net energy (energy of retention) but also know the energy lost as heat from the animal body and thus we can compare different feedstuffs for their nutritive value.

2. BY BOMB CALORIMETER. The energy value of feeds is usually expressed in nutrition in terms of the kilocalorie and traditionally designated as large calorie. The trend, however, is slowly moving away from the use of the term calorie toward the more accurate practice of using kilocalorie by its own name.

Since Lavoisier's classic experiments on the origin of animal heat, it has been known that foods burned outside the body produce the same amount of heat as foods oxidised by the slow processes of intermediary metabolism. If, then, foods are burned and heat produced is measured, the quantity of heat expressed in kilocalories represents the *gross energy* value *of combustion* of the food. The instrument used to determine heat of combustion is known to all students of nutrition as the Bomb calorimeter. In this the food is ignited and the heat of combustion calculated from the rise in temperature of the surrounding water placed in a jacket inside the calorimeter. The data obtained regarding gross energy content of any feed stuff are precise physical measurements which represent the total energy available on oxidation. They do not represent the physiological values for the energy available to the tissues. Since the food is not completely digested and absorbed from the alimentary canal, and oxidation in the tissues is not always complete, some losses of energy are inevitable.

Thus, merely energy content of any feed does not mean the actual utilisation of that energy by the animal system. Feeds are assessed by their ability to promote energy retention in the body. To determine the energy retention, the intake of energy and losses of energy as heat in faeces, urine and as combustible gas are determined.

3. CALCULATING TDN FROM DIGESTIBILITY TRIAL AS AN INDEX OF ENERGY CONTENT OF FEED. In a number of countries including India, energy value of the feed is expressed in terms of TDN which is the abbreviation for total digestible nutrients. TDN is simply a figure which indicates the relative energy value of a feed to an animal. It is ordinarily expressed in kg or in per cent. TDN can be determined only by a digestion trial where the per cent digestible nutrients are

computed on the fresh basis directly by multiplying the percentage of each nutrient, present in the feed ingredient in question (protein, fibre, N-free extract and fat) by their corresponding digestion coefficient. The value is then arrived at by adding together as below:

per cent digestible crude protein =
per cent digestible crude fibre =
per cent digestible N-free extract =
per cent digestible crude fat ×2.25 =

per cent of TDN=

To approximate the greater calorific value of fat, which contains approximately 2.25 times as much energy as carbohydrates, the percentage of digestible fat or ether extract is multiplied by 2.25. This is the result of their chemical composition. Fats contain larger ratio of carbon plus hydrogen to oxygen, i.e., fats are in a lower stage of oxidation and are, therefore, capable of yielding more energy when oxidised. It may be interesting to note that the burning of 1 gram of hydrogen produces over 4 times as much heat as does the burning of 1 gram of carbon.° The formula for TDN is thus written as follows:

Per cent of TDN=Dig. Prot. %+Dig. fibre %+Dig. NFE %+(Dig. Ether Extract % × 2.25).

Total digestible nutrients is not an actual total of the digestible nutrients in a feed. In the first place, it does not include the digestible mineral matter as no direct energy is obtained from them. Secondly, the digestible fat is multiplied by 2.25 before being included in the TDN figure. The latter step is necessary to allow for the extra energy value of fats compared to carbohydrates and proteins. As a result of this step, feeds high in fat will sometimes exceed 100 in percentage TDN. (Animal fat, 175 per cent; Maize oil, 172 per cent; Dried whole milk, 110 per cent TDN content).

Since protein has a higher calorific value than carbohydrate, why has no adjustment for protein been made in the digestible protein figure? This is because losses of energy in the urine due to the excretion of nitrogen make digestible protein approximately equivalent to digestible crude fibre and digestible NFE as source of energy.

A limitation of TDN as a measure of feed energy is that it does not account for certain losses such as combustible gases and the heat increment which has been discussed before in this chapter. These losses are considerably larger for roughages than for concentrates and thus a kilogram of TDN in roughage has considerably less value for productive purposes than a kilogram of TDN in concentrates. TDN then tends to over-evaluate roughages and under-evaluate concentrates as a measure of energy for ruminants. 0.5 kg TDN in maize, better hays and poor roughages yield 1.0, 0.75 and 0.50 therm respectively.

To arrive at the quantity of energy available from a certain amount of TDN, the general accepted value is as follows:

1 kg. TDN = 4400 kcal Digestible energy
= 4.40 kcal per gram of TDN
1 kg. TDN= 3520.00 kcal Metabolisable energy.
= 3.52 kcal ME per gram of TDN.
1 kg TDN = 0.869 SE (Starch Equivalent)

It is also not very difficult to calculate the total energy value from a given value of TDN, since when the individual per cent digestible nutrients are multiplied by Atwater's physiological fuel value and on adding up, the calorific value is obtained. The Atwater's physiological fuel values although are not applicable in the case of ruminants because of low digestibility in comparison to human being, but yet the following values are still in use in calculating the calorific value of TDN.

*Atwater's Physiological fuel value (ME)*

| | |
|---|---|
| Carbohydrate | 4.0 kcal/gram |
| Fat | 9.0 kcal/gram |
| Protein | 4.0 kcal/gram |

## FACTORS AFFECTING THE TDN VALUE OF A FEED

**A. The Percentage of Dry Matter.** Water can in no way contribute in a positive way to the TDN value of a feed. The more water present in a feed, the less there is of other nutrients. Since the TDN value depends on the amount of carbohydrate, fat and protein, and not on water as such, any feed having less of water is expected to have more of TDN. Silage is low in TDN compared to hay mainly because of a difference in water content.

**B. The Digestibility of Dry Matter.** TDN results from the digestible portion of the nutrients present in a feed. Mineral oil has a high gross energy value, but it cannot be digested by the animal and so has no digestible energy or TDN value. Lignin would fall in similar category. Feeds high in fibre are, in general, low in digestibility and relatievly low in TDN.

**C. The Amount of Mineral Matter in the Digestible Dry Matter.** Since mineral compounds contribute no energy to the animal as such they have no TDN value. Salts like limestone and defluorinated phosphate are all digested by the animal but would have 0.0 TDN values.

**D. The Amount of Fat in the Digestible Dry Matter.** In calculating TDN, the digestible fat is multiplied by 2.25 as reasons mentioned earlier. Consequently, the more digestible fat a feed contains, other things being equal, the greater will be the TDN value. In feeds high in fats such as dried whole milk, TDN values may even exceed 100 per cent. A pure fat which has a coefficient of digestibility of 100 per cent would theoretically have a TDN value of 225 per cent × 2.25.

**4. ENERGY VALUE FROM CHEMICAL COMPOSITION.** Our present system of proximate analysis was developed by Henneberg and Stohmann (1868) at the Weende Experiment Station in Germany. After almost 100 years in 1965 Dr. P.J. Van Soest of U.S.A developed another method of partitioning carbohydrate portion of plant origin. At present both the systems of chemical analysis of feed are in practice in almost all the nutritional laboratories of the world.

From the gross-chemical composition of the feed sample, obtained by either of the methods, the amount of energy yielding groups of nutrients, carbohydrate, ether extract and protein are estimated. Once the amount of each component is known, estimation of the expected amount of heat of combustion can easily be made out by multiplying appropriate factors. The heats of combustion for individual carbohydrates, proteins and fats differ somewhat. The gross energy yield of sucrose, for example, was determined by Atwater to be 3.96 kcal/gram whereas starch yielded 4.23 kcal/gram. Energy yield of butterfat was found to be 9.21 kcal/gram and that of lard, 9.48 kcal/gram. For practical use, individual figures were averaged to apply to the major food stuffs (carbohydrate, fat and protein) as gross energy of food, i.e., heat of combustion.

*Atwater's average Gross Energy value factors*

| | | |
|---|---|---|
| Carbohydrate | — | 4.15 kcal/gram |
| Fat | — | 9.4 kcal/gram |
| Protein | — | 5.65 kcal/gram |

Since the gross energy value of food stuff does not represent the energy actually available to body cells, some potential energy therefore never enters the body and is excreted in the faeces. In this connection, Atwater made a large number of experiments in which he analysed the faeces of three young American men for periods lasting for 3–8 days. The following digestibility figures were obtained by him.

| | |
|---|---|
| Carbohydrates | 98 per cent digestible |
| Fats | 95 per cent digestible |
| Proteins | 92 per cent digestible |

*N.B: For digestible coefficient divide each digestible per cent value by 100.*

From this the "*Atwater's factor*" for the available energy (digestible energy, DE) has been formulated. The calorific values of the three nutrients were multiplied by those corresponding digestible coefficients to get the physiological values as below:

*Atwater's Digestible energy value factors*

| | |
|---|---|
| 1 gram carbohydrate | $= 4.15 \times 0.98 = 4.0$ kcal |
| 1 gram fat | $= 9.4 \times 0.95 = 9.0$ kcal |
| 1 gram protein | $= (5.65 \times 0.92) = 5.20$ kcal |

After digestion and absorption, carbohydrates and fats in human beings are completely oxidised to carbon dioxide and water in the process of cellular metabolism as in the calorimeter. Protein, on the other hand, is less efficient to be completely oxidised by the cell. In biological systems, urea, uric acid, creatinine, and other nitrogenous compounds derived from protein are excreted in the urine. Many observations of the heat of combustion of urine have shown that it contains unoxidised material equivalent to 7.9 kcal/gram of nitrogen. The value when expressed in terms of protein becomes 1.25 kcal (by dividing 7.9 with 6.25). This energy represents metabolic loss and must be subtracted from the "digestible" protein. After considering this point, Atwater has given factors for Metabolisable energy which is also known as physiological fuel value as below:

*Atwater's Physiological fuel value factors*

| | |
|---|---|
| Carbohydrate | $4.15 \times 0.98 = 4.0$ kcal/gram |
| Fat | $9.4 \times 0.95 = 9.0$ kcal/gram |
| Protein | $(5.65 - 1.25 \times 0.92) = 4.0$ kcal/gram |

It has already been mentioned that these values are not suitable for calculating energy values of ruminants feed as the per cent digestibility of feed components is always poor and moreover, the loss of energy in the urine is significantly higher in comparison to human beings.

Estimation of energy value of feeds obtained by multiplying the per cent composition with the appropriate Atwater's fuel value factors are thus a crude procedure for ruminants. In order to have a more precise estimate of nutritive value, the feed must be fed to the particular animal species involved (thus undergo a biological evaluation) for estimation of metabolisable energy.

## D. EVALUATION OF PROTEIN QUALITY

### (A) FOR NON-RUMINANTS

As discussed before, protein quality can be evaluated from the amount of digestibility, but there we do not know the efficiency with which the absorbed protein is utilised by the body. Since protein of different sources might have equal digestibility and may differ in their utilization by the body, different methods of evaluating protein have been formulated.

**1. Protein Efficiency Ratio (PER).** It is a measure of weight gain of a growing animal divided by protein intake.

$$PER = \frac{\text{Weight gain (gm)}}{\text{Protein intake (gm)}}$$

The PER was used as early as 1917 by Osborne and Mendal in their studies establishing differences in protein quality. It has most often been applied to studies in growing rats, but is also applicable to studies with human infants.

As carried out with rats to compare specific proteins or protein sources, a nitrogen free, otherwise adequate basal diet is used in which the protein sources to be compared are included for different groups of young animals.

It is the simplest method for evaluating protein quality since it requires only an accurate measure of dietary intake and weight gain. However, the method requires the strict adherence to certain conditions: (i) the calorie intake must be adequate; (ii) protein must be fed at an adequate but no excessive level since at high levels of dietary protein, weight gain does not increase proportionately with protein intake.

The greatest sources of error in the PER method lies in the use of weight gain as sole criterion of protein value. Weight gain cannot be assumed to represent proportional gain in body protein under all conditions.

To make a standard it has been suggested to test the protein level at 10 per cent dietary level—a level well below the level of protein ordinarily obtained in most protein rich foods.

PER is not characteristic of protein alone as it varies with different animals and condition in different laboratories.

**2. Biological Value (BV).** Technically, the term is defined as that proportion of the digested (and absorbed) protein that is not excreted in the urine, i.e., per cent of the absorbed nitrogen retained by the body for maintenance and/or growth. A balance trial is conducted in which nitrogen intake and urinary and faecal excretions are measured and the results are used to calculate the BV as follows:

$$BV = \frac{\text{N intake} - (\text{faecal N} + \text{urinary N})}{\text{N intake} - \text{faecal N}} \times 100$$

$$BV = \frac{\text{Retained Nitrogen}}{\text{Absorbed Nitrogen}} \times 100$$

This simplified formula measures the biological value of protein for growth purposes only. A more useful measure is one that takes account of maintenance as well. This can be accomplished by considering the metabolic and endogenous losses separately from the total faecal and urinary excretions. Biological value of dietary protein in the above sense can be expressed by the Thomas-Mitchell equation:

$$\text{per cent BV} = 100 \times \frac{\text{N intake} - (\text{faecal N} - \text{MFN}) - (\text{urinary N} - \text{EUN})}{\text{N intake} - (\text{faecal N} - \text{MFN})}$$

were MFN=*metabolic faecal nitrogen* and EUN=*endogenous urinary nitrogen.*

It will be seen that the total faecal nitrogen is corrected for the metabolic faecal nitrogen (i.e., that portion not a diet residue) and likewise the endogenous urinary nitrogn is deducted from the total urinary excretion in order to eliminate the so called wear and tear nitrogen losses that would occur even in the absence of dietary intake. If the correction is not made, i.e., MFN and EUN are not considered as in the previous case, BV obtained is designated apparent biological value.

In Thomas-Mitchell determination, it is, of course, necessary to determine the nitrogenous excretions on a nitrogen free diet or with rations containing small amounts of proteins which

**Table 152**

**Calculation of BV of a protein for maintenance and growth of the fat***

| | |
|---|---|
| Food consumed daily (gm) | 6.00 |
| Nitrogen in food (%) | 1.043 |
| Daily nitrogen intake (mg) | 62.6 |
| Total nitrogen excreted daily in urine (mg) | 32.8 |
| Endogenous nitrogen excreted daily in urine (mg) | 22.0 |
| Total nitrogen excreted daily in faeces (mg) | 20.9 |
| Metabolic faecal nitrogen excreted daily (mg) | 10.7 |

$$BV = \frac{62.6 - (20.9 - 10.7) - (32.8 - 22.0)}{62.6 - (20.9 - 10.7)} \times 100 = 79$$

*The example is taken from H. H. Mitchell, 1924, J. boil Chem. 58, 873.

are known to be practically 100 per cent digested in order to obtain values for metabolic faecal and endogenous urinary nitrogen. Using this procedure the metabolic nitrogen has been found to be approximately 0.1 gm for man, pigs and rats per 100 gm. dry matter consumed and 0.5 gm for ruminants.

Table 153

Biological values of the Protein of human food**

| *Animal food* | *BV* | *Vegetative food* | *BV* |
|---|---|---|---|
| Whole milk | 80 | Potato | 67 |
| Whole egg | 94 | Wheat | 67 |
| Egg white | 83 | Oats | 65 |

**The example is taken from H. H. Mitchell, The Protein Values of Foods in Nutrition, *J. Home Econ.*, 19, 122, 1927.

From the Table 153 it is evident that animal proteins always have more BV than vegetative proteins. This is due firstly, to the fact that the animal proteins are composed of well distributed essential amino acids and secondly, they are in right amount and in proper ratio, required for animal growth. So we can reach a definite conclusion that a protein in which all the essential amino acids are present in sufficient amounts and in proper ratio will show a high biological value in non-ruminants.

1. The B.V. does not apply to ruminants because of the ability of the rumen to synthesise amino acid from a variety of nitrogen compounds.

2. The criticism levelled against B.V. include, as can be seen from the equation, the method of judging protein quality refers only to combined functions of maintenance (meaning replacement of existing protein) and growth (formation of new tissues) but not for production.

3. The difficulties encountered in the measurement of metabolic and endogenous nitrogen fractions. This is more difficult in poultry where they excrete urine and faeces together.

4. It is of utmost importance to maintain some optimum protein levels of all the experimental feeds which are to be compared. Such rations are often adjusted to 10 per cent protein. Excess or lower nitrogen intake affects the determined value. Thus B.V. of the same protein might change depending on N-intake.

5. Adequate non-nitrogenous sources to provide energy and also of minerals and vitamins should be present in all test diets.

**3. Net Protein Utilisation (NPU).** This is the percentage of dietary protein which is converted into body protein.

$$\text{NPU} = \frac{\text{Retained Nitrogen}}{\text{Intake of Nitrogen}} \times 100$$

Nitrogen retention may be estimated by carcass analysis. The method combines in a single index, both the digestibility and the biological value of protein.

$$NPU = BV \times Digestibility$$

The method is much less laborious but time consuming than determining BV or nitrogen balance, but is limited to those animals that are available for carcass analysis.

**4. Nitrogen Balance.** Nitrogen balance study is commonly made to evaluate protein quality in non-ruminants as well as in ruminants. The method has been described under Ruminants (B).

**5. Nitrogen balance index**

It is essentially the same as biological value. It may be determined from the slope of the line when nitrogen balance is plotted against absorbed nitrogen. More simply, nitrogen balance index may be calculated from the following equation :

$$\text{Nitrogen Balance Index} = \frac{B-B_0}{A}$$

where B is nitrogen balance; $B_0$ is nitrogen balance when nitrogen intake is zero; and A is absorbed nitrogen. Since $B_0$ represents metabolic nitrogen, the nitrogen balance index is a measure of dietary nitrogen retained.

**6. Net protein ratio (NPR)**

The NPR assay simply represents the weight gain of a group of experimental animals (rats) fed the test diet plus the weight loss of a similar group fed a protein-free diet, the total divided by the weight of protein consumed by the first group. The method is an attempt to avoid the fundamental criticism of PER method by making allowance for maintenance.

## Other chemical methods

**7. Crude protein (CP)**

Chemically the protein of a feed is calculated from its nitrogen content, determined by a modification of classical Kjeldahl technique. Two assumptions are made in calculating the protein content namely, (1) all the nitrogen of the feed is present as protein, (2) all the feed protein contains 16 per cent nitrogen. The result is thus expressed in terms of crude protein.

Regarding principles of estimation the total nitrogen from true protein and non-protein substances present in the sample is oxidised to $(NH_4)_2SO_4$ by digestion with concentrated $H_2SO_4$. The digest is made alkaline with concentrated NaOH and the $NH_3$ is distilled into a saturated solution of boric acid. The ammonium borate produced is titrated with standard HCl. The amount of nitrogen obtained is multiplied by 6.25 to arrive at the CP content of the sample.

**8. True protein**

Determined by precipitating with cupric hydroxide or by heat coagulation in cas es of some plant mater al. The protein is then filtered and the residue is treated like Kjeldahl determination.

## (B) FOR RUMINANTS

**Estimation of DCP (Digestible Crude Protein).** It is the most common way of expressing the protein value of feed for ruminants. As discussed previously, the term crude protein includes both the true proteins as well as non-protein nitrogenous compounds such as amides, amino acids, nitrogenous glucosides, alkaloids, ammonium salts and others present in feed stuff. For ruminants, since the non-protein nitrogenous compounds can serve to provide the essential amino acids as a result of microbiological synthesis, distinction between true and crude protein of feeds seems no longer worthwhile.

From simple chemical analysis of the feed the amount of crude protein (true protein + non protein nitrogenous compounds) can easily be known, but the quantity present does not provide enough information on how well it is utilised in the body. Only on a digestion trial when we know the per cent absorbed, this provides some real clue about the usefulness of crude protein present in a feed stuff.

*To find out the per cent digestibility of crude protein (DCP) multiply the digestibility coefficient of that protein with the crude protein content of the feed stuff.*

Such trials give figures for "*apparent*" and not "*true*" digestibility owing to the presence of metabolic nitrogen in the faeces, which is not derived directly from the feed but comprises substances originating in the body, such as residues of the bile and other digestive juices, epithelial cells abraded from the alimentary tract by the feed passing through it, and bacterial residues. The apparent figures are thus lower than the true values, but since the loss of the *metabolic faecal nitrogen* is inevitable, it is better to ignore while expressing nitrogen digestibility. Usually no attempt is made to determine the true digestibility, and the values we see are all apparent values.

In general the most common practice of evaluation of food protein in ruminants is based firstly on the finding out of crude protein content. By running a digestibility trial as discussed earlier, the DCP values are then obtained. For concentrates, digestibility coefficient values are readily available in the literature, which are then used to find out the values of DCP. Roughages, due to low protein content may have sometimes negative digestible crude protein value due to greater importance of metabolic feacal nitrogen. As such a typical equation as is commonly used for both grass, hays and silages is given below:

$$\text{Per cent DCP} \quad (\%CP \times 0.9115) - 3.67$$

At present not only the protein values of ruminant feed stuff are tabulated as DCP but also the protein requirements of the animal are expressed as digestible crude protein requirements.

**Nitrogen Balance Experiment.** The method is applicable to determine the protein quality in ruminants as well as in non-ruminants. By applying the same technique the biological value (BV) of protein for non-ruminants is also estimated. The technique is equally in use to determine the protein requirements for various body functions in all classes of livestock.

The experimental technique is similar to that of a digestion trial except that in this case adequate provision for collection and analysis of urine and of any nitrogenous product such as milk should be made. When the experiment is conducted only to know the utilisation efficiency of the dietary nitrogen in terms of gaining or losing of nitrogen by the body, faeces and urine may be collected and analysed together for the sake of simplicity of the procedure. When the experimentar desires to find out simultaneously the BV of the nitrogen and digestibility separately, the collection of faeces and urine must be made separately using metabolic crate as described before.

The method actually involves an accurate account of the amount of nitrogen consumed through feed and excretion through faeces, urine and brushings (hair, feathers etc.) This must be collected and analysed under controlled conditions. Furthermore, any product for example, milk or eggs, will also need to be recorded and used as the case may be for nitrogen content.

**The method involves determination of the amount of endogenous urinary as well as that of metabolic faecal nitrogen, both of which either may by calculated from the existing formulae (See Protein Metabolism) or may be obtained by conducting actual trials which are time consuming. Feed is withheld from animals so that their bodies enter into a catabolic condition. The nitrogen excreted in the urine and faeces during this period represents the nitrogen lost through metabolic process, the values thus obtained are accordingly known as *endogenous urinary nitrogen* (EUN) and *metabolic faecal nitrogen* (MFN)**

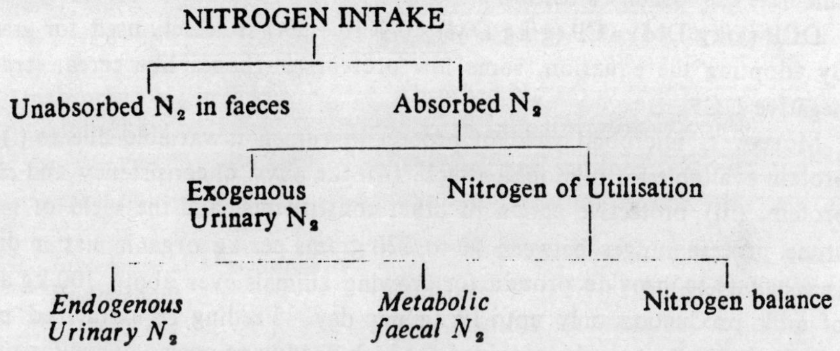


**These values are then substracted from the total nitrogen values obtained in the collection of the urine and faeces during the collection period of the balance trial. Exogenous urinary nitrogen and faecal nitrogen from feed are determined by the following equations :**

1. Exogenous Urinary Nitrogen = total urinary nitrogen minus endogenous urinary nitrogen
2. Faecal Nitrogen from feed = total faecal nitrogen minus metabolic faecal nitrogen

When the daily nitrogen intake is less than the total outgo from the body, the animal in that case, is in *negative nitrogen balance*. If the nitrogen intake equalled the outgo, the animal is in *nitrogen equilibrium*.

In practice, this condition can hardly be observed. An excess of intake over outgo will represent a *positive nitrogen balance*, involving a deposition and storage of protein in the body.

To measure the quality of protein of a particular feed, care must be taken that the protein is fed at an adequate amount but not at an extra high level since with a higher protein intake (than the required), there will be more of excretion. Thus it will be difficult to compare the protein quality of various feeds.

## THE NEW CONCEPT TO DETERMINE REQUIREMENTS OF PROTEINS IN RUMINANTS

The method most widely used for expressing the ruminant's requirement for protein and the extent to which a certain feed could meet these requirements is one based on the measurement of *digestible crude protein* (DCP). Since this method was considered to give too much weight to non-protein nitrogen, another concept of *protein equivalent* (PE) introduced in 1925, where non-protein nitrogen fraction was assumed to be fully digestible but to have half the value of digestible true protein.

$$PE = \frac{\% \text{ Dig. Crude Protein} + \% \text{ Dig. True Protein}}{2}$$

In 1960, the method was found to underestimate the value of the non-protein nitrogen of silages etc., and the use of DCP was again proposed for feeds of ruminants.

With this conception, determination of DCP by means of digestibility trial of large number of feeds gradually become difficult particularly for roughages, which unlike concentrate feeds, have variable composition and for this regression equations for DCP on CP are used to calculate the former as below :

DCP (g/kg DM) = CP (g/kg DM) × 0.9115 − 36.7 is widely used for grasses hays and silages. By adopting the equation, some low protein roughages like cereal straws are found to have negative DCP.

Moreover, microbial yield of protein in rumen is variable due to (i) surface area of feed protein available for microbial attack, (ii) the physical consistency and chemical nature of the protein, (iii) protective action of other constituents, and the yield of microbial protein from crude protein ranges between 90 to 230 grams per kg organic matter digested. This amount is adequate to provide protein for growing animals over about 100 kg and to maintain levels of milk production only upto 10 kg per day. Feeding of extra feed protein (true proteins) per se obviously must be provided for high producing cows. Thus for providing protein needs if we rely much on DCP (which contains NPN + true protein) without caring the amount of true protein, high yielders will thus be affected.

As a result for many years there has been considerable dissatisfaction with this method.

In an attempt to overcome some of the disadvantages accociated with DCP system, protein requirements for ruminants were expressed as *Available Protein*, which is the crude protein of a define biological value that would have to be absorbed from the gastrointestinal tract to meet requirements for maintenance and production. Unfortunately the system has also number of limitations. It assumes that the faecal loss of N can be divided into a component of indigestible feed N and the other protein which represents unabsorbed secretions of N-containing compounds i.e. metabolic faecal N. In fact, faecal N consists mainly of microbial nitrogen and no such division is possible and to some extent, of biological value is in doubt. For these reasons a new conceptual approach has been made to the problems of meeting the protein requirements of ruminants particularly for high yielders.

**The New Approach**

In ruminants, as in other animals, the needs of the tissues are met by amino acids absorbed from the small intestine. The ideal system for calculating the nitrogen requirements of ruminants must provide, therefore, estimates of the total and individual amino acids absorbed from the small intestine. These amino acids are supplied partly by microbial protein synthesised in the rumen and partly by dietary protein which has escaped fermentation in the rumen (bypass protein). The value of dietary urea or similar NPN sources depends entirely on degradation to ammonia in the rumen by microbes and the subsequent use of this ammonia foı microbial protein synthesis. The extent of the synthesis depends on the energy available to the microorganisms. Dietary protein also is degraded in the rumen by microbial attack ; the pathways of this degradation are poorly understood but the nitrogenous products include peptides, amino acids and ultimately $NH_3$. These products are used for the synthesis of microbial protein and there is evidence that mixed bacteria growing in the rumen incorporate considerable amounts of preformed amino acids as well as $NH_3$ when the diet contains protein. It is possible that this results in better microbial growth than the use of $NH_3$ alone but, as a net effect for the host animal, good dietary protein which is degraded in the rumen is used inefficiently.

Degradability of dietary proteins in the rumen varies among different natural protein sources and with different processing treatments.

$$\text{Degradability} = 1 - \frac{\text{Dietary protein entering duodenum}}{\text{total dietary protein intake}}$$

That part which escapes degradation (bypass protein) supplements microbial protein in providing a source of amino acids for digestion and absorption in the small intestine of the host animal.

The new system thus takes care of the amount of microbial as well as the amount of "bypass protein" requirement of ruminants i.e., proportion of degradable and undegradable amount of protein for ruminants.

Burroughs et.al in 1975 of Iowa State in U. S. A. proposed "*Metabolisable Protein*" (MP) system and Urea fermentation potential (UFP).

*Metabolisable protein is defined as the quantity of protein digested or amino acid(s) absorbed in the post ruminal portion of the digestive tract of cattle and other ruminants and is available for use at tissue level.* It consists partly of dietary ture protein which has escaped degradation in the rumen but which has been broken down to amino acids and are subsequently absorbed from the small intestine. Microbial protein, synthesised in the rumen, similarly contributes to metabolisable protein. This is illustrated in page 574

In this instance 1000 gm of dietary protein yields 750 g of MP, but this depends upon the validity of certain assumptions particularly the proportion of dietary crude protein present in non-protein form, the degradability of dietary true protein, and the efficiency of synthesis of microbial protein, which is determined by the supply of readily available energy for micro-organisms (Fig. 84 ).

Thus MP supplied by different diets is estimated by taking into account (i) extent of degradation of feed protein in the rumen, (ii) the amount of microbial protein synthesised in the rumen and the (iii) digestibility of these components in the small intestine. Potential

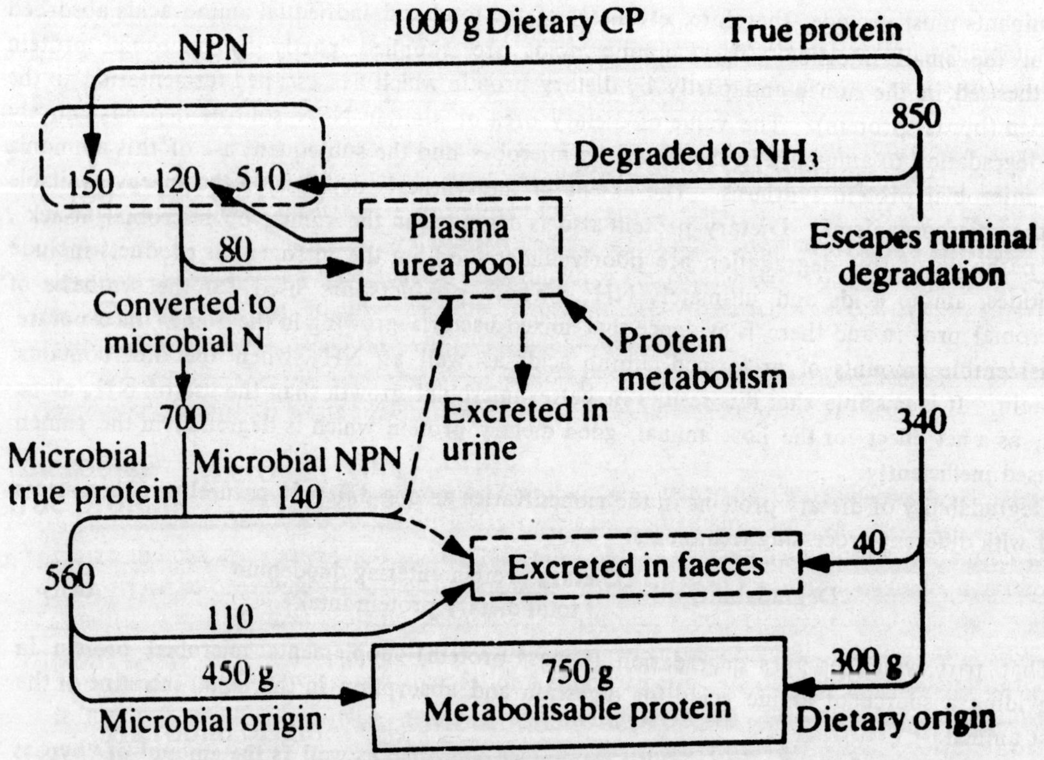


Fig. 84 Calculation of "Metabolisable Protein" of diet.

microbial protein synthesis in the rumen is estimated by assessing, from the TDN content of the diet, the energy available for this purpose.

*Urea fermentation potential* (*UFP*) *is a term used to indicate the amount of urea that can be utilised in a ruminant ration.* A positive UFP value of a feed represents the estimated grams of urea per kg. of feed dry matter consumed that can be used for ruminal synthesis of microbial protein.

**Factors involved in the New Approach**

The general scheme of the new approach is to calculate the amount of amino acid N of microbial origin that could be retained in the body for tissue synthesis when the maximal rate of fermentation of a particular energy input is achieved. This amount of amino acid N is compared with the total tissue needs for the particular energy input. Two alternatives present themselves :

1. If the amount of microbial amino acid N available to the tissues is greater than the tissue needs, then the nitrogen requirement is the amount of degraded N needed by the rumen microorganisms ;
2. If the microbial amino acid N is less than the tissue needs, then the difference must be supplied by amino acids from undegraded dietary protein.

For practical calculation of N requirements simple summary equations can be derived as follows :

(a) Rumen degradable N (RDN) requirement (g/day) = 1.25 ME

(b) Amino acid N supplied to the tissues (TMN) by microbial synthesis from RDN (g/day) = 0.53 ME

(c) If total tissue N requirement, calculated by the factorial method (TN) is greater than TMN, then Undegraded dietary N (UDN) requirement (g/day) = 1.91 TN − 1.00 ME where ME is metabolisable energy requirement.

Total dietary N requirement is thus the sum of the RDN and UDN requirements.

In a proposed ration, the weights of degradable N (RDN) and undegraded N (UDN) are calculated, and these are compared with the RDN and UDN requirements of the animal.

1. If the UDN requirement of the animal is greater than the UDN content of the ration, then additional protein must be given to correct the deficiency of UDN and the weight of RDN supplied by the new ration must be calculated.

2. If the RDN requirement of the animal is greater than the RDN content of the ration, then the deficiency could be made up by urea. Alternatively, if the deficiency arises after correcting for a deficiency of UDN by supplementary protein, a source of protein of higher degradability could be used.

It is suggested that feed tables should contain values for rumen-degradable protein and undegradable protein by multiplying N with 6.25 factors rather than N as used while explaining the principles.

## SOME IMPORTANT FACTS RELATED TO THE CONCEPT

### 1. Microbial N yield in the Rumen and Quality

For each kg of organic matter fermented, approximately 30 gm N is taken up by rumen bacteria as protein and nucleic acids.

Regarding quality of microbial protein the following points may be noted :

1. Diet does not affect the amino acid composition of individual species of bacteria or protozoa
2. Biological value of rumen bacteria & protozoa are same i.e., about 0.8 but the digestibility of bacterial protein is lower, 0.74 compared to 0.91 for protozoal protein.
3. Protozoa numbers are higher on high roughage diets than on concentrate diets.
4. Microbial protein contains 20% nucleic acid which has no value for animals.

### 2. Proportion of Total microbial N present as amino acid N

A value of 0.80 has been adopted for calculating N requirements. In using this factor, it must be borne in mind that the value used subsequently for efficiency of utilisation of absorbed N derived from bacteria should refer to as amino acid N and not to total N.

### 3. Apparent absorbability in the small intestine of amino acids derived from microbial & dietary protein

A value of 0.75 for efficiency of utilisation of apparently absorbed amino acid N from the small intestine has been adopted for both cattle and sheep.

**4. Extent of degradation of dietary protein in the rumen**

While the rumen contains a potent supply of proteases and deaminases, all feed proteins are not degraded to the same degree as is shown below. The figures represent degradable percent.

| | | | | | |
|---|---|---|---|---|---|
| Urea | — | 100 | Soybean meal | — | 60 |
| Casein | — | ·90 | Lucerne hay | — | 60 |
| Cotton seed meal | — | 70 | Maize | — | 40 |
| Groundnut meal | — | 65 | Fish meai | — | 30 |

As expected, urea is 100% degradable like soluble casein. Plants are highly variable but maize, with its high content of insoluble *zein*, is only 40% degraded. Casein a high quality protein largely converted to microbial protein, while much of fish meal, also of high quality largely passes intact into small intestine.

Proteins which are generally ( but not necessarily) more soluble considered to be more degradable. The competition between passage and rumen digestion for potentially digestible substrate determines the proportion of unfermented feed passing to the omasum and abomasum. This passage (bypass protein) is important in regard to potentially digestible true protein since it will deteirmine the proportion of unaltered dietary protein and amino acids reaching peptic digestion.

Moreover, when feed proteins are treated by mild heat, or chemicals such as formaldehyde or tannin, decreases rumen microbial attack by manipulating the solubility and thus increase the amount of bypass protein in the same way as described above.

**Conclusions**

As it stands now, the new conception to deteirmine requirements of protein in ruminants makes certain questionable assumptions, and suffer the major disadvantage that no satisfactory method exist for routinely determining protein degradability The general approach although highly commendable but it should wait some more time to be introduced in regular practice after the validation under field conditions.

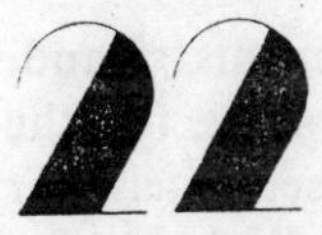

# METHODS TO FIND OUT NUTRITIVE REQUIREMENTS FOR BODY PROCESSES AND PRODUCTIVE FUNCTIONS

*The Chapter has been discussed as per following arrangements*

*General*

*Feeding Standards for Maintenance*

A. Energy Requirement for Maintenance
   1. By Basal and Fasting Metabolism
   2. From Feeding Trials

B. Protein Requirement for Maintenance
   1. Estimation of Protein Requirement from EUN and MFN
   2. Nitrogen Balance method as a measure of protein Maintenance
   3. Feeding Trial Method to determine protein Maintenance.

*Feeding Standards for Growth*

A. Energy Requirement for Growth
   1. By Feeding Trials
   2. By the Factorial Method

B. Protein Requirement for Growth
   1. Factorial Method
   2. Nitrogen Balance Method
   3. Feeding Trials

*Protein Requirement for Reproduction*
*Energy Requirement for Reproduction*
*Protein Requirement for Lactation*
*Energy Requirement for Lactation*
*Protein Requirement for Work*
*Protein Requirement for Bulls*

Nutritive requirements are the statements of the amount of nutrients required by animals that should support normal function. A rough distinction between requirement and allowance is that, the allowance is greater than the requirement by a safety margin designed principally to allow variations in requirement among the individual animals. These requirements or allowances for different purposes, such as growth, fattening, lactation of different species are generally laid down in Tables known as feeding standards or Tables of requirements. Standards may be given separately for each function of the animal or as overall figures for the combined functions. The requirements of dairy cows, for example, are given separately for maintenance, pregnancy and for milk production but those for growing chickens are for maintenance and growth combined. Requirements may be expressed in quantities of nutrients or in dietary proportions. Thus the phosphorus requirement of a 50 kg pig might be expressed as 11 g. phosphorus per day or as 0.5% phosphorus in the diet. The exact amount of nurtrient requirement is used mainly for animals given exact quantities of feed, the expression as per cent of the diet is used for animals fed to appetite.

When the standard is set to represent the needs of the average in a population, many will require more than the figures stated, and many will require less. The individual stockman does not know whether the average requirements are below or above the requirements of his animals. For this reason feeding standards should be considered as guides to feeding practice and the stockman should make finer adjustment of food intake to animal performance. The standard which is revised from time to time, guides the stockman for an average requirement of feed for his livestock. The object in this section will be to discuss the scientific basis for feeding standards and to describe briefly how they are determined.

## FEEDING STANDARDS FOR MAINTENANCE

An animal is in a state of maintenance when the amount of nutrients in the feed will maintain the animal in equilibrium i.e., its body composition remains constant and is not growing, working or giving no product as milk or mutton or egg. This minimum demand of feed is referred to as the maintenance requirement. If this need is not met, animals are forced to draw upon their body reserves to meet their nutrient requirements for maintenance, commonly revealed by a loss in weight and to various other undesirable consequences. The knowledge of this maintenance requirement of farm animals is of utmost importance to find out the total requirements of feed for animals under various conditions such as pregnancy or yielding certain quantity of milk or doing certain amount of work. The procedure involves the summing up of the requirements of each function on top of maintenance requirement. The starting point of finding maintenance requirement is the fasting catabolism.

### A. Energy Requirements for Maintenance

#### (I) BASAL AND FASTING METABOLISM

The term Basal Metabolism or Basal Metabolic rate refers to the heat production of an animal resting in a thermally neutral environment (temperature range in which environmental temperature does not stimulate normal metabolism, approximately 25°C) and in a post-absorptive state (that is after the digestion and absorption of the last food ingested has stopped). During this rest period although the animal will be doing no external or digestive work nor will it have any emotional excitement, still it will carry on a variety of internal processes which are essential to life. These processes include respiration, circulation, maintenance of muscular tonus, production of internal secretions, etc. In the absence of food, the nutrients required to support these activities must come from the break-down of body tissues itself.

The heat production can be determined by direct calorimetry, or by indirect calorimetry. The conditions of the animals which are essential for measuring metabolic rate are as follow:

1. *Good nutritive conditions*—this implies that the previous diet of the subject has been adequate, especially as regards to energy and protein. Poor state of previous nutrition tends to decrease the basal heat production.

2. *Environmental temperature*—temperature of about 25°C specified as one which is above the critical and below the point of hyperthermal rise, thus avoids tissue breakdown.

3. *Relaxation on bed prior to and during measurement*—by this way the minimum muscular activity can be achieved. This is very difficult for any kind of animal other than man.

4. *Post-absorptive state*—a state when the process of digestion or absorption disappears. It is reached by an overnight starvation in case of human, but for ruminants it may require about three or four days. This condition can hardly be fulfilled by any ruminants, hence it is measured after a starvation period of about 5 hours. Because of the fact that the last two conditions cannot be fulfilled and a modification is recommended for ruminant animals, hence the term *resting metabolism* is used in place of basal metabolism

An animal in the resting state accomplishes little or no work in the physical sense of the word. All of the energy released, even that needed to carry out vital functions of the body is degraded to heat and lost to the environment. Under these circumstances the intensity of energy metabolism can be estimated either by calculating heat production from the exchange of respiratory gases (indirect calorimetry) or by measuring the heat which is lost from the body by radiation, conduction, convection and evaporation (direct calorimetry).

*Direct Calorimetry*

This is simple in theory, difficult in practice. Sensible heat loss (heat of radiation conduction) from the animal body can be measured with two general types of calorimeters, adiabatic and gradient. The insensible heat (latent heat of water vapourized from the skin and the respiratory passages) is estimated by determining in some way the amount of water vapour added to the air which flows through the calorimeter. For this, rate of air flow and change in humidity is measured.

1. ADIABATIC CALORIMETERS

In this type an animal is confined in a chamber constructed in such a way that heat loss through the walls of the chamber is reduced to near zero. This is attained by a box within a box. When the outer box or wall is electrically heated to the same temperature as the inner wall, heat loss from the inner wall to the outer wall is impossible. Water circulating in a coil in such a chamber absorbs the heat collected by the inner wall; the volume and change in temperature of the water can be used to calculate sensible heat loss from the animal body. The construction and operation are complicated and very expensive.

2. GRADIANT CALORIMETERS

Calorimeters of this type allow the loss of heat through the walls of the animal chamber. The outer surface of the wall of the calorimeter is maintained at a constant temperature with a water jacket; the temperature gradient is measured with thermocouples which line the inner and outer surfaces of the wall. By the use of appropriate techniques it is possible to measure separately the radiation component of the sensible heat loss.

*Indirect Calorimetry*

Because the animal body ultimately derives all of its energy from oxidation, the magnitude of energy metabolism can be estimated from the exchange of respiratory gases. Such measurements of heat production are more readily accomplished than are measurements of heat dissipation by direct calorimetry. A variety of techniques are available for measuring the respiratory exchange; all ultimately seek to measure oxygen consumption and $CO_2$ production per unit of time.

1. OPEN CIRCUIT SYSTEM

Devices allow the animal to breath atmospheric air of determined composition; the exhaust air from a chamber or expired air from a mask or cannula, is either collected or else metered and sampled and then analyzed for $O_2$ and $CO_2$ content. Analysis of gases has been accomplished with chemical and volumetric or manometric techniques. More recently methods of analysis based on physiological properties of gases have been developed. Oxygen for example, can be determined by its paramagnetic effect or with mass spectrometer; $CO_2$ can be measured by infra-red absorption or thermal conductivity.

2. CLOSED CIRCUIT SYSTEM

Devices require the animal to rebreathe the same air. $CO_2$ is removed with a suitable absorber which may be weighed before and after use to determine its rate of production. The use of oxygen by the animal body decreases the volume of the respiratory gas mixture, and this change in volume is used as a measure of the rate of oxygen consumption. Oxygen used by the animal is then replaced by a metered supply of the pure gas. Both $O_2$ consumption and $CO_2$ production must be corrected for any differences in the amounts present in the circuit air at the beginning and end of the experiment. Methane is allowed to accumulate in the circuit air, and the amount present is determined at the end of the experiment by drawing the air sample over platinized Kaolin or a similar substance at red heat. Methane is oxidized and determined from the $CO_2$ produced.

Respiratory exchange can thus be measured with or without any animal chamber. In later case the subject is fitted with a face mask, which is then connected to either a closed or an open circuit for determining $O_2$ consumption alone or both $O_2$ consumption and $CO_2$ produced. This method is suitable for short periods of measurements.

**Interpretation of the RQ**

From our previous discussion we know that the *R.Q. is the ratio between the oxygen consumed and the $CO_2$ given off, i.e.*

$$R.Q. = \frac{\text{Volume of } CO_2}{\text{Volume of } O_2}$$

*Energy Values of $O_2$ and $CO_2$ at different R. Q.*

| R.Q. | kcal per litre $O_2$ | kcal per litre $CO_2$ | kcal per gram $CO_2$ |
|---|---|---|---|
| 0.70 | 4.686 | 6.694 | 3.408 |
| 0.75 | 4.739 | 6.319 | 3.217 |
| 0.80 | 4.801 | 6.001 | 3.055 |
| 0.85 | 4.863 | 5.721 | 2.919 |
| 0.90 | 4.924 | 5.471 | 2.785 |
| 0.95 | 4.985 | 5.247 | 2.671 |
| 1.00 | 5.047 | 5.047 | 2.569 |

The measurement of respiratory exchange and the calculation of heat production thus represented constitutes procedure of indirect calorimetry to measure basal metabolism of energy.

**Units of reference in fasting metabolism**

Heat production or basal metabolism rate varies with body size. Rubner developed the concept, referred to as the *surface area law*, that the heat given off by all warm blooded animals is directly proportional to their body surface and that, expressed on this basis, heat production is constant to body surface for all species. The surface area on the other hand is very difficult to measure, and methods were therefore devised for predicting it from their fractional or decimal power of body weight. In 1964 an international conference of scientists concerned with the energy metabolism of farm animals decided to standardize the expression of fasting metabolism on ¾ power of body weight i.e., Kg. $W^{0.75}$ because of the close relationship between metabolism and metabolic body weight.

**Table 154**

**Some typical values for the fasting metabolism of adult animals of various species**

| Animal | Live weight (kg) | Fasting metabolism (kcal/day) Per kg. $W^{0.75}$ |
|---|---|---|
| Cow | 500 | 71 |
| Pig | 72 | 52 |
| Man | 70 | 70 |
| Sheep | 50 | 56 |
| Fowl | 3 5 | 73 |
| Rat | 0 29 | 71 |

The fasting metabolism of adult animals of species ranging in size from rat to cow has an average value of 70 kcal per Kg. $W^{0.75}$ per day, but there are considerable variations from species to species.

**Table 155**

**Metabolic Body size (kg. $W^{0.75}$) for various body weights**

| $W_{kg}$ | $W_{kg}^{0.75}$ | $W_{kg}$ | $W_{kg}^{0.75}$ | $W_{kg}$ | $W_{kg}^{075}$ | $W_{kg}$ | $W_{kg}^{0.75}$ |
|---|---|---|---|---|---|---|---|
| 1·0 | 1.0 | 100 | 31.62 | 210 | 55.16 | 440 | 96.07 |
| 3 | 2.28 | 105 | 32.80 | 220 | 57.10 | 460 | 99.33 |
| 5 | 3.34 | 110 | 33.97 | 230 | 59.06 | 480 | 102.33 |
| 10 | 5.62 | 115 | 35.12 | 240 | 60.98 | 500 | 105.74 |
| 15 | 7.62 | 120 | 36.26 | 250 | 62.87 | 520 | 108.89 |
| 20 | 9.46 | 125 | 37.38 | 260 | 64.75 | 540 | 112.02 |
| 25 | 11.18 | 130 | 38.50 | 270 | 66.61 | 560 | 115.12 |
| 30 | 12.83 | 135 | 39.60 | 280 | 68.45 | 580 | 118.19 |
| 35 | 14.39 | 140 | 40.70 | 290 | 70 28 | 600 | 121.23 |
| 40 | 15.91 | 145 | 41.79 | 300 | 72.08 | 620 | 124.20 |
| 45 | 17.37 | 150 | 42.86 | 310 | 73.88 | 640 | 127.20 |
| 50 | 18.80 | 155 | 43.93 | 320 | 75.66 | 660 | 130.20 |
| 55 | 20.20 | 160 | 44.99 | 330 | 77.42 | 680 | 133.20 |
| 60 | 21.56 | 165 | 46.04 | 340 | 79.18 | 700 | 136.10 |
| 65 | 22.89 | 170 | 47.08 | 350 | 80.92 | 750 | 143.30 |
| 70 | 24.20 | 175 | 48.11 | 360 | 82.65 | 800 | 150.40 |
| 75 | 25.49 | 180 | 49.14 | 370 | 84.36 | 850 | 157.40 |
| 80 | 26.75 | 185 | 50.16 | 380 | 86.07 | 900 | 164.30 |
| 85 | 27.98 | 190 | 51.17 | 390 | 87.76 | 950 | 171.10 |
| 90 | 29.22 | 195 | 52.18 | 400 | 89.44 | 1000 | 177.80 |
| 95 | 30.43 | 200 | 53.18 | 420 | 92.78 | 1050 | 184.50 |

**Basal metabolism of various body weights are nowadays determined from the formula**

$$BM\ (kcal) = 70W_{kg}^{0.75}$$

**The coefficient 70 represents an average value for the kilocalories of basal heat produced per unit of metabolic size in experiments with groups of adult mammals. It should be noted that the above formula applies only in case of adult animals whose growth is complete.**

## (2) ENERGY REQUIREMENT BY FEEDING TRIALS

In this method an attempt is made to determine the amount of feed in terms of energy which is sufficient to maintain constant weight for an extended period. The value so obtained may be expressed in terms of TDN by inclusion of a digestion trial or may be calculated from the average digestion coefficients. This inclusion of metabolic trial helps to calculate the results in terms of ME. As live weight is the sole criterion of exactness of this method, it should be noted that the weight should remain constant over an extended period for direct application into practice. If for any reason there be gain in weight or loss, necessary correction in intake should accordingly be made for such loss or gain in weight. Correction figures as proposed by Knott and associates (1934) are shown below:

Pounds gained × 3.53 = TDN required for gain
Pounds lost × 2.73 = TDN equivalent to loss.

Such corrections are, however, only approximate since the nature of tissue gained or lost is difficult to assess, e.g., if the accumulation of water, which has no feed equivalent, be responsible for weight gain, then the use of the above correction factor for gain will be meaningless. The object, therefore, is to use these correction factors as minimum as possible for reasons as already stated above. Another defect of this method is that constancy of weight does not necessarily mean the integrity of body tissue or in other words the weight maintenance does not mean the energy maintenance. This defect, however, can be eliminated by inclusion of slaughter test which, however, adds to the cost of experiment and at the same time may not be practicable for all classes of stock.

Garrett and coworkers (1959) deduced the following formulae expressed in terms of TDN, DE, ME and NE requirements from a comprehensive feeding trial which included metabolic trials to measure both faecal and urine losses and the loss of methane was calculated. Slaughter data were also obtained.

$$\left.\begin{array}{ll}\text{Pounds TDN/days} & = 0.036\ W^{0.75} \\ \text{DE (kcal)/day} & = 76\ W^{0.75} \\ \text{ME (kcal)/day} & = 62\ W^{0.75} \\ \text{NE (kcal)/day} & = 32\ W^{0.75}\end{array}\right\}\ W = \text{Body weight in pounds.}$$

Most of the data on energy maintenance requirement was based on feeding trial carried out for an extended period to obviate criticism as to constancy of live weight vis-a-vis integrity of tissues.

**B. Protein Requirements for Maintenance**

It has been already discussed elsewhere that loss of protein continually occurs through wear and tear of body tissues, for renewal of hairs, nails, feathers etc., and if the losses are not compensated promptly by proper amount of protein either in the form of tissue protein or NPN substances, the animal will rundown in condition and its reproducing ability or productivity will be adversely affected. The losses of body protein in the animal when kept on a low protein or protein free ration although adequate in other nutrients usually occurs through urine and faeces but losses may also occur, although in negligible amount, through shedding of hairs, loss of nail, skin etc. The loss which occurs through urine is known as EUN or *endogenous urinary nitrogen* loss and loss which occurs through faeces is called MFN or *metabolic faecal nitrogen* loss.

EUN: Here the loss of nitrogen is due to the catabolism incidental to maintenance of the vital tissues of the body, which can be measured at the minimum urinary excretion on a nitrogen free otherwise adequate (particularly energy adequacy) diet. It is so likely that the quantity of nitrogen thus lost through urine will be dependent on the body size. However, this loss like energy loss is not directly proportional to body weight but to $W^{0.75}$ where W is the body weight in kg. The value of EUN for a cow weighing 450 kg is 13 gm daily. Experiment in Indian cows has shown that the value of EUN is about 0.02-0.03 gm/kg body weight.

Faecal nitrogen consists of two parts: undigested food nitrogen and another part known as MFN which comprises residues originated from the body, e.g., residues of bile, digestive enzymes, epithelial cells derived from the alimentary tract from friction of food materials passing through it and undigested bacteria.

MFN: Metabolic faecal nitrogen unlike EUN is not proportional to body weight but rather this value is dependent on the amount of feed ingested. There is also species difference. Mukherjee, Kehar and Sen (1943) have determined the value of MFN to be 0.35 gm per 100 gm dry matter intake but the value 0.5 gm per 100 gm of dry matter ingested is now in common use. The value will be lower with rations low in roughage and higher where roughage alone will be fed.

## 1. ESTIMATION OF PROTEIN REQUIREMENT FOR MAINTENANCE FROM ENDOGENOUS URINARY AND METABOLIC FAECAL NITROGEN (THE FACTORIAL METHOD)

From the above discussion it is evident that the minimum protein requirement of an adult for maintenance must be met by supplying digestible protein required to compensate losses through EUN and MFN plus losses for adult growth in an otherwise adequate diet. In practice, however, a larger amount is given to afford a margin of safety for variation of requirement from animal to animal arising out of variable wastage in metabolism like loss of nitrogen in hair etc., which being very negligible can also be omitted for all practical purposes or an account may be taken from an estimate of 0.02 $W^{0.73}$ gm nitrogen loss per day in cattle.

*Example*: A cow weighing 450 kg body weight and consuming 7 kg dry matter will excrete 13 gm of EUN everyday and 35 gm of MFN totalling 48 gm in all. The loss of nitrogen in adult like growth and renewal of hair, nails in cattle is practically negligible. Thus, $48 \times 6.25 = 300$ gm protein loss is evidenced. Now to arrive at the protein requirement, this value has to be converted to digestible or absorbed protein but absorbed protein is not utilized with 100% efficiency because the efficiency of utilization depends on the biological value of protein which is about 70% in ruminants.

Therefore, $100/70 \times 300 = 428$ gm or say 0.43 kg is the amount of true digestible protein required for just maintenance. As the requirement of protein in the feeding standard is given in the form of apparent digestible protein, say DCP, the value of MFN in terms of protein should be deducted from the figure of true digestible protein. Therefore, 0.430 kg—$(6.25 \times 0.035) = 0.22$ kg is the value expressed in DCP. Now this value is increased by 25% to provide margin of safety which thus becomes 0.28 kg. DCP—a value which has been recommended in the Table of feeding standards.

It will appear from the above that in the calculation of protein requirement, first the value of MFN has been included but subsequently the same value has been subtracted for converting true digestible protein to apparent digestible protein or say DCP. The reason for this is to allow the wastage of amino acids incurred in the synthesis of metabolic faecal protein.

From the above, the following formulae may be deduced for estimating the total digestible protein, e.g.

$$\text{Total digestible protein} = (\text{EUN} + \text{MFN} + \text{S}) \times 6.25 \times \frac{100}{\text{B.V.}}$$

In cattle, S for the loss of nitrogen in hair etc., may be determined from an estimate of 0.02 $W^{0.73}$ gm nitrogen loss per day. This value may, however, be omitted, for all practical purposes as the amount is very negligible.

B.V.=Biological value of protein which for an adult cattle fed on different ration is estimated at 70. This true digestible protein may be converted to DCP by procedure as enumerated above.

Since the value of MFN is depenent on dry matter intake and is likely to differ from animal to animal, they pose a problem in tabulating requirements. To obviate this difficulty a formula has been evolved where the MFN factor has been eliminated to express the requirement as AP (available protein). The difference between AP and DCP is that in AP determination, "Protein wasted in synthesizing MFN estimated from the figure for B.V." has been subtracted. The formula is shown below:

$$AP=(EUN+S)\times 6.25\times 100/B.V.$$

where,

AP=Available protein

EUN=Endogenous Urinary Nitrogen

S=Loss of Nitrogen in hair and scurf.

However, this may not be considered as the minimum protein requirement, for other factors are to be considered for arriving at the recommended value for practical feeding. The relation of EUN to basal metabolism has been clearly established and by now wealth of reliable data on basal metabolism have been determined and found highly satisfactory for practical consideration. In practice, the actual determination of EUN value on a nitrogen free diet is difficult, if not impossible, since most animals refuse to eat a sufficient amount of a nitrogen free diet for any extended period. Therefore, it would always be wise to derive values of protein requirement on the basis of a fairly constant relationship of EUN to basal metabolism.

This procedure has been adopted by FAO and WHO in its 1965 report. The formula for the adult is shown below:

$$R=(UB+FB+S)\times 1.1$$

where, R=requirement of nitrogen per kg body wt. per day

UB=basal urinary nitrogen loss

FB=basal faecal nitrogen loss

S=Nitrogen loss from skin (integumental and mild sweating)

Factor 1.1. represents an addition of 10 per cent "to allow for the stress of ordinary life". $R\times 6.25$ is the requirement in terms of reference protein which is defined in the report.

## 2. NITROGEN BALANCE METHOD AS MEASURE OF PROTEIN MAINTENANCE

The protein requirement as determined by nitrogen balance studies is a satisfactory and reliable measure. In this method, rations containing different levels of protein but adequate in all other respects are fed to the animals and the minimum protein intake capable of enforcing nitrogen equilibrium in a well-nourished animal is said to be the maintenance requirement of protein. It is important that animals chosen for such determination must be in a good state of protein nutrition at the start. Minimum intake capable of maintaining nitrogen equilibrium is also very important since unnecessarily high intake may also result in protein equilibrium showing the false maintenance requirement. On the contrary, in a protein depleted animal, equilibrium may also be established by intake level which is not enough for maintaining the needed protein reserves. The minimum level of intake capable of maintaining these reserves denotes the actual requirement of protein.

Large number of animals should be used for the study over an extended period to offset individual variation etc. The value so determined must be set at a higher level in practice to cover individual and other variations as well as difference in biological value of different feed combinations.

### 3. FEEDING TRIAL TO DETERMINE MAINTENANCE REQUIREMENT OF PROTEIN

Rations containing different levels of protein but otherwise adequate in energy and other nurtrients are fed to determine the amount of intake capable of maintaining an adult non-producing animal in sufficiently good condition for an extended period without loss of weight or otherwise. Data obtained from slaughter tests (although very difficult to perform in adult cattle) are very helpful to determine the integrity of the nitrogenous tissues.

## FEEDING STANDARDS FOR GROWTH

### A. Energy requirement for growth

### 1. FROM FEEDING TRIALS

The data of energy requirement for growth shown in the feeding standard are based on the results of feeding trials. Here the experimental animals in groups throughout the growth period are fed at different levels of energy intake so as to determine the optimum level most suited to normal growth and development without being unnecessarily high. The energy so found may be expressed in terms of any desired measure of energy. TDN data are most common in such studies by inclusion of digestion trial or by use of average coefficients of digestibility.

Several formulae have been developed in growth studies for obtaining energy requirement in calves for the combined maintenance and growth.

$$f=0.0553\ W^{\frac{2}{3}}\ (1+3.805\ g).$$

**(After C.F. Winchester, Energy requirement for beef calves for maintenance and growth, *U.S Deptt. Agr. Tech. Bull. 1071*, 1953).**

Where, $f$=TDN in lbs.
$W$=Body wt. in lbs.
$g$=Daily gain in lbs.

The expression of $0.0553\ W^{\frac{2}{3}}$ denotes maintenance requirement where the expression $(1+0.805\ g)$, denotes growth requirement at specific rate of gain expected or desired. Table of requirements showing maintenance requirement at different body weights and combined growth and maintenance requirement at varying rate of daily gain (1/2 to 2 lb. or 0.23 to 0.91 kg) has been provided, Garrett and associates developted formula of requirement of energy for growth:

$$TDN = 0.36\ W^{\frac{3}{4}}(1+0.57\ g)$$

$$DE = 76\ W^{\frac{3}{4}}(1+0.58\ g)$$

$$ME = 62\ W^{\frac{3}{4}}(1+0.60\ g)$$

$$NE = 35\ W^{\frac{3}{4}}(1+0.45\ g)$$

**(Garret, Meyer and Lofgreen. The comparative energy requirement of sheep and cattle for maintenance and gain, *J. Animal Science*, 18 : 547, 1959).**

2. BY THE FACTORIAL METHOD

The principle of energy requirement for growth is that the energy of the tissue formed is determined first and the value of basal metabolism increased by an activity factor is added to it. Thus the requirement of energy is determined at any given period by the expected rate of gain and the average body weight during the period in question. Data from slaughter experiment in respect of fat and protein provides the figure for computing the calories for expected rate of gain while the body weight data provide the basis for arriving at the required energy for basal metabolism. An activity increment over the energy required for basal metabolism has to be considered. The data of basal metabolism and activity factor is to cover the maintenance requirement. Thus the sum of calories of basal metabolism+activity increment factor+growth tissue formed is the estimated energy requirement expressed as net energy which in turn can be converted to ME or DE or TDN by the appropriate factors.

In practice, however, all results of energy requirement found out by the factorial method suffer from certain uncertainties (e.g., gain in terms of fat and protein may vary according to genetic make up and nutritional regime of the experimental animals) which, therefore, should be supported by tests in feeding trial before putting in into practice.

**B. Protein requirement for growth**

Protein plays a vital role in growth as well as in production and reproduction. As such, a comprehensive knowledge is desirable as to the requirement of protein for various physiological purposes.

Young calves require relatively larger proportion of protein for rapid growth. As the animals grow older, the amount of protein requirement is proportionately lower. This is primarily due to growth in the beginning of life being protein in nature followed by growth of tissues of less protein and more fat.

Therefore, the requirement of protein for growing animal will primarily depend on the size of the animal and the rate of new tissue formed i.e. the growth rate. However, it must be noted that usually the rate of growth is determined by increase in body weight but this suffers from the flaw that increase in body weight also includes skeletal growth, retention of water and deposition of fat. Fortunately the latter form of growth in a growing animal does not contribute to any great extent and the growth in new tissue formed is mostly protein in nature and for this purpose, in practice, the requirement of protein is given for any species or breed according to body weight. Requirements of protein in the feeding chart are based on careful experiments of established growth rate of different breeds within a species at different ages. The skeletal growth has also been determined and subtracting this skeletal growth from body weight gain, the synthesis of new tissues, protein in nature, can be estimated and the knowledge of such estimate helped to calculate the amount of protein required for the particular growth.

While calculating such requirements for different body weights, it should be noted that there are two opposite factors in operation. The metabolic body size increases as the animal gets older and, therefore, the maintenance requirement also increases with the increase in age. The other factor is that the growth rate continues to decrease after attainment of a particular age which is different in different species or different breeds within the same species and such growth rate completely ceases at adult stage. Quite likely, therefore, the requirement of protein is higher in very young animals per unit weight basis and the requirement continues to diminish as the animal becomes older until maintenance requirement is reached.

## 1. FACTORIAL METHOD

The amount of protein required for maintenance is determined first. The value thus obtained is added to the amount of protein required for growth (or say gain in weight) plus losses in metabolism.

The maintenance needs can be determined directly on the basis of endogenous urinary nitrogen or calculated from the basal energy metabolism and later corrected for metabolic faecal nitrogen losses. The amount required for the growth tissue formed can be estimated from the slaughter data as shown by Blaxter and Mitchell (1948).

*Example*: A calf weighs 70 kg and consumes 2 kg dry matter per day. Its EUN and MFN would be appoximately 3.5 g and 7.0 gm respectively. The slaughter tests reveal that the amount of nitrogen deposited in the tissue will be 16 gm per day for a calf gaining at the rate of 0.5 kg per day.

Theoretically, the sum of nitrogen excreted as EUN and MFN plus the amount of nitrogen deposited in the body as growth tissue should be supplied in the diet for proper protein nutrition. Thus $3.5+7.0+16.0=26.5$ gm nitrogen $\times 6.25=166$ gm protein should be supplied in the diet. The biological values of protein for body building activity in growing animals is taken for only 65% as against 70% in adults in consideration of rumen function which is not fully developed in a growing animal and that there is greater loss of feed nitrogen in urine. Thus the amount of true digestible protein will be $100/65\times 166=255$ gm. As the feeding standards Table show the requirement of protein in terms of apparent digestible protein say, DCP, the value of MFN in terms of protein should be deducted from the figure of true digestible protein. Therefore, $255—(6.25\times 7)=211$ gm or 0.21 kg is the minimum requirement of DCP for a calf weighing 70 kg and growing @ 0.5 kg per day.

## 2. NITROGEN BALANCE METHOD FOR ESTIMATING OF PROTEIN FOR GROWTH

The protein requirement may also be determined by nitrogen balance studies and is said to be an exact measure of actual requirement of protein. In this method, calves are raised on equal amounts of dry matter and on isocaloric rations which contain different levels of protein and the minimum intake of protein which provides maximum retention is taken as the estimate of requirement. However, in such studies, the animals must be making satisfactory rate of growth during the study. Large number of animals should be taken for the study over an extended period to offset animal variation, difference in body weight and nitrogen balances Recommendations for practice, however, should be set at a higher level to cover individual variation and difference in biological value of the ration.

3. FEEDING TRIALS FOR ESTIMATING PROTEIN NEED FOR GROWTH

In this method, the rations containing different levels of protein are fed to determine the minimum level required to give the maximum rate of growth. The nature of growth thus obtained may be further tested by slaughter tests for assessing the integrity of the nitrogenous tissues.

**Protein requirement for reproduction**

Adequate provisions must be made for the growth of the foetus as well as for the mother for onset and continuance of good milk flow on calving. This extra provision has to be given in addition to maintenance requirement during last third period of pregnancy. Failure of adequate provision will undernourish the dam and the calf is born weak and undersized. Milk yield will be low and poor in vitamin content.

The requirement for gestation as proposed by Sen & Roy is 0.14 kg DCP and 0.7 kg TDN in addition to maintenance requirement and their recommendations do not refer to the size of the cow. Morrison feeding standard recommended such requirement with reference to size of the cow as shown below:

| | | DCP | TDN |
|---|---|---|---|
| Small cow | — | 0.50-0.55 lb. | 5.5 lb. |
| 1000 lb cow | — | 0.55-0.60 lb. | 5.5-6.0 lb. |
| Large cow | — | 0.65-0.70 lb. | 6.5-7.0 lb. |

**Energy requirement for reproduction**

The energy requirement for reproduction consists of the energy stored in the new tissue formed plus the energy expended in the process. During the last three months of the gestation, the growth of the foetus is very rapid. Thus in practice, most pregnant animals must be given a sufficient energy allowance to enable them to gain some weight during the period as a whole, with special attention given to the last quarter when the specific needs are felt. The aim should be to have the animals in good flesh at parturition without being too fat.

The amount of energy stored in the foetus and its membrane, had been calculated to range from 235 kcal in the 7th month to 940 kcal in the 9th month pregnancy. At the same time, the BMR of the dam is also increased during this period. Towards the end of the gestation period, the total energy requirement for maintaining the dam as well as for the normal growth of the foetus has been calculated to be 21 Mcal of ME. In other words, an extra quantity of 10 Mcal of ME will have to be provided (over maintenance requirement) for pregnancy needs. The recommendation of Sen and Roy to provide 0.7 kg TDN to meet the energy requirement during the last quarter for pregnancy is too low when we calculate the value on the basis that *1 kg TDN supplies 3.6 Mcal of ME.*

**Energy requirement for lactation**

The energy standard for lactation may be derived either by using formulae or by factorial method. The formula is based on the statistical interrelationships between milk constituents to calculate the gross energy content from the percentage of a single constituent since as fat (F) i.e.

$$\text{kcal per kg milk} = 304.8 + 114.1 \times F$$

Assuming fat content of a sample of milk 4.5%, the gross energy content of 1 kg of milk will thus be equivalent to $304.8 + (114.1 \times 4.5) = 818.25$ kcal.

A more recent formula of Cornell University workers may also be cited here where it incorporates solids not fat also.

$$\text{kcal per kg milk} = 92.25\ F + 49.15\ SNF - 56.40$$

For a milk having a fat percentage of 4.5 and an SNF of 8.75 per cent, this formula gives a value of 788.68 kcal per kg of milk.

Apart from formula, energy liberated per kg of milk may also be derived by two other methods. The gross energy is determined either by bomb calorimetry or by a detailed chemical analysis; the amounts of protein, fat and carbohydrate which are then multiplied by their individual calorific values.

The efficiency of conversion of feed ME into energy content of milk is 70%; so that for providing sufficient energy the calorific value of milk is multiplied by $100 \div 70 = 1.43$. For producing 1 kg of 4.5% fat corrected milk, the requirement thus becomes 788.68 (value obtained by applying Cornell University formula as above) multiplied by 1.43 which becomes 1127.8 kcal or 1.13 Mcal. Indian workers found the average value to be 1.23 Mcal of ME. It will thus be seen that a safety margin of about 10% is allowed for practical feeding schedules. The values that are now mostly considered is that of feeding standards by Sen and Roy where the TDN values corresponding to ME figures are also given for various fat percentages of milk per kg. It may be mentioned that this allowance for milk production is to be added to the maintenance requirement in order to calculate the total need of a lactating animal.

**Protein requirement for lactation**

Extensive studies have been made to determine the amount of protein required for milk production. Milk is rich in protein.

It is obvious, therefore, that the animal must be provided with sufficient quantity, in addition to maintenance requirement, in order to able to cope with the continuous drain of protein from its body. It has been shown that the lactating animal can efficiently convert food protein into milk protein.

Results of various studies have shown that provision of 1.25 times as much protein as secreted in the milk will be sufficient for milk production. This allowance should be given in addition to maintenance requirement. This extra provision of protein for milk production will, therefore, depend on the amount of mlik produced. However, experiments have also shown that cows of very good milk yield may yield somewhat more milk and fat when the protein allowance is greater than the above but provision of more than 1.50 to 1.60 times greater amount of protein than secreted in the milk has not been found to increase the milk yield. Although protein requirement for milk produced, unlike energy requirement is not dependent theoretically on the fat percentage of milk, but for practical feeding purposes, the amount of protein being supplied to animals yielding higher fat content should be increased slightly so as to maintain the proper nutritive ratio for the maximum utilization of all the nutrients in the diet. Accordingly NRC recommendation furnishes 135 to 145 per cent protein of that secreted in the milk in addition to maintenance requirement. The committee report suggests that although lower intakes than the above have resulted in excellent production in several experiments, they may not yield as much under many conditions. Liberal allowances therefore, are justified as general recommendation. From economical stand point, the extra cost of high protein feeds may sometimes offset the benefit achieved through such liberal allowance.

**Protein requirement of work**

Increased muscular activity results in nutrients being oxidized in the system. All the organic constituents of food are capable of being oxidized and utilized as energy sources. As long as supply is adequate, the working animal is to draw sources of carbohydrates and fat to meet the energy need. If the supply is inadequate, body fat will be drawn upon first and in the last stage, the protein tissues may be broken down to furnish energy for work as it is now accepted that the protein is not the normal fuel of muscular work and that no protein catabolism or extra wear and tear of tissues occurs during work. Therefore, theoretically no extra protein is required to be supplied as long as the ration provides sufficient carbohydrate and fat for extra energy required for work. From the stand point of an efficient ration for work, however, other considerations appear more important than the question as to whether the protein requirement is actually increased during work or not. During hard work, the need for energy may be almost doubled and unless the protein content of the ration is simultaneously increased, the nutritive ratio becomes wide. As a result efficiency of energy utilization will be poorer since digestibility will be depressed by wide ratio and metabolic heat losses will also be increased. Naturally, therefore an efficient ration in all respects will demand inclusion of additional protein along with energy for maintaining the proper nutritive ratio (as in lactating animals having different fat content mentioned earlier) for increased muscular activity although the additional protein may not be specifically required for muscular activity.

Quantitative requirement of the working animals in respect of protein at different body weights is shown in Tabular form under the heading "*Feeding Standards for Cattle*".

**Protein requirement of bulls**

Comparatively little studies have been made to work out the requirement of bulls in service. A bull requires more nutrients to maintain body weight than a dry cow of comparable body weights. For a bull in service, there should be adequate provision of protein which is dependent on the number of service per week. Assuming that number of services is 4 in a week, the requirement of protein of a bull may be calculated at about 40% more DCP than comparable body weights of a dry cow.

# 23

# NUTRITIONAL AND METABOLIC DISORDERS OF LIVESTOCK

Nutritional deficiency diseases may be brought about by (1) too little feed, (2) diets that are too low in one or more nutrients, and (3) imbalance of nutrients.

Metabolic disease on the other hand is a disturbance of the internal homeostasis of the body, brought about by an abnormal change in the rate of one or more critical metabolic processes. This definition unites two important concepts. Firstly, metabolic disease involves an abnormal change in the internal environment of the body and secondly, this change must be brought about by an alteration in the dynamic equilibrium of metabolism.

Unfortunately, several nutritional and metabolic disorders frequently occur. Accordingly, successful animal feeders must be prepared to cope with these problems. This chapter is devoted to a brief discussion of some of the major metabolic and nutritional disorders of common livestock.

## Milk fever

*Synonyms*

Parturient paresis, Hypocalcaemia

*Species affected*

Cattle, Sheep, Goat (occasionally)

*Cause*

Low blood calcium and phosphorus with an increase in magnesium concentration. Deficiency or too much calcium in the ration can cause this condition. In milking cows, the Ca : P ratio should not exceed 2 : 1.

**Table 156**

**Blood serum concentration of cows in various metabolic states**

| State | Blood Serum, mg/100 ml | | |
|---|---|---|---|
| | Calcium | Phosphorus | Magnesium |
| Normal | 9.4 | 4.6 | 1.7 |
| Normal at parturition | 7.7±0.9 | 3.9 | 3.0±0.5 |
| Milk fever | | | |
| Stage 1 | 6.2±1.3 | 2.4±1.4 | 3.2±0.7 |
| Stage 2 | 5.5±1.3 | 1.8±1.2 | 3.1±0.8 |
| Stage 3 | 4,6±1.1 | 1.6±1.0 | 3.3±0.8 |

*Symptoms*

1. Commonly occurs in high producing cows soon after calving. Rarely occurs at first calving.
2. Less of appetite is the first symptom.
3. Constipation and general depression followed by nervousness and finally collapse.
4. Head is usually turned back.

*Treatment*

Injection of a calcium salt in the form of $CaCl_2$, Ca lactate, Ca gluconate or other Ca salts to elevate blood serum Ca above the concentration of the 5 or 6 mg/ml that is associated with the onset of tetany.

*Prevention*

1. *Calcium-phosphorus ratio and amounts.* Approximately a 2.3 : 1 Ca : P ratio. Feed a ration that contains 0.5-0.7 per cent Ca and 0.3-0.4 per cent P.
2. *Calcium shock treatment.* 10-14 days before calving, feed a Ca-deficient ration with a Ca : P ratio 1 : 2. This activates the cow's calcium-mobilising mechanism for drawing calcium from the bones, with the result that it is functioning before calving and milk fever is avoided.
3. *High Vitamin D.* This consists in feeding 20 million units of vitamin D/cow/day starting about five days before calving and continuing through the first day post-partum, with a maximum dosage period of seven days.

*Remarks*

Contrary to the common name, milk fever, body temperature is not elevated. In fact, a decrease in body temperature is very common.

## Grass tetany

*Synonyms*

Grass staggers, Hypomagnesaemic tetany.

*Species affected*

Cattle, Sheep.

*Cause*

Magnesium deficiency. The total Mg. in the body of an adult cow is approximately 200 g, 70 per cent of which is in the skeleton where it is relatively unavailable, about 29 per cent is in the soft tissue of the body, and only 1 per cent circulates in the extracellular fluids which is equivalent to 2 gm in a normal cow. Grass tetany is liable to occur if concentration in the blood plasma drops from the normal of 2.5 mg/100 ml to less than 1 mg/100.

*Symptoms*

Generally occurs during the first two weeks of pasture season. Nervousness, twitching of muscles (usually of head and neck), head held high, accelerated respiration, high temperature, gnashing of the teeth and abundant salivation and finally death.

*Treatment*

Intravenous injection of a solution of calcium and magnesium salt by a veterinarian, keep animals quiet after treatment.

*Prevention*

A salt lick of 10 parts each of magnesium sulphate and calcium disphosphate with 80 parts of salt will aid in prevention. Also, a mixture of two parts magnesium oxide to one part salt as the only source of salt is effective.

*Remarks*

Affected animals show low blood magnesium, often low serum calcium. Treated cattle may be aggresive on arising; so be careful!

## Ketosis

*Synonyms*

In cattle the disease is known as: (a) *acetonemia*, (b) *cow fever*, (c) *post-parturient dyspepsis*, (d) *hypoglycemia ketosis*. In sheep it has been called (i) *lambing sickness*, (ii) *twin lamb disease*, (iii) *sleepy sickness*, (iv) *pregnancy disease*, (v) *pregnancy toxaemia.*

*Species affected*

Cattle, sheep and goat.

*Cause*

It results from an input/output imbalance in emergency metabolism, and is liable to occur when energy requirements reach a peak, as for example in late pregnancy in sheep or in full

**Table 157**

**Blood changes in Clinical Ketosis**

| Component | Normal | Ketosis |
|---|---|---|
| | ...... mg/100 ml ...... | |
| Blood | | |
| Glucose | 52 | 28 |
| Ketones (total) | 3 | 41 |
| Plasma | | |
| Free fatty acids | 3 | 33 |
| Triglycerides | 14 | 8 |
| Free cholesterol | 29 | 15 |
| Cholesterol esters | 226 | 150 |
| Phospholipids | 174 | 82 |

**Source :** Digestive Physiology & Nutrition of Ruminants, Vol. 2 by D. C. Church. O & B Books Inc. Coravallis, the U.S.A.

lactation in cows. In both the cases the need for glucose is especially high. The entire glucose needs of milk production and of the developing foetus have to be synthesised in the liver. Should the pathways of gluconeogenesis become overloaded then the whole system of energy metabolism is in jeopardy and liable to breakdown, leading to Ketosis.

*Symptoms*

Affected cows will show loss of appetite, reduced rumen activity, dullness, decrease in milk production with high fat content, production of a peculiar sweetish chloroform like odour of acetone that may be present in the milk and urine.

In ewes and goats, symptoms include grinding of teeth, dullness, weakness, frequent urination and trembling when exercised—with the final stage being complete collapse, followed by death in 90 per cent of the cases.

*Treatment*

Cattle: 250-500 gm. of either propylene glycol or sodium propionate daily, with the dose divided into two doses for treatment for 5 to 10 days. Add a dose to the grain if a cow is eating, otherwise give it as a drench. Intravenous injection of glucose (500 ml of 50 per cent glucose solution) is a rapid way of raising the blood sugar level.

Sheep and goat: 100 cc of propylene glycol may be given orally twice daily.

*Prevention*

1. Care must be taken to prevent excessive fattiness in cows at calving.
2. After calving the amount of concentrates may be increased along with good quality roughages.
3. In problem herds, feeding 50 cc of propylene glycol or sodium propionate daily may be helpful.

*Remarks*

Cows having ketosis in one lactation are more prone to this disorder in later lactations.

## Bloat

*Species affected*

Ali ruminants.

*Cause*

When animals are fed excessive amounts of legume forages, frothy bloat develops due to the interaction of soluble forage proteins, rumen microbes and the animal itself. In such conditions the developed gases comprising $CO_2$ and methane are not eliminated. Not all legumes present an important bloat problem for example trefoils, sweet clovers, *kudju*, peas, soybeans, crimson clover usually are not bloat producing forages. Recently it has also been noted that when ruminants are fed high concentrate rations, there is an increase of slime producing bacteria in rumen and the slime traps fermentation gas and produces bloat.

*Symptoms*

First observed as distention of the rumen on the left side in front of the hipbone. This is followed by distension of the right side, protrusion of the anus, respiratory distress, cyanosis of the tongue, struggling and death if not cured.

*Treatment*

Mild cases may be home treated by: (i) keeping the animal on its feet and moving, and (ii) drenching cattle with (a) 500 to 1000 ml mineral oil or (b) 25 to 50 ml of poloxalene.

Severe cases of bloat should be treated by a veterinarian. Puncturing of the rumen should be the last resort.

*Prevention*

The incidence is lessened by:—

1. Avoiding feeding of excessive legume forages.
2. Feeding dry forage along with green forage.
3. Avoiding a rapid fill from an empty start.
4. Keeping salt and water conveniently accessible at all times.

*Remarks*

Bloat conditions are relatively unknown in wild ruminants or in domestic animals on the range. The occurrence is likely to be the result of man's interference through mismanagement of the normal balance between plant and animal.

**Parakeratosis**

*Synonym*

*Greasy skin disease.*

*Species affected*

Swine.

*Cause*

(1) High Ca level in the diet, above 0.8 per cent and (2) low zinc level in the diet.

*Symptoms*

Reduce appetite and growth, diarrhoea and vomiting. It affects pigs of one to five months old.

*Treatment*

Add about 200 gms of zinc carbonate or about 450 gms of zinc sulphate heptahydrate per ton of feed.

*Remarks*

## Goiter

*Synonyms*

*Big neck, iodine deficiency.*

*Species affected*

All farm animals including man.

*Cause*

A failure of the body to obtain sufficient iodine from which the thyroid gland can form thyroxine.

*Symptoms*

Goiter is the most characteristic symptom in human, calves, lambs and kids. There may be reproductive failures and weak offsprings that fail to survive. Pigs may be born hairless and show edema of shoulders and neck.

*Prevention*

In iodine deficient areas, feed iodized salt (containing 0.01% potassium iodide) to all form animals throughout the year.

## Osteomalacia

*Species affected*

All species

*Cause*

1. Inadequate phosphorus or calcium
2. Lack of vitamin D in confined animals
3. Incorrect ratio of calcium to phosphorus

*Symptoms*

Phosphorus deficiency symptoms are depraved appetite (gnawing on bones, wood, or other objects, or eating dirt); lack of appetite, stiffness of joints, failure to breed regularly, decreased milk production and an emaciated look.

Calcium deficiency symptoms are fragile bones, reproductive failures and lowered lactations.

Mostly matured animals are affected during pregnancy and lactation. Low birth weight in lambs is associated with inadequate transfer of mineral across the placenta.

*Treatment*

1. Sufficient natural feeds that contain sufficient quantities of calcium and phosphorus.
2. Feed a special mineral supplement. If this disease is far advanced, treatment will not be successful.

***Prevention***

1. Feed balanced rations, and allow animals free access to a suitable phosphorus and calcium supplement.
2. Increase the calcium and phosphorus content of feed through fertilizing the soils.
3. Vitamin D therapy may be of some assistance.

## White muscle disease

***Synonyms***

Muscular dystrophy in sheep, stiff lamb disease.

***Species affected***

Calves and lambs.

***Cause***

1. Selenium and vitamin E deficiency; it may be lack of availability of vitamin E or the presence of any inhibitor.
2. Mouldy feeds increase incidence.

***Symptoms***

Calves stand or lie with protruded tongue, fighting for breath against a severe edema. It seems that more calves than lambs develop foetal heart damage. Affected calves show pathological lesions similar to those of "stiff lambs" namely whitish areas in the heart and other muscles. Affects calves from birth to three months of age.

***Treatment***

Injection of selenium and tocopherol (Vit. E). Confine affected calves or lambs to a stall and give plenty of rest.

***Prevention***

Feed 500 gms of linseed meal per cow during last two months of pregnancy as it contains high selenium. Commercial Vitamin E may be incorporated to the ration of the new born animals according to direction.

## Acidosis

***Synonyms***

Lactic-acidosis.

***Species affected***

Cattle, sheep.

***Cause***

Acidosis is caused by an increase in lactic acid producing bacteria and the rapid production of lactic acid. It commonly occurs when there is a sudden shift from a high roughage to a high concentrate ration. However, cattle maintained on high energy rations may be in a marginal state of acidosis due to the formation of lactic acid by the rumen flora. Thus ingredient changes, poor mixing of grain in the ration, or faulty feeding can produce acute acidosis.

*Symptoms*

Marginal acidosis is characterised by poor performance and inconsistent feed ingestion. If ingredient changes or erratic feeding persists, acute acidosis may result, creating laminitis and eventually "ski shoe" cattle. In severe cases, the rumen becomes immobilised, followed by increased pulse and respiration rate, variable rectal temperature, sunken eyes, loss of dermal elasticity (dehydration), staggering, coma and death.

*Treatment*

(1) Removal of rumen contents and replacement by contents of an animal on a normal ration; (2) feeding a high level of an antibiotic to suppress lactic acid producing bacteria; (3) drenching (or intravenous injection) with a solution of sodium bicarbonate to restore the acid-base balance; (4) daily intra-muscular administration of antihistamines and cortical steroids for each of several days to help prevent intoxication and laminitis.

*Prevention*

Prevention consists in avoiding erratic feeding and abrupt ration changes.

## Nitrate poisoning

*Synonyms*

Oat hay poisoning, cornstalk poisoning.

*Species affected*

Primarily cattle, buffalo, sheep, horses. Ruminants are most susceptible because of the conversion of nitrates to nitrites in the rumen.

*Cause*

Forages (vegetative part) of most grain crops namely oats, wheat, jowar, barley, rye, maize, especially (1) when under stress such as drought, insufficient sunlight, or after spraying with weed killer (herbicide); or (2) following heavy nitrate fertilisation of soils (commercial, green manure crop, barnyard manure). Some nitrate may be formed after forage is stacked. Inorganic nitrate or nitrite salts or fertiliser left where animals have access to them, or where they may be mistaken for salt.

*Symptoms*

Accelerated respiration and pulse rate; diarrhoea; frequent urination, loss of appetite; general weakness; trembling; staggering gait; frothing from mouth; lowered milk production; abortion; blue colour of the mucous membrane, muzzle, and udder due to lack of oxygen in blood; death within four-and-a-half to nine hours after consuming nitrates. Blood from affected cows will look brown instead of the normal red colour. Nitrates oxidise ferrous haemoglobin (oxyhaemoglobin) to ferric haemoglobin, (methaemoglobin) which is not an efficient oxygen transporter. The animal essentially suffocates for lack of oxygen to tissues. When three-fourths of the oxyhaemoglobin is converted to methaemoglobin, the animal will die.

*Treatment*

A 4 per cent solution of methylene blue (in a 5 per cent glucose or a 1.8 per cent sodium sulphate solution) administered by a veterinarian intravenously at the rate of 100cc/500 kg liveweight.

*Prevention*

More than 0.9 per cent nitrate (dry basis) may be considered as potentially toxic in feed, which should be analysed when in question. Nitrate poisoning may be reduced by: (1) feeding high levels of grains and other high energy feeds (molasses) and vitamin A, (2) limiting the amount of high nitrate-feeds, (3) ensiling forages which are high in nitrates (fermentation reduces some nitrates to gas).

*Remarks*

Nitrate form of nitrogen does not appear to cause the actual toxicity. During digestion, the nitrate is reduced to nitrite, a far more toxic form (10 to 15 times more toxic than nitrates). In cows and sheep, this conversion takes place in the rumen, in a horse it is in the caecum. A lethal dose varies with: (1) nutritional state, size and type of animal; and (2) the consumption of feed other than nitrate containing material. Methods of reporting nitrates (dry basis) in rations in relation to death losses follow:

| | Potentially lethal levels | |
|---|---|---|
| | (%) | (ppm) |
| Nitrate ($NO_3$) ... ... | over 0.9 | 9,000 |
| Nitrate nitrogen ($NO_3N$) ... | over 0.21 | 2,100 |
| Potassium nitrate ($KNO_3$) ... | over 1.5 | 15,000 |

**Table 158**

Major nutritional deficiency symptoms.

| Nutrient | Clinical symptoms[a] |
|---|---|
| Protein | Kwashiorkor or with low energy, marasmus, black hair turns red and is brittle (H); poor productivity, low fertility, birth of underweight young with poor livability, poor milk production, low blood albumin and/or blood urea, unkempt appearance. |
| Lysine | White barring of primary wing feathers (T). |
| Other amino acids | No specific symptoms have been observed in farm animals. |
| Essential fatty acids | Poor growth (YC, YS, YCh), skin lesions (YC, YS). |
| Carbohydrates | No specific symptoms unless associated with low energy intake. |
| Energy | Low productivity, loss of body weight, stillborn young, poor or nil milk production, poor fertility. Usually associated with deficiencies of other nutrients such as protein and minerals such as P. |
| Water soluble vitamins | |
| Thiamin | Beriberi, edema, heart failure (H); polynuritis (YCh); opistothonus, anorexia, high blood pyruvic acid; blindness (C) |
| Riboflavin | Facial dermatitis, insomnia, irritability (H); lesions of the eye, anorexia, vomiting, birth of weak or stillborn young (S); curled-toe paralysis (YCh); diarrhea, loss of hair (YC, YSh). |
| Niacin | Pellegra (H); diarrhea, vomiting, dermatitis around the eye (YCh), poor growth. |
| Pyridoxine | Convulsions, anorexia, poor growth, brown exudate around eyes (YS); abnormal feathering (YCh). |
| Pantothenic acid | Poor growth, graying of hair in some species; dermatitis, embryonic death (YCh); loss of hair, enteritis, goose-stepping, incoordination in walking (YS). |
| Biotin | Dermatitis, perosis (YCh, YT). |
| Choline | Perosis, fatty liver (YCh, YT); abnormal gait, reproductive failure in females, hemorrhagic kidneys, fatty liver (S). |
| Folacin | Anemia, gastrointestinal disturbances, impaired coordination (H); anemia in other species. |
| Cobalamin | Anemia, poor feathering, perosis (YCh); low hatchability, fatty livers, enlarged hearts (Ch, T); rough hair coats, incoordinated hind leg movements, anemia, abortion, other reproductive problems (S). |
| Vitamin C | No problems in domestic animals; scurvey (H). |
| Fat-soluble vitamins | |
| Vitamin A | Xeropthalmia, night blindness, permanent blindness (all species); diarrhea, convulsions, high cerebrospinal fluid pressures (Y); incoordination, reproductive failure in males, abortion or birth of weak or dead young (C). |

Table 158 (*Contd.*)

| | |
|---|---|
| Vitamin D | Rickets in young, osteomalacia in adults, lameness and sore joints, crooked legs, spontaneous fractures of long bones (Y); negative mineral balance, low bone ash (A). |
| Vitamin E | Nutritional muscular dystrophy (Y), fetal reabsorption, sterility, testicular atrophy (C, CH, T), liver necrosis (YS), fragile red blood cells (YS, YSh); encephalomalacia, exudative diathesis (YCh). |
| Vitamin K | Slow blood clotting; subcutaneous hemorrhages. |
| Macrominerals | |
| Calcium | Rickets, osteoporosis, poor growth; muscle cramps, convulsions (H). |
| Phosphorus | Rickets (Y), osteoporosis (A), anorexia, pica, low fertility. |
| Magnesium | Anorexia, poor productivity, tetany; weak crooked legs (S). |
| Potassium | Muscular weakness, paralysis (H); abnormal electrocardiograms; unsteady gait, weakness, pica. |
| Sodium | Anorexia, muscle cramps, mental apathy (H); dehydrated appearance; craving for salt, weight loss. |
| Chlorine | Depressed growth. |
| Sulfur | Reduced gain or loss of weight (C, Sh), loss of wool (Sh). |
| Trace Minerals | |
| Chromium | Impaired ability to metabolize glucose. |
| Cobalt | Primarily ruminants; symptoms similar to cobalamin; emaciation, anemia, fatty degneration of the liver. |
| Copper | Anemia; when coupled with high Mo and/or sulfate, swayback or enzootic neonatal ataxia, loss of pigment in hair or wool (C, Sh); bone abnormalities, cardiovascular lesions, reduced egg production, reproductive failure. |
| Flourine | Excessive tooth decay (H). |
| Iron | Anemia and associated poor productivity; very common in young pigs. |
| Manganese | Lameness and shortening and bowing of the legs, enlarged joints (Y); perosis (YCh, T); reduced egg shell thickness (ACh, T); weakness, poor sense of balance; crooked calf disease (C); poor fertility (C). |
| Molybdenum | Reduced growth rates (not common). |
| Nickel | Prenatal mortality, unthriftiness, decreased growth rate (YCh, T, YS), poor N retention (YSh). |
| Selenium | Nutritional muscular dystrophy (Y), exudative diathesis (YCh, T); liver necrosis (YS); heart failure (YC); retained placenta (AC). |
| Zinc | Poor growth, anorexia, parakeratotic lesions on head, neck, belly and legs (C, Sh, S); perosis, abnormal feathering (YCh, T); poor testicular development, slow wound healing (H, other species). |

'Y, young; A, adults; H, humans; C, cattle; Ch, chickens; S, swine; Sh, sheep; T, turkeys.

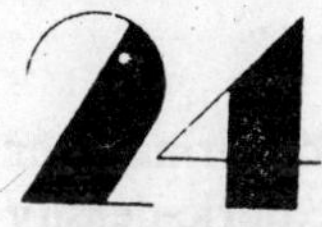

# LABORATORY ANIMAL DIETS

Extensive nutrition research with most common laboratory animals plus fish, poultry, swine, sheep, goats, horse and cattle has produced diets capable of adequately nourishing these animals during growth, gestation, lactation, work, maintenance and most other conditions of stress.

Commercial diets, where applicable, provide the most uniform economical nutrition. Some variation will occur since processing methods vary and ingredients from the same agricultural area vary from year to year depending on the crop conditions, processing changes and storage conditions. Working ingredient specifications, however, minimise variation; thus, nutrition intake can be almost standardized.

## A. Types of Diets

Many kinds of diets ranging from mixtures of almost pure chemical nutrients to combinations of natural ingredients and by-products are available. These extremes and combinations in between have been fed successfully to many species of animals.

### 1. *Pure Chemical Nutrient Diets*

Pure chemical nutrient diets are mixtures of almost pure vitamins, minerals, fatty acids, carbohydrates and amino acids mixed togther and supplied with deionized or distilled water. These are expensive and generally used under highly controlled conditions and usually for short periods.

### 2. *Purified Diets*

Purified diets consist of mixtures of sources of ingredients that are relatively constant and generally include chemically pure salts and vitamins, sucrose, fats with known compositions, and proteins such as casein and refined soyabean proteins with known amino acid compositions. Purified diets are less expensive than pure chemical diets and can generally be used for most nutrition studies. These diets are useful since specific nutrients can be decreased in the basic diet and then added back in graded levels and the comparative levels fed simultaneously with the specific nutrient as the major variable.

### 3. *Commerical Diets*

Commercial diets designed and tested for their ability to provide the precise nutrients needed by specific animal species are available. These include diets for various ages and conditions within some species. Some of these diets have included a relatively unchanging formula through the years, although slight changes in nutrient content have occurred based on commerical ingredient changes due to processing, time of year and other incompletely controlled factors.

4. *Therapeutic-type Diets*

Several therapeutic-type diets are available for stress conditions encountered normally or intentionally produced and include low-sodium diets for cardiac control, low caloric-density diets, and some with anorexigens for obesity control. Others contain low levels of protein to help prevent kidney nitrogen overload in specific circumstances.

## B. Dietary Additives

In addition to the 45 plus nutrients needed by animals, diets contain many additives and naturally occurring materials and are present in the feed as a result of ingredient composition or production, processing, storage or packaging. Each additive has a purpose. Some enhance nutrient availability, protect against disease, add flavour and aroma, enhance colour and retard oxidation.

In general antioxidants help protect against the oxidation of fats in the diet and in the animal's body and enable fats to perform their biological role in the body. Oxidation of double-bond fatty acids produces short-chain fatty acids and aldehydes. These peroxides are powerful oxidising agents and tend to destroy vitamins A, D, E, and K in the diet. Natural antioxidants, including tocopherols, are widely distributed in vegetable oils. Commercial antioxidants include BHT (butyl hydroxytoluene), BHA (butyl hydroxyanisole), NDGA (nordihydro guaiaretic acid) santoquin, ascorbic acid, gallic acid and propyl gallate.

Colour additives are used by food manufacturers to maintain uniform appearance with changing ingredient quality and present an attractive product appearance to the food purchaser. *Animals are influenced little by colour, since most are colourblind.*

Nitrates and nitrites are permitted at a level of 200 ppm in processed feeds and help maintain bright colour which also prevent growth of undersirable toxin producing orgnaisms. If these are added at higher level there will be conversion of nitrate to nitrites which will prevent the iron of haemoglobin carrying normal quantities of oxygen.

Flavouring agents help maintain feed acceptability, particularly for animals taught to be accustomed to a variety of feeds.

Nonnutrient sweeteners, anticaking materials, acidity and alkalinity agents, bacteriostats and fungistats are added to animal diets.

## C. Feeding Methods

The ways in which diets are fed may be a critical factor when feed intake and weight gains or obesity are considered. Several feeding methods are discussed below :

1. *Ad Libitum vs Restricted Feeding*

When the feed intake of animal is restricted by any method, the process is called *controlled feeding*, while unrestricted feed intake is termed *ad libitum* feeding. Both methods of feeding have advantages for some animals. *Ad libitum*-fed animals tend to fluctuate in their daily feed intake and are influenced by general environmental variation, diet acceptability, and changing physiological needs. Restricted or controlled feeding may be necessary for some studies, such as livability. On the other hand the evaluation of *ad libitum* feed consumption may be an important factor since feed intake is related to activity, obesity, digestibility and environment. Generally where a specific dietary ingredient or nutrient is being compared at various levels, it is necessary to use controlled feeding to restrict variation to that single factor and not to the varying intake of total feed. When the controlled intake of two or more animals is governed by the consumption of the animal eating the least, the method is termed *equalized paired feeding*. This usually places most stress on the superior diet, which produces most gains and subsequently a greater demand on nutrients for maintenance. Controlled feed intake (animals are fed on nutritionally adequate diets but slightly, less than the daily ration) is particularly useful in production units with some species such as cattle, poultry, hogs and dogs that tend to overeat as adults.

2. *Controlling Feed Intake*

The method of offering feed influences feed intake; most species prefer moist feed more than extremely dry feed, particularly if dust is present. Adding controlled levels of moisture is one way of increasing food intake in most domestic animals and some laboratory animals. With most dry diets, the addition of one part by weight of water to two parts by weight of dog food will increase food consumption by approximately 20%. The addition of 20% of the diet as meat will increase total nutrient intake by another 20%. These methods are useful when increasing nutrient intake during the stress of lactation and hard physical work.

Feed intake outside these parameters can be controlled by offering measured quantities of food or placing predetermined portions in the digestive tract.

3. *Single vs Pair or Group Feeding*

Some animals, such as puppies, will consume about 20% less feed when housed alone than when housed with a littermate; when one starts to eat, the other usually joins. With older dogs, a tendency may develop for one dog to guard the food container and restrict the pen-mate's feed consumption. This can be alleviated by providing an extra feeder out of guard distance. Group feeding does not provide individual feed consumption data. Many factors influence feed intake, such as, density, composition, moisture, texture, processing. It is also influenced by the animal's condition, including the status of the gums, teeth, digestive tract, hormone levels, state of activity, production, metabolic age.

## TABLE—A*

### Housing and environment

| SPECIES (weight) | | SPACE per ANIMAL: Single floor area | Minimal height | Group or loose housing | TEMPERATURE °C: Room/Cage | Pen/free ranging | R.H % | Ventilation changes/hr | B. T. U. Animal/hr |
|---|---|---|---|---|---|---|---|---|---|
| MONKEY | < 7 Kg | 0.40 m² | 0.9 m | 2-3 m² | 22-25 | 18-29 | 45-60 | 10-15 | 60-200 |
| (Macaque) | > 15 Kg | 0.75 m² | 1.2 m | perches | | | | | |
| CAT | | 0.28 m² | 0.76 m perch | 0.56 perches | 20-22 | 15-25 | 45-60 | 10-18 | 25-30 |
| RAT | < 150 g | 150 cm² | 18 cm | fem+litter | 20-25 | 15-29 | 50-55 | 10-20 | 40 |
| | > 150 g | 250 cm² | | 800 cm² | | | | | |
| CHICKEN | | | | | 65-70 | 12-27 | 45-70 | 5-15 | 30 |
| DOG | < 12 Kg | 0.75 m² | 0.8 m | 1.5 m² | 13-21 | 5-25 | 45-55 | 8-12 | 80-150 |
| | > 15 Kg | 1.20 m² | 0.9 m | 2.0 m² | | | | | |
| GERBIL | | 116 cm² | 15 cm | pair+litter 900 cm² | 15-24 | 0-30 | 40-50 | 8-10 | 4.0 |
| MOUSE | < 20 g | 65 cm² | 13 cm | fem+litter | 22-25 | 20-30 | 50-70 | 8-12 | 0.6 |
| | > 20 g | 100 cm² | 15 cm | 160 cm² | | | | | |
| GUINEA PIG | < 350 g | 300 cm² | | 500 cm² | 16-20 | 13-31 | 50-60 | 4-8 | 5.6 |
| | > 350 g | 650 cm² | | 800 cm² | | | | | |
| HAMSTER | | 100 cm² | fem+litter 18 cm | 900 cm² | 21-24 | 20-30 | 45-65 | 6-10 | 2.5 |
| RABBIT | < 4 Kg | 0.37 m² | 0.38 m | fem+litter | 16-20 | 10-28 shade | 40-50 | 10-20 | 30-40 |
| | > 4 Kg | 0.46 m² | | 0.93 m² | | | | | |

B. T. U. - British Thermal Unit

## TABLE — B*

### Parameters of reproduction in common laboratory aminals

| | Rat | Mouse | Syrian hamster | Cat | Gerbil | Rabbit | Guinea pig | Dog |
|---|---|---|---|---|---|---|---|---|
| **Male** | | | | | | | | |
| Age at pairing (weeks) | 10-11 | 6 | 6-8 | 7-9** | 10-12 | 6-9** | 3** | 10-12** |
| Duration of E.R.A.*(month) | 6-9 | 6-9 | 12-15 | 5-7+ | 12-18 | 3-6+ | 2.5-3+ | 5-7+ |
| **Female** | | | | | | | | |
| Age at pairing (weeks) | 10-11 | 6 | 6-8 | 7-8** | 10-12 | 6-7** | 3** | 12-14** |
| Duration of E.R.A.(months) | 6-9 | 9-12 | 9-12 | 5-8+ | 12-15 | 1-3+ | 1.5-2.5+ | 4-5+ |
| Type of estrous cycle | Polyestrous | Polyestrous | Polyestrous | Polyestrous | Polyestrcus | Polyestrcus | Polyestrous | Monoestrous |
| Length of estrous cycle (days) | 4-5 | 4-5 | 4 | 14-21 | 4-6 | No regular cycle | 13-18 | 21-28 |
| Breeding season | All year | All year | All year, with decrease Oct-Feb. | Jan-Oct. | All year | All year with decrease in summer and winter | All year | Biannual, usually spring and fall |
| Length of gestation (days) | 20-22 | 19-21 | 16-17 | 64 | 24-26 | 31 | 63 | 63 |
| Litter size at birth (mean) | 8 | 8 | 7 | 4 | 5 | 7 | 3 | 6 |
| (range) | 7-14 | 6-12 | 6-9 | 1-8 | 4-8 | 6-10 | 1-6 | 4-8 |
| Wt. of young at birth (g) | 5-6 | 1-3 | 2 | 95-140 | 3 | 30-70 | 85-90 | Variable |
| Weaning age (days) | 21 | 21 | 21 | 6-7@ | 21 | 6-8@ | 2-3@ | 6-8@ |
| Weaning wt (g) | 40-50 | 10-12 | 35-40 | 703-800 | 11-18 | 800-1500 | 180-240 | Variable |
| Return of estrous after parturition | Post-partum estrous, regular cycle at end of lactation | Post-partum estrous, regular cycle at end of lactation | Past-partum estrous, regular cycle end of lactation | 4th week of lactation | Post-partum estrous | 4th week of lactation | Post-partum estrous then regular cycle | Next breeding season |

*E. R. A. Economic Reproductive Ability
** = Months
@ = Weeks
+ = Years

TABLE — C*

**Heamatological and electrolyte values**

Mean values and ranges

| SPECIES | R B C x $10^6$/mm³ | Hb g/100ml | P C V ml% | Blood vol. ml/Kg | W B C x $10^3$/mm³ | Sodium mEq/l | Potassium mEq/l. | Inorganic phosphorus mg/100ml | Calcium mg/100ml |
|---|---|---|---|---|---|---|---|---|---|
| MONKEY | 5 | | | | | | | | |
| (M. fascicularis) | 4-6 | 10-12 | 35-43 | 55-75 | 5-10 | 146-152 | 4-5 | 5-5.4 | 9.5-10 |
| | 7.3 | 10.5 | 40.5 | | 17.0 | 151 | 4.8 | 6.3 | 10.7 |
| CAT | 5-10 | 8-15 | 24-45 | 45-75 | 5-20 | 147-156 | 4-6 | 4.5-8.1 | 5-13 |
| | 8.5 | 14.2 | 45.9 | | 9.8 | 147 | 6.2 | 7.9 | 11.5 |
| RAT | 6-10 | 11-17 | 40-50 | 50-65 | 5-13 | 140-156 | 5.4-7.0 | 3-11 | 5-14 |
| | 3.1 | 10.1 | 34.3 | | 19.7 | 155 | 5.3 | 7.0 | 16.8 |
| CHICKEN | 2-4 | 7-13 | 25-45 | 60-90 | 9-31 | 148-163 | 4.6-6.5 | 6.2-7.9 | 9-24 |
| | 6.8 | 17.0 | 53.6 | | 12.6 | 147 | 4.5 | 4.2 | 9.9 |
| DOG | 5.5-8.5 | 12-18 | 37-59 | 75-100 | 6-18 | 135-180 | 3.5-6.7 | 2-9 | 2.9-11.7 |
| | 8.5 | 15.0 | 47.0 | | 10.2 | — | 3.3-6.3 | 3.7-8.2 | 3.7-6.2 |
| GERBIL | 7-10 | 10-17 | 43-52 | 60-85 | 7-22 | | | | |
| | 6.5 | 13.5 | 40.8 | | 8.6 | 144 | 6.0 | 4.9 | 9.9 |
| RABBIT | 5-8 | 8-17 | 31-50 | 45-70 | 3.0-12.5 | 138-160 | 3.7-6.8 | 2.3-6.9 | 5.6-12 |
| | 5.2 | 14.3 | 43.6 | | 11.2 | 123 | 5.0 | 5.3 | 10.2 |
| GUINEA PIG | 3-7 | 11-17 | 37-50 | 65-90 | 6-17 | 120-149 | 3.8-7.9 | 3-7.6 | 5.3-12 |
| | 7.2 | 16.4 | 50.8 | | 8.1 | 131 | 5.0 | 5.7 | 9.9 |
| HAMSTER | 4-10 | 13-19 | 39.59 | 65-80 | 5-11 | 106-146 | 4.0-5.9 | 3.4-8.2 | 5-12 |
| | 9.2 | 11.1 | 41.8 | | 13.6 | 136 | 5.3 | 6.0 | 6.4 |
| MOUSE | 7-13 | 10-14 | 33-50 | 70-80 | 6-17 | 128-186 | 4.9-5.9 | 2.3-9.2 | 3.2-8.5 |

TABLE — D*

**Clincal biochemistry reference values**

Mean values and ranges

| SPECIES<br>x̄ range | Glucose<br>mg/100m | B. U. N[1].<br>mg/100ml | Cholesterol<br>mg/100ml | Total<br>Protein<br>g/100ml | Albumin<br>g/100ml | S.G.O.T[2]<br>I.U./l | S.G.P.T.[3]<br>I.U./l | Alkaline<br>phosph.<br>I.U./l |
|---|---|---|---|---|---|---|---|---|
| MONKEY<br>(M. fasciculars) | 60-90 | 18-28 | 100-150 | 7.5-8.7 | 2.4-3.4 | 34-56 | 21-39 | 15-35 |
| | 117 | 26 | 105 | 6.0 | 2.8 | 18 | 19 | 12 |
| CAT | 60-145 | 20-30 | 75-150 | 4.5-8 | 2-4 | 7-29 | 9-30 | 3-21 |
| | 75 | 14.5 | 27 | 7.6 | 3.7 | 63 | 24 | 87 |
| RAT | 50-135 | 5-29 | 10-54 | 4.7-8.2 | 2.7-5.1 | 46-81 | 18-30 | 57-128 |
| | 164 | 2.0 | 96 | 6 | 2.7 | 148 | 13 | 35 |
| CHICKEN | 125-200 | 0.5-6 | 52-148 | 5-7 | 2-3.5 | 88-208 | 10-37 | 25-44 |
| | 86 | 16.5 | 189 | 6.8 | 3.4 | 52 | 37 | 17 |
| DOG | 64-120 | 8-22 | 95-275 | 5.7-7.8 | 2-4 | 33-75 | 16-67 | 7-25 |
| | 94 | 21 | — | 7.9 | 3.1 | — | — | — |
| GERBIL | 40-140 | 17-31 | 90-130 | 5-17 | 2.5-4.5 | — | — | 12-37 |
| | 132 | 18.5 | 26 | 6.8 | 3.3 | 71 | 65 | 130 |
| RABBIT | 78-155 | 9-32 | 20-83 | 5-8 | 2.5-4 | 42-98 | 49-79 | 90-170 |
| | 92 | 23.5 | 30 | 5.2 | 2.6 | 47 | 42 | 70 |
| GUINEA PIG | 82-107 | 9-32 | 16-43 | 5-6.8 | 2.1-3.9 | 27-68 | 25-59 | 55-108 |
| | 69 | 22 | 53 | 7.1 | 3.3 | 100 | 24 | 17 |
| HAMSTER | 33-118 | 12-26 | 10-80 | 4-8 | 2.5-4 | 38-168 | 12-36 | 3-31 |
| | 89 | 19.5 | 64 | 6.2 | 3 | 36 | 13 | 19 |
| MOUSE | 63-176 | 14-28 | 26-82 | 4-8.6 | 2.5-4.8 | 23-48 | 2-24 | 10-28 |

1. Blood Urea Nitrogen.
2. Serum Glutamic Oxaloacetic Transaminase.
3. Serum Glutamic Pyruvic Transaminase.

TABLE—E*

**Recommended dietary allowances for different animal species**

| Animal species | Nutrient (percentages) | | | |
|---|---|---|---|---|
| | Protein | Carbohydrate | Fat | Fibre |
| Cat | 30-40 | NE | 25-30 | NE |
| Chicken | 15-20 | 60 | 1 (EFA) | NE |
| Dog | 20-25 | 60 | 10 | NE |
| Guinea pig | 18 | 45-48 | 4.7 | 10 |
| Hamster | 15 | 60 | 5 | 3 |
| Monkey | 15 | 61.8 | 5 | 3-5 |
| Mouse | 21.2 | 60.7 | 7.6 | 5.5 |
| Rabbit | 16-20 | 48 | 5-10 | 11 |
| Rat | 20 | 60 | 5 | 5 |

NE — Not essential, EFA-Essential fatty acid.

Salt mixture (4%) and vitamin mixture (1%) should be added to these diets to meet the requirements of minerals and vitamins of these species.

TABLE - F*

**Composition of stock diets**

| Ingredients | Diet I (%) | Diet II (%) |
|---|---|---|
| 1. Wheat flour | 15 | 62 |
| 2. Roasted bengalgram dhal | 58 | 28 |
| 3. Groundnut flour | 10 | — |
| 4. Skim milk powder | 5 | — |
| 5. Casein | 4 | 1 |
| 6. Refined oil | 4 | 5 |
| 7. Salt mixture | 4 | 4 |
| 8. Vitamin mixture | 0.2 | 0.2 |
| 9. Vitamin C | — | 0.05 |

Diet I is for rats, mice and hamsters.

Diet II is for monkeys, rabbits and guinea pigs.

An extra amount of 20 g of sprouted bengalgram, 15 g groundnuts and one banana a day for monkeys; 20 g sprouted bengalgram and 50 g lucerne grass for rabbits and 25 g of sprouted bengalgram and 25 g of lucerne grass for guinea pigs.

## TABLE—G*

### Composition of mineral mixture (g/100 g of salt mixture)

| | | | |
|---|---|---|---|
| 1. | Calcium carbonate $CaCO_3$ | — | 38.1400 |
| 2. | Cobalt chloride $CoCl_2.6H_2O$ | — | 0.0023 |
| 3. | Cupric sulfate $CuSO_4.5H_2O$ | — | 0.0477 |
| 4. | Ferrous sulfate $FeSO_4.7H_2O$ | — | 2.7000 |
| 5. | Magnesium sulfate $MgSO_4.7H_2O$ | — | 5.7300 |
| 6. | Manganese sulfate $MnSO_4.H_2O$ | — | 0.4010 |
| 7. | Potassium iodide KI | — | 0.0790 |
| 8. | Potassium phosphate monobasic $KH_2PO_4$ | — | 38.9000 |
| 9. | Sodium chloride NaCl | — | 13.9300 |
| 10. | Zinc sulfate $ZnSO_4.7H_2O$ | — | 0.0548 |

**Dry and grind to a fine powder before weighing. Grind in a mortor a portion of NaCl with KI. Grind together the reminder of NaCl with other salts. Finally, add the NaCl-KI mixture. Store in a cool dry place.**

### Composition of vitamin mixture

**One g of vitamin mixture contains the following :**

| | | | |
|---|---|---|---|
| 1. | Vitamin A+ | — | 2000 IU |
| 2. | Vitamin D+ | — | 200 IU |
| 3. | Vitamin E | — | 10 IU |
| 4. | Vitamin K (Menadione) | — | 0.5 mg |
| 5. | Thiamine | — | 0.5 mg |
| 6. | Riboflavin | — | 0.8 mg |
| 7. | Pyridoxine | — | 0.5 mg |
| 8. | Calcium pantothenate | — | 4.0 mg |
| 9. | Niacin | — | 4.0 mg |
| 10. | Inositol | — | 10.0 mg |
| 11. | Para aminobenzoic acid | — | 10.0 mg |
| 12. | Biotin | — | 40.0 $\mu$g |
| 13. | Folic acid | — | 0.2 mg |
| 14. | Vitamin $B_{12}$ | — | 3.0 $\mu$g |
| 15. | Choline chloride++ | — | 200.0 mg |

**Mix all the above ingredients and add sufficient amount of starch to make up to 1 g.**

**+ Vitamin A and D are available as commercial preparation, vanitin. Add appropriate volume of this concentrate to the oil before mixing it with the diet.**

**++ Prepare a 50% (W/W) mixture of choline chloride with starch and add at 0.2% level at the time of preparation of the diet.**

**Store in a cool, dark and dry place.**

**Source :** ***A Manual of Laboratory Techniques,*** **National Institute of Nutrition, Indian Council of Medical Research, Hyderabad 500 007, 1983**

## GLOSSARY OF TERMS RELATED TO ANIMAL NUTRITION

**ABATTOIR** A slaughterhouse.

**ABOMASUM** The fourth compartment of ruminant stomach, also known as true stomach.

**ABSCESS** A collection of pus in any part of the body.

**ABSOLUTE ZERO** The zero point on the absolute temperature scale—273.2°C.

**ABSORPTION** The passage of materials across a biological membrane.

**ACETIC ACID** One of the volatile fatty acids with the formula $CH_3COOH$. Commonly found in silage, rumen contents, and vinegar.

**ACETONEMIA** (ketosis) A condition characterised by an abnormally elevated concentration of ketone (acetone) bodies in the body tissues and fluids.

**ADAPTATION** The adjustment of an organism to a new or changing environmental condition.

**ADF (acid detergent fibre)** Fiber extracted with acidic detergent in a technique employed to help appraise the quality of forages.

**ADDITIVE** An ingredient or a combination of ingredients added to the basic feed mixture or parts thereof for a specific purpose, like, to increase feed ingestion or as an aid for digestion or added to produce more desirable consumer products or to alter metabolism. Generally additives are themselves non-nutrients and are added in micro quantities, thereby requires a thorough mixing.

**ADIPOSE** Of a fatty nature.

**AD LIBITUM** As desired by the animal.

**ADRENAL GLAND** One of the endocrine glands of the body, located near the kidney.

**AERIAL PART** The above-ground part of a plant.

**AEROBIC** A term usually applied to microorganisms that require oxygen to live and reproduce.

**AFTERBIRTH** The membranes expelled from the uterus following delivery of a foetus.

**ALANINE** One of the nonessential amino acids.

**ALFALFA LEAF MEAL** The powdered form of dried alfalfa (lucerne) leaves. When leaves are collected reasonably free from other crop plants or weeds, the meal on an average contain about 20 per cent crude protein and less than 18 per cent crude fibre.

**ALFALFA MEAL** The ground product obtained from the dried alfalfa plant as a whole (stem containing leaves).

**ALFALFA STEM MEAL** The ground meal obtained from aerial portion of the plant from which leaves have been excluded.

**ALIMENTARY** Having to do with feed or food.

**TEMPERATURE AMBIENT** The prevailing or surrounding temperature.

**AMINO ACID** Any one of a class of organic compounds which contain both the amino $(NH_2)$ group and the carboxyl (COOH) group.

**AMMONIATED** Combined or impregnated with ammonia or an ammonium compound.

**AMYLASE** Any one of several enzymes which aid in the hydrolysis of starch to maltose, for example, pancreatic amylase (amylopsin) and salivary amylase (ptyalin).

| | |
|---|---|
| **Anabolism** | The conversion of simple substances into more complex substances by living cells. Constructive metabolism. |
| **Anaerobic** | Living or functioning in the absence of air or molecular oxygen. |
| **Anemic** | Lacking in size and/or number of red blood cells. |
| **Animal Protein Factor (APF)** | The same compound which was once recognised as an unidentified growth factor present in animal feeds found absolutely essential for poultry and swine growth. It is now known to be the same as Vitamin $B_{12}$. |
| **Antibiotic** | Originally defined as a compound produced by a microorganism that inhibits the reproduction, or causes the destruction, of other microorganisms. The term now has been extended further and defined as a compound produced by a microorganism or a plant, or a close chemical derivative of such a compound that is toxic to microorganisms from a number of other species. |
| **Antibody** | Substance produced in the body that acts against disease. |
| **Antigen** | A high-molecular-weight substance (usually protein) that, when foreign to the bloodstream of an animal, stimulates the formation of a specific antibody and reacts specifically *in vivo* or *in vitro* with its homologous antibody. |
| **Antioxidant** | Substances having the property of protecting other substances from oxidation such as Vitamin E protects unsaturated fatty acids by oxidising themselves. |
| **Apparent Digestible Energy (DE)** | The food intake gross energy minus fecal energy. Also called apparent absorbed energy, or apparent energy of digested food. |
| **Arachidoni : Acid** | A 20-carbon unsaturated fatty acid having four double bonds. |
| **Arginine** | One of the essential amino acids. |
| **Artificially Dried** | Dried by other than natural means. Dehydrated. |
| **Ascorbic Acid** | Same as vitamin C, the antiscorbutic vitamin. |
| **Ash** | The incombustible residue remaining after incineration at 600°C for several hours. |
| **Aspartic Acid** | One of the nonessential amino acids. |
| **Asphyxia** | Suffocation or the suspension of animation as the result of suffocation. |
| **Aspirated** | Removal of light materials from heavier material by use of air. |
| **Atom** | A particle of matter indivisible by chemical means. It is the fundamental building block of the chemical elements. The elements, such as iron and sulphur, differ from each other because they contain different kinds of atoms. There are approximately six sextillion (six followed by 21 zeros, or $6 \times 10^{21}$) atoms in an ordinary drop of water. An atom consists of a dense inner core (the nucleus) and a much less dense outer domain of electrons in motion around the nucleus. Atoms are electrically neutral. |
| **Atomic Number** | The number of p .ons in the nucleus of an atom and also its positive charge. |
| **Atomic Weight** | The mass of an atom relative to other atoms; the atomic weight of any element is approximately equal to the total number of protons and neutrons in its nucleus. |
| **Atrophy** | A wasting away of a part of the body. |

**Avidin** A protein in egg albumen which can combine with biotin to render the latter unavailable to the animal.

**Balanced Ration** The ration will contain a combination of feed ingredients which will provide all essential nutrients in proper amount and proportion based upon the standard recommendations for a particular species under a specified physiological condition such as during growth, pregnancy or in production where the quality and quantity of the products are also considered.

**Barley Hulls** The outer covering of barley.

**Barley Feed** The by-product obtained during the manufacture of pearl barley from clean barley.

**Barley Mixed Feed** The products that obtained during the milling of barley flour from clean barley. The compound is mostly composed of the outer covering of the barley (hulls) with coarsely ground barley particulars.

**Basal Metabolism** Heat production of an animal during physical, digestive and emotional rest at about 25°C. The animal should have an adequate previous nutritive status.

**Beer Molasses** Apart from cane sugar, beet is also utilised for the manufacture of sugar, the product is known as beet sugar. During this process a by-product is obtained known as beet molasses which carries the same specifications as cane molasses except relatively high in protein (6.6% *vs.* 4.4%).

**Beet Pulp** A fibrous by-product of beet sugar industry.

**Bile** A greenish-yellow fluid formed in the liver, stored in the gall bladder (except in the horse which has no gall bladder), and secreted via bile duct into the upper small intestine. It functions in digestion.

**Biological Half-Life** The time required for a biological system, such as a human or an animal, to eliminate by natural processes half the amount of a substance (such as radioactive material) that has entered it.

**Biological Value** The efficiency with which a protein furnishes the proper proportions and amounts of the essential amino acids. A protein which has a high biological value is said to be of good quality.

**Blood Meal** Blood which has been dried firstly by passing live steam until the temperature reaches 100°C, the process ensures sterilisation and causes blood to clot. It is then drained, pressed to expel occluded serum, dried again by steam heating and finally ground. The compound contains about 80 per cent protein but deficient in leucine.

**Bomb Calorimeter** An instrument used for determining the gross energy content of a material.

**Bone Ash** Ash obtained by burning bones with free access to air.

**Bone Charcoal** Bone black is the product obtained by charring (partial burning) of bones in closed retorts (a container generally of glass with a long tube, in which substances are decomposed by heat).

**Bone Meal, Raw** Dried and ground bone meal obtained from undecomposed bones which have first been boiled in hot water.

**Bone Meal Steamed** The ground product sterilised by cooking undecomposed bones with steam under pressure.

**Bran** The pericarp or seed coat of grain removed during processing.

**Brewer's Dried Grain** The grain products are the residue which remains after most of the starches and sugars have been removed from the barley malt alone or in combination with other cereal grain products in the beer industry. The compound has got about 25 per cent crude protein. In view of a high fibre content the product is seldom fed to swine or poultry.

**Brewer's Dried Yeast** Dried, non-fermentative non-extracted yeast belonging to the species *Saccharomyces cerevisiae* obtained as a by-product in the process of brewing beer. It contains about 42 per cent crude protein. The compound is a valuable source of many of the B group of Vitamins and also relatively rich in phosphorus.

**Buffer** Any substance that can counteract changes in free acid or alkali concentration.

**Buttermilk (Dried)** The dried form of sour liquid left after the butterfat in milk has been made into butter.

**Butyric Acid** One of the volatile fatty acids with the formula $CH_3CH_2CH_2COOH$. Commonly found in rumen contents and poor quality silage.

**Calcification** Process by which organic tissue becomes hardened by a deposit of calcium salts.

**Calcite** Calcium carbonate, $CaCO_3$, with hexagonal crystallisation, an acceptable source of Ca.

**Calorie (Small)** The amount of energy as heat required to raise one gram of water to 1°C (precisely from 14.5° to 15.5°C). This is equivalent to 4.185 g.

**Calorimeter** An instrument for measuring energy.

**Carcass** The body of dead animal less the viscera and usually the head, skin and lower leg.

**Carcinogenic** Cancer producing.

**Cardiovascular** Pertaining to the heart and blood vessels.

**Carotene** A yellow organic compound that is a precursor of vitamin A.

**Cartilage** The gristle or connective tissue attached to the ends of bones.

**Catabolism** The conversion of complex substances into more simple compounds by living cells. Destructive metabolism.

**Catalyst** A substance that speeds up the rate of a chemical reaction but is not itself used up in the reaction.

**Cellulose** A polysaccharide having the formula $(C_6H_{10}O_5)_n$, found in the fibrous portion of plants. Low in digestibility. It has been shown to consist of a large number (200 to 2000) of β-glucose units joined together in a non-branched chain of 1, 4-glycoside bonds which are non-responsive to any enzyme secreted by mammalian tissue. However, it is utilised to a limited extent, by the microorganisms which inhabit the rumen.

**Chlorophyll** The green colouring matter present in growing plants.

**Cholesterol** The most common member of the sterol group.

**Choline** One of the B vitamins.

**Chopped** Reduced in particle size by cutting.

**Chuni** Chuni means "Churna". The compound consists primarily of the broken pieces of endosperm including germ and a portion of husks obtained as by-product during the processing of pulse grains for human consumption

| | |
|---|---|
| | for example arhar chuni, masur chuni, mung chuni etc. The compound is valued as a concentrate feed due to being comparatively low in fibre and more in energy and protein content in comparison with roughages. |
| COCONUT OILCAKE | The product is obtained after removal of oil from dried coconuts by a mechanical extraction process. |
| COEFFICIENT OF DIGESTIBILITY | The percentage value of a food nutrient that has been absorbed. For example, if a food contains 10 g of nitrogen and it is found that 9.5 g has been absorbed, the digestibility is 95 per cent. |
| COENZYME | A partner required by some enzymes to produce enzymatic activity. |
| COFFEE MEAL | Ground coffee beans after extraction of oil. |
| COFFEE PULP | The outer covering of the coffee berry. It has about 17.5 per cent protein but poor palatibility. |
| COLLAGEN | The main supportive protein of connective tissue. |
| COMBUSTION | The combination of substances with oxygen accompanied by the liberation of heat. |
| COMPLETE RATION | A single feed mixture into which has been included all of the dietary essentials, except water of a given class of livestock. |
| CONCENTRATE | Feeds having crude fibre less than 18 per cent while T.D.N. is over 60 per cent on air dry basis. Usually contain one or more nutrients in a concentrated form. |
| CONGESTION | Excessive accumulation of blood in a part of the body. |
| CONVULSION | A violent involuntary contraction or series of contractions of the voluntary muscles. |
| COPRA MEAL | The product is what remains after the dried edible portion of coconuts have been subjected to fat extraction and ground. The relatively low quality of its protein and its relative high content of fibre restrict its use in rations for swine and poultry. |
| COTTON SEED HULLS | The outer protective covering of cotton seeds. |
| COTTON SEED OIL CAKE | Residue which remains after mechanical pressing of clean cotton seed, composed, principally of the kernel with such unavoidable portions of the hull and fibre as may be left in course of expression of oil. |
| DECORTICATED COTTON SEED OIL CAKE | The product obtained after mechanical pressing of clean, mature and unhulled cottonseed from which maximum oil has been extracted. |
| UNDECORTICATED CRAB MEAL | It is the undecomposed ground dried waste of the crab and contains the shell, viscera, and part or all of the flesh. It must contain not less than 25 per cent protein. |
| CREATININE | A nitrogenous compound arising from protein metabolism and secreted in the urine. |
| CRIMPED | Having been passed between rollers with corrugated surfaces. |
| CRUDE FIBRE | The more fibrous, less digestible portion of a feed. Consists primarily of cellulose, hemicellulose and lignin. |
| CRUDE PROTEIN | Total ammoniacal nitrogen × 6.25, based on the fact that feed protein on the average contains 16.0 per cent nitrogen. |
| CUD | A bolus of previously eaten food which has been regurgitated by a ruminant animal for further chewing. |

**Curie (Ci)** — The basic unit to describe the intensity of radioactivity in a sample of material. The curie is equal to 37 billion ($3.7 \times 10^{10}$) disintegrations per second. It is also a quantity of any nuclide having one curie of radioactivity.

**Cyanocobalamin** — Same as vitamin $B_{12}$.

**Cystine** — One of the nonessential amino acids. It is sulphur containing and may be used to meet in part the need for methionine.

**Decortication** — Removal of the bark, hull, husk, or shell from a plant seed, or root. Also, removal of portions of the cortical substance of a structure or organ, as in the brain, kidney, and lung.

**Deficiency Disease** — A disease resulting from an inadequate dietary intake of some nutrient.

**Defluorinated** — Having had the fluorine content reduced to a level which is nontoxic under normal use.

**Dehydrated** — Having had most of the moisture removed through artificial drying.

**Dermatitis** — Inflammation of the skin.

**Desiccate** — To dry completely.

**Dextrin** — An intermediate polysaccharide product obtained during starch hydrolysis.

**Dicoumarol** — A chemical compound found in spoiled sweet clover and lespedeza hays. It is an anticoagulant andcan cause internal hemorrhages when eaten by cattle. The trade name is Dicumarol.

**Digestible Energy** — That part of the gross energy of a feed which does not appear in the faeces.

**Digestion** — The processes involved in the conversion of feed into absorbable forms.

**Digestion Coefficient** — (coefficient of digestibility) The difference between the nutrients consumed and the nutrients excreted expressed as a percentage.

**Disaccharide** — Any one of several so-called compound sugars which yield two monosaccharide molecules upon hydrolysis. Sucrose, maltose, and lactose are the most common.

**Dispensable Amino Acid** — Basically the same as nonessential amino acid.

**Dry Matter** — That part of feed which is not water, sometimes referred to as total solids. This is the sum of the crude protein, crude fat, crude fibre, nitrogen free extract and ash.

**Dried Citrus Pulp** — The material is the residue from the processing of citrus fruit into juices and canned fruit. After extraction of the fruit or juice, lime water is added to minimise acidity and the pulp and peelings are then dried.

**Dried Silk Warm Pupae** — The product obtained by drying the boiled cocoons after reeling; removing outer chitinous covering followed by washing.

**Dried Tomato Pomace** — A dried product composed of tomato skins, pulp and crushed seeds. (Pomace means the crushed pulp of fruits pressed for juice.)

**Distiller's Dried Grains.** — In the manufacture of alcohol and other distilled liquors from maize rye or wheat, the soluble materials are extracted leaving the residue. This residue after filtration is sold as wet or dried distiller's grains. The material is rich in crude protein (20-25 per cent), lipid (5-8 per cent) and crude fibre (5·8 per cent). In view of its fibre content the grain is seldom fed to swine or poultry.

DISTILLER'S DRIED GRAIN WITH SOLUBLES — Distiller's grains always contain small amount of liquor after distilling off. When the material is spray dried to produce a light brown powder of variable composition it will be termed as "distillers' solubles". These are often mixed with distillers' grains and dried together to yield a material sold as distillers' dried grains with solubles or dark grains.

EDEMA — Swelling of a part of or of the entire body due to an accumulation of an excess of water.

ELEMENT — Any one of the fundamental atoms of which all matter is composed.

EMACIATED — An excessively thin condition of the body.

EMULSIFY — To disperse small drops of one liquid into another liquid.

ENCEPHALITIS — An inflammation of the brain that results in various central nervous system disorders.

ENDEMIC — Occurring in low incidence but more or less constantly in a given population.

ENDOCRINE — Pertaining to internal secretions.

ENDOGENOUS — Originating from within the organism.

ENDOMETRIUM — The mucous membrane that lines the uterus.

ENERGY — The capacity to perform work.

ENSILAGE — The same as silage.

ENTERITIS — Inflammation of the intestines.

ENZYME — One of a class of organic compounds, formed by living cells, capable of producing or accelerating specific organic reactions. An organic catalyst.

EPIDEMIC — When many people in a given region are attacked by some disease at the same time.

EPITHELIAL — Refers to those cells that form the outer layer of the skin and other membranes.

ERGOSTEROL — One of the sterols which upon exposure to ultraviolet light is converted to vitamin $D_2$.

ESSENTIAL AMINO ACID — Any one of several amino acids that are needed by animal and cannot be synthesised by them in the amount needed and so must be present in the protein of the feed as such.

ESSENTIAL FATTY ACID — A fatty acid that cannot be synthesised in the body or that cannot be made in sufficient quantities for the body's needs. Linoleic acid is essential for humans.

ESTROGENS — Estrus-producing hormones secreted by the ovaries.

ETIOLOGY — The causes of a disease or disorder.

EXCRETA — The products of excretion—primarily faeces and urine.

EXOGENOUS — Originating from outside of the organism.

EXPELLER PROCESS — A process for the mechanical extraction of oil from seeds, involving the use of a screw press.

EXTRINSIC FACTOR — A factor coming from or originating from outside an organism.

EXTRUDED — As applied to feed—having been forced through a die under pressure.

**Exudative Diathesis** Symptom of vitamin-E deficiency in poultry. It is characterised by an accumulation of fluid in subcutaneous fatty tissue.

**Factor** In nutrition, any chemical substance found in feed.

**Fattening** This is the deposition of unused energy in the form of fat within the body tissues.

**Fatty Acid** Any one of several organic compounds containing carbon, hydrogen, and oxygen which combine with glycerol to form fat.

**Fauna** The animal life present. Frequently used to refer to the overall protozoal population present.

**Feather Meal** Product resulting from the treatment under pressure of clean, undecomposed feathers from slaughtered poultry, free of additives and/or accelerators. Not less than 80 per cent of its crude protein content must consist of "digestible protein".

**Fibrous** High in content of cellulose, hemicellulose and/or lignin.

**Fibrinogen** A soluble protein present in the blood and body fluids of animals that is essential to the coagulation of blood.

**Fish Meal** Product obtained by drying followed by grinding of clean, undecomposed fish from which the oil portion might or might not have been extracted.

**Fish Oil** Oil extracted from undecomposed dried fish.

**Fish Scrap** Consists mostly of unedible portion like bones and some viscera of fish.

**Fish Solubles** Products obtained by concentrating the 'stickwater' or clarified liquor, which consists of dissolved, dispersed fish protein particles along with minerals, B-complex vitamins and some unknown growth factors. The material is obtained as a by-product during fish meal production.

**Flaked** Rolled or cut into flat pieces.

**Flora** The plant life present. In nutrition it generally refers to the bacteria present in the digestive tract.

**Fodder** The entire above-ground part of nearly mature corn or sorghum in the fresh or cured form.

**Folacin** Same as folic acid. One of the B vitamins.

**Forage** Crops used in the whole plant form (except roots) at pasture, hay, silage, or green chop for feeding purposes.

**Fortify** Nutritionally, to add one or more nutrients to a feed.

**Galactose** A hexose monosaccharide found especially in ripe fruits and honey. Obtained along with glucose from suçrose hydrolysis. Commonly known as fruit sugar.

**Gall Bladder** A membranous sac lying next to the liver of all farm livestock (except the horse) in which bile is stored.

**Gastric Juice** A clear liquid secreted by the wall of the stomach. It contains hydrochloric acid and the enzymes rennin, pepsin and gastric lipase.

**Gelatin** An organic colloidal substance made from animal bones, skins or hide fragments. Used in leather finishes to produce a touch film on the leather. Glue is an impure form of gelatin.

**Gluconeogenesis** Formation of glucose from protein or fat.

**Glycogenesis** Conversion of glucose into glycogen.

| | |
|---|---|
| GLYCOGENOLYSIS | Conversion of glycogen into glucose. |
| GLYCOLYSIS | Conversion of carbohydrate into lactate by a series of catalysts. The breaking down of sugars into simpler compounds. |
| GLUTAMIC ACID | One of the nonessential amino acids. |
| GLYCOGEN | A polysaccharide with the formula $(C_6H_{10}O_5)_n$ which is formed in the liver and muscle and depolymerised to glucose to serve as a ready source of energy when needed by the animal. Known also as animal starch. |
| GOITER | An enlargement of the thyroid gland located in the neck. Sometimes caused by an iodine deficiency. |
| GOSSYPOL | A substance present in cotton-seed and cotton-seed meal which is toxic to swine and to certain other nonruminant animals. |
| GRAVID | Pregnant. |
| GROAT | Grain from which the hulls has been removed. |
| GROUNDNUT OIL CAKE | The oilcake obtained after the mechanical extraction of oil from decorticated groundnut kernels. |
| GROUNDNUT SKIN | The product comprises mostly the outer skin covering of the groundnut kernel along with varied proportion of groundnut kernels (exclusive of hulls). |
| GUAR MEAL | Guar is a legume, and the meal, a by-product from the preparation of guar green obtained by removing most of the endosperm from whole guar beans. |
| HAY | The aerial part of finer-stemmed forage crops stored in the dry form for animal feeding. |
| HAYLAGE | Low-moisture silage (35 to 55 per cent moisture). Grass and legume crops are cut and wilted in the field to a lower moisture level than normal for grass silage, but the crop is not sufficiently dry for baling. |
| HEAT INCREMENT | The heat which is unavoidably produced by an animal incidental with nutrient digestion and utilisation. Was originally called work of digestion. |
| HEXOSAN | A hexose-based polysaccharide having the general formula $(C_6H_{10}O_5)_n$. Cellulose, starch, and glycogen are the most common. |
| HISTIDINE | One of the essential amino acids. |
| HYDRAULIC PROCESS | A process for the mechanical extraction of oil from seeds, involving the use of a hydraulic press. Sometimes referred to as the old process. |
| HYDROGENATION | The chemical addition of hydrogen to any unsaturated compound. |
| HYDROLYSIS | The splitting of a substance into the smaller units by its chemical reaction with water. |
| HYPERTENSION | An abnormally high tension—usually associated with high blood pressure. |
| HYPERTHYROIDISM | Overactivity of the thyroid gland. |
| INTRINSIC FACTOR | A chemical substance in normal stomach juice necessary for the absorption of vitamin $B_{12}$. |
| IODINATED CASEIN | Milk protein (casein) that has been treated with iodine. It has the same physiological effect as thyroxine (hormone produced by the thyroid gland). It is commonly referred to as thyroprotein and is sometimes used to stimulate cows to secrete more milk. |
| ION | An atom or a group of atoms (molecules) carrying an electric charge, |

which may be positive or negative. Ions are usually formed when salts, acids, or bases are dissolved in water.

**IRRADIATED DRIED YEAST** Dried nonfermentative yeast of the botanical classification Torulopsis or Saccharomyces which has been separated from the medicine in which it was propagated. Once dried the material is exposed to ultraviolet rays in order to produce its antirachitic value.

**IRRADIATION** The act of treating with ultraviolet light.

**JEJUNUM** The middle portion of the small intestine which extends from the duodenum to the ileum.

**KERATIN** A sulphur-containing protein which is the primary component of epidermis, hair, wool, hoof, horn, and the organic matrix of the teeth.

**KERNEL** A dehulled seed.

**KERATOSIS** Any horny growth, such as a wart, causing the cornification, or hardening, of the epithelial skin layers.

**LACTIC ACID** An organic acid, one form (CHOH. $CH_2$. COOH) of which is commonly found in sour milk, sauerkraut, and silage. Other forms enter into body metabolism.

**LEGUME** Refers to those crops that can absorb nitrogen directly from the atmosphere through bacteria that live in their roots. The clovers and alfalfa are common examples of legumes.

**LIGNIN** An indigestible compound which along with cellulose is a major component of the cell wall of certain plant materials such as wood, hulls, straws, and overripe hays.

**LIMITED FEEDING** Feeding animals to maintain weight and growth but not enough to fatten or increase production. Feeding animals less than they would like to eat.

**LIMITING AMINO ACID** The essential amino acid of protein that shows the greatest percentage deficit in comparison with the amino acids contained in the same quantity of another protein selected as standard.

**LINOLEIC ACID** An 18-carbon unsaturated fatty acid having two double bonds. It reacts with glycerol to form linolein. This is an essential fatty acid.

**LINSEED OIL CAKE** The residual product left after extraction of oil by mechanical means from matured linseed.

**LIPIDS** A broad term for fats and fat-like substances.

**LIVER AND GLANDULAR MEAL** These are obtained by drying and grinding liver or liver and other glandular tissue from slaughtered mammals.

**LYMPH** The slightly yellow, transparent fluid occupying the lymphatic channels of the body.

**MALT SPROUTS** The product is obtained by removing the developing buds of malted barley and the mixing together with malt hulls or any other parts of malt.

**MAIZE BRAN** The bran, which essentially comprises the husk (pericap and testa) is the outer coating of the maize kernel (a grain or seed) with varying proportion of the starchy part of the germ (the rudimentary form from which a new plant is developed).

**MAIZE GERM CAKE** The cake obtained after extraction of oil from maize germ.

**MAIZE GERM OIL CAKE (MEAL)** Solvent extraction of oil of maize germ cake.

**Maize Gluten Meal** The product is the dried residue from maize after the removal of the larger part of the starch and bran by the process employed in the wet milling manufacture of maize starch.

**Maize Grit** The fine to medium sized crushed maize grain with little or none of the bran or germ.

**Meal** A feed ingredient having a particle size somewhat larger than flour.

**Meat Meal** The finely dried ground residue from mammal tissues exclusive of hair, hoof, horn, stomach contents and hide trimmings, except in such traces as may occur unavoidably in good factory practice.

**Megacalorie** 1,000 kilocalories or 1,000,000 calories.

**Metabolism** The sum total of the chemical changes in the body, including the building up (anabolic, assimilation) and the breaking down (catabolic, dissimilation) processes. The transformation by which energy is made available for body uses.

**Metabolite** Any substance produced by metabolism.

**Metabolizable Energy** Digestible energy minus the energy of the urine and fermentation gases.

**Meihionine** One of the essential amino acids. It is sulphur containing and may be replaced in part by cystine.

**Micro Ingredient** Any ration component normally measured in milligrams or micrograms per kilogram or in parts per million.

**Molasses** A thick, viscous, usually dark coloured, liquid product containing a high concentration of soluble carbohydrates, minerals, and certain other material.

**Mustard Oil Cake** The cake obtained after extraction of the oil from whole mustard and rape seeds by a mechanical extraction process.

**Mycotoxin** A fungus or bacterial toxin. Sometimes present in feed material.

**Net Energy** This is that part of metabolisable energy over the use of which the animal has complete control. It is metabolisable energy minus the heat increment.

**Net Protein Ratio** The difference between the average final body weight of a test group of animnls fed a protein diet and that of a control group receiving a protein free diet, divided by the amount of protein taken by the test group.

**Nitrogen-Free Extract** That part of feed dry matter which is not crude protein, crude fat, crude fibre, or ash. It consists mostly of sugars and starches. Sometimes referred to as NFE.

**Nonprotein** Any one of a group of ammoniacal nitrogen containing compounds which are not true proteins. Urea is a common example.

**Nutrient** Any chemical compound having specific functions in the nutritive support of animal life.

**Nutriture** Nutritional status.

**Oat Feed** A kind of by-product consisting of fraction of oat grains, hulls and also dust. The product is obtained during milling of table cereals from clean oats. The crude fibre percentage does not exceed 25 per cent.

**Oat Hulls** The outer covering of threshed oats obtained during the milling of table cereals.

**Oatmeals or Rolled Oats** Obtained in the manufacture of rolled oat kernels or rolled oats and consists of broken rolled oat kernels and floury portions of the oat kernels with only such quantity of finely ground oat hulls as is unavoidable in the usual process of commercial milling.

**Oat Groats** These are oat grains from which the hull has been removed. In other words, these are oat kernels. Since most of the feeding value of oat grain is found in the kernel, oat groats are very high in feeding value.

**Osmosis** The passage of a solute or a solution through a semi-permeable membrane toward effecting an equalisation of th concentration of fluids on the opposite sides of the membrane.

**Ossification** The process of bone formation.

**Osteomalacia** A weakening of the bones due to a calcium, phosphorus, and/or vitamin D deficiency.

**Osteoporosis** An abnormal porousness of bone as the result of a calcium, phosphorus, and/or vitamin D deficiency.

**Oxidation** Chemically, the increase of positive charges on an atom or the loss of negative charges. There may be a loss of one electron (univalent 0) or two electrons (divalent 0). The combining of oxygen with another element to form one or more new substances. Burning is one kind of oxidation. Also called oxydation.

**Oyster Shell Flour** Oyster shell is a hard shell of a shell fish found especially on the bottom of the sea. It contains calcium to the extent of 37-40 per cent. The material is sold either as dried shell or in dried powdered form.

**Pancreas** A large, elongated gland located near the stomach. It produces pancreatic juice which is secreted into the upper small intestine via the pancreatic duct.

**Pancreatic Juice** A thick, transparent liquid secreted by the pancreas into the upper small intestine. It contains the enzymes pancreatic amylase, pancreatic lipase, and trypsin; also the hormone insulin and glucagon.

**Parakeratosis** Any abnormality of the outermost horny layer of the skin.

**Pellets** Compacted particles of feed formed by forcing ground material through die openings.

**Phagocytes** Any cell that can ingest particles or cells that are foreign or harmful to the body.

**Plasma** The colourless fluid portion of the blood in which the corpuscles are suspended.

**Poultry Hatchery By-product** A mixture of eggshells, in fertile and unhatched eggs, culled chicks which have been cooked, dried and ground with or without removal of part of the fat.

**Poultry Manure Meal** Pasteurised ground chicken manure free from other foreign materials, the dehydrated form contains about 2.5 per cent nitrogen.

**Precursor** A compound that can be used by the body to form another compound.

**Prehension** The seizing (grasping) and conveying of food to the mouth.

**Pre-mix** A uniform mixture of one or more microingredients and a carrier, used in the introduction of microingredients into a larger mixture.

| | |
|---|---|
| PROSTAGLANDINS | A large group of chemically related 20-carbon hydroxy fatty acids with variable physiological effects in the body. |
| PURIFIED DIET | A mixture of the known essential dietary nutrients in a pure form that is fed to experimental (test) animals in nutrition studies. |
| PUTREFACTION | The decomposistion of proteins by microorganisms under anaerobic conditions. |
| RADIOACTIVE | Giving off atomic energy in the form of alpha, beta, or gamma rays. |
| RADIOISOTOPE | A radioactive form of an element. |
| RANCID | A term used to describe fats that have undergone partial decomposition. |
| RATION BALANCED | A balanced ration is one which will supply the various nutrients in such proportions as will properly nourish a given animal when fed in proper amounts for a 24 hour period. |
| RED MEAT | Meat that is red when raw. Red meat includes beef, veal, pork, mutton, and lamb. |
| RENNIN | The milk-curdling enzyme present in the gastric juice of milk-consuming animals. |
| RETICULOENDOTHELIAL SYSTEM | A widely spread network of body cells concerned with blood cell formation, bile formation, and engulfing or trapping of foreign materials, which includes cells of bone marrow, lymph, spleen, and liver. |
| RICE BRAN | The material consists primarily of the seed coat and germ which are removed from rice grain in the manufacture of polished rice for human consumption. In view of its relatively high content of fat and fibre and its frequent lack of palatability, the use of rice bran is usually limited to not over approximately one third of the ration concentrates. |
| RICE HULLS | The outer covering of rice obtained during the milling of rice. |
| RICE POLISH | The material obtained during the polishing of rice kernels after initial removal of hulls and bran. |
| ROLLED | Compressed into flat particles by having been passed between rollers. |
| ROUGHAGE | Any feed high (over about 20 per cent) in crude fibre and low (under about 60 per cent) in TDN, on an air-dry basis. Opposite of concentrate. |
| RYE | Rye (*Secale cereale*) is a hardy cereal grass widely grown for its grain and straw. The grain or seeds of this plant are used for making flour and whisky and as feed for livestock. Like wheat, rye should be crushed or coarsely ground for feeding animals. The grain is not commonly given to poultry. |
| RYE BRAN | The coarse outer covering of the rye kernel as removed in the usual processes, other than scouring. |
| RYE MIDDLINGS | Consists of a small proportion of fine bran particles, germ and a large proportion of low grade fibrous flour as separated in the usual process of flour milling. The crude fibre content does not usually exceed 5 per cent. |
| SAFFLOWER MEAL WITHOUT HULLS | This is what remains after most of the hull and the oil has been removed from safflower seed. Protein content is more than 40 per cent but the quality is not as good as that of soybean oil meal. |

**Sarcoma** A tumor of fleshy consistency—often highly malignant.

**Sedentary** Sitting most of the time.

**Serum** The colourless fluid portion of blood remaining after clotting and removal of corpuscles. It differs from plasma in that the fibrinogen has been removed.

**Sesame Oil Meal** The meal is produced from what remains following the extraction of oil from til (sesame) seed. The cake is high in protein and calcium.

**Shorts** A by-product of flour milling consisting of a mixture of small particles of bran and germ, the aleurone layer, and coarse flour.

**Solvent Extracted Cotton Seed Meal** Cotton seed meal consists of dehulled mechanically fat extracted ground to a meal. When the product is subjected to hexane or any other solvent extraction, the residue will be termed as solvent extracted. Cotton-seed meal is an excellent high protein feed for ruminants. However, it may kill the growing swine if included in the ration at levels over 9 per cent because of a toxic factor known as *gossypol*.

**Solvent Extracted Coconut Oilcake** The meal is the residue remains after removal of most of the oil from dried meal of coconut by any solvent extraction process. Solvent extraction differs from mechanical extraction of oil in that the former removes most efficiently lipid portions of the cake (meal). This meal is also known as copra meal.

**Solvent Extracted Groundnut Oilcake** The meal is the product obtained after extraction of most of the oil by solvent extraction process from either groundnut cake of expeller variety or directly from clean hulled groundnut kernels.

**Solvent Extracted Linseed Meal** The product is obtained by processing the linseed cake of expeller variety of the ground linseed grain through solvent extraction method. The product thus obtained may also be termed as deoiled linseed cake as the solvent extraction method is highly efficient in removing most of the oil portion.

**Solvent Extracted Mustard Cake** The product is obtained by treating the mechanically extracted (ghani or expeller variety) cake through solvent extraction process, thus the cake will be made devoid of any significant oil.

**Solvent Extracted Rice Bran** The product is the result of the treatment of rice bran through solvent extraction method and thereby removal of rice oil from rice bran. Product commonly known as deoiled rice bran.

**Solvent Extracted Safflower Oilcake** The residue obtained after extracting the oil by solvent extraction process from whole safflower seed or safflower cake originally obtained by either ghani or as an expeller variety.

**Solvent Extracted Sal Seed Meal** The meal obtained by extraction of oil from decorticated and flaked *sal* seed kernels through solvent extraction process, thereby reducing the oil percentage of the remaining meal to a negligible amount.

**Solvent Extracted Soybean Oilcake** The meal is devoid of fat which has been extracted by solvent process and has been ground and sometimes pelleted to suit livestock feeding.

**Shrimp Meal** Same as crab meal.

**Substrate** A substance upon which an enzyme acts. Same as *zymolyte*.

**Supplement** A semi-concentrated source of one or more nutrients used to enhance

| | |
|---|---|
| | the nutritional adequacy of a daily ration or a complete ration mixture. |
| SYNDROME | A medical term meaning a set of symptoms that occur together. |
| TAPIOCA CHIPS | Thin sliced pieces of tapioca tubers in dried condition. |
| TAPIOCA FLOUR | Tapioca has different names in different parts of the world. The English speaking territories refer to it as cassava or cassava root; in Latin America it is known as manoica. The dried tapioca root meal contains about 1.8 per cent crude protein, 1.3 per cent fat, 85 per cent nitrogen-free-extract and 1.0 per cent fibre. |
| TAPIOCA SPENT PULP | The pulp has everything except the starchy portion of the tapioca tubers which has been removed. |
| THROMBOSIS | The obstruction of a blood vessel by the formation of a blood clot. |
| TOCOPHEROL | Any of the four different forms of an alcohol which is also known as vitamin E. |
| TOXIC | Of a poisonous nature. |
| TRACER ELEMENT | A radioactive element used in biological and other research to trace the fate of a substance. |
| TRACE MINERAL | Any one of several mineral elements that are required by animals in very minute amounts. Same as micromineral. |
| UREA | A white, crystalline, water-soluble substance with the formula $CO(NH_2)_2$. It is the most extensively used source of nonprotein nitrogen for adult ruminant animal feeding. |
| UREASE | An enzyme which acts on urea to produce carbon dioxide and ammonia. It is found in the jackbean and the soybean, and is produced by certain microorganisms in the rumen. |
| VFA | (Volatile fatty acids) Commonly used in reference to acetic, propionic, and butyric acids produced in the rumen of cattle, goats, and sheep, in the cecum of sheep, the cecum and colon of swine, the colon of the horse, and the cecum of the rabbit. |
| VILLI | Small thread-like projections attached to the interior side of the wall of the small intestine. |
| VISCERA | The organs of the great cavities of the body which are normally removed upon slaughter. |
| WHEAT BRAN | The material consists of the seed coat of wheat which is removed in the manufacture of wheat flour. It is used in livestock feeding primarily as a source of bulk, as mild laxative and as a source of phosphorus. |
| WHEAT GERM MEAL | Consists chiefly of wheat germ mixed with some bran and middlings or shorts. It must contain not less than 25 per cent crude protein and 7 per cent crude fat. The product must be obtained in the usual process of commercial milling. |
| WHEAT MIDDLINGS | Consists of fine particles of wheat bran, wheat shorts (a by-product of milling that consists of bran, germ and coarse meal) and some of the offal from the "tail of the mill" and must contain not more than 9.5 per cent crude fibre. |

| | |
|---|---|
| XANTHINE | An intermediate in the metabolism of purines; related to uric acid. |
| XEROPHTHALMIA | Dry infected eye condition caused by lack of vitamin A. |
| XYLOSE | A 5 carbon aldehyde sugar that is not metabolised by the body. |
| ZEIN | A protein of low biological value present in maize, deficient in lysine and tryptophan. |
| ZYMOGEN | The inactive form of an enzyme. |

# INDEX

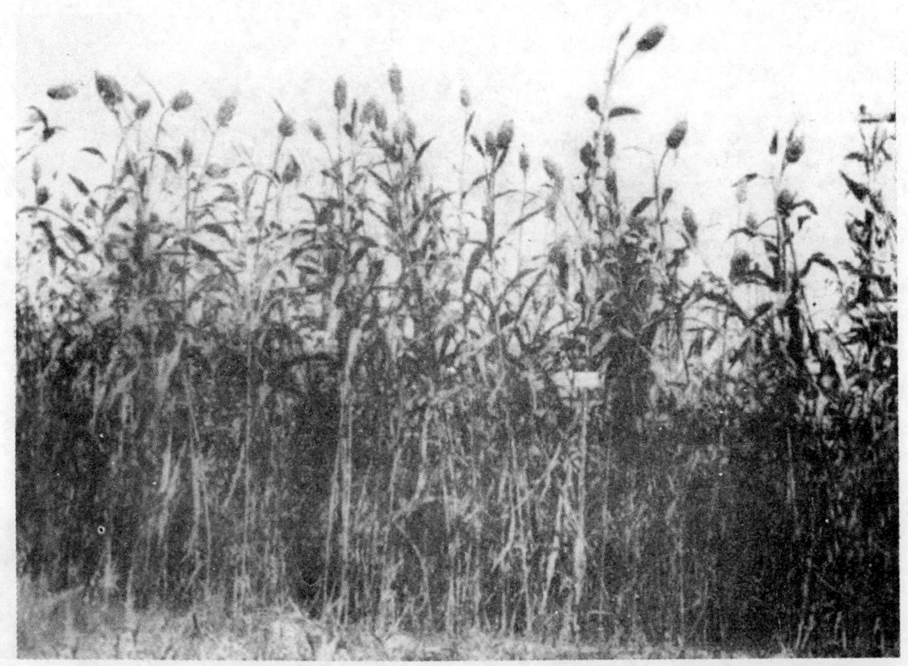

Jowar a non legume *kharif* fodder, most commonly grown throughout the country.

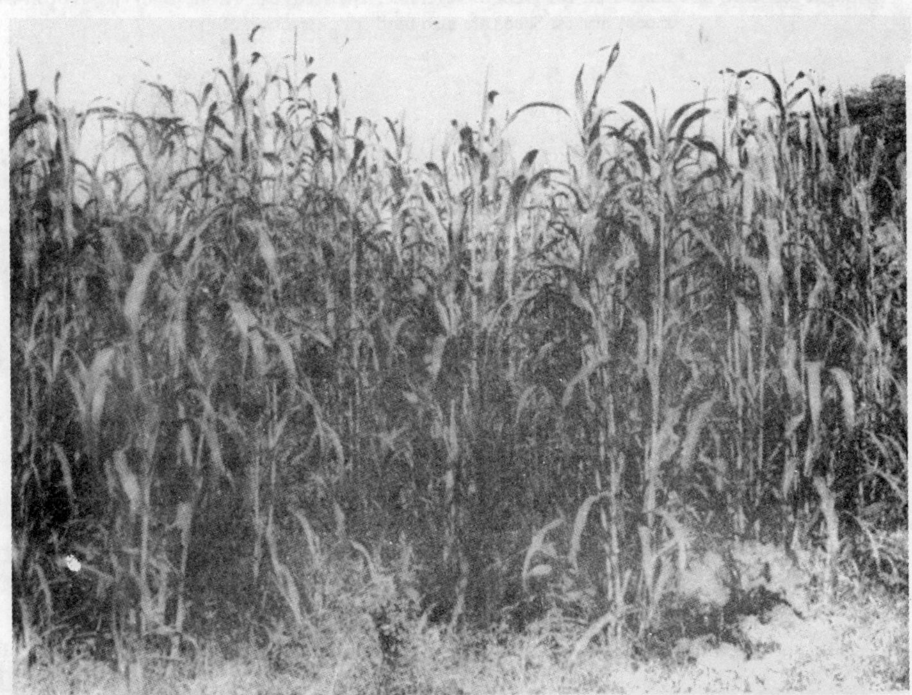

Bajra or Pearl millet or Indian millet grown in drier areas. Has a rapid rate of growth and matures quickly when the rains come. The first cutting is done 50-80 days after sowing followed by subsequent cuttings after 35-40 days. For good regrowth the cutting height is preferred to be 15 cm from the ground.

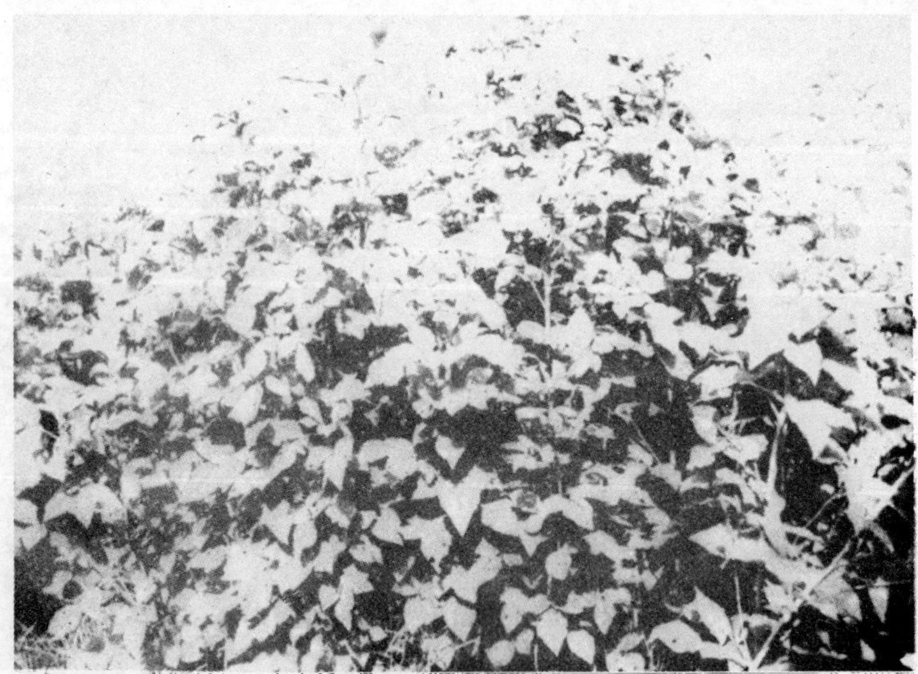

Gaur or Cluster bean is a nutritious fodder crop grown extensively throughout northern India. Drought resistant, also cultivated for grain or vegetable. The seeds can be fed to all classes of livestock except horses. Seeds are also used for extraction of gum.

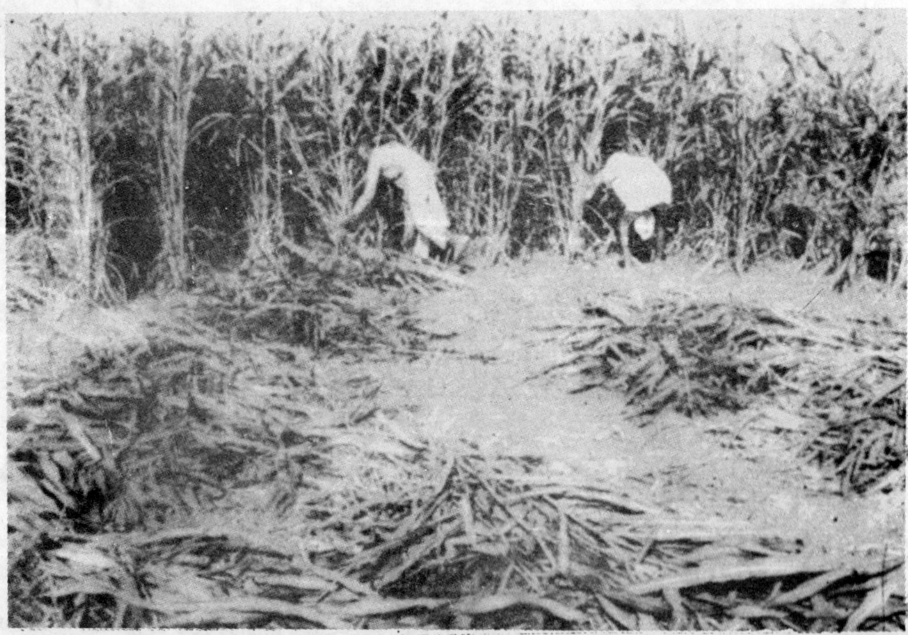

Teosinte or *Makchari* grown as a high yielding fodder crop in many areas. It is an inter-generic cross between maize and chari. When sown in February-March it will be ready for first cut in May-June. The second and third cuttings will be ready in August and November respectively. The cutting height should be from 10 to 15 cm from the ground.

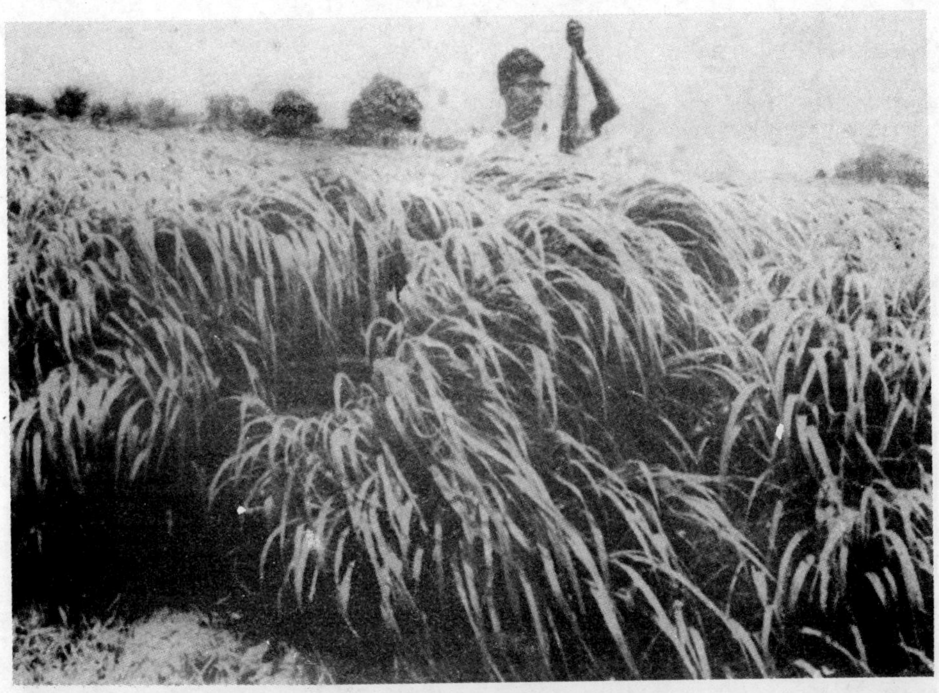

***Pennisetum pedicellatum*** **(Dinanath grass) showing luxurious growth at 120 DAS (days after sowing).**

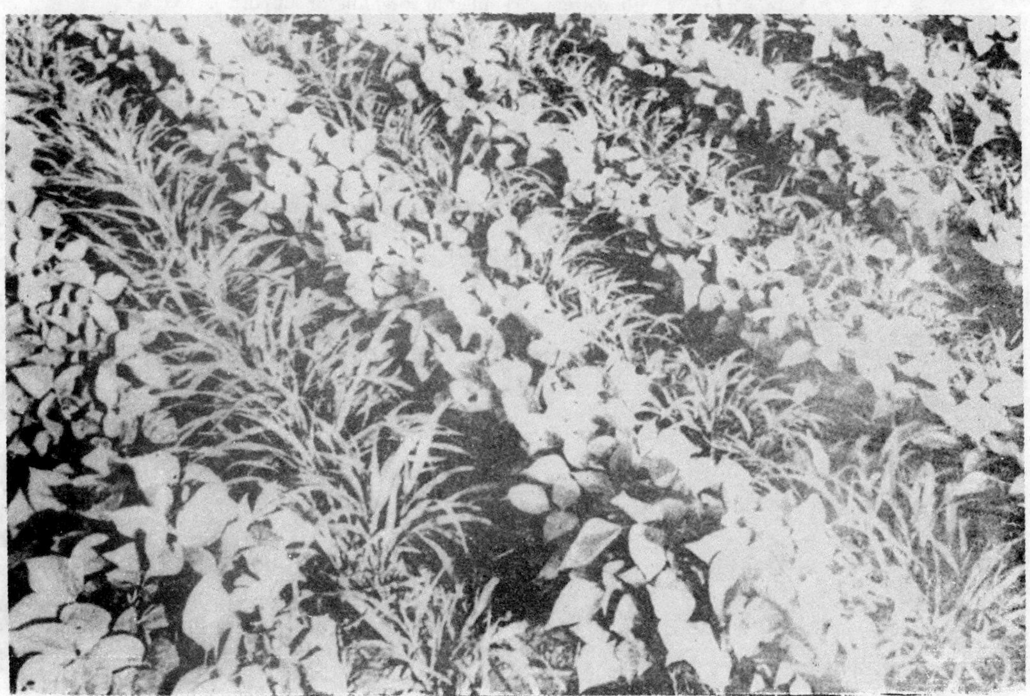

A mixture of maize along with cowpea, which is leguminous. Feeding of mixed forages provide nutrient in best form and ratio to our livestock.

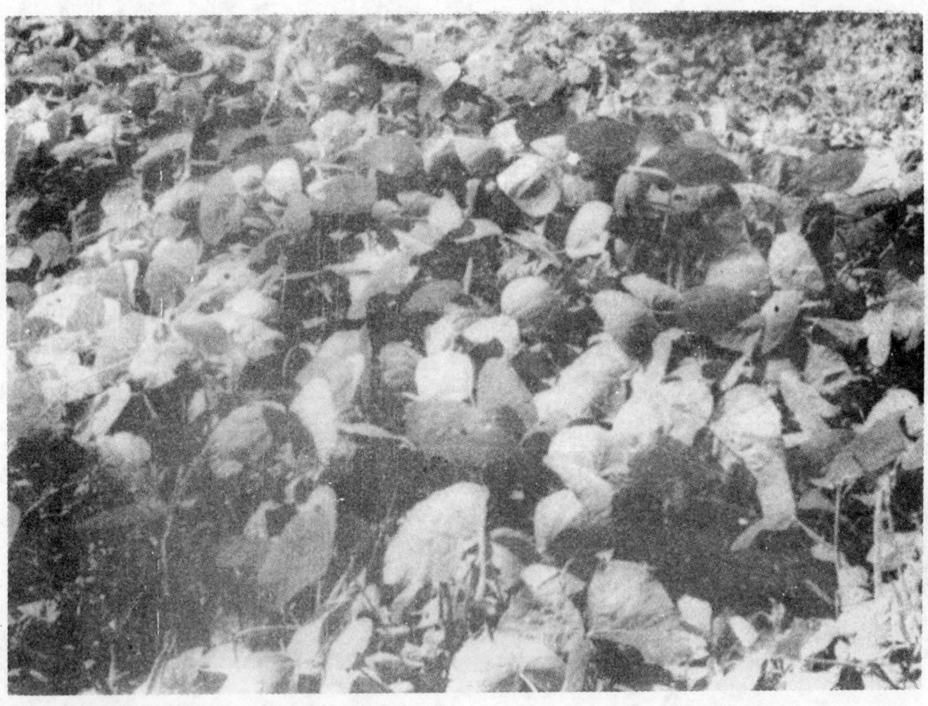

Velvet beams, *Stizolobium* spp. are a group of vigorous-growing annuals belonging to several species and to hybrids between them. Grown as long wires (3-15m) but bushy types also exists. Mostly grown as mixed forage with maize, pearl millet or sorghum for support.

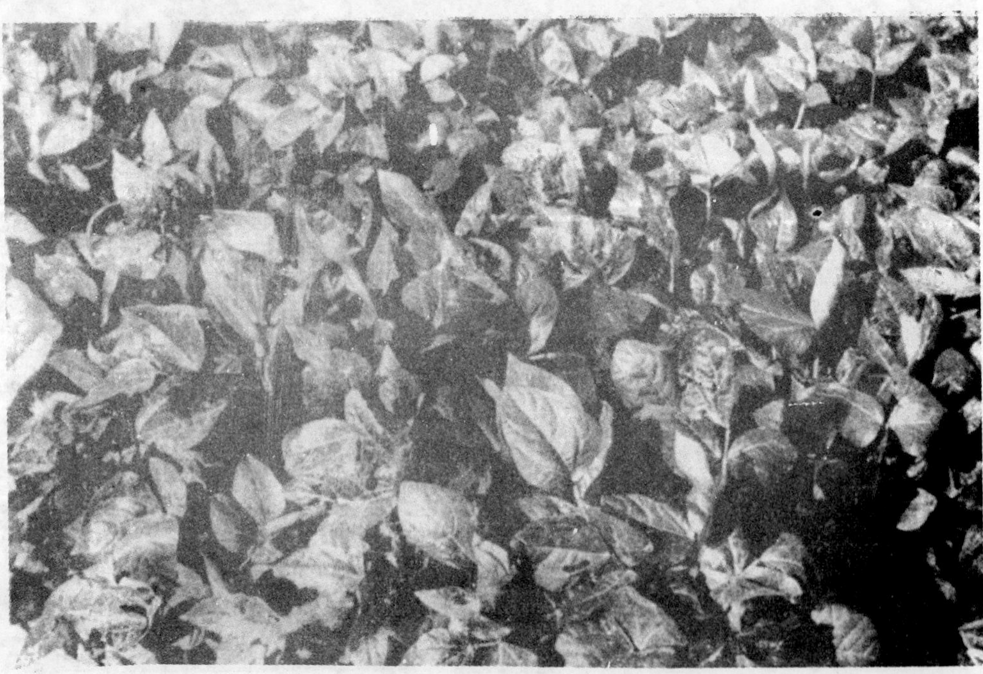

Cowpea is a high yielding leguminous *kharif* forage crop requires very little of irrigation, grows faster, has tremendous nutritive value.

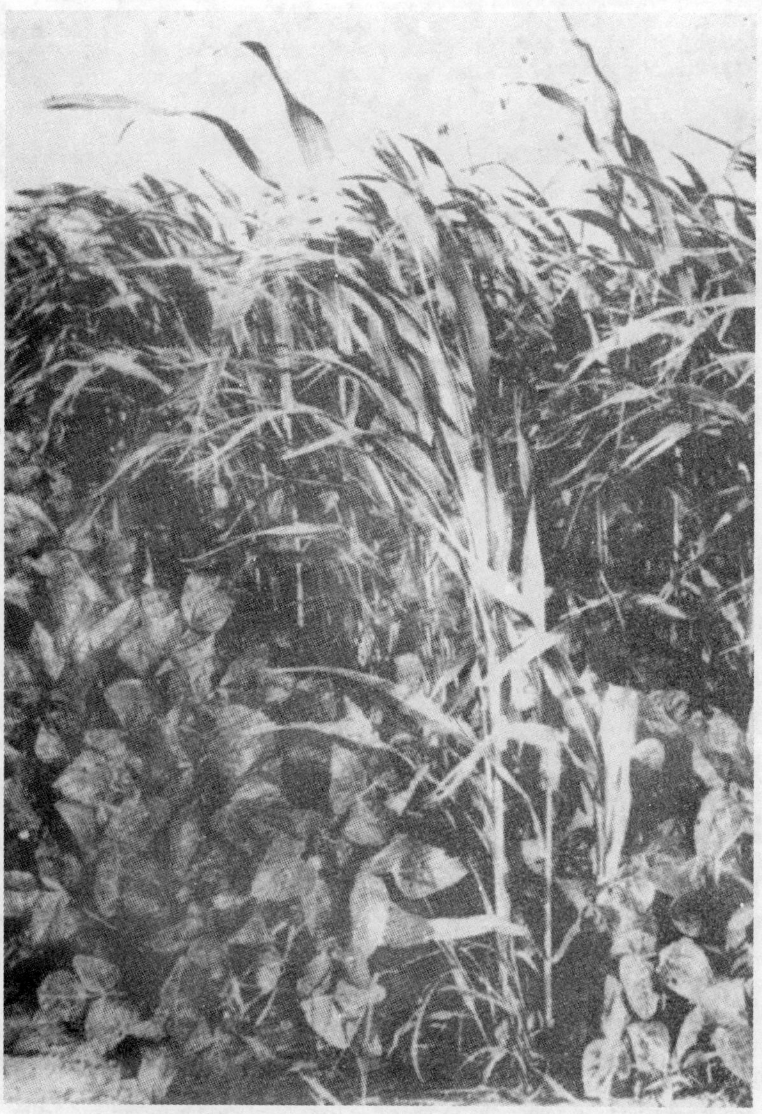

Photo shows a unique combination of Jowar and Cowpea grown together on alternate rows. Luxuriant growth assures the economy and brings health of the herbivores.

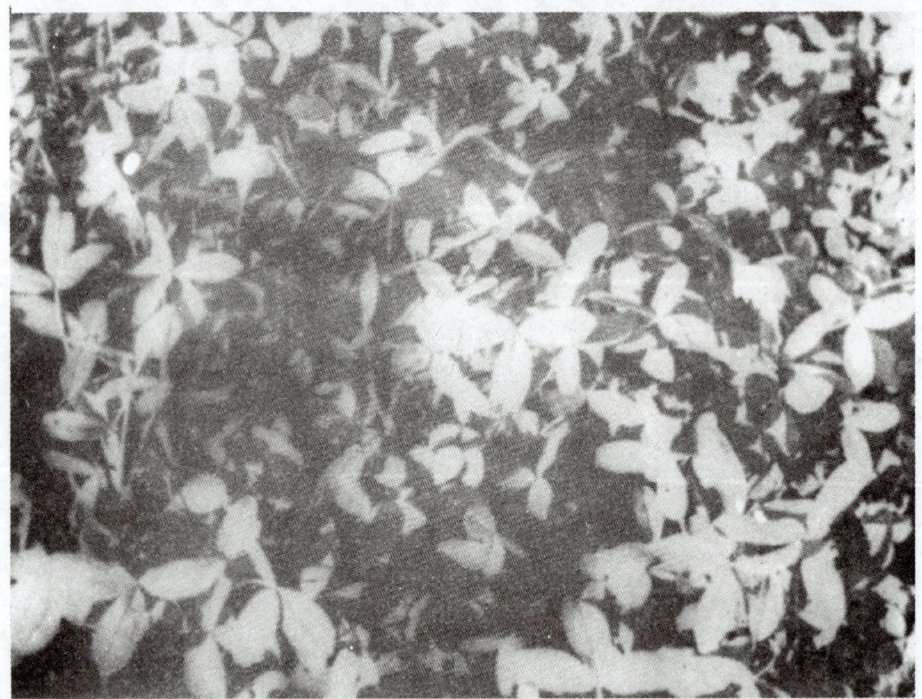

Berseem is one of the most important cultivated forages of India. Highly palatable and may be cut everal times a season for use as green fodder or hay. The highest yield of protein with a relatively low yield of fibre is obtained if the plant is cut at a height of about 40 cm.

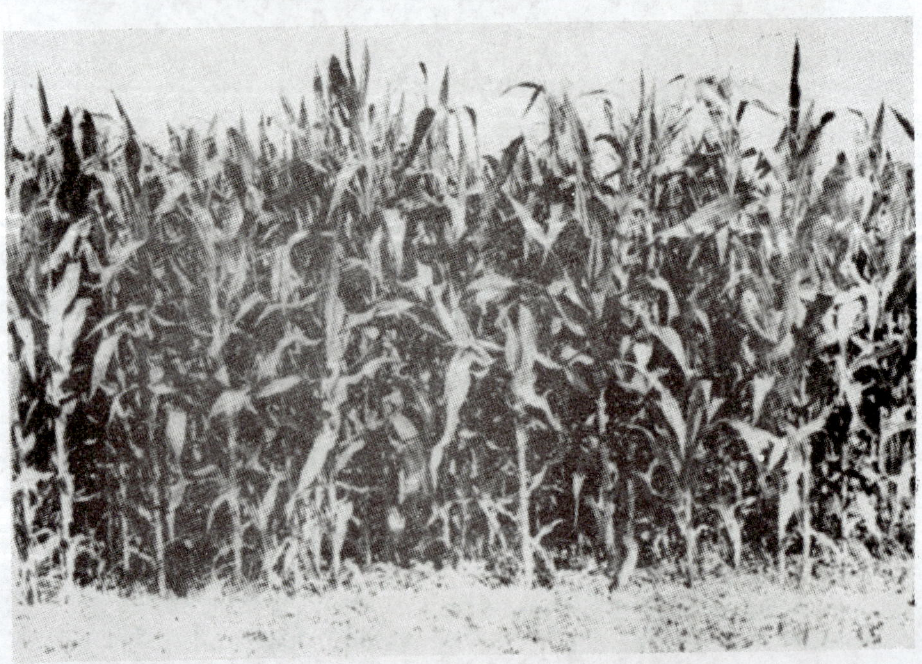

Maize crop is very popular among the farmers due to its dual use for fodder and grains. The green portion of the plant left after removing cobs is also used as forage. When grown for forage alone harvesting is best at the milk stage, when the leaves are still green and tender.

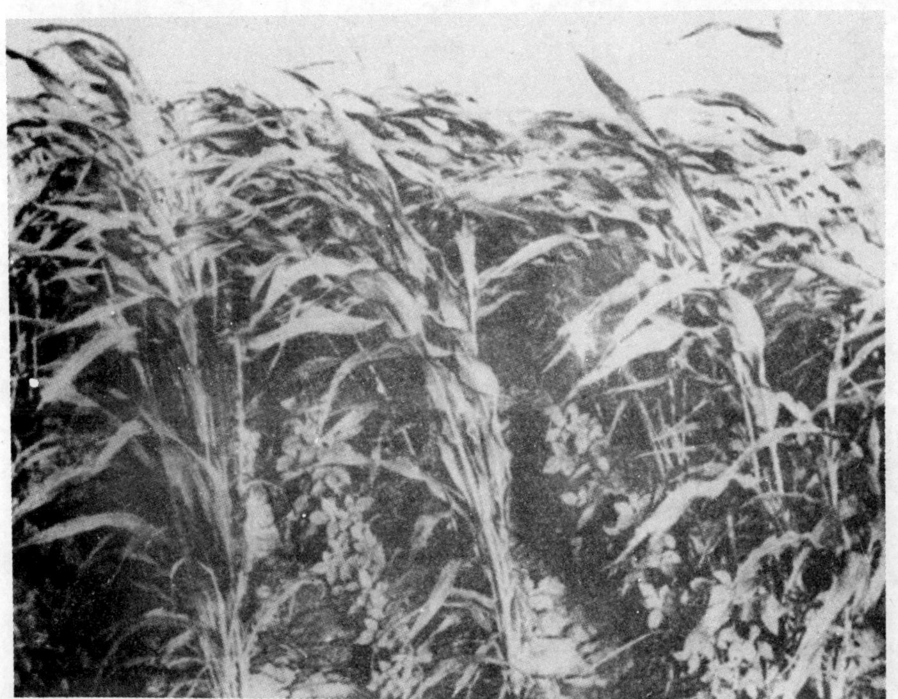

Photo shows alternate line of maize and *Phaseolus calcaratus* a wonderful combination of graminacious and leguminous family grown together.

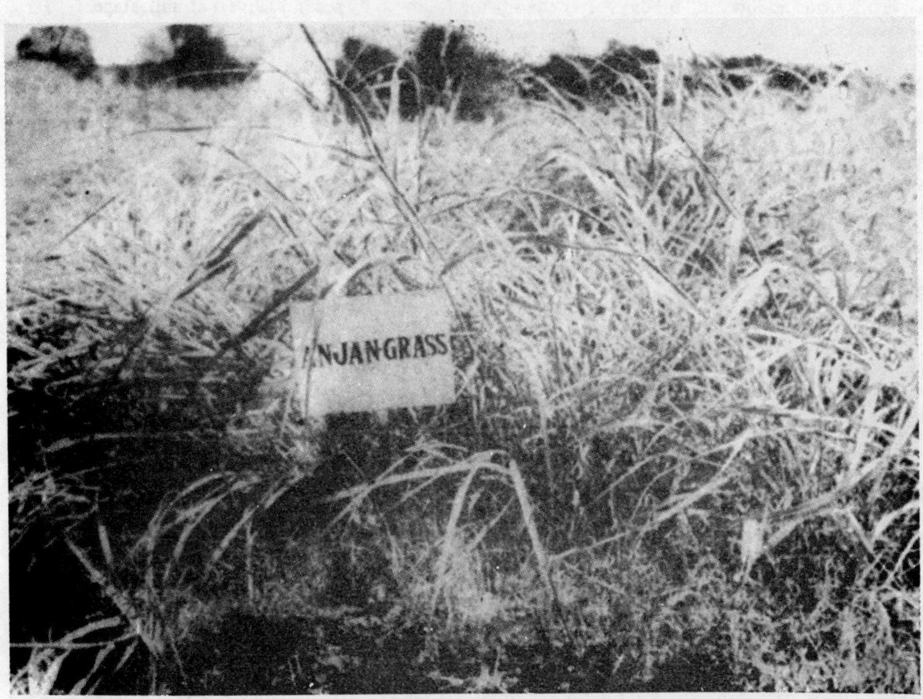


Anjan Grass also known as Blue buffalo grass, African Foxtail found on many soil types but sensitive to waterlogging. The forage has high protein content and digestibility when young but with age the quanlity declines

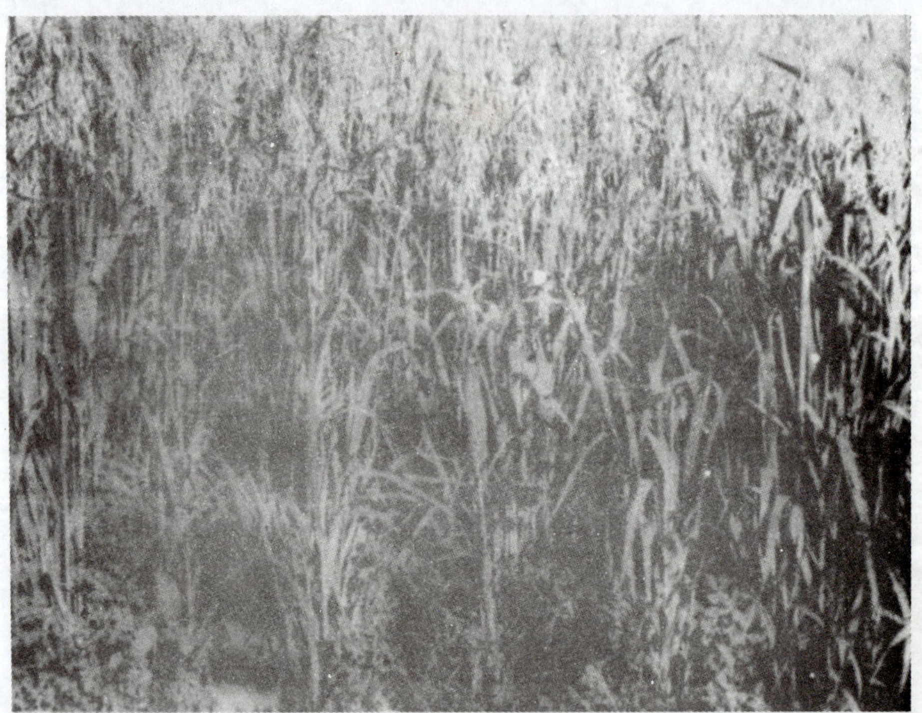

Oats are extensively grown in all the regions of the country where wheat or barley is taken. The crop is used for forages as well as for grains. Among promising high yielders are varieties of HFO-114, O-S-6, O-S-7 etc. The fodder is harvested at 50 per cent flowering stage in one cut crop. In two cut crop the first harvest is made at about 50-60 days after the sowing followed by second harvest at milk stage.

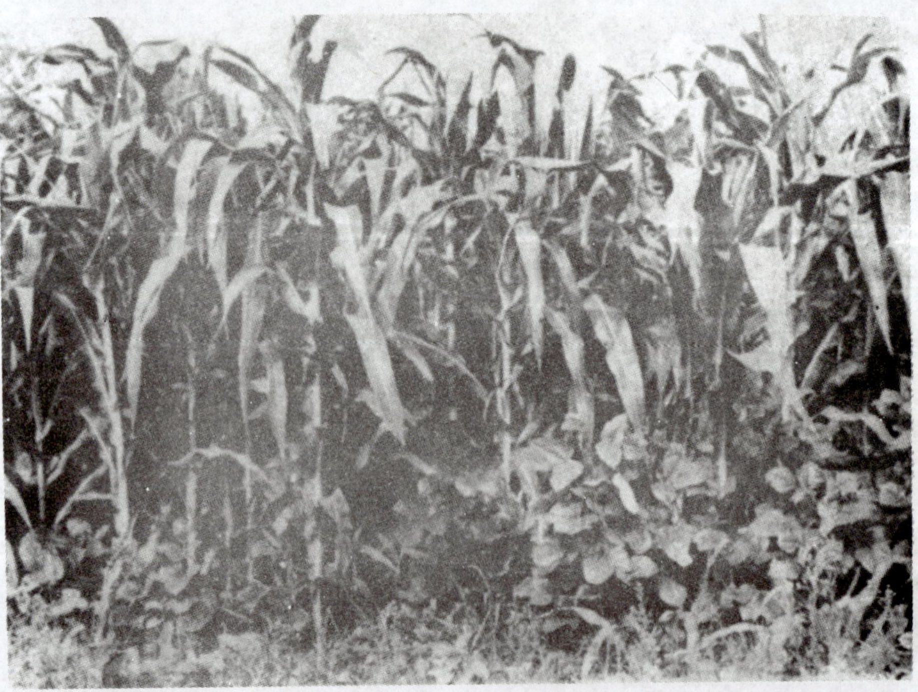

A mixture of *Pennisetum pedicellatum*, commonly known as Dinanath grass, a graminaeceous ***kharif*** forage crop along with Cowpea which is leguminous grown on alternate rows

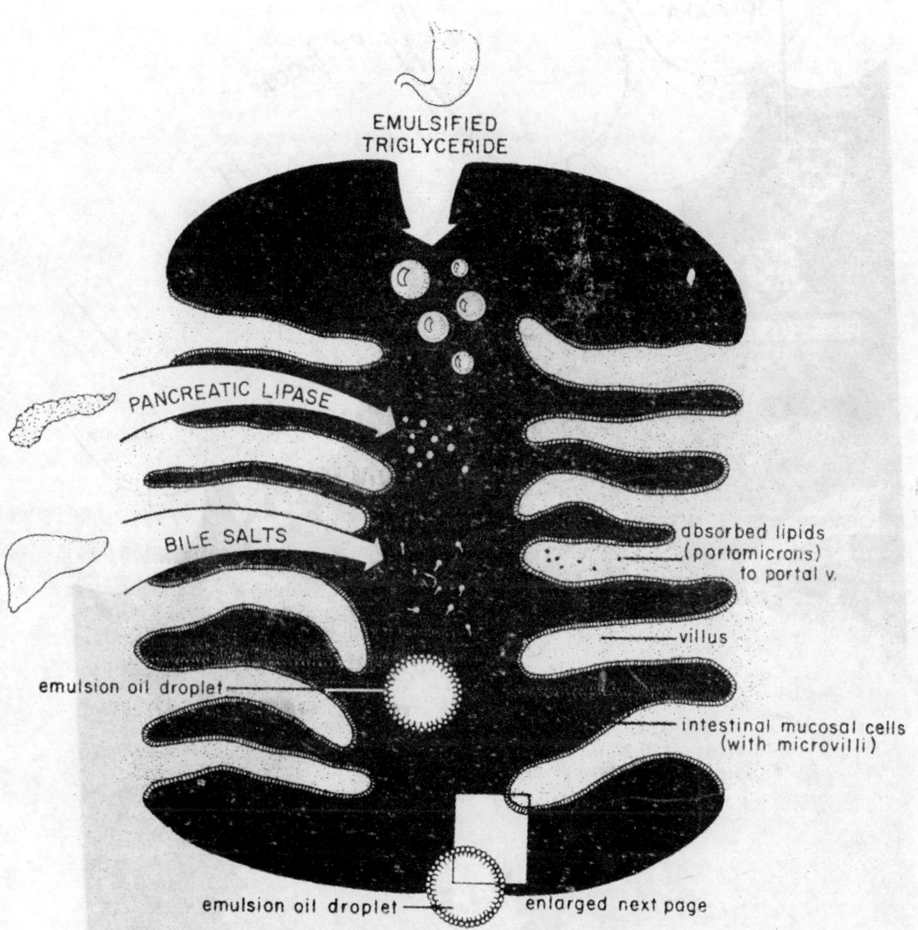


Intraluminal section of the duodenum showing initial stages of fat digestion.

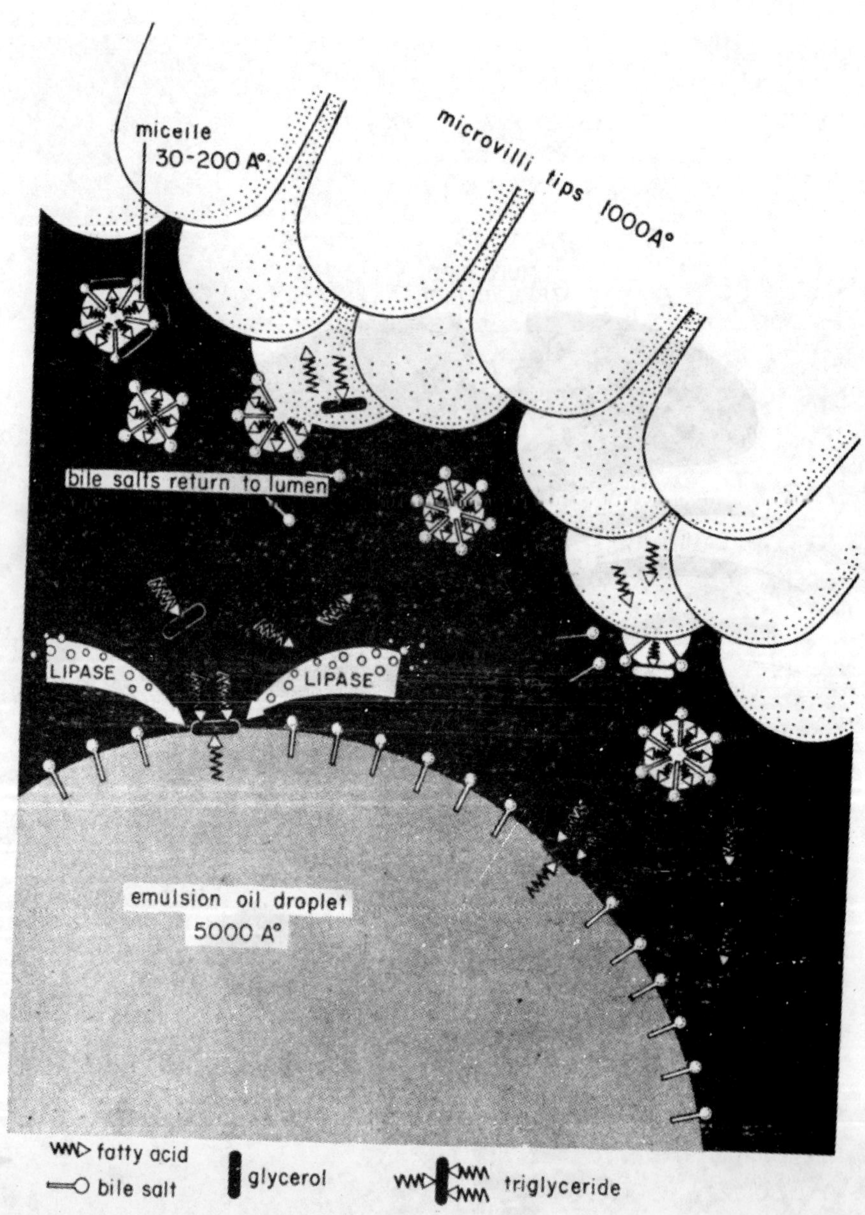


Enlarged section showing the relationship of the emulsion droplet, lipase, micelles, and the tips of the microvillus during fat digestion and absorption.